We dedicate the book to our wives and children
Donna Cox and Debbie Roper
Dermot and Catriona Cox
Louis, Adam, Susannah, and Anthony Roper

Preface

As a medical student entering the clinical years, you will find that talking to and examining patients is rather different from analysing the Kreb's cycle (or whatever fancy biochemistry you get up to these days).

The purpose of this book is to allow you to make the transition from scholar to hands-on physician as smoothly as possible. It is about those techniques in history and examination that need to be practised and cannot be learned just by studying. These clinical skills are described in the style of a tutor teaching at the patient's bedside. Common difficulties encountered are faced head on, not just ignored, and solutions are suggested. Whether you are a veteran, albeit a neurotic one, about to take your Finals, or a fresh-faced third year (or possibly first year) starting your first clinical attachment, this book is on your side.

Good luck!

Niall Cox and T. A. Roper

Acknowledgements

All illustrations by **Dr T. A. Roper**, except the cartoons by Paul Brown, Medical Illustration Leeds. Photography by Tim Vernon, Mark Hinchcliffe, and Medical Illustration Leeds.

We acknowledge the following individuals for providing slides: Dr Andrew Catto, Consultant Physician in Medicine for the Elderly at Leeds General Infirmary (Figs 4.7, 5.2, 6.2, 6.5, 6.7, 6.9, 6.11, 6.36, 6.40, 6.41, 9.1, 9.2, 11.3, 11.16–11.18, 11.20, 11.45,12.13, 12.15(a), 12.19, 13.3(b), 13.4, 13.40, 14.8, 14.9, 14.12, 14.13, 14.17, 14.19); Dr Michael Darby, Dr Hilary Moss, and Dr Rod Robertson, Consultant Radiologists at Leeds Teaching Hospitals (Figs 16.7–16.9, 16.16, 16.19–16.21, 16.24(a), 16.25–16.28, 16.30–16.33, 16.35, 16.41, 16.44, 16.50–16.53, 16.56, 16.59); Mr Paul Finan, Consultant Surgeon in Colorectal Surgery at Leeds General Infirmary (Figs 7.12–7.16, 13.9); Dr Douglas Chalmers, Consultant Physician in Gastroenterology at Leeds General Infirmary (Figs 5.7, 6.6, 6.10, 6.12, 13.37, 13.38, 14.18(a), 14.20); Dr Alexander Fraser, Consultant Physician in Rheumatology at Leeds General Infirmary (Figs 13.3(c) and (d), 13.28, 13.39); Pam Giles and Claire Brewster, Nurses on Coronary Care Unit at St James Hospital, Leeds (Figs 15.19, 15.29, 15.38, 15.42, 15.46, 15.48, 15.54, 15.55); Dr Mike Henry, Consultant Physician in Respiratory Medicine at Leeds General Infirmary (Figs 16.36, 16.45); Dr Martin Muers, Consultant Physician in Respiratory Medicine at Leeds General Infimary (Figs 5.1, 13.3(a)); and Dr Peter Sheridan, Consultant Physician in Endocrinology (retired) at St James Hospital Leeds and Seacroft Hospital (Figs 4.3, 6.3, 6.4, 6.8, 6.13, 6.19, 11.21, 11.22, 12.2, 12.11, 12.14, 12.15(b), 12.16–12.18, 13.5, 13.7, 14.1–14.4, 14.6, 14.7, 14.10, 14.14, 14.15). All other radiographs courtesy of the X-Ray Museum at St James Hospital and all other electrocardiograms provided by Dr Greg Reynolds, Consultant Cardiologist at Leeds General Infirmary.

Thanks to Dr Andy Brown for finding rheumatology slides and contributing the GALS assessment section in Chapter 13 as well as for further advice. Thanks to all our models: Kathryn Richardson, Debbie Roper, Tom Mwambingu, Namal Perera, Julie Forster, Joni Walker, Alistair Walling, Helen Parkinson, and Holly. And thanks finally to all the staff at Oxford University Press, especially Georgia Pinteau, Catherine Barnes, and Laura Johnstone for bringing this project to fruition.

Contents

Contributors

Most authors were chosen shortly after passing their MRCP examinations when their clinical skills were arguably at their peak. All were chosen for their love and enthusiasm for teaching.

Emma E. B. Burton
SHO in General Medicine
Leeds General Infirmary
Leeds, UK

Niall Cox
Consultant in Medicine for the Elderly
Dewsbury and District Hospital
Yorkshire, UK

Chris Gale
SPR in Cardiology
Yorkshire rotation
Yorkshire, UK

Richard Gale
SPR in Ophthalmology
Yorkshire rotation
Yorkshire, UK

Yasir Kasmi
SHO in Psychiatry
Leeds Teaching Hospitals
Leeds, UK

Catriona Morrison
SPR in Geriatric and General Medicine
Yorkshire rotation
Yorkshire, UK

T. A. Roper
Consultant in General and Geriatric Medicine
St James University Hospital
Leeds, UK

Anita Sainsbury
SPR in Gastroenterology
Yorkshire rotation
Yorkshire, UK

Aravamuthan Sreedharan
SPR in Gastroenterology
Yorkshire rotation
Yorkshire, UK

Permissions

Fig. 4.1 The cardiac cycle. Reproduced by permission of Oxford University Press from **Fig. 15.11** (p. 286), *Human physiology: the basis of medicine*, by G. Pocock and C. Richards (1999).

Fig. 4.12 The jugular venous pressure waveform. Reproduced by permission of Oxford University Press from **Fig. 15.13** (p. 306), *Human physiology: the basis of medicine* (2nd edn), by G. Pocock and C. Richards (2004).

Fig. 8.5 The dermatomes of the upper limbs. Adapted by permission of Oxford University Press from **Fig. 1(a)** and **(b)** (pp. 21.110 and 21.112), *Oxford textbook of medicine* (2nd edn, Vol. 2), edited by D. J. Weatherall *et al.* (1987), reproduced by permission of Oxford University Press from *Brain's clinical neurology* by R. Bannister.

Fig. 8.8 Spasmodic torticollis. Reprinted from **Fig. 6.52** (p. 6.18), *Atlas of Clinical Neurology* (2nd edn), by G. David Perkin, Fred Hochberg, and Douglas C. Miller (1993), Mosby Publications, with permission from Elsevier.

Fig. 9.3 Carpal tunnel syndrome. Reprinted from **Fig. 2.39** (p. 2.17), *Atlas of Clinical Neurology* (2nd edn), by G. David Perkin, Fred Hochberg, and Douglas C. Miller (1993), Mosby Publications, with permission from Elsevier.

Fig. 10.1 The anatomy of the lumbar region demonstrating the termination of the spinal cord. Reproduced by permission of Oxford University Press from **Fig. 6.5** (p. 67), *Neurology*, by M. Donaghy (1997).

Fig. 10.2 Dermatomes of the legs and lower body. Adapted by permission of Oxford University Press from **Fig. 1(a)** and **(b)** (pp. 21.110 and 21.112), *Oxford textbook of medicine* (2nd edn, Vol. 2), edited by Weatherall, D. J. *et al.* (1987), reproduced by permission of Oxford University Press from *Brain's clinical neurology* by R. Bannister.

Fig. 10.3 Hereditary sensory motor neuropathy (Charcot Marie Tooth disorder). Reprinted from **Fig. 2.2** (p. 2.2), *Atlas of Clinical Neurology* (2nd edn), by G. David Perkin, Fred Hochberg, and Douglas C. Miller (1993), Mosby Publications, with permission from Elsevier.

Fig. 10.16 Eliciting the plantar reflex. Reproduced by permission of Oxford University Press from **Fig. 2.35(a)** (p. 31), *Neurology*, by M. Donaghy (1997).

Table 11.4 Contrasting symptoms of cardiovascular and neurological causes of blackout with modifications for the older patient. Adapted from **Table 3** (p. 21) *Epilepsy in elderly people* by Raymond Tallis (1995), Martin Dunitz, with permission.

Fig. 11.27 IIIrd nerve palsy. Reprinted from **Fig. 14.38(a)–(d)** (p. 14.13), *Atlas of Clinical Neurology* (2nd edn), by G. David Perkin, Fred Hochberg, and Douglas C. Miller (1993), Mosby Publications, with permission from Elsevier.

Fig. 11.28 VIth nerve palsy. Reprinted from **Fig. 14.38(a)** and **(b)** (p. 11.4), *Atlas of Clinical Neurology* (2nd edn), by G. David Perkin, Fred Hochberg, and Douglas C. Miller (1993), Mosby Publications, with permission from Elsevier.

Fig. 11.39 Xth nerve palsy. Reprinted from **Fig. 14.63(a)** and **(b)** (p. 14.22), *Atlas of Clinical Neurology* (2nd edn), by G. David Perkin, Fred Hochberg, and Douglas C. Miller (1993), Mosby Publications, with permission from Elsevier.

Fig. 11.41 XIIth nerve palsy. Reprinted from **Fig. 14.67** (p. 14.23), *Atlas of Clinical Neurology* (2nd edn), by G. David Perkin, Fred Hochberg, and Douglas C. Miller (1993), Mosby Publications, with permission from Elsevier.

Fig. 12.1 Anatomy of the thyroid. Reproduced by permission of Oxford University Press from **Fig. 12.12** (p. 227), *Human physiology: the basis of medicine*, by G. Pocock and C. Richards (1999).

Fig. 15.2 Normal electrocardiogram trace. Reproduced by permission of Oxford University Press from **Fig. 15.9** (p. 304), *Human physiology: the basis of medicine*, by G. Pocock and C. Richards (1999).

Fig. 15.3 Electrocardiogram trace associated with chest lead position. Reproduced by permission of Oxford University Press from **Fig. 15.7** (p. 300), *Human physiology: the basis of medicine*, by G. Pocock and C. Richards (1999).

CHAPTER 1

Introduction: about this book

Chapter contents

Clinical skills—what are they?

Clinical skills are the skills needed to practise clinical medicine. So when a patient comes to the doctor with a problem, the doctor has two main tasks:

(1) to **make a diagnosis** by evaluating the patient's symptoms (taking a history), carrying out the relevant examination, and then performing or arranging investigations;

(2) to organize **treatment** aimed at improving the patient's condition.

History, examination, investigation (these first three aimed at diagnosis), and treatment comprise the clinical skills.

The aim of this book

Clearly, the area of clinical skills represents a vast subject requiring a wealth of both factual knowledge and technical expertise.

This book focuses on those aspects of clinical skills that need to be practised and cannot be learned just by studying—particularly history and examination (the key diagnostic skills). It is a book for medical students and the description of various techniques is aimed at someone who has not done them before. Common difficulties encountered are discussed and solutions suggested.

Difficulty factor

Proficiency in clinical skills is hard won over many years. In the same way that we easily forget that we used stabilizers before we learnt to ride a bicycle, doctors will not always remember the difficulties they encountered when they first dealt with patients. This may give you the impression that history and examination should be easy—and in turn may result in frustration and self-doubt if (and when) you find that they are not. In a sense, it is reassuring to know that **some skills are difficult and come only with practice.** Consider examination of the jugular venous pressure (JVP). As a student, I remember doctors waxing lyrical about the triple waveform—yet I could not see a single ripple. I spent hours scouring books for the answer, to no avail. If I had only known that the JVP can be very difficult to assess, then I would have known to put my difficulties down to inexperience and set about the business of examining JVPs until I became proficient.

Throughout this book, clinical signs are given a mark out of 10 (a **difficulty factor** (DF)) to give the student some idea of how much practice is needed to get it right. Thus, if difficulties are being experienced with a sign that we have given a DF of 4/10, it is likely that a basic error is being made, which should be easily corrected. If problems are being experienced with a sign given a DF of 9/10, there still may be a basic error but the chances are it is lack of practice that is the problem. Please note that DF is a subjective mark given by the authors and entirely arbitrary. It is not found in other books and teachers will not be familiar with it. Symptoms are not given DFs: here the difficulty depends very much on what is causing the symptom rather than the symptom itself.

CHAPTER 2

About the wards

Chapter contents

Introduction

This chapter provides a brief overview of the system in which undergraduates work in the UK. Apologies are made to readers from other countries to whom some of this may not be applicable.

It is the aim of all medical schools that their students acquire an adequate knowledge of medicine and learn to apply this knowledge to help patients with their problems—to become good doctors. The best way to learn medicine is to talk to and examine as many patients in as many different situations as possible and to combine this with reading books about the relevant symptoms, signs, and conditions you have seen. You will spend most of your time in hospitals but hopefully a fair proportion with general practitioners as well.

Clinical work

During your clinical student years, you will move around the local hospitals spending roughly a month at a time working in different specialties. For each attachment, you will be assigned to a particular 'consultant firm', which includes the consultant and their junior doctors, for example, house officers and registrars. Clinical teaching may be time-tabled or informal.

Time-tabled clinical teaching takes three main forms.

1. **Group teaching**. This is where a doctor takes a group of between two and 10 students to a patient. One student is picked out (usually at random) to either take a history or perform an examination. Try not to avoid being picked out. You may be afraid

and embarrassed by being put in the spotlight but your fear will only worsen if you continue to hide. These sessions (which may be infrequent) should not be missed as it is here that the doctor most easily imparts their hard-won knowledge.

2. **Out-patient teaching**. Here you will either sit in with a doctor while they do clinic or see patients yourself and then tell (present) their story to the doctor.
3. **Ward rounds**. This is where the consultant and their team go round the ward evaluating their patients. Students are usually expected to attend but ward rounds are becoming increasingly business like (due to pressure of time) and their vast teaching potential is often untapped.

Informal clinical teaching

Most of your time during a clinical attachment is unsupervised. Lingering around a ward wasting time or just staying at home may be tempting, but is clearly counter-productive. A systematic approach to this unsupervised time should be adopted: twice as much will be learnt in half the time.

1. To learn history taking, take histories from patients on the ward and present them either verbally or in written form to a doctor for criticism.
2. Once you have seen a patient, make sure you follow their progress; find out what tests they have undergone, what diagnoses are made, what treatment they receive, and whether it works.
3. To learn examination technique, join a fellow student or students and visit patients in twos or threes (if you go alone you never quite get the critical atmosphere required).
4. As finals approach, this self-teaching may escalate into an unsavoury game of 'patient hunting'. 'There's a spleen on ward 136B' will be a common whisper (Fig. 2.1). Sometimes, it is an important clinical skill to know when not to examine.

This fame business is not what it's cracked up to be.
SPLEEN

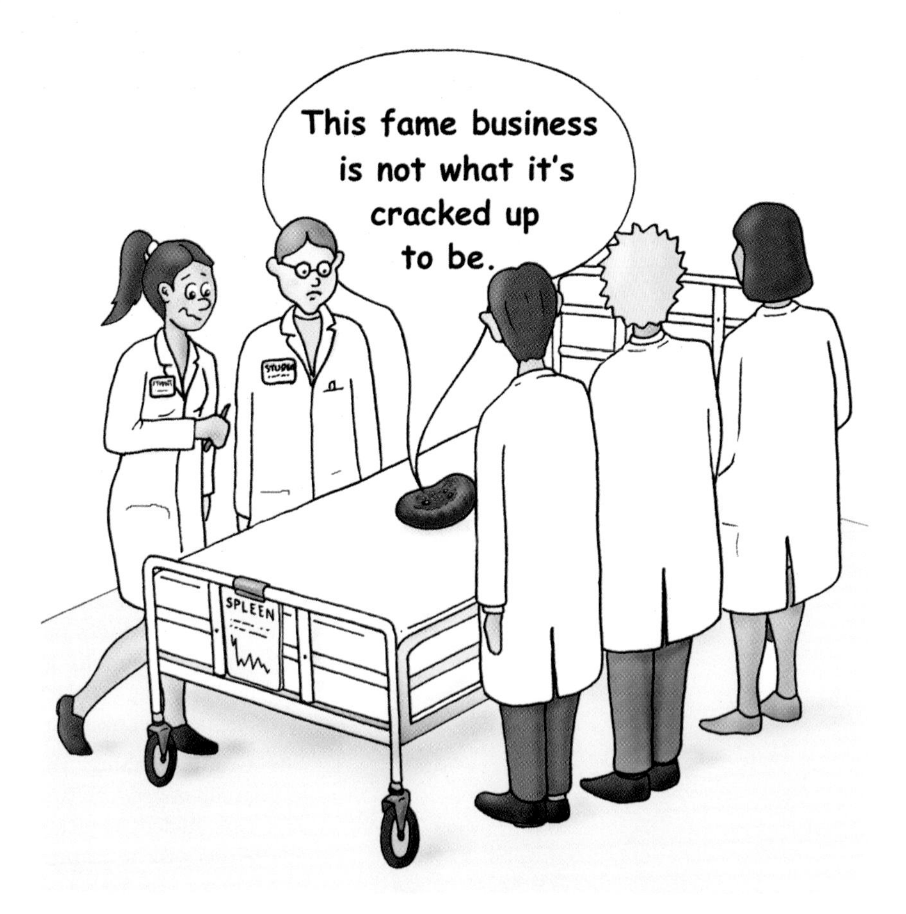

Fig 2.1 The price of fame.

5. The ward staff may be very busy; it is very easy to feel a bit like a spare part. Be enthusiastic—if you show willing and are courteous to both the junior doctors and the nurses, you will soon be made very welcome.
6. Simply 'shadowing' the house officer can be extremely rewarding. Be as helpful as you can; this will give them more time to discuss issues with you.

Patients' feelings

Patients vary in their responses to involvement in student teaching. Sometimes, medical students get themselves a bad reputation because of the 'patient hunting' just mentioned. However, most patients quite enjoy involvement with students. Not only does it relieve the boredom of hospital but often students are the only 'doctors' who have enough time to listen to **all** a patient's complaints and worries. Remember always to treat patients courteously and thank them when you have finished.

Chaperones

Rules relating to chaperones mostly apply to men examining women (although as time goes by, protocol may demand chaperones in other situations). There should always be a woman present who could be doctor, student, or nurse when any group of students or doctors is examining a female patient. So if your group contains only men, you will need to enlist the chaperoning skills of a friendly (but usually busy, so be patient!) female nurse.

Clinical skills centres

Many medical schools now have clinical skills centres where students can practise many techniques such as use of the stethoscope or ophthalmoscope or inserting intravenous cannulae (venflons). Videos, computers, and mannikins (dummy patients) are used. These are excellent for practising techniques but do not fool yourself into thinking you can learn all you need without seeing real patients.

Keypoints

- Unsupervised time can be frustrating but be focused and enthusiastic and your time will be highly productive.

CHAPTER 3

General aspects of history-taking and examination

Chapter contents

Introduction

When a patient consults their doctor about a problem, the doctor evaluates which conditions might be causing their symptoms. To do this they use three techniques:

(1) they discuss the patient's complaints with them (history taking);

(2) they do any relevant physical examination;

(3) they perform or arrange appropriate investigations.

General aspects of the first two techniques—history and examination—are discussed in this chapter.

History taking

What is a history?

The patient's history is the story of their problems. It has two main components:

(1) the patient's actual 'raw' complaint(s);

(2) further information gleaned by the doctor.

The aims are

(1) to lead to a diagnosis—the doctor's fundamental objective;

(2) to evaluate the impact of patient's symptoms on their lives.

Sometimes the history will produce a clear diagnosis but often there is a range of possibilities—this is known as differential diagnoses.

How to take a history

There are two main elements of history taking:

(1) developing a rapport with the patient—the 'bedside manner';

(2) evaluating the patient's complaint(s) in detail.

The 'bedside manner'

A doctor's bedside manner is their approach or attitude to the patient and is important for several reasons:

1. **Compassion.** When a patient sees any health professional, they are often at a low ebb psychologically. It is clearly important that they are made to feel at ease for humanitarian reasons.
2. **Confidence.** A good bedside manner tends to increase the patient's confidence that they are being cared for properly and so makes them feel more settled.
3. **Doing your job.** The more at ease the patient is, the more likely they are to feel free to tell you all their problems. The more information the patient gives you, the more likely you are to get the right diagnosis—and the correct diagnosis provides the key to effective treatment.

How to adopt a good 'bedside manner'

Many students try to be friendly, smiley, and jokey and many patients like this—to a point. But patients will often interpret joviality as evidence that you do not know what you are doing; a few patients will take exception to any frivolity where their health is concerned.

My own very personal belief is that the best style is slightly authoritative, yet open to questions; kind and thoughtful; and reassuring but not misleading.

1. Shake the patient's hand whilst introducing yourself. Say something like 'Hello, I'm Michaela Quinn, a third-year medical student. Do you mind if I have a few words with you about why you had to come into hospital?'
2. Mostly your patient will be sitting down. Do not stand towering over them. Ask permission to sit down next to them at a sociable distance—not too far, not too near.
3. Avoid appearing too busy to listen. Patients often imagine that doctors have a lot of more serious cases to deal with. If you appear rushed, they will hesitate to bother you with what they might feel are their 'trivial problems'.

CASE 3.1

Problem. I'm not sure about shaking hands. Is it not a bit old fashioned?

Discussion. Shaking hands can be reassuring when visiting teacher, car salesman, or doctor and is strongly recommended.

Evaluating the patient's complaint(s) in detail.

The aims are

(1) to look for clues that will lead to a diagnosis—so that appropriate treatment can be started;

(2) to determine the effects of symptoms on the patient's life—so that strategies can be put in place to support them; for example, an old person with joint pains may no longer be able to get to the shops and may need someone to help with her shopping.

How to evaluate the patient's complaints in detail

A major part of the history involves asking questions directly relating to the patient's complaint(s). First of all, ascertain what the patient's basic complaint is (known as the presenting complaint). Then find out more details about this complaint; for example, when it started, how long have they had it for (this is known as the history of the presenting complaint).

Other important information should be obtained:

- drug history
- family history
- social history
- any other symptoms.

This is often a complicated business. Assessing even the simplest of complaints can be a major challenge and is the focus of the next few pages.

The presenting complaint

You need to define the problem that is troubling the patient and why they have come to see you. Ask 'What was the problem that brought you into hospital?' The patient may well answer with a diagnosis such as 'a heart attack'. If so, you need to focus on symptoms: ask questions like 'How did it affect you?' or 'What did it feel like?'

TABLE 3.1 History of presenting complaint: a patient with headache

Presenting complaint
Headache
Further details of main complaint
Duration: 3 h
Onset: sudden, at its worst within a minute
Site: back of head
Severity: 10 out of 10
Character: dull
Precipitating factors: came out of blue while watching TV
Relieving factors: paracetamol no good, co-codamol partial relief
Previous similar symptoms: no previous headaches.
Other symptoms in the affected system
Dizziness: no
Diplopia: no
Hearing loss: no
Weakness: no
Syncope: fell to the ground at some point early on, not sure if blacked out
Questions relevant to possible causes
Subarachnoid haemorrhage must be a possibility. This may also cause vomiting and is more common in people with high blood pressure, so
Vomiting: twice
High blood pressure: no
Fffects of the symptoms on the patient's life
Not really relevant given short timescale

History of the presenting complaint

To evaluate the presenting complaint(s) further, you need to ask questions aimed at working out the cause and effects of the symptom(s). This is known as the history of the presenting complaint. An example is given in Table 3.1.

What to ask

1. Find out more about the symptom(s) themselves. Ask about
    - site
    - duration/onset
    - severity (if necessary, ask patient to rank pain out of 10)
    - character
    - precipitating factors
    - relieving factors
    - previous similar symptoms.

    The importance of these features varies widely for different symptoms. It requires considerable experience and knowledge to know how much detail to go into for each symptom and which are the most useful questions for each symptom. Try to avoid 'leading questions'. There is a danger that suggestible patients may lead you up the wrong avenue in their attempts to be helpful: if the patient has chest pain and you suspect angina, you may wish to find out if the pain is brought on by exertion. Avoid the temptation to ask 'Does walking bring the pain on?' but instead say 'Does anything seem to bring the pain on?' Then, if the patient says 'yes', ask 'What brings on the pain?' This will guarantee an authentic answer. If however you find that your patient is vague or is having difficulty then it is reasonable to be more direct and ask 'Does walking bring on the pain?'

2. Find out about other symptoms in the affected system. Thus, if a patient complains of coughing up blood (haemoptysis), this is a respiratory symptom so also ask about cough, phlegm, breathlessness, wheeze, and chest pain.
3. Ask questions about possible causes. In the patient with haemoptysis, you need to be thinking about what might cause this and also what other questions you should ask about these causes. So if you think of pulmonary embolism, you ask about recent operations, pleuritic chest pain, or leg swelling—or you may think of lung cancer and ask about weight loss and smoking.

Tip

Asking about previous episodes is quite useful. For instance, a patient may present with a severe occipital headache—suggestive of a subarachnoid haemorrhage (bleeding into the brain). If he tells you he has had a similar headache seven times in the last year without major ill effect, this is less likely to represent subarachnoid haemorrhage than if he tells you he has no previous headaches.

CASE 3.2

Problem. I don't have any problem talking to patients. However I do find that often the patient talks a lot without giving me the information I need but when I butt in to find out more about their main complaint, I can't help feeling very rude.

Discussion. Some, but by no means all, patients are bursting to tell you about all their problems. They will switch from one problem to another dipping in and out of the past, apparently at random, describing diagnoses that don't seem to fit to their symptoms. It is tempting to stop such patients at each turn and demand clear details. However, this can be a little unfriendly so early on in the interview. It may be best to give such a patient a free rein for 2 or 3 minutes. Don't ask them many questions. Just listen while you give them a chance to have their say. After that time, the patient's complaints can be summarized back to them and suggestions made as to how you're going to proceed. For example, 'So you're a diabetic on insulin but you've been quite well recently until 5 days ago. Then you started to feel sickly and off your food. This morning you've developed some pain in your tummy and vomited twice. Now, I need to ask you some more questions about your tummy pain ... '

Tip

It is useful to ask 'When were you last well?' and '... then, what happened?'

4. Find out about the effects of the symptoms on the patient's life. Ask how the symptoms have affected their lifestyle; for example, whether they have had to miss work or give up hobbies or whether they are unable to do their shopping.

Past medical history

There are two main reasons for delving into the past.

1. If the patient has a long-standing disease, there is a strong chance that any new symptom could relate to this.
2. Past history is useful in deciding how active a patient (and their doctor) might want the doctors to be with their treatment. If, for example, you consider two different patients both with lung cancer and one has a long-standing severe disability due to stroke whereas the other is previously well, there may well be a difference in their attitudes to chemotherapy or radiotherapy.

What to ask

It is surprising how some patients can forget their past so you may have to probe quite a bit to find out about previous problems. Ask 'Do you suffer from any long-term health problems?' and 'Have you been in hospital before?'

Ask specifically about these common important conditions:

- heart attack
- angina
- stroke
- high blood pressure
- rheumatic fever
- tuberculosis
- diabetes
- epilepsy
- jaundice
- chronic bronchitis/emphysema
- anaemia
- stomach ulcers
- operations
- allergies.

When the patient says 'yes' to any of these, you must try to verify the diagnosis. For example, if the patient admits to having previously suffered a stroke, ask 'How did the stroke affect you?'

Alcohol intake and smoking can be included in the past medical history (students usually include these in the social history). It is important to know the full history of alcohol intake and smoking: a patient may tell you he does not smoke or drink but may admit he smoked 40 per day until yesterday and drank 40 pints of beer per week until 2 years ago.

Tip

It is better to ask about 'high blood pressure' than 'hypertension', which most patients understandably think is a nervous complaint.

Drug history

A drug history is very important because of the following.

1. Drug side-effects may cause all or part of the patient's problem. As an example, if a patient has recently developed diarrhoea, it is important to know if they have recently had a course of antibiotics.
2. Before adjusting treatment or starting any new treatments, you need to know what the patient is taking already.
    1. In cases where a patient is already taking medication for a condition, you need to know the current doses. Prescribing frusemide 80 mg for a patient's deteriorating heart failure will not help much if this is the dose they are already taking.
    2. You need to make sure the old and new treatments will not cause problems when used together. So, if you want to start a patient on a non-steroidal anti-inflammatory drug such as diclofenac, it is important to know whether they are taking an anti-coagulant such as warfarin. If so, the risks of diclofenac causing bleeding from the stomach are greatly increased.
3. The medication list also helps to give an idea of what diseases a patient is suffering from. So if the patient is taking mesalazine, this suggests that the patient has inflammatory bowel disease.

What to ask

Patients are often unsure about their medications and the more they take (polypharmacy) the more difficult it is for the patient to remember them. Equally, the more medications a patient takes, the more chance there is of adverse drug interactions—so you need to be thorough.

Ask the patient 'Are you taking any tablets, inhalers, or drops for anything?' If yes, ask if they've got their medication with them.

1. If they have, go through the boxes or bottles individually reading the labels. These will usually give the name of the tablet, the dose, and how often the patient is taking them. Often the label is out of date, or the patient's adherence to their medication regime is imperfect so check with the patient what they think they should be taking, the dose, and the frequency. Record their responses.
2. If they have not, the patient may have a list of medications. Again, go through this with the patient checking each medication as you go.

Tip

When asking patients about drugs, do not use the word 'drugs'. To many patients 'drugs' suggests cocaine, heroin, and so on. Instead, you should enquire about 'tablets', 'medicines' or 'inhalers'.

Patients are often unsure of their current medication. This is especially so in hospital where drugs are often changed. The drugs will be written on a drug chart, which is usually at the end of the patient's bed. If the patient cannot give you a good drug history, look at the drug chart. The format of the drug chart varies from hospital to hospital. Ask one of the nurses or doctors on the ward how to interpret it. If you are not sure about any of the drugs, look them up in the *British national formulary*, which is an invaluable guide to drugs and usually available on the ward.

Family history

Family history may sometimes give a clue to the cause of the patient's problems. Ask the following.

1. 'Has anyone in your family had similar problems?'
2. 'Do any diseases run in the family?'
3. 'Did anyone in your family die young—and if so, how?'

It can be difficult to decide how much detail to take. For instance, in a woman with haemoptysis, it may not be particularly helpful to know that the woman's sister has a stomach ulcer.

Social history

This helps to build up a general picture of the patient: what they were like in the past and how the current illness is affecting them. Ask about the following.

1. **Marital status and children.** Ask briefly about the family's state of health. It is particularly important in frail elderly patients to get an idea whether family will be able to care for the patient if needed.
2. **Occupation (or previous occupation if unemployed or retired).** Some occupations may bring increased risk of certain illnesses: shipbuilders may suffer from asbestos-related diseases. Some occupations may find particular problems more troublesome: lorry drivers with epilepsy must give up their job. If the patient has had multiple jobs, you may not have time to discuss the ins and outs of all of these. Focus on the current job and on any jobs that may have involved exposure to toxic materials.

3. **Where they live.** Some patients will live in a nursing home, a residential home, or an old people's home suggesting that they are no longer able to look after themselves. In the UK, an old people's home is also known as a Part III home and is council run. A residential home is the equivalent in the private sector. Those patients who are more disabled are looked after in nursing homes (nearly always private). Occasionally, you may hear of 'EMI homes': these are for elderly, mentally infirm patients.
4. **How your patient's condition restricts them and what help they have in coping with any restrictions.** Who does the shopping? Who collects the pension? It is often said that if an old person is able to collect their own pension they are probably coping reasonably well. Who does the washing and cleaning? Do they have a home help, a warden, or meals-on-wheels?

Some patients may consider these questions intrusive. If so, it is best just to skip on to the systematic questions.

Systematic questions

It is often possible to miss important symptoms from the history because you forget to ask or the patient neglects to mention them. Systematic questioning is something of a dredging system but acts as a fail-safe mechanism to make sure you do not miss anything vital. Often you will only turn up minor things but occasionally it can be something important. For instance, in a patient with haemoptysis you may have forgotten to ask about breathlessness.

Ask about the following symptoms:

- general
  - weight loss
  - anorexia
  - night sweats
  - itch
- cardiovascular
  - oedema
  - palpitations
  - chest pain
  - breathlessness
  - orthopnoea
  - paroxysmal nocturnal dyspnoea
  - dizziness
  - syncope
- respiratory
  - cough
  - phlegm
  - wheeze
  - haemoptysis
  - chest pain
  - breathlessness
- abdominal
  - heartburn
  - nausea
  - vomiting
  - haematemesis
  - indigestion
  - abdominal pain
  - diarrhoea
  - constipation
  - rectal bleeding
  - jaundice
  - dysphagia
- genitourinary
  - dysuria
  - haematuria
  - frequency
  - nocturia
  - incontinence
- locomotor
  - joint pains
  - stiffness
  - central nervous system
  - dizziness
  - diplopia
  - hearing loss
  - weakness
  - syncope.

You will learn more about these symptoms in the relevant chapters.

Your chances of working out the diagnosis depend on

(1) your knowledge of possible causes of the symptom(s);

(2) your ability to ask relevant questions to establish which conditions are more likely;

Tip

The aim is to get through the systematic questions quickly but without missing anything.

Tip

Before finishing your history it is always worth asking 'Is there anything else you think I might have missed out?' Just in case!

CASE 3.3

Problem. I thought I'd cracked history taking yesterday when I saw a patient with chest pain. I got a really good history and diagnosed angina, which turned out to be correct. But today I was really disappointed. I didn't know where to start with my patient who complained of dizziness.

Discussion. When you start your clinical attachments, the doctors will likely send you off with the apparently casual instruction: 'Go and take a history from Mrs Smith'. This can lead you to expect history taking to be easy. Don't become disheartened when you inevitably find it difficult.

CASE 3.4

Problem. I saw a patient with chest pain yesterday. I felt fairly confident that the pain was cardiac and knew that it was important to find out how long the pain lasted. But the patient couldn't tell me. Then I got criticised by the doctor for not finding out.

Discussion. Although medical knowledge is clearly important in determining how good your history is, dogged perseverance is equally important. In this sort of situation, give the patient options: 'Does the pain last a few seconds, 5 minutes, half an hour, a few hours, a few days?'. Usually the patient will get the idea and give you a rough duration.

Note that 'a long time' or 'not very long' mean next to nothing.

CASE 3.5

Problem. My patient came in feeling sickly and vomiting but she has a multitude of other complaints and I realize I've ended up being side-tracked by these.

Discussion. It is very easy to lose sight of your main objective—to establish the cause of the patient's most important complaints. Patients often like to dwell on the past and to be fair to them, we doctors like to ask them all sorts of questions not directly related to the presenting complaint. It's no wonder that sometimes we all miss the point.

At all times, keep a focus on the patient's main problem.

(3) the patient's ability to answer your questions;

(4) whether the history is typical for the condition causing it;

(5) whether the patient has a common condition.

Clearly, your knowledge of different symptoms and conditions will vary as will the features of the conditions that individual patients demonstrate. Thus, your success in establishing a diagnosis will vary greatly from patient to patient. You will always do better with patients whose conditions you know about and who present with classical features.

Despite this you can always approach each case in a systematic way evaluating duration, severity, precipitating factors, and so on even if you're not sure of the relevance of the answers.

Examination

Examining the patient often provides important information with regard to

(1) the diagnosis causing the patient's symptoms;

(2) the severity of their condition.

In this chapter, it is not the intention to give an overview of examination technique. All the techniques used are different and are described individually throughout the book. Here the aim is to prepare students for the process by which they will be taught examination skills.

System routines

The most commonly used method of teaching and learning examination technique is visiting patients and examining a system such as the cardiovascular or respiratory system. These system routines have some advantages.

1. They allow the teaching of examination techniques to be divided into logical, manageable chunks.
2. They allow the doctor to assess the students' ability both to elicit a range of signs—normal and abnormal—and then to tie them together to make a rational diagnosis.

They are not without their faults.

1. They are somewhat artificial—for example, a patient suffering from breathlessness requires assessment of both the cardiovascular and respiratory systems.
2. There is an unwritten rule that no history should be taken—mainly so that the patient does not spoil

CASE 3.6

Problem. I've been talking to an 81-year-old man for several minutes but I can't work out what he is complaining of. What might the problem be?

Discussion. The problem may simply be a lack of focus on either you or your patient's part. However, you must consider the alternative possibilities that the patient is confused or suffering from speech problems. As regards speech problems, the patient may be unable to express himself (expressive dysphasia) or unable to understand the spoken word (receptive dysphasia). Expressive and receptive dysphasia may co-exist. They are caused by neurological disease, most commonly stroke. First, assess the patient's word-finding ability. Ask 'Do you mind if I ask you a few questions to test your speech?' Show the patient some common objects—such as a watch, a strap, a buckle, a tie, or a pen—and ask them to name them. Difficulty suggests expressive dysphasia. Next, assess the patient's ability to understand the spoken word. Ask him to follow some instructions. Start off simple: 'close your eyes, please ... put out your tongue'. Move on to more complicated instructions: 'lift your right arm up in the air ... touch your nose with your left index finger'. Resist the temptation to show the patient what you mean—the aim is to assess language abilities. Difficulty following instructions suggests receptive dysphasia.

If the patient's language skills seem reasonably preserved, move on to assess for confusion. It's best to use the same questions for all patients. Patients should be questioned about the following 10 items; their answers are used to calculate the abbreviated mental test score (see Hodkinson 1972):

(1) their age;

(2) their birthday;

give the patient an address to remember and ask them to remember it for a few minutes ('42 West Street' is traditionally used);

(3) what year it is;

(4) what month it is;

(5) what time it is (to the nearest hour);

(6) where they are;

(7) the date of the start of the First World War;

(8) the monarch—ask 'Is there a king or queen in England these days?' and then check they've got the name right, 'What's her name?';

(9) Count backwards from 20 to 1 (give the patient a start to show what you mean 20, 19, 18 ...);

(10) ask if they can remember the address (42 West Street).

Give a mark for each correct answer. No half marks should be given for being close. The score out of 10 gives you some idea of the patient's ability to provide a relevant history.

If the patient scores three or less, he is very confused. History is likely to be very difficult and you will need to rely on any third parties you can find such as relatives if available, nurses, the medical notes including the general practitioner's letter, and casualty records.

If the patient scores between four and six and six, much of the patient's history may be unreliable and you must bear this in mind, particularly if certain parts of the story seem difficult to put together. Again, it is wise to consult any third parties who may have knowledge of the patient's illness.

If the patient scores seven or more, you should be able to obtain useful information from the patient. I suggest you quickly go through all the systematic questions for clues noting any positive symptoms. Once you have got all these, then go back over them in more detail.

---

the learning opportunity by inadvertently giving you the answer. This is rather unrealistic. In their daily work, a doctor would be negligent not to take a history prior to examining the patient.

There are some general rules that apply when examining systems.

1. **Be courteous at all times.** The patient is doing you a favour and you should treat them accordingly. Make all efforts not to hurt the patient—though it may be impossible to completely avoid inflicting pain, for example, when assessing for tenderness.
2. **Introduce yourself.** Always introduce yourself to the patient and shake hands. Say something like

CASE 3.7

Problem. Yesterday, I examined for a collapsing pulse when examining the cardiovascular system and the consultant criticized me saying it was superfluous. So today, I omitted checking for a collapsing pulse from the examination and another doctor told me I was wrong. Can they not make their minds up?

Discussion. Often it is the order and content of the routines that are the source of most problems for the student. Every book and doctor suggests different orders—the student is never quite sure which is correct. For example, some doctors insist that you check for a collapsing pulse (p. 37) every time you do the cardiovascular examination. Others feel this is wasting time unless you find other signs of aortic regurgitation (p. 68)—the condition that usually produces this sign.

Each system routine is an abbreviation of all the possible tests (there may be hundreds) that might be done for that system. There is no agreement on exactly how a particular routine should be abbreviated. Don't waste time scouring books for the perfect routine that will win Honours with every examiner. What is really important is that you know **why** you are doing what you're doing. If you can justify why you have done something, no one can complain. In this book routines have been suggested for the various systems. While these routines may not satisfy all teachers all the time, they will always give you a strong pass.

'Hello, I'm Leonard McCoy, a third-year medical student' (extend hand for shaking).

3. **Ask permission.** You should ask the patient for permission to carry out whatever examination you are doing: 'Do you mind if I examine your heart and pulses?' Sometimes the patient will either not hear you or may misunderstand you. If so, do not just ignore this. Ask permission again until it is clearly given.
4. **Left side of the bed.** Always examine from the left side of the bed (patient's right side). This is simply a matter of tradition. If the patient's bed is right up against the wall you will have to move it rather than examine from the right side of the bed (Fig. 3.1).
5. **Correct positioning is essential.** For most systems the patient should be in a particular position, such as lying flat for the abdomen or sitting at 45° for the cardiovascular system. You should get the patient into the correct position before commencing examination. If the patient misinterprets your instruction do not get flustered—just ask again! It is easy to feel you are wasting time but positioning is important. Get it right! (Sometimes, though, your patient will be confused or frail and unable to co-operate; then you will need to compromise.)

Tip

Learn how to adjust the headrest on hospital beds!

6. **The general look.** There is much emphasis on taking a general look at the patient before examining them. The idea here is that students adopt a holistic approach to the patient and avoid tunnel vision, which it is all too easy to develop. Unfortunately many students waste time taking some kind of vague gormless look at the patient. The general look is the impression obtained prior to examining. So in the respiratory system the general look involves looking for cyanosis, tachypnoea, a sputum pot, and a nebulizer while you are introducing yourself, positioning, and waiting for the patient to undress.
7. **Always inspect.** No matter what you are examining, good inspection is essential. Students may worry about wasting time during inspection and rush it. Alternatively, they may look slow and ponderous because they are not sure what they are looking for.
8. **The hands.** The cardiovascular, abdominal, and respiratory system examinations all begin with the hands. Get off to a good start by knowing what you are looking for in the hands when you start these examinations: cardiovascular—clubbing, splinters, and nicotine staining; respiratory—clubbing, cyanosis, flap, and nicotine staining; abdomen—leuconychia, palmar erythema, Dupuytren's, spiders, and flap.
9. **Use easily identifiable signs to guide you with more difficult ones.** For instance, if you palpate an irregular pulse and a tapping apex beat and hear a loud first heart sound (all relatively easily identifiable signs of mitral stenosis—p. 64), you should auscultate intently for the more difficult opening snap and mid-diastolic murmur of mitral stenosis. Think again about difficult signs you have

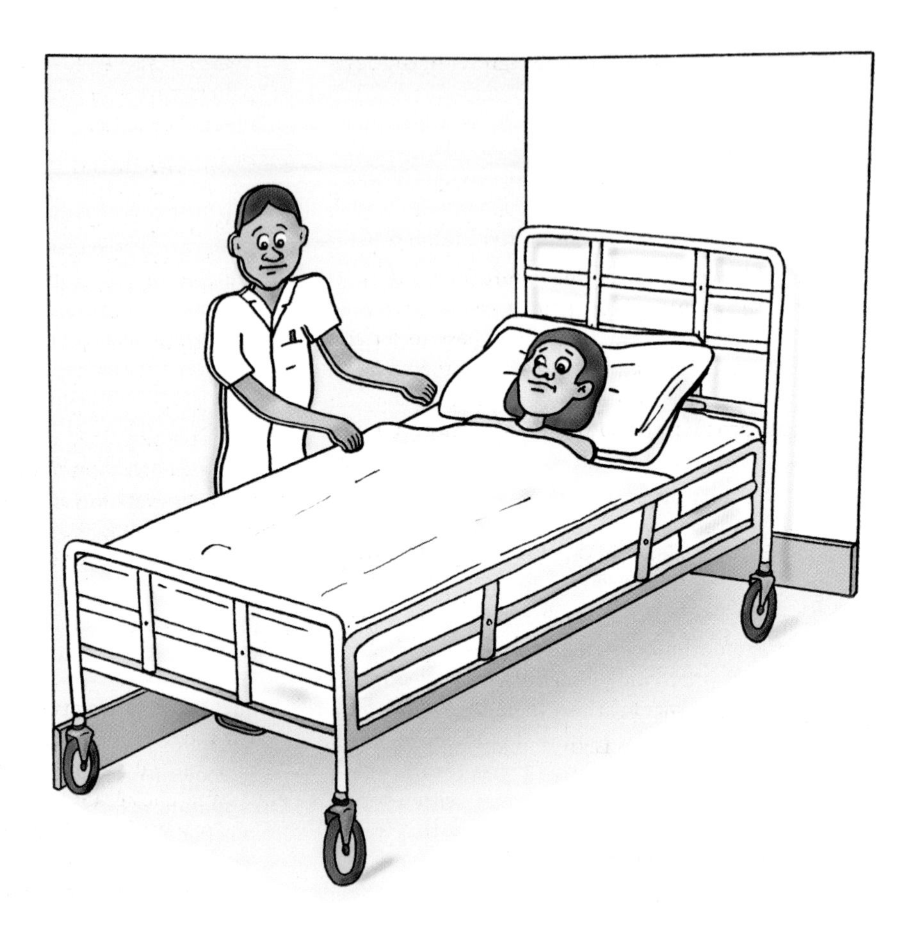

Fig. 3.1 Examining from the left side.

found if easier signs contradict them. For instance, if you find chest expansion by palpation (a difficult sign) is reduced on one side but percussion and breath sounds (easier signs) are normal, you need to reconsider whether expansion really was reduced.

Tip

Experience normal as well as abnormal. Approach the fitter patients on your ward and ask for permission to examine them. Only by getting a feel for what is normal will you be able to identify abnormalities.

Tip

One step at a time. When practising unsupervised, take your time to examine for individual signs—pulse, jugular venous pressure, tendon reflexes, and so on. Once you are getting the hang of these, practise combining signs into systems examinations.

Writing it down

Why write it down?

When working as a doctor, you should make a note in the patient's records every time you see them or receive some new medical information such as test results. This is for two main reasons.

1. No matter how good your memory, you will not be able to remember the subtleties of the patient's clinical features in a week's time.
2. The medical care of any individual patient is shared by a number of doctors who may all be called to attend the patient at different times and without the initial doctor being available. Thus, it is important that doctors record in the notes all their findings and what they believe to be the diagnosis so that the next doctor who sees the patient does not have to start from scratch.

It should not be forgotten that when patients make complaints or legal action against doctors, the written record in the notes carries great weight with the adjudicating parties.

How to write it down

1. Write the history down in rough as you go along and fill in bits as the patient gives them. Structure your history in headings such as presenting complaint, history of presenting complaint, and so on (see Case 3.8 below), so people can follow your clerking more readily. Often it is best to let the patient have their say about the past medical history (which they may often dwell on more than the present problem) or social history before talking about the main complaint.

CASE 3.8

Problem. When I look in the medical notes, there seem to be all sorts of abbreviations that I don't understand. What are they?

Discussion. Rightly or wrongly, it is traditional to use various abbreviations to demarcate different parts of the history:

PC—presenting complaint.

HPC—history of presenting complaint.

PMH—past medical history

DH—drug history

SH—social history

FH—family history

SQ—systematic questions, SE—systems enquiry.

You will also notice various other abbreviations. Any abbreviations can cause confusion and in an ideal world should not be used but some are so commonplace that you should be familiar with them:

SOB—short of breath

PND—paroxysmal nocturnal dyspnoea

od—once daily, bd—twice daily, tds—three times a day, qds—four times a day, nocté—at night

O/E—on examination

°—no, as in °murmurs = no murmurs

a/c/j—anaemia/cyanosis/jaundice

club/lymph—clubbing/lymphadenopathy

HS—heart sounds.

2. There is no need to write down everything the patient says as much will not be relevant to their medical condition.
3. Often, when taking the history you will miss important facts about the main complaint. It is always wise to leave a space on your sheet of paper at the end of the history of the presenting complaint so that you can fill in additional features as you go along. You might not have thought of lung cancer as a cause of the haemoptysis but when you asked about smoking you realized it was a possibility. Indeed, many relevant parts of the history may not occur to you until you have examined the patient. It may be that in a lady with haemoptysis that the diagnosis of lung carcinoma occurs to you only when you find clubbing (p. 84)—and only then do you remember to ask about anorexia and weight loss.

Presentation

Why present?

As a doctor, you will never know everything about your patient's condition. Medical practice is a constant round of second opinions. Whether as a house officer telling your consultant about a patient just admitted to hospital or a professor asking for ideas from a specialist in another field, you will need to be able to pass on the important facts about your patient to other health professionals. In your early years as a doctor, this is nearly always done by simple word of mouth. Thus presenting your findings on history and examination is an essential part of working as a medical student.

How to present

History

Your opening line is the presenting complaint. Give a brief statement describing the patient's name, age, occupation, and mode of admission and the main symptom and its duration. In one sentence, this gives an overview of the problem: 'Mrs Jones is a 62-year-old retired teacher, admitted via the general practitioner with a 2-day history of coughing up blood.'

Next, you elaborate on the presenting complaint—this is the history of presenting complaint (HPC). The HPC is meant to be an account of how the patient's symptoms have developed over a period of time and should include anything you think relevant to the main complaint. 'Two days ago Mrs Jones coughed up around a teaspoonful of dark red blood. This has recurred six times over the last 2 days. It has never happened previously. She normally suffers from a cough with occasional white phlegm. She has felt breathless over the last 6 months and her exercise tolerance has fallen from being very active to 20 yards. She hardly ever gets out of the house now. She has no orthopnoea or wheeze and no chest pain—pleuritic or otherwise. She had a spontaneous deep vein thrombosis 4 years ago. She used to smoke 30 per day until 2 years ago. She also admits to 2 stone weight loss and increasing anorexia over the last 6 months. She has been constipated in the last few weeks.'

Here, the following have been described:

(1) the main complaint—haemoptysis;

(2) other respiratory symptoms and how they have affected the patient;

(3) risk factors for possible causes (previous deep vein thrombosis is a risk factor for pulmonary embolism and smoking is a risk factor for lung cancer);

(4) other symptoms that give a clue to the cause of the main complaint, that is, weight loss and anorexia suggest lung cancer.

To do this, included are elements gleaned from the past medical history, the social history, and the systematic questions. This is an inexact science and different people will consider different features to be important. For example, here constipation has been mentioned in the HPC. This is probably not related to the main complaint and many people would not mention it here. But there is a chance that the constipation is related to hypercalcaemia secondary to a possible lung cancer—hence it can be considered reasonable to mention it in the HPC.

Having presented the HPC, run through the rest of the history: past medical, family, drug, and social histories and systematic questions. Mention negatives only where relevant. Keep it flowing. Use phrases such as 'In the past, Mrs Jones had a myocardial infarction ... ' rather than 'Past medical history: Mrs Jones had a myocardial infarction ... '.

It is said that you should always use the patient's own words—however, this may not be useful unless something very striking is said.

Examination

It is traditional that the student presents what they find on examination. Just as it is important to start the examination confidently, so it is essential to finish with a good presentation.

1. **Leave presentation to the end.** It is often difficult to decide whether to present as you go along or to wait until you have finished. In general, I suggest that you save presentation until you have finished examining and have all the information together.
2. **Use the end of your examination to think about your presentation.** As you come close to finishing examining the patient, focus your mind on what you have found, what you think the diagnosis is and what you're going to tell the examiner.
3. **Do not wait to be asked.** Once you have finished examining, stand up straight and present your findings!
4. **If you suspect a particular diagnosis, say so.** 'Mrs Smith has aortic stenosis as shown by a low volume pulse, a forceful but non-displaced apex beat, and an ejection systolic murmur radiating to the carotids. Jugular venous pressure was normal.'
5. **Stick to your guns.** Teachers often enjoy teasing students (they have got to get their fun somehow!) by querying findings even when they are correct. So it is important you stick to your guns. You should back down only if you are shown something that convinces you that you are wrong.

Answering doctors' questions

After presenting a case to a doctor, they will often ask you questions. These tend to follow a couple of themes:

(1) questions relating to the cause of your individual findings;

(2) questions relating to how you might deal with a patient with a particular symptom, sign, or condition.

Clearly, a certain amount of factual knowledge is required but just as important is a good system. There are some useful general rules to help you make the most of your knowledge.

Questions relating to the cause of your individual findings

A reasonable classification and an emphasis on common pathology are more important than the exact answer. Thus, when asked 'What are the causes of a pleural effusion?' a student might give a very comprehensive list: 'pneumonia, pulmonary emboli, nephrotic syndrome, systemic lupus erythematosus, rheumatoid arthritis, cardiac failure, bronchial carcinoma, lymphoma, mesothelioma, sub-phrenic abscess, Meig's syndrome, and hepatic failure.' However, such an answer implies little understanding of how pleural effusion occurs and no understanding of which causes are more likely. However, such understanding is paramount when it comes to actually managing such a problem. A much more preferable, though less comprehensive, answer might be 'pleural effusion may be classified into transudates and exudates. Transudates have protein content less than 30 g/l and are often bilateral. Exudates have protein content more than 30 g/l and tend to be unilateral. Transudates are commonly caused by cardiac failure. Exudates are commonly caused by lung malignancy, infection, or infarction.'

Questions relating to how you might deal with a patient with a particular symptom, sign, or condition

Here, the key is ABC (airway, breathing, circulation) for emergencies and history, examination, and investigation for non-emergencies. Thus, when asked 'How would you manage a patient having a myocardial infarction?' students are inclined to say 'thrombolysis ... oxygen ... analgesia ... '. A better answer is 'First of all, I would ascertain that the patient was conscious and breathing, with a palpable pulse. Presuming this to be the case, I would immediately insert an intravenous cannula (venflon) and give high-dose oxygen. Then, I would give intravenous analgesia (such as diamorphine) and an intravenous anti-emetic (such as metoclopramide). Next, I would give aspirin, provided the patient was not allergic to it and intravenous streptokinase, provided there were no contraindications.'

When asked 'How would you manage a patient with jaundice?' students are inclined to say 'ultrasound scan ... liver biopsy ... blood count ... '. A better answer is 'I would attempt to establish a diagnosis. First I would take a history—Does the patient drink alcohol? Have they had abdominal pain? Have they started new drugs recently? Next, I would examine the patient—Are the sclerae jaundiced? Are there signs of chronic liver disease? Is there an abdominal mass? Is there hepatomegaly? Then I would investigate—liver function tests, urinary urobilinogen, bilirubin, and ultrasound scan of abdomen.'

Keypoints

- The prime aim of history and examination is to arrive at a diagnosis or to produce possible differential diagnoses.
- A good bedside manner allows patients to more easily impart information to the doctor.
- Knowledge, experience, and perseverance together are essential for a good history.
- History taking may produce a morass of information. In all this, it is absolutely vital you are clear what the patient's main problem is.
- Always introduce yourself to the patient and shake hands.
- There is no perfect systems routine for examining systems.
- When managing emergencies, think 'airway, breathing, circulation'.
- When managing non-emergencies, think history, examination, investigation'.

Reference

Hodkinson HM. Evaluation of a mental test score for assessment of mental impairment in the elderly. *Age and Ageing* 1972; **1**:233–7.

CHAPTER 4

Cardiovascular system

Chapter contents

Introduction

The cardiovascular system comprises the heart and the vascular system—arteries, veins, and capillaries. It is of great importance because it is affected by several very common and potentially serious diseases, in particular coronary artery disease, which causes angina, myocardial infarction, and congestive cardiac failure. Furthermore many non-cardiac diseases produce cardiovascular effects—fast heart rate, low blood pressure, and excess vascular fluid.

In this chapter, you will learn what questions to ask patients with cardiovascular diseases and how to examine the cardiovascular system. Two of the most important cardiovascular investigations, the chest X-ray and the electrocardiogram (ECG), are discussed in chapters of their own (Chapters 15 and 16).

Symptoms

Chest pain

Chest pain is a very common symptom. It is important for several reasons: it is common, it may signify unpredictable and dangerous diseases, and patients, understandably, can get very anxious about it. Thus, you should have a good idea how to assess it. Although discussed in this (cardiac) chapter, chest pain is not always due to heart problems. Common and important causes are given in Table 4.1 and this discussion is confined to these.

Stable angina, unstable angina, and myocardial infarction all occur mostly in patients with coronary artery disease. In coronary artery disease, lipid deposits (atherosclerosis) in the walls of the coronary arteries produce narrowing of the arteries. This results in reduced blood flow to and hence hypoxia of the heart—ischaemic heart disease. High-risk groups for coronary artery disease include smokers and ex-smokers and patients with hypertension (high blood pressure), diabetes mellitus, hyperlipidaemia (*high-per-lipid-ee-mia*), or a family history of coronary artery disease.

TABLE 4.1 Common and important causes of chest pain

Common causes of chest pain	
Cardiac (coronary artery disease)	Stable angina, unstable angina, myocardial infarction, pericarditis
Respiratory	Infective pleurisy, pulmonary embolism
Upper gastro-intestinal	Gastro-oesophageal reflux disease, oesophagitis
Musculoskeletal	Viral infection of muscles, muscle strain
No cause found	Very common
Other less common but important causes of chest pain	
	Pneumothorax, aortic dissection

In stable angina, the narrowed coronary arteries can cope when the patient is resting, but when the heart needs more oxygen, as when the patient is walking, it cannot get enough oxygen—ischaemia (*iss-key-mia*). This ischaemia is felt as pain (angina). Because the pain is predictable the angina is said to be 'stable'. Stable angina may also occur in other conditions such as anaemia (because of reduced oxygen-carrying capacity of the blood) or thyrotoxicosis (increased oxygen demand from the tissues) (see p. 333). Unstable angina occurs when a thrombus forms on the diseased arterial wall but does not totally occlude (block) it. Such a thrombus may resolve or may go on to occlude the artery resulting in a myocardial infarction, hence 'unstable'. A myocardial infarction is usually due to a thrombus completely blocking off one of the coronary arteries so that an area of heart muscle actually dies—this is also known as a 'heart attack'.

Pericarditis (*perry-card-eye-tiss*) is an inflammation of the pericardial sac. It is commonly caused by viruses or occurs shortly after a myocardial infarction. Other rare causes are chronic kidney failure (uraemia), underactive thyroid (hypothyroidism), and tumours. Infective pleurisy (*ploor-issy*) occurs when pneumonia involves the pleural sac. Pulmonary embolism (*em-bo-liz-em*) is where a thrombus lodges in one of the pulmonary arteries often resulting in an area of pulmonary infarction. It commonly follows a thrombus in the leg veins (deep venous thrombosis) which detaches from the wall of the vein and reaches the pulmonary arteries via the right atrium and ventricle. Gastro-oesophageal reflux occurs when stomach acid refluxes back up from the stomach into the oesophagus. When this acid reflux causes mucosal damage, which is visible with an endoscope (camera test), this is called oesophagitis (*os-offer-jye-tiss*). Muscular pain may be due to muscular strain of the intercostal muscles or a viral infection of the muscles. Pneumothorax (*new-mo-thore-axe*) is where air gets into the pleural sac, usually resulting in a degree of lung collapse. Aortic dissection (*ay-or-tick dis-sex-shun* or *dye-sex-shun*) is where a tear occurs in the wall of the ascending aorta or the arch of the aorta.

This split in the wall of the aorta may spread to involve other arteries.

What to ask

This can be broken down into three sections: (1) questions about the pain itself, (2) questions about potential causes of the pain, and (3) questions about other cardiac symptoms.

Questions about the pain itself

As with any symptom, your questions should initially be open, for example, 'tell me about this pain' but there are certain key facts you need to establish.

> **Tip**
>
> Watch out for non-verbal clues. If the patient clenches their fist over the sternum in an effort to describe the pain, think cardiac. If they make an upward scooping movement of the hand over the chest, this may signify oesophageal pain 'trying to come out'.

1. Was this a single bout of pain or were there several?
2. How long did it last? You need an answer in seconds, minutes, hours, and so on. 'Not long' or 'forever' can mean anything. The patient may be reluctant to hazard what may be a misleading guess. Reassure them that you only need an estimate. If necessary (and it often is) give options: 'Did it last 2 seconds, 5 minutes, 1 hour, 5 hours ... ?'
3. Did anything bring it on? Ask specifically about exercise (such as walking) and breathing in. Pain worsened by inspiration is known as 'pleuritic pain'.
4. Did anything make it better? Ask about the effect of rest and treatments. Ask specifically about whether the patient uses a tablet or spray under their tongue. This is glyceryl trinitate (GTN); it usually relieves the pain of stable angina.

> **Tip**
>
> Relief by glyceryl trinitate (GTN) or rest is a very useful diagnostic point suggestive of stable angina but make sure you agree with the patient's assessment. Often, the patient will tell you that GTN helps the pain but it will turn out that the chest pain continued unabated for 20 min after taking GTN before resolving. It is very hard to say if this is really a response to GTN—which should occur within 5 min.

5. Where was the pain? Ask specifically about radiation (spread) of the pain to arms, neck, and jaw.
6. What kind (character) of pain was it? It may be easiest to give options: knife like, tight, burning, heavy, or aching.

> **Tip**
>
> Some patients may mix up 'sharp' and 'severe': the pain may actually be heavy but because it is severe, the patient describes it as sharp.

7. Onset? Was this gradual with a slow build-up or was the worst pain at the start?

You may notice that severity does not come into this list of questions even though myocardial infarction pain is often very severe. However, severity is so subjective and so difficult to quantify it is really not worth spending too much time on. Furthermore, many myocardial infarction pains are quite mild—indeed chest pain is absent in 25% of cases.

Questions about potential causes of the pain

The answers to your questions about the pain may lead you to suspect certain diagnoses. Ask about associated symptoms and risk factors relevant to the condition(s) you suspect. If these are present, it increases your index of suspicion.

Questions about other cardiac symptoms

You should always ask about the other cardiac symptoms—whether the patient also had breathlessness, palpitations, dizziness, or syncope around the time of the chest pain and also whether they have a tendency to ankle swelling.

Stable angina is suggested by a pain lasting 1–30 min brought on by exertion and relieved by rest or GTN within a minute or two. The pain is usually in the centre of the chest and may radiate into the arm(s), neck, or jaw. The character is usually tight or aching but it can be heavy or burning; knife-like pain is rare.

> **Tip**
>
> Be careful with the smoking history. When asked 'Do you smoke?', patients are inclined to answer 'no', carelessly omitting the fact that they stopped yesterday (the day of their admission with chest pain). Always ask 'Did you ever smoke?', 'When did you stop?', and 'How many did you smoke—two per day, 20 per day, 60 per day?'.

Associated symptoms are breathlessness, palpitations, and belching. Risk factors are family history, smoking, hypertension, diabetes mellitus, hyperlipidaemia, and previous cardiac history.

In unstable angina, two patterns are possible. The patient's stable angina deteriorates so that they have more severe angina after less and less exertion—with the character of the pain similar to their normal stable angina. This is also known as 'crescendo angina'. Alternatively, angina may occur at rest—often with the pain coming and going. It is unusual for pain to be present continuously for longer than half an hour but it may last several hours on and off. Associated symptoms are nausea and vomiting, belching, sweating, breathlessness, and palpitations. Risk factors are as for stable angina.

Tip

When taking a family history, younger relatives with cardiac histories are more important. If a younger sister died aged 40 from a myocardial infarction it is more significant than a grandfather dying aged 85. Ask about bypass operations. These are fairly hard second-hand evidence of cardiac disease.

The pain of myocardial infarction is traditionally said to be 'heavy and pressing' but it is just as often tight, burning, or aching. The pain quickly builds in severity and involves the central chest possibly radiating into the arm(s), neck, or jaw. The pain usually lasts for over half an hour. Associated symptoms are nausea and vomiting, belching, sweating, breathlessness, and palpitations. Risk factors are as for stable angina.

Tip

When a patient with chest pain is also suffering from nausea, vomiting, or sweatiness, these associated symptoms greatly increase the chance that the patient is having a myocardial infarction.

Tip

A very important risk factor in a patient with prolonged chest pain is a previous history suggestive of stable angina. Patients may tell you they have got angina. Do not just accept this. They may have been diagnosed by the plumber. You must go through the history and convince yourself.

Pericarditis produces a knife-like sternal pain, which is constant and may last for days. The pain may be eased by sitting forward and worsened by breathing in. Associated symptoms depend on the cause. A viral cause is associated with influenza-like symptoms such as feeling hot and cold, sweating, musculoskeletal pains, a cough, phlegm, and a sore throat. If the cause is a recent myocardial infarct, associated symptoms will be as described previously.

Infective pleurisy typically produces a knife-like pain worsened by inspiration. It lasts for days and occurs anywhere on the chest especially the sides and back. Associated symptoms are a cough, phlegm, feeling hot and cold, sweating, and musculoskeletal pains. Risk factors are previous history, contacts, and history of chest disease.

Pulmonary embolism produces a sudden-onset knife-like pain, usually, but not always, worsened by inspiration and it may occur anywhere on the chest. The site may change from hour to hour. Duration may be minutes to days. Associated symptoms are breathlessness, haemoptysis (*he-mop-ta-sis*), and leg swelling (suggestive of deep venous thrombosis in the leg). Risk factors are recent immobility or operation, previous history of pulmonary embolism, or deep venous thrombosis.

Tip

The patient may have more than one type of chest pain. Try to separate them out and analyse them individually.

Gastro-oesophageal reflux disease and oesophagitis tend to result in a pain that is retrosternal and burning, that is made worse by citrus fruits and spicy foods and sometimes by bending over, and that is eased by milk and antacids. It may last from a few minutes to several hours. It tends to be recurrent. It may occasionally be relieved by GTN, where this reduces oesophageal spasm through its muscle-relaxant properties. Associated symptoms are nausea, vomiting, and abdominal pain. Risk factors are smoking and alcohol consumption.

Muscular pain tends to be knife like, it may occur anywhere on the chest, and it may be increased by movement but this is very variable. It may come and go or it may last weeks. A risk factor is recent unusual physical activity.

Pneumothorax produces a sharp chest pain, which is worse on inspiration and usually localized to one area.

CASE 4.1

Problem. Your patient is a 73-year-old woman. She has burning chest pain but somehow seems more unwell than you might expect for someone with heartburn or oesophagitis. Why might this be?

Discussion. The patient may be having a myocardial infarction! It is often said that angina pain is tight, myocardial infarct pain is heavy, and oesophageal pain is burning. This is true: 95% of burning chest pain is oesophageal and only 5% is cardiac. However, cardiac chest pain may be burning or aching so that perhaps 30% of patients with myocardial infarction describe their pain as burning.

CASE 4.2

Problem. You're seeing a 50-year-old man with chest pain just arrived in the casualty department. He doesn't look well, yet after several minutes you've only got the answers to a couple of questions and you're starting to panic.

Discussion. Your approach to the history should alter according to the situation. In this emergency situation, you must combine your history with examination (pulse and blood pressure especially), arranging an electrocardiogram, inserting a venflon (a little plastic tube inserted into the vein with help from a needle that allows treatment to be given) (see Fig. 17.4), and giving treatment (oxygen, analgesia, aspirin, and thrombolytic drugs). Such a scenario makes precise detail in the history both less important and more difficult to achieve. The key questions should address (1) duration and character of the pain, (2) effect of inspiration, (3) presence of nausea and sweating, (4) smoking, diabetes, and hypertension, and (5) previous cardiac history. If you believe the patient is having a myocardial infarction, you will need to ask about possible reasons where treatment with aspirin or thrombolysis (*throm-bo-lie-sis or throm-bol-iss-iss*) might be dangerous—such as a recent gastrointestinal bleed.

More commonly, the student will see the patient either a few days after this event or when they are describing less severe, more intermittent symptoms not currently present. Here a more comprehensive history is both achievable and expected.

Breathlessness is an associated symptom. Risk factors are previous pneumothorax and recent chest injury.

For aortic dissection, see Case 4.3.

Sometimes, an exact diagnosis of the cause of the chest pain is impossible. The history can never be 100% conclusive. This is even more the case if the patient is vague or through anxiety exaggerates their symptoms (usually by lengthening them) so making them sound less cardiac. Therefore, doctors often confine themselves to confirming or excluding the more serious causes, such as cardiac ischaemia or infarction and pulmonary embolism or more treatable causes, such as infective pleurisy. This limited aim is not often explained well to the patient who can be understandably annoyed or worried to be sent home from hospital with no diagnosis for a chest pain deemed severe enough to require admission.

CASE 4.3

Problem. Your patient is a 40-year-old man. He looks very unwell and is complaining of severe chest pain together with pain between the shoulder blades, yet the electrocardiogram shows no sign of myocardial infarction. Why might this be?

Discussion. Consider aortic dissection. This is where a tear occurs in the wall of the aorta. This often produces a sudden searing pain in the chest and between the shoulder blades. The pain of dissection is worst at onset as opposed to the more gradual build-up of pain in myocardial infarction. This split in the wall of the aorta may spread to involve other arteries. In around half of all cases, the left subclavian artery is involved but not the right—resulting in a reduced left radial pulse. The dissection may occasionally involve the aortic valve producing signs of aortic regurgitation (10%) and there may be evidence of a left pleural effusion (3%). Risk factors include hypertension, pregnancy, and Marfan's syndrome. In around 1% of cases, the dissection may involve the coronary arteries—producing signs of a myocardial infarction. This is important because thrombolysis (clot busting), which is used in the treatment of myocardial infarction, is dangerous in aortic dissection, where it makes the bleeding worse. **Thus, all patients with an apparent myocardial infarction should have their pulses compared prior to giving thrombolysis.**

Keypoints

- Chest pain has multiple causes, not just cardiac causes.
- The most important causes are cardiac causes, pulmonary embolism, and aortic dissection.
- Your approach to taking a chest pain history depends greatly on the urgency of the situation.
- Various features in the history of chest pain point to or away from certain diagnoses but no single feature or group of features can exclude or conclusively diagnose any chest pain.
- There are two main types of question: those about the pain itself and those about potential causes of the pain.
- Onset, duration, site, character, precipitating factors, and relieving factors are the most important features when asking about the pain itself.
- Duration is useful in deciding whether a particular cardiac pain represents angina or myocardial infarction.
- Pain lasting just a few seconds or continuously for longer than 24 h is rarely cardiac.
- Cardiac pain is usually central, not left sided.
- Relief by rest or glyceryl trinitate and aggravation by exertion are probably the best ways of diagnosing stable angina.
- The character of myocardial infarction pain is quite non-specific.
- Associated symptoms such as sweating or nausea are important in deciding how likely it is for prolonged chest pain to be due to a myocardial infarction.
- Aggravation by inspiration suggests a pleuritic or pericarditic pain.
- The electrocardiogram is very helpful in diagnosing myocardial infarction.

Breathlessness

Like chest pain, breathlessness (dyspnoea) (*dis-knee-a*) is a very common symptom. You should be confident in evaluating patients with breathlessness. Common and important causes are listed in Table 4.2 and this discussion is confined to these. Breathlessness is a symptom of many conditions, not just cardiac conaditions. It could equally be discussed under a respiratory system heading.

TABLE 4.2 Common and important causes of breathlessness

Cardiac	Cardiac failure which may be acute (associated with angina or myocardial infarction) or chronic; angina equivalent
Respiratory	Asthma, pneumothorax, pneumonia, bronchitis, bronchiectasis (*bron-key-eck-ta-sis*), chronic obstructive pulmonary disease, pulmonary fibrosis, pulmonary embolism
Non-cardiorespiratory	Anaemia, hyperventilation including diabetic ketoacidosis, overweight

1. Cardiac failure is where the heart is unable to pump enough blood to meet the demands of the body tissues. Fluid accumulates throughout the body. In the lungs, this results in pulmonary congestion and oedema (*ee-dee-ma*) so causing breathlessness.

Tip

Be careful when using the terms ‘heart failure’ or ‘cardiac failure’ to patients. Take time to explain that the heart has not ground to a complete halt but rather it is not working as well as it should.

2. Angina equivalent is caused by coronary artery disease in the same way as angina, the difference being that the primary symptom is breathlessness rather than pain.
3. Asthma is where the bronchial airways are obstructed (usually reversible to some extent).
4. For pneumothorax, see p. 119 and Figs 16.43 and 16.44.
5. Inflammation of the lungs is usually caused by infection. It may affect the bronchi alone (bronchitis) or may also affect the alveoli (pneumonia). In bronchiectasis, the primary problem is dilated bronchi; these are prone to infection.
6. Chronic obstructive pulmonary disease (COPD) occurs when there is longstanding airways obstruction, which is mostly irreversible. It may be a sequela (*see-quill-ee*) of either chronic bronchitis, emphysema (*em-fi-seem-ya*), or both (most common). Chronic bronchitis is defined as sputum production for most days in 3 months of 2 successive years. Emphysema is defined

on a histological basis as dilated air spaces but clinically is a disease of smokers associated with minimal previous sputum production.

7. Patients with pulmonary fibrosis have widespread fibrosis of the lungs. It may be idiopathic (*id-ee-owe-path-ick*) or result from autoimmune disease, dust exposure (asbestos or coal), or drugs (such as amiodarone (*am-ee-owe-da-roan*)).
8. For pulmonary embolism, see Fig 16.45.
9. Anaemia is where a patient's haemoglobin level is low. This may result in 'high-output' cardiac failure.
10. Hyperventilation is where breathing is excessive, more than is necessary to maintain oxygen and carbon dioxide levels. It is usually a reaction to anxiety where hyperventilation results in a respiratory alkalosis but occasionally it is a response to metabolic acidosis as in renal failure or diabetic ketoacidosis (*key-toe-acid-owe-sis*).

What to ask

As with chest pain, your approach to the history depends greatly on the situation. If your patient has just come through the casualty department doors and is in distress, your history need not be so comprehensive and you will need to combine it with examination (especially pulse, blood pressure, respiratory rate, chest, and temperature), inserting a venflon, arranging or doing tests (such as arterial blood gases, chest X-ray, ECG, and blood count), and giving treatment (oxygen, diuretic, steroids, and bronchodilator depending on the cause). The questions can be broken down into three sections: (1) questions about the breathlessness itself, (2) questions about other cardiac and respiratory symptoms, and (3) questions about potential causes of the breathlessness.

Questions about the breathlessness itself

Your questions should initially be open, for example, 'tell me about this breathlessness', but there are certain key facts you need to establish.

1. When did the breathlessness start? Are we talking about a single bout or recurrent bouts of breathlessness (acute) or has the breathlessness been present for some time (months or years)?—chronic? If the latter, has there been a recent deterioration?—acute-on-chronic?
2. How bad is it? How disabling is it? What can the patient not do that they used to be able to do? This may be obvious, the patient may be breathless at rest but if not, it is best to ask how much exercise they can do. Get a specific answer—a flight of stairs, 10 yards, 100 yards, a mile—or their metric equivalents. Patients may find this difficult. Ask if they get out much. If so, do they walk to or around the shops, to the pub, and so on? Try to get a comparison with normal, say a few months ago.
3. Do they get breathless lying flat (orthopnoea) (*or-thop-knee-a*)? If so, do they regularly prop themselves up in bed and how many pillows do they use? Orthopnoea suggests a more severe degree of breathlessness. It is more typical of cardiac breathlessness but also occurs in patients with respiratory causes.
4. Does the patient suffer from paroxysmal nocturnal dyspnoea? This is where the patient wakes up at night feeling breathless. There may or may not be a story of the patient either sitting over the side, getting out of bed, or putting their head out of the window for a breath. Again, this is more suggestive of cardiac breathlessness but by no means an absolute rule.
5. What treatment have they previously had for their breathlessness and did it work?

Questions about other cardiac and respiratory symptoms

Ask about chest pain, palpitations, dizziness or syncope, and ankle swelling. Also ask about the main respiratory symptoms—cough, phlegm, haemoptysis, and wheeze.

Questions about potential causes of the breathlessness

Hopefully, your previous questions will have given you some idea of what the diagnosis is, so obtain further information about what you think are the likely causes. Ask about associated symptoms and risk factors relevant to the condition(s) you suspect.

The answers to these questions should give you some idea of the cause. It is simplest to divide causes into acute, chronic, and acute-on-chronic.

Acute

1. **Angina equivalent**. Breathing difficulties lasting 1–30 min brought on by exertion and relieved by rest or GTN within a minute or two. Associated symptoms are palpitations and belching. Risk factors are a family history, smoking, hypertension, diabetes mellitus, and hyperlipidaemia.
2. **Stable angina with cardiac failure.** Breathlessness and chest pain lasting 1–30 min brought on by exertion and relieved by rest or GTN within a

minute or two. The pain is usually in the centre of the chest and may radiate into the arm(s), neck, or jaw. The pain is usually tight or aching but can be heavy or burning; knife like pain is rare. Associated symptoms are palpitations and belching. Risk factors are as for angina equivalent.

3. **Myocardial infarction with cardiac failure.** Sudden-onset acute breathlessness at rest, which may be severe. Associated symptoms are chest pain, nausea and vomiting, belching, sweating, and palpitations. Risk factors are as for angina equivalent.
4. **Asthma.** Intermittent bouts of breathlessness, especially in young people, which may be severe. It responds to bronchodilators in either inhaler or nebulizer form. Associated symptoms are wheeze and a dry cough. Risk factors are a history of allergy and a family history.
5. **Pneumothorax.** Sudden-onset breathlessness in (often young) people who were usually not breathless previously. An associated symptom is pleuritic chest pain. A risk factor is a history of chest disease.
6. **Pneumonia and bronchitis.** Gradual-onset breathlessness but of short duration (days). Associated symptoms are a cough, phlegm, feeling hot and cold, and pleuritic chest pain. Risk factors are a previous history, contact with patients with a similar illness, and a history of chest disease.
7. **Pulmonary embolism.** Sudden-onset breathlessness, which may be severe. May be eased by lying flat (see Case 4.6). Associated symptoms are pleuritic chest pain, breathlessness, haemoptysis, and leg swelling suggesting deep venous thrombosis. Risk factors are recent immobility or operation and a previous history of pulmonary embolism or deep venous thrombosis.
8. **Hyperventilation.** Sudden-onset breathlessness. An associated symptom is anxiety. Risk factors are uncontrolled diabetes, acute renal failure, and anxiety.

Chronic

1. **Cardiac failure.** Chronic breathlessness with orthopnoea, with or without paroxysmal nocturnal dyspnoea; responds to diuretics. An associated symptom is ankle swelling. Risk factors are ischaemic heart disease (myocardial infarction or angina), smoking, hypertension, and valvular heart disease.
2. **COPD.** Long history of breathlessness with orthopnoea; may respond to bronchodilators, antibiotics, or steroids. Associated symptoms are a cough, phlegm, and wheeze. A risk factor is smoking.
3. **Bronchiectasis.** Long history of breathlessness associated with producing large amounts of sputum. Associated symptoms are a cough and copious phlegm. Risk factors are childhood measles or whooping cough and smoking.
4. **Pulmonary fibrosis.** Long history of breathlessness with orthopnoea. An associated symptom is a cough. Risk factors are smoking, coal mining, asbestos exposure, and amiodarone treatment.
5. **Pulmonary embolism.** Occasionally multiple pulmonary emboli may cause chronic breathlessness. See previous text for associated symptoms and risk factors.
6. **Anaemia.** Chronic breathlessness. An associated symptom is fatigue. Risk factors are chronic bleeding—overt or occult. Ask specifically about non-steroidal anti-inflammatory drug use.
7. **Hyperventilation.** Gradual-onset breathlessness, especially in renal failure. An associated symptom is the tingling of fingers and toes. Risk factors are diabetes and kidney failure.

Acute-on-chronic

All the acute causes commonly occur in patients with chronic diseases causing breathlessness. Thus, in many patients with breathlessness the onset is 'acute-on-chronic'. Acute cardiac problems tend to occur in patients with chronic cardiac disease and acute respiratory problems tend to occur in patients with chronic respiratory disease.

CASE 4.4

Problem. My patient is very breathless, so much so he can't answer my questions. What should I do?

Discussion. Hopefully, the patient has a companion who can help with history. If not, use the history the patient can give you along with clues from any medication he may have with him and examination findings to come to a diagnosis. You may have to give treatments such as nebulizers and diuretics without being entirely sure they are appropriate. Do not delay.

CASE 4.5

Problem. A 23-year-old man arrives in the casualty department. He is so breathless he cannot speak; his friend tells you he is an asthmatic. But when you listen to his chest with the stethoscope, he seems to be getting good amounts of air into and out of his lungs. What might be going on? What sign and which test will help you to decide?

Discussion. The patient may be hyperventilating. It is not surprising that some asthmatic patients may misinterpret their own symptoms and work themselves into a hyperventilation frenzy. Beware of making this diagnosis lightly: your patient's anxiety may be well founded and they could be having a severe asthmatic attack. The patient's heart rate may be helpful. If the patient's heart rate is above 120 beats/min, his symptoms are unlikely to just be caused by anxiety. Never diagnose hyperventilation without checking arterial blood gases. If PO_2 is greater than 10.6 kPa and pH is greater than 7.45, hyperventilation is likely. A low PCO_2 may occur both in asthma and hyperventilation.

CASE 4.6

Problem. Your patient is a 75-year-old man who had a hip operation 10 days ago. He has a past history of cardiac failure. All was going well until today when he developed a sudden onset of breathlessness eased by lying flat. What might be happening?

Discussion. Although the patient has had cardiac failure in the past you should be thinking of pulmonary embolism. The breathlessness of pulmonary embolism may be unusual because sometimes it is eased by lying flat, which increases right ventricular filling and hence cardiac output. In this patient, the post-operative timing is typical of a pulmonary embolism. Ask about leg swelling (suggesting deep venous thrombosis).

Ankle or leg swelling

See also text discussing examination of ankle oedema (p. 57) and examination of sacral oedema (p. 62). Patients may complain of leg or ankle swelling. Leg or ankle swelling may be caused either by fat or by abnormal accumulation of fluid within the subcutaneous tissues (peripheral oedema). Patients do not tend to complain of leg swelling when the cause is fat as the onset is so gradual and the cause clear. However, when build-up of fluid occurs within the tissues, this can be quite rapid and hence noticeable to the patient.

CASE 4.7

Problem. The patient is an 80-year-old man complaining of severe breathlessness on a background of chronic breathlessness. How do you decide whether he has chronic cardiac failure or chronic respiratory disease?

Discussion. This is a common problem and nowhere near as simple as it might sound. Ask about indicators of heart disease such as chest pain and previous history of angina or myocardial infarction. Ask about indicators of respiratory disease such as a cough and phlegm along with a previous history of chest disease. Oedema points slightly towards cardiac failure. Wheeze points slightly towards chest disease. Both groups tend to be smokers. Ask about medications. If the patient is mostly on bronchodilators, respiratory causes are more likely whilst diuretic therapy suggests cardiac failure. Physical examination and the chest X-ray are helpful. Often though the conditions may co-exist or it is difficult to decide which condition is present—as demonstrated by the high number of patients on both types of treatment.

Keypoints

- Try to decide if breathlessness is acute, chronic, or acute-on-chronic.
- Get an idea of how disabling the breathlessness is.
- Orthopnoea and paroxysmal nocturnal dyspnoea are said to suggest cardiac causes but may also occur in respiratory causes.
- Response to diuretics suggests a cardiac cause.

Classification of peripheral oedema

Peripheral oedema may be generalized or localized (see Table 4.3). Generalized oedema is caused by fluid overload or hypoproteinaemia (where a reduction in plasma osmotic pressure causes leakage of fluid across the capillaries). In generalized oedema, gravity dictates where the fluid collects so in a normally ambulant patient, fluid tends to initially collect around the ankles. The

TABLE 4.3 Causes of peripheral oedema

Generalized (usually results in bilateral oedema)	
Fluid overload	Heart failure, oliguric renal failure, iatrogenic (*eye-at-roe-jen-ick*)*
Hypoproteinaemia	Gastrointestinal malabsorption, protein malnutrition, liver cirrhosis (*si-roe-sis*), nephrotic (*nef-rot-ick*) syndrome
Localized (often results in unilateral oedema)	
Chronic venous insufficiency (varicose veins)	Usually bilateral
Venous obstruction	Venous thrombosis, tumour
Increased capillary permeability	Injury, infection
Lymphatic obstruction	Lymphoedema (Milroy's congenital hypoplasia of lymphatic vessels†, tumour)
Postural	Standing for long periods

* Iatrogenic: caused by a doctor's intervention.

† *William Forsyth Milroy (1855–1942), American physician.*

most common serious cause of ankle swelling is the generalized oedema of cardiac failure. However, ankle oedema is caused by many other conditions (Table 4.3), the most common being postural oedema exacerbated by incompetent venous valves. So be careful before diagnosing cardiac failure on the basis of ankle swelling alone.

What to ask

If the patient has bilateral ankle swelling, evaluate for a cardiac cause. Ask about chest pain, breathlessness, previous angina, myocardial infarction, and smoking. Remember also to ask about varicose veins.

Keypoints

- Bilateral ankle swelling is a feature of heart failure but also occurs in many other situations.
- Ask about other cardiac history and varicose veins.

Palpitations

What are they?

Palpitations are an awareness of the patient's own heart beating.

What are they due to?

Palpitations may be due to sinus tachycardia (*tacky-cardia*), ectopic beats (extrasystoles) (*extra-sis-toe-lees*), or arrhythmias (*ay-rith-me-as*).

Palpitations due to sinus tachycardia are a normal response to exercise and may occur in various conditions, particularly infections and stress. Ectopic beats are cardiac beats that do not originate from the sinoatrial (*sigh-no-ay-tree-al*) node. They are often one-off abnormal beats of minimal significance but may sometimes be caused by coronary ischaemia. Arrhythmias are abnormal heart rhythms lasting for more than a few beats. They are usually caused by electrical problems in the heart. Sometimes, the primary problem may be ischaemia, which damages the electrical pathways. They may be worsened by electrolyte imbalance.

You will come across palpitations in three main situations.

1. The patient has noticed occasional 'missed beats'. This is rarely important and is usually due to ectopic beats.
2. The palpitations are a minor part of a more serious situation such as when the patient is suffering a myocardial infarction
3. The patient is suffering from intermittent bouts of prolonged palpitations, which are their main symptom.

It is this third scenario that I will now discuss. Common causes are shown in Table 4.4.

When taking a history you are aiming to decide the following.

What the patient means by palpitations

Some patients will use the term 'palpitations' in an apparently knowledgeable way but when you ask them you will find they are talking about a chest pain, indigestion, or even a shaking feeling. Ask 'Do you get a feeling of your heart beating in your chest?'

TABLE 4.4 Common causes of palpitations

Common types of palpitations	Features
Sinus tachycardia	Fast, regular, gradual onset and end
Atrial arrhythmias	
Atrial tachycardia	Fast, regular, abrupt onset and end
Supraventricular tachycardia	Fast, regular, abrupt onset and end
Atrial fibrillation	Fast, irregular, abrupt onset and end
Atrial flutter	Fast, regular or irregular, abrupt onset and end
Ventricular arrhythmias	
Ventricular tachycardia	Fast, regular, abrupt onset and end, tendency to blackout
Multiple ectopic beats	
Atrial or ventricular	Slow, irregular

Are the palpitations caused by sinus tachycardia or an arrhythmia? If it is an arrhythmia, is it ventricular tachycardia or atrial fibrillation or is it due to ischaemia?

Find out what the palpitations are like.

1. Are the beats fast, slow, regular, or irregular?

Tip

Patients may find it difficult to describe the speed and regularity of palpitations. Ask them to tap the rhythm out on a desk or table. If necessary, give them a demonstration of what you mean.

2. Was the onset of the palpitations sudden or gradual (see Table 4.4)?
3. Ask about blackouts.
4. Was there any chest pain? Did the pain precede the palpitations?
5. Ask about potentially avoidable precipitating factors: exercise, stress, and alcohol. These can all cause sinus tachycardias or precipitate other arrhythmias.

A gradual onset suggests sinus tachycardia whereas an abrupt onset suggests an arrhythmia. However, patients often find it difficult to decide how suddenly the palpitations started. Irregular palpitations suggest atrial fibrillation (*fib-rill-ay-shun*). Ventricular tachycardia is important as it may be life threatening. Usually it results in a markedly reduced cardiac output so palpitations are not felt and blackout occurs instead. Sometimes, though, the patient may feel palpitations and there may be associated blackouts (dizziness may be associated with any type of palpitation). Arrhythmias may result in reduced cardiac output and so patients may develop cardiac ischaemia with angina. However, sometimes ischaemia is actually the primary problem. If the pain precedes the palpitations, then ischaemia is likely to be the primary problem. If the palpitations precede the pain, ischaemia is likely to be secondary. It has to be said that patients do not always find this differentiation easy.

How troublesome the palpitations are to the patient

Apart from ventricular tachycardia, atrial fibrillation, and arrhythmias due to ischaemia, most other types of arrhythmia are quite benign, more troublesome than life threatening. You should find out how much trouble they cause. Ask how often the palpitations happen,

CASE 4.8

Problem. My patient complains of palpitations. Could this be due to her high coffee intake?

Discussion. Contrary to popular opinion, caffeine rarely causes a sinus tachycardia. In fact, most of the evidence points to a bradycardia. Caffeine does cause a sensation of tremulousness and this can be mistaken for palpitations.

Keypoints

- Make sure you and the patient are on the same wavelength when using the word 'palpitations'.
- Ask about speed of onset, rate, regularity, chest pain, blackouts, precipitants, and effects on quality of life.
- Gradual onset and ending suggests sinus tachycardia.
- Irregularity suggests atrial fibrillation.
- When palpitations are accompanied by blackouts, think about ventricular tachycardia.
- If chest pain occurs find out whether it precedes or follows the palpitations.

how long they last, and whether they stop the patient doing things they would otherwise like to?

Syncope

Syncope is discussed in Chapter 11.

The importance of examining the cardiovascular system

The clinical approach to examining the cardiovascular system has changed greatly in recent decades. First, rheumatic (*room-attic*) heart disease is now much rarer in Western countries. Rheumatic heart disease causes valvular heart disease, which in the past caused considerable illness and death in relatively young people. These valvular lesions produced specific physical signs so that, with good technique, the physician could make diagnoses using clinical examination. Valvular heart disease has not gone completely but it is rarer, especially the distinctive lesions produced by rheumatic heart disease. Second, the development of new investigations has meant that most, if not all, examination techniques can be equalled by 'tests'. For example, a cardiac monitor can be used to assess pulse rate and rhythm, a chest X-ray (Chapter 16) can be used to check for heart failure, and an echocardiogram (echo) can be used to evaluate heart valves.

Despite these changes, skill in cardiovascular system examination remains extremely important. Why? The ability to examine pulse rate and rhythm, blood pressure, jugular venous pressure, and basal lung crackles is absolutely essential in managing acutely unwell patients, while clinical assessment of valvular lesions remains an important part of medical work. And remember you may not always have access to technology when you really need it.

The key to examining the cardiovascular system is practice. By getting a feel for normality you can quickly tell when something is not quite right. As elsewhere in the book, a difficulty factor (DF) has been assigned to each sign. This gives some general idea of how difficult a test is and how much practice is needed. Examining the cardiovascular system may seem daunting initially but with practice becomes quite easy.

Many cardiac lesions produce signs that are best described in relation to the 'cardiac cycle', which will

Keypoints

- With practice, examining the cardiovascular system becomes easy.

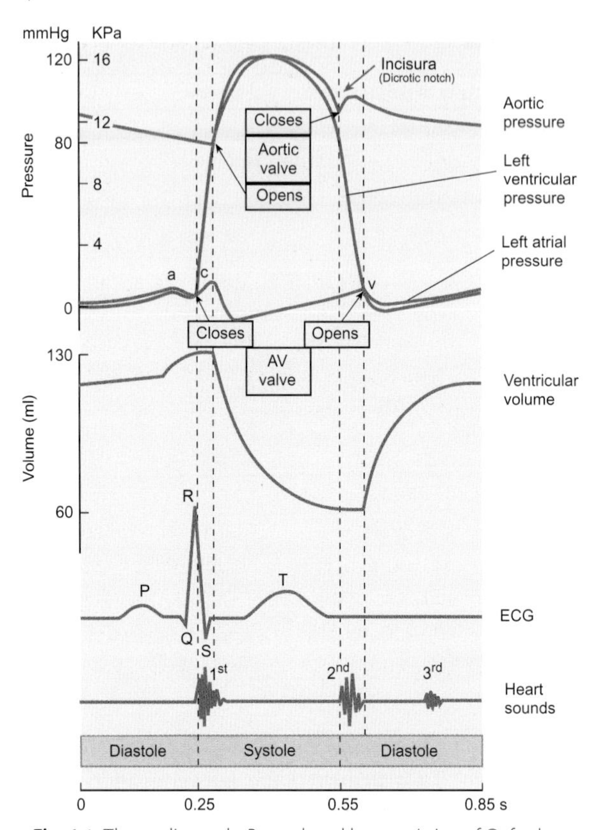

Fig. 4.1 The cardiac cycle. Reproduced by permission of Oxford University Press from **Fig. 15.11** (p. 286), *Human physiology: the basis of medicine*, by G. Pocock and C. Richards (1999).

be briefly described (see Fig. 4.1). Do not waste time trying to learn this off by heart now. Use it as a reference for the rest of the chapter. The cardiac cycle can be divided into ventricular systole (*sis-toe-ly*) (contraction) and diastole (*die-ass-toe-ly*) (relaxation). At the start of diastole, all heart valves (mitral, tricuspid (*try-cuss-pid*), aortic, and pulmonary) are closed. This is the period of isovolumetric (*ice-so-vol-you-metric*) relaxation. 'Isovolumetric' means that the volume of blood in the ventricles remains constant. Next, the mitral and tricuspid valves open and blood pours from the atria into the relaxed ventricles. Initially, this flow of blood is fast (period of rapid ventricular filling), then it slows down (period of reduced ventricular filling). Then the atria contract to force a further small bolus of blood into the ventricles (atrial systole). Now, the ventricles begin to contract and the mitral and tricuspid valves are forced shut. There is a short period of isovolumetric contraction before the aortic and pulmonary valves are forced open. Blood is now ejected from the ventricles. Initially this is fast (period of rapid ventricular ejection), then it slows down (period of reduced ejection). As the contraction ends, the aortic and pulmonary valves shut again and diastole begins with the period of isovolumetric relaxation.

As with all systems, a routine has been used to discuss the various physical signs. This has the advantage of simulating how students are taught and examined. Like all routines, it is an abbreviation of all the signs you might possibly look for. Routines are not perfect, for instance, rare tests such as inspection for splinter haemorrhages are included in this cardiovascular system routine while important tests such as blood pressure measurement are excluded.

Cardiovascular system examination summary

This summary contains many terms that you will not understand on first reading. These terms are explained in the next section 'Cardiovascular examination in detail'.

1. Introduce yourself to the patient and ask for permission to examine.
2. Ask the patient to get on to the bed (if not already on the bed). You may need to help!
3. Ask the patient to remove all garments covering chest and arms. For female patients, offer to cover the chest with a sheet or towel.
4. Arrange the patient so that their chest is at 45°.
5. While doing 1–4, be having a 'general look'. Is the patient distressed, for example?
6. Inspect both hands and fingernails for splinter haemorrhages (DF 5/10), clubbing (DF 8/10), and tar staining (DF 1/10).
7. Palpate right radial pulse for pulse rate (DF 3/10) and rhythm (DF 6/10). Palpate right and left radial pulses together and compare (DF 8/10). Check for collapsing pulse (DF 6/10).
8. Inspect face for malar (*may-lar*) flush (DF 7/10) and xanthelasmata (*zan-the-laz-matta*) (DF 2/10). Inspect eyes for corneal arcus (*ark-us*) (DF 2/10). Inspect conjunctivae for anaemia (DF 9/10). Inspect tongue for cyanosis (*sigh-an-owe-sis*) (DF 9/10).
9. Palpate right carotid pulse for pulse character (DF 8/10).
10. Inspect right internal jugular vein for jugular venous pressure (DF 9/10). Check for hepatojugular reflux (DF 8/10).
11. Take sheet off chest (female patients). Inspect praecordium (*pre-cord-ee-yum*) in general and specifically for scars, cardiac impulse, and any other abnormal pulsations (DF 5/10).
12. Palpate at apex for apex beat, assessing position and character (DF 9/10). Palpate for left parasternal impulse (DF 9/10) and aortic and pulmonary thrills (DF 6/10).
13. Auscultate (DF 8/10)—whilst palpating carotid pulse to time any murmur. Listen with
    - diaphragm at mitral area (move to axilla if systolic murmur heard)
    - bell at apex with patient lying on their left-hand side
    - bell at tricuspid area (normal patient position)
    - diaphragm at tricuspid area
    - diaphragm at pulmonary area
    - diaphragm at aortic area
    - diaphragm at right, then left carotid
    - diaphragm over lower left sternal edge with patient sat forward with breath held in expiration
    - diaphragm to auscultate over lung bases.
14. Palpate for ankle or shin oedema over lower anterior tibia (DF 3/10).
15. Consider looking for other signs such as—radiofemoral delay and pulsatile liver.
16. Wash your hands.
17. Now say 'I would like to check the blood pressure'. Pause briefly and then present findings.

Cardiovascular system examination in detail

Getting started

1. Introduce yourself to the patient and ask for permission to examine.

1. Put out your hand to shake the patient's hand.
2. Say something like 'Hello, I'm William Osler, third-year medical student. Do you mind if I examine your heart and pulses?' Do not just say 'heart'! The patient will wonder what you are up to when you start looking at his hands!

2. Ask the patient to get on to the bed (if not already on the bed). You may need to help!

Usually, this will be no problem, but if the patient is unable to get on to the bed, offer your assistance and if necessary ask for the assistance of trained nurses.

3. Ask the patient to remove all garments covering chest and arms. For female patients, offer to cover the chest with a sheet or towel.

The cardiovascular system is examined with the patient's chest bare (Fig. 4.2). It is best to get this sorted out at the start of the examination—and in female patients offer to cover the chest up with a sheet or towel till you get to examination of the chest itself.

At least one woman (such as medical student or nurse) must be present to act as a chaperone.

4. Arrange the patient so that their chest is at 45°.

The cardiovascular system is examined with the patient sitting so that the upper part of their body is at 45°to the horizontal; the patient's neck should be **relaxed** against the pillow (Fig. 4.2), primarily to facilitate examination of the jugular venous pressure (p. 40). You may need to adjust the bed's headrest to get the patient in the correct position.

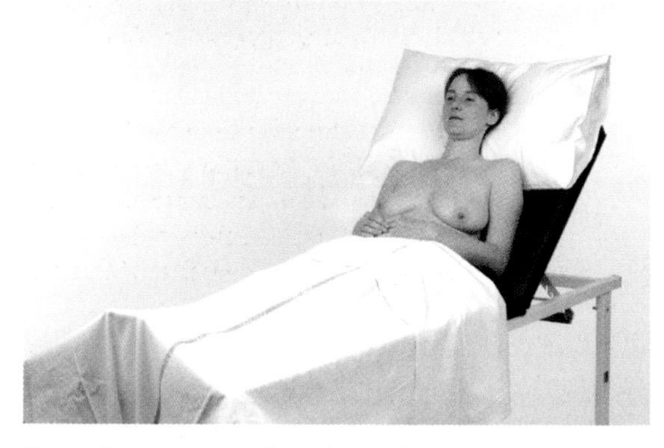

Fig. 4.2 Patient exposure for cardiovascular system examination.

CASE 4.9

Problem. I don't feel quite right asking women to bare their chests especially when the first part of the cardiovascular examination doesn't involve the chest.

Discussion. Students, quite understandably, are often unsure if this is appropriate. Such doubt can create a confidence problem—not a good thing at this early stage of the cardiovascular examination. I suggest you say something like 'Ideally, it's best if I examine you with your chest bare. Is that all right? I can cover up your chest with a sheet for part of the examination.' Give the patient opportunity to refuse. If she refuses (unusual), do not take this as a slight, just get on with the examination as best you can.

Tip

Get to know how to work the headrests on hospital beds.

5. While doing 1–4, be having a 'general look'. Is the patient distressed, for example?

See p. 15 for more details on 'general look'.

1. Patient distress suggests severe illness.
2. A venflon suggests recent chest pain (the venflon is in case analgesia or resuscitation are required) or heart failure (requiring intravenous diuretics). Rarely, the venflon is being used to give intravenous antibiotics in patients with infective endocarditis (p. 63).
3. A monitor suggests recent chest pain or arrhythmia.
4. A malar flush (p. 37) suggests *mitral stenosis (my-tral-sten-owe-sis)* (p. 64).
5. Tachypnoea (*tack-kip-nia*) suggests heart failure (pp. 68–9).
6. Cyanosis suggests hypoxia.
7. Forceful neck pulsations may indicate aortic regurgitation (p. 67).

Tip

Always remember that the general look is something you do while sorting other things out. Do not stand back to have an aimless gawp.

Hands

6. Inspect both hands and fingernails for splinter haemorrhages (DF5/10), clubbing (DF8/10), and tar staining (DF1/10).

Splinter haemorrhages

What are they?

These are small haemorrhages within the nailbed under the nail.

Significance

Inspection for splinter haemorrhages is included in the cardiovascular system examination because they occur in patients with infective endocarditis (p. 63), which is infection of the heart. Infective endocarditis affects the heart mainly by damaging the valves. It may also cause widespread inflammation of small vessels (vasculitis). Vasculitis in the nailbed may be followed by haemorrhage—producing splinter haemorrhages. However, 90% of patients with infective endocarditis do not have 'splinters'. Furthermore, they are more commonly caused by minor trauma to the nails. When due to trauma, they are much more common in fingers than in toes and occur particularly in manual workers.

How to examine

Splinter haemorrhages usually look like dark pen marks under the nail (Fig. 4.3), though occasionally they are bright red. They lie parallel to the long axis of the nail. Though they are small, they are relatively easy to see if you look carefully. Be careful, they may occur in just one nailbed. It is said that splinter haemorrhages due to endocarditis are more commonly seen in the proximal part of the nail, though hard evidence for this is lacking.

1. Take the patient's right hand.
2. Stoop down to inspect the nails.
3. Combining thoroughness and speed, carefully inspect all the nails of the right hand.
4. Do the same for the left hand.

The main trouble with finding splinter haemorrhages is that because they are rare, students may find themselves just going through the motions so that when they do occur, they miss them. Avoid complacency!

Clubbing

Clubbing is mainly seen in respiratory disease and is therefore discussed in detail on p. 84. However, it may be seen very rarely in cardiovascular disease—cyanotic congenital heart disease and infective endocarditis (p. 63). Clubbing is a late feature of infective endocarditis, so if clubbing is due to this, there will be other more convincing features of infective endocarditis present.

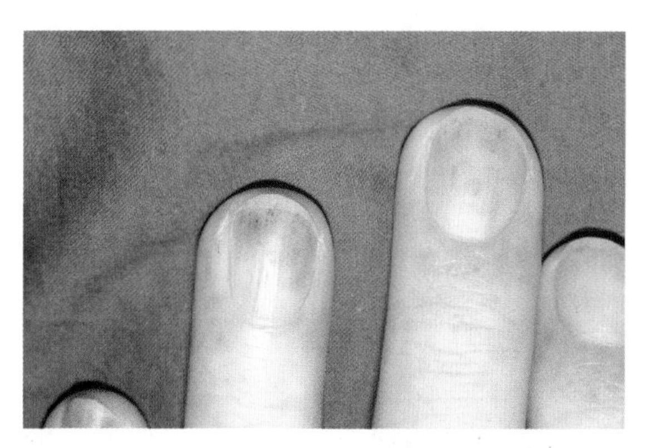

Fig. 4.3 Splinter haemorrhages: small dark longitudinal marks in nail bed.

Tar staining

Tar staining is easily recognizable as a yellowish discolouration of the fingers caused by cigarettes. It raises the possibility of coronary artery disease, which may cause angina, myocardial infarction, arrhythmias, and heart failure (nicotine is colourless).

> **Keypoints**
>
> Splinter haemorrhages are usually caused by trauma but also occur in 10% of patients with infectious endocarditis.

Radial pulse

7. Palpate right radial pulse for pulse rate (DF 3/10) and rhythm (DF 6/10). Palpate right and left radial pulses together and compare (DF 8/10). Check for collapsing pulse (DF 6/10).

Palpate right radial pulse for pulse rate and rhythm

The right radial pulse is used to assess pulse rate and rhythm. These are both extremely important signs. Pulse character (p. 39) is better assessed at the carotid pulse though you may get a sense of it at the radial pulse.

Rate

Normal pulse rate is 60–100 beats/min. A slow pulse rate (<60 beats/min) is known as bradycardia (*braddy-card-ia*). For causes, see Table 4.5. A fast pulse rate (>100 beats/min) is known as tachycardia. For causes, see Table 4.6. Tachycardia in resting patients is always abnormal.

Rhythm

Pulse rhythm is either regular or irregular. The normal rhythm of the heart is known as sinus rhythm because it is controlled by the sino-atrial node. Normally, the heart speeds up during inspiration and slows down in expiration. This is because during inspiration the normal tone of the vagus nerve (which slows the heart) is inhibited leading to an increase in heart rate. During expiration, vagal tone returns, slowing the heart. In

TABLE 4.5 Major causes of bradycardia

Common	Normal finding in fit young people, β-blocker drugs
Less common	Heart block, hypothyroidism

TABLE 4.6 Major causes of tachycardia

Exercise
Anxiety
Pyrexial illness
Hyperthyroidism
Drugs (β2 agonists—salbutamol, etc.)
Hypovolaemic (*high-poe-vole-ee-mick*) shock (as in gastrointestinal bleeding)
Arrhythmias

most patients over 40 years, this 'irregularity' is subtle and the pulse feels regular. In younger patients, the pulse may feel irregular—known as 'sinus arrhythmia'. This is a misleading term as an arrhythmia is defined as an abnormality of cardiac rhythm of any type—whereas sinus arrhythmia is quite normal.

Causes of an irregular pulse are shown in Table 4.7. An irregular pulse may be 'regularly irregular' or 'irregularly irregular'. With the former, there is some consistency to the irregularity such as every fourth beat is missed or the rate varies with respiration in a consistent fashion. With the latter, there is no pattern. It is difficult to differentiate between the different causes of an irregularly irregular pulse clinically. An ECG (p. 413) is required. However, the effect of exercise may be helpful. Often (but not always), ventricular ectopic beats may be abolished by exercise so that the pulse becomes regular. If the irregular pulse is due to atrial fibrillation, then exercise will not make the pulse more regular.

What is the pulse deficit?

This is a term you may hear mentioned. In atrial fibrillation, not only is the rhythm irregular, but the strength of the pulse is irregular too. This is because the ventricle contracts randomly and may not always be completely filled when ejection occurs. Sometimes, the amount of blood the left ventricle ejects (stroke volume) is so low that no pulse is felt at the radial artery. Thus, if you listen to the heart with a stethoscope while feeling the pulse, the rate on auscultation may be faster than at the radial pulse. For example, the rate might be 126 beats/min at the apex compared to 116 beats/min at the wrist. This difference is termed a 'pulse deficit'—in this case 10 beats/min.

TABLE 4.7 Causes of an irregular pulse

Regularly irregular pulse
Sinus arrhythmia
Wenckebach (*when-key-back*) second-degree heart block*
Irregularly irregular pulse
Atrial fibrillation (most common)
Multiple ventricular ectopic beats
Atrial flutter with variable block

* Karel Frederik Wenckebach (1864–1940), Dutch physician.

How to examine

The radial pulse is felt on the radial side of the flexor surface of the forearm just a few centimetres proximal to the wrist (Fig. 4.4).

1. Hold the patient's right hand with your right hand.
2. Then, use the tips of both the index and middle fingers of your left hand to palpate the pulse.
3. Once you have found the radial pulse you must time it; use your watch and count the beats over 20 s. Then multiply by 3 to give beats/min.
4. Whilst counting the rate, you should also be concentrating on the pulse rhythm. Is it regular or irregular? If it is irregular, is it irregularly irregular or regularly irregular?

Palpate right and left radial pulses together and compare

Significance

The right and left radial pulses may differ in the following circumstances:

(1) in acute aortic dissection (p. 25);

(2) in proximal arterial disease such as atherosclerosis of the axillary artery or stricture of the axillary artery following angiography.

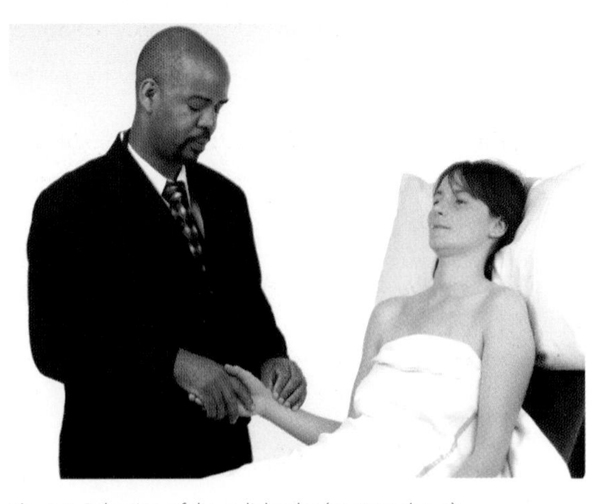

Fig. 4.4 Palpation of the radial pulse (see text above).

CASE 4.10

Problem. I've examined a well-looking 25-year-old man but couldn't palpate the radial pulse.

Discussion. Perhaps, it isn't there (congenital anomaly)—but usually this is because you've missed the pulse. Occasionally, the student puts their fingers down on the patient's wrist in the right place but then moves them—away from the pulse—when they do not feel the pulse immediately. When you feel for the radial pulse, wait for at least 10 s in any one position before palpating somewhere else. Usually, you will feel the pulse if you just wait. Then, if you want, you can move your fingers to where you sense the pulse is stronger.

CASE 4.11

Problem. The rhythm seems generally regular but you have noticed one slight irregularity.

Discussion. This is either a ventricular or atrial ectopic beat—so the rhythm is 'sinus rhythm with occasional ectopic beats'.

How to examine

Keep your fingers on the right radial pulse and simultaneously feel the left radial pulse with your right hand (Fig. 4.5). Compare the strength of both sides.

Check for collapsing pulse

Pulse character (p. 39) is normally best assessed at the carotid pulse (or the brachial (*brake-key-al*) pulse in children). However, the radial pulse can be used to assess for a collapsing pulse.

Significance

A collapsing pulse is a sign of aortic regurgitation (p. 67). (In the context of valvular lesions, 'regurgitation' and 'incompetence' mean the same thing.)

How to examine

1. Ask the patient if they have any pain in the shoulder.
2. If not, use your left hand to raise the patient's right arm whilst holding their wrist with your fingers (do not keep your fingers specifically on the pulse) (see Fig. 4.6).
3. If you feel the pulse vibrating back down your fingers, this is a collapsing pulse.

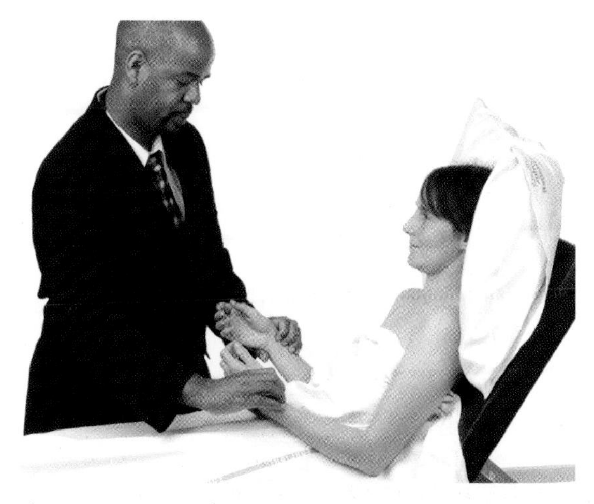

Fig. 4.5 Comparing pulses.

CASE 4.12

Problem. I always think the pulses are asymmetrical!

Discussion. It is more awkward to feel the left pulse and this may produce an (incorrect) impression of asymmetry. **Take your time**. Make sure you are happy with how you are palpating before moving on.

Face, eyes, and tongue

8. Inspect face for malar flush (DF 7/10) and xanthelasmata (DF 2/10). Inspect eyes for corneal arcus (DF 2/10). Inspect conjunctivae for anaemia (DF 9/10). Inspect tongue for cyanosis (DF 9/10).

Malar flush

Malar flush, also known as mitral facies (*face-ease*), is found in mitral stenosis. It refers to rosy cheeks with something of a bluish tinge. It is caused by dilation of the capillaries of the cheek, which in turn is secondary to pulmonary hypertension. Most patients with rosy cheeks do not have mitral stenosis!

Xanthalesmata and corneal arcus

Xanthalesmata and corneal arcus are both signs of hyperlipidaemia. Xanthalesmata are little yellowish papules (fatty deposits), usually around the eyes. They nearly always suggest hyperlipidaemia.

Corneal arcus (sometimes known as arcus senilis (*sen-ill-iss*)) is a grey ring around the outer margin of the iris (again due to fat deposits) (see Fig. 4.7). This is usually a normal finding in the elderly. In patients <50 years, though, it is suggestive of hyperlipidaemia.

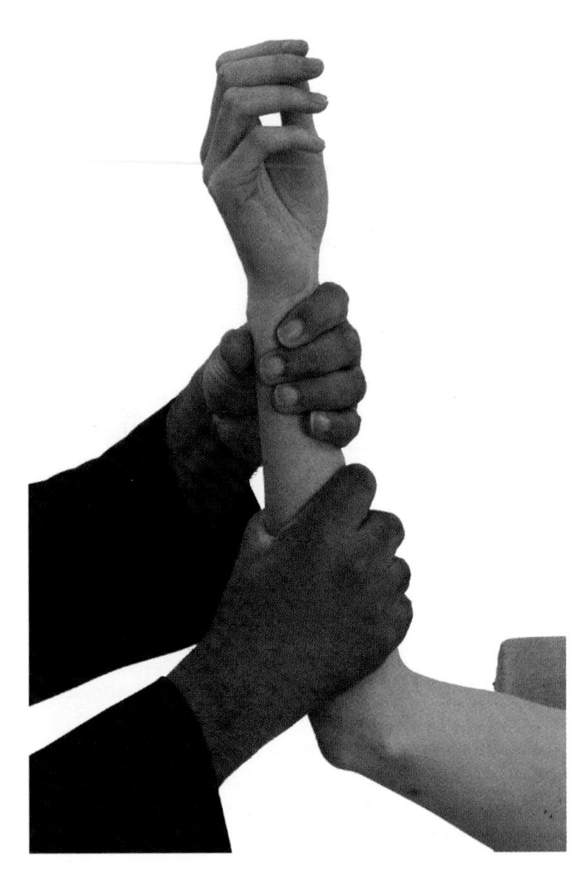

Fig. 4.6 Palpating for collapsing pulse. Hold up patient's left arm with your right holding the flexor surface of the wrist with your fingers.

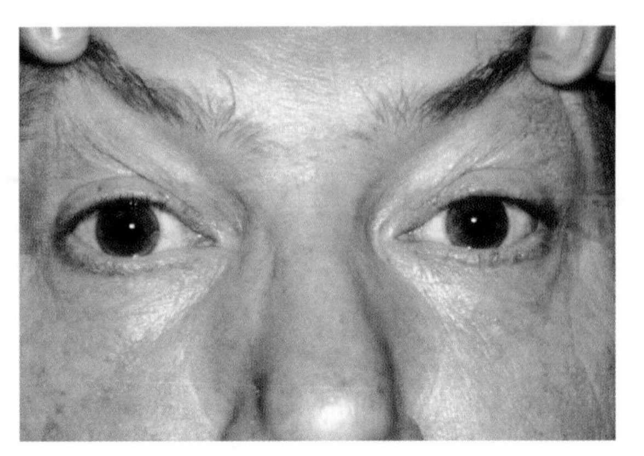

Fig. 4.7 Corneal arcus.

Keypoints

- Bradycardia may be normal.
- Tachycardia has multiple causes and is often not due to cardiac pathology.
- While counting pulse rate, concentrate also on rhythm.
- Sinus arrhythmia becomes less marked with age.
- Atrial fibrillation is the most common cause of an irregularly irregular pulse but an elecrocardiogram is required to decide the cause.
- Never forget to compare right and left radial pulses; always consider aortic dissection in patients with apparent myocardial infarction.
- When testing for a collapsing pulse, hold the whole wrist—not just the pulse.

Anaemia

Significance

Anaemia may be a cause of heart failure or angina and hence is included in the cardiovascular examination. Skin colour is a poor reflection of the haemoglobin level. Anaemia is best looked for in the conjunctivae of the lower eyelid. Even then, this is quite a crude test and experienced physicians are often wrong.

How to examine

1. Ask the patient's permission: 'Can I pull down your eyelid?'
2. Use your right index finger to gently pull down the right lower eyelid to expose the conjunctiva and inspect (Fig. 4.8).
3. Normally, the anterior part of the conjunctiva is a brighter red compared to the posterior portion. In anaemic patients, this distinction is lost (Fig. 4.8).

Cyanosis

See p. 90.

Causes

When examining the cardiovascular system, you are looking for central cyanosis. The most common cardiovascular cause is pulmonary oedema. Pulmonary oedema may come on suddenly usually due to coronary ischaemia or myocardial infarction or may be chronic due to valvular lesions or left ventricular systolic dysfunction. Right-to-left cardiac shunts are a very rare cause of cyanosis.

How to look for central cyanosis

See p. 90.

(a)

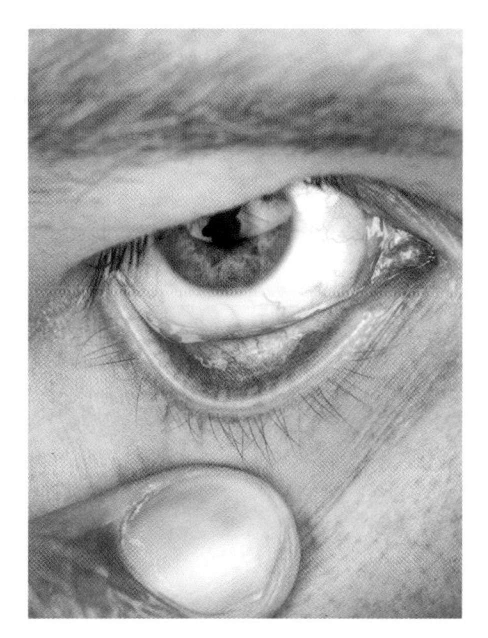

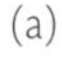

(b)

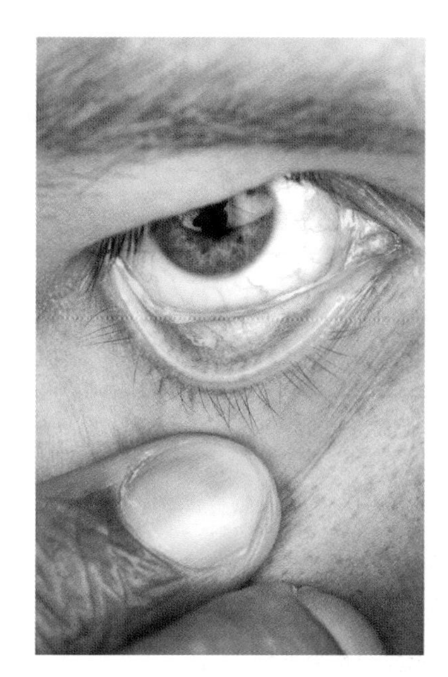

Fig. 4.8 Examining for anaemia in (a) normal patient, (b) anaemic patient (see text).

Keypoints

- Skin colour is a poor reflection of anaemia; examine the conjunctivae but even this is not always reliable.

Carotid pulse

9. Palpate right carotid pulse for pulse character (DF 8/10).

What is pulse character?

You may have heard the terms 'volume' and 'character' interchanged. There is a subtle difference between the two. When you feel a pulse, you get a sensation of the power of the pulse. This is pulse 'volume', which depends on the cardiac stroke volume. Pulse volume may be altered not only by cardiac lesions but also by other states, especially low blood pressure (hypotension). Students usually find assessment of volume quite simple but assessment of character is trickier. Character relates not only to the power of the pulse but also to how slowly or quickly it achieves its power. Abnormal pulse character is more indicative of a valvular lesion. Because it is often subtle, character is best assessed at the carotid pulse—the nearest accessible artery to the heart.

Significance

Abnormal pulse character is a characteristic feature of aortic valve disease (p. 68):

(1) **aortic stenosis**—slow rising, plateau pulse;

(2) **aortic regurgitation**—fast rising (waterhammer), fast falling (collapsing) pulse;

(3) **mixed aortic valve disease**—'bisfiriens' (biss-firienz) pulse—double impulse pulse;

(4) other conditions may occasionally affect the pulse character, one rare example being **hypertrophic obstructive cardiomyopathy**—jerky pulse.

See Fig. 4.9.

How to examine

See Fig. 4.10. The carotid pulse is not always easy to find.

1. Ask the patient to turn their head to the left-hand side. Make sure the patient's head is lying back against the pillow so that their neck is relaxed. If the neck is not relaxed, ask your patient to 'sink down into the bed' (just asking the patient to relax usually makes them go rigid).
2. Next, warn your patient: 'I am going to feel your pulse in the neck and it will be slightly uncomfortable.'

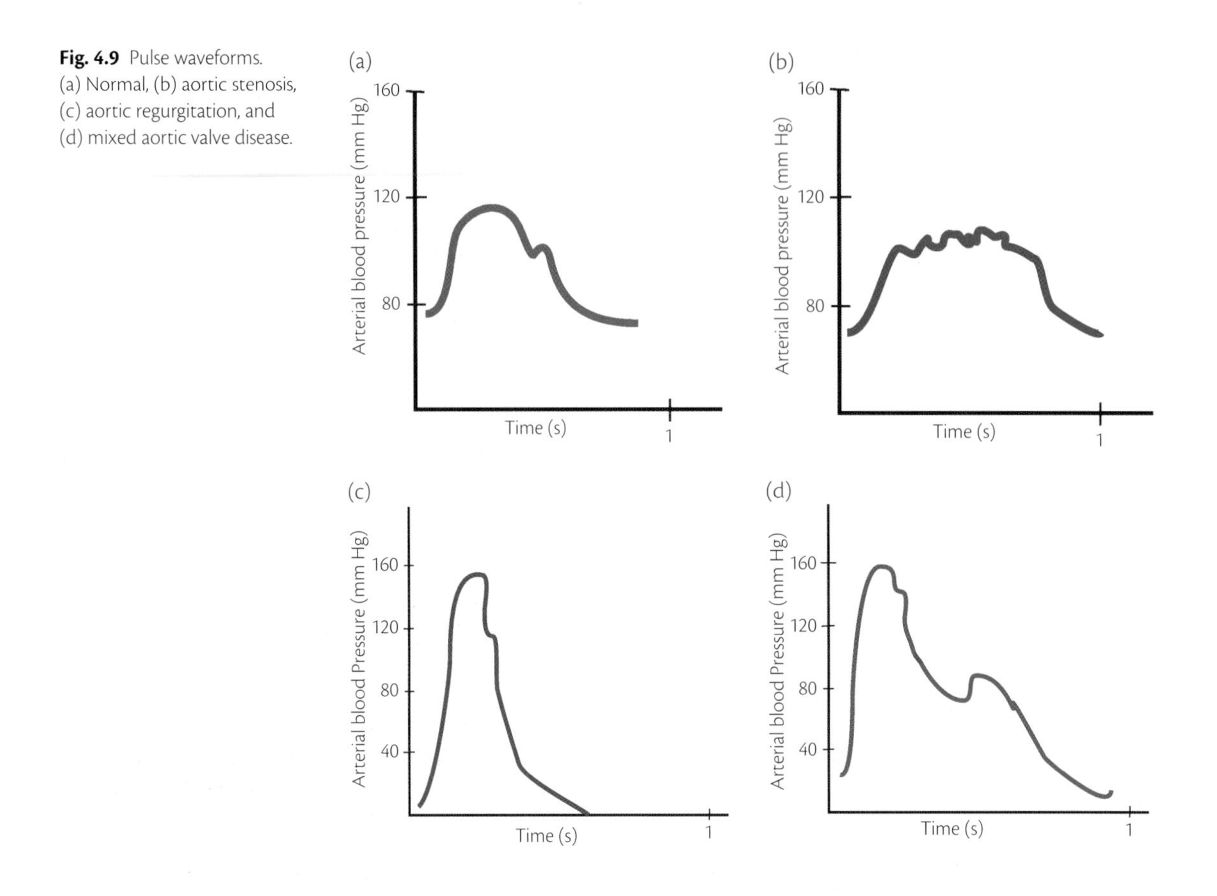

Fig. 4.9 Pulse waveforms. (a) Normal, (b) aortic stenosis, (c) aortic regurgitation, and (d) mixed aortic valve disease.

3. Use your left thumb and place it **gently** against the thyroid cartilage (Adam's apple).
4. **Gently** move the thumb laterally and posteriorly until you no longer feel the cartilage. Usually the carotid pulse is palpable just here.
5. Decide on pulse volume and how quickly it rises and falls.

Practise feeling normal pulses; only then will you be confident in diagnosing an abnormality. If unsure about the character, consider whether there are other signs of aortic valve disease. If so, the likelihood of pulse abnormality is increased.

Jugular venous pressure

10. Inspect right internal jugular vein for jugular venous pressure (DF 9/10). Check for hepatojugular reflux (DF 8/10).

The right atrial pressure is an important indicator of cardiac or pulmonary disease but clearly it cannot be measured directly at the bedside. However, the right atrium communicates with the right internal jugular vein so that the pressure within the right internal jugular vein gives an accurate indication of right atrial pressure. Thus, assessment of jugular venous pressure is an essential part of routine medical practice.

Unfortunately, the internal jugular vein can be very difficult to examine and this can be very frustrating for the student. Do not be alarmed! Everyone experiences difficulties in assessing the jugular venous pressure. **Practice is everything!**

In the next few pages, jugular venous examination will be reviewed, with a focus on anatomy, physiology, significance, and examination technique.

Anatomy

The internal jugular vein lies quite deep in the root of the neck between the sternal and clavicular heads of sternocleidomastoid (*stern-owe-clyde-owe-mast-oid*). It travels deep underneath the medial aspect of sternocleidomastoid towards the ear (Fig. 4.11). The external jugular vein lies lateral to the sternocleidomastoid muscle and is more superficial so it is much easier to see.

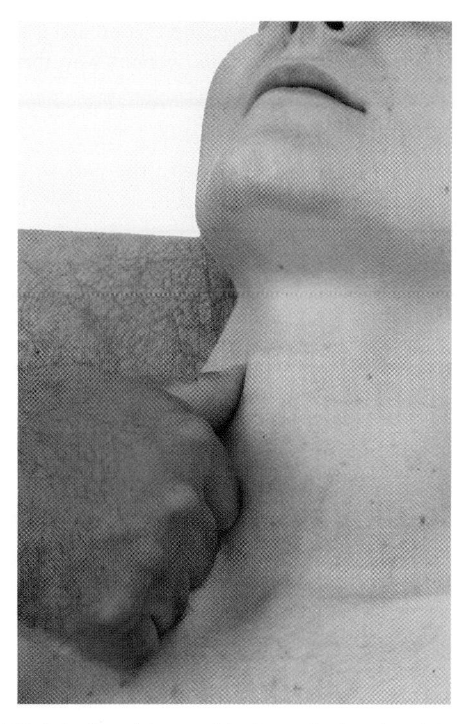

Fig. 4.10 Palpation of the carotid pulse: neck relaxed, use left thumb (see text)..

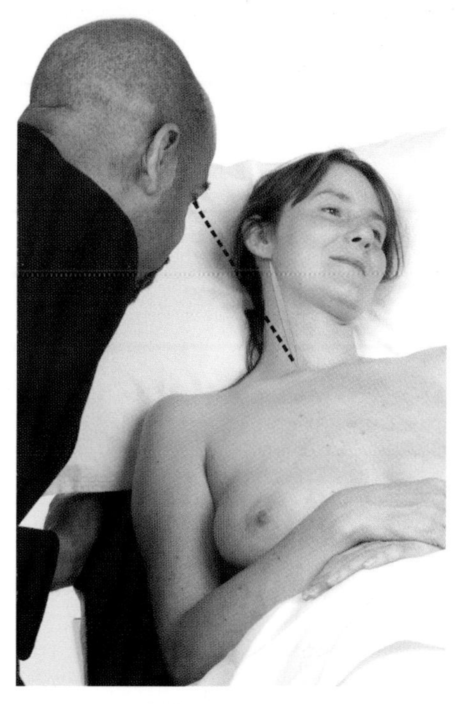

Fig. 4.11 Inspection of the jugular venous pressure waveform. Patient at 45°. Neck relaxed against pillow and turned to the left. Delineate internal and external jugular veins and root of neck.

Keypoints

- Abnormal pulse volume may occur in non-cardiac disease.
- Pulse character abnormalities are important indicators of cardiac disease—usually aortic valve disease.
- Pulse character is a tricky sign; students' most common mistake is to say character is abnormal when it is not—usually because they are describing volume, not character.

Physiology

The right atrial pressure (and so jugular venous pressure) varies through the cardiac cycle. It is worth revising how

(1) in ventricular systole the tricuspid valve is closed and the right atrium fills passively;

(2) as the ventricle relaxes in diastole, the tricuspid valve opens and blood flows passively from the atrium into the ventricle;

(3) the right atrium then contracts and squeezes further blood into the ventricle;

(4) the right atrium then relaxes, the tricuspid valve closes and ventricular systole starts again.

The jugular venous waveform is shown in Fig. 4.12. There are three stages at which pressure increases (known as A, C, and V waves) and two stages at which pressure decreases (known as X and Y descent).

1. The A wave is caused by right atrial contraction.
2. The X descent is due to right atrial relaxation.
3. There is a slight blip in the X descent, known as the C wave. The exact cause of this is unclear. It may be due to the tricuspid valve flicking back into the right atrium at the start of the systole or may possibly be caused by the carotid artery pulsation.
4. The V wave follows. This is due to passive atrial filling (with the tricuspid valve closed).
5. The Y descent occurs during ventricular diastole when the tricuspid valve opens and blood flows passively from the atrium to the ventricle.
6. The A wave then represents atrial contraction again.
7. The normal right atrial pressure at the top of the A wave is 7 cm water.

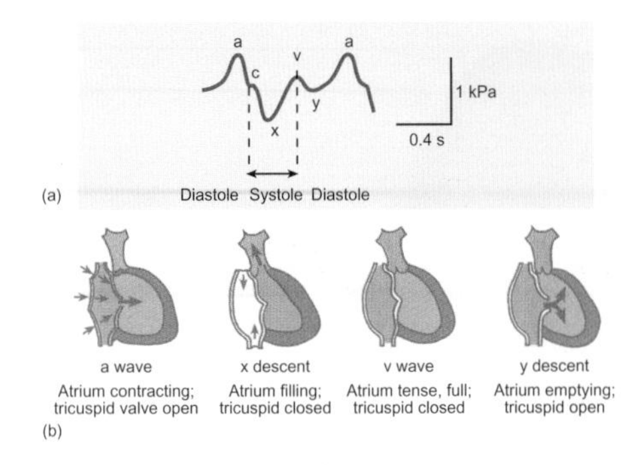

Fig. 4.12 The jugular venous pressure waveform. Reproduced by permission of Oxford University Press from **Fig. 15.13** (p. 306), *Human physiology: the basis of medicine* (2nd edn), by G. Pocock and C. Richards (2004).

Significance

An elevated jugular venous pressure is most commonly due to right heart failure. This is usually secondary to left heart failure, which in turn is caused by ischaemic heart disease or occasionally mitral valve disease. Right heart failure may also be secondary to pulmonary disease—cor pulmonale (*core-pull-ma-nail-ee*). In the case of pulmonary emboli, cor pulmonale may present acutely. Other important causes of elevated jugular venous pressure are given below.

1. **Fluid overload.** This may be due to kidney failure or excess intravenous fluids.
2. **Tricuspid regurgitation.** The tricuspid valve does not shut properly so the internal jugular pressure reflects the right ventricular pressure; when the right ventricle contracts, the jugular venous pressure is very high (giant V wave).
3. **Complete heart block.** Here, there is atrioventricular dissociation so that the atrial and ventricular contractions are not related in time. Atrial contraction may occur when the tricuspid valve is shut, so producing a large venous pulsation, known as a 'cannon A' wave. These are irregular, reflecting the fact that sometimes the tricuspid valve is shut and sometimes it is open when the right atrium contracts.
4. **Superior vena caval obstruction.** See Fig. 5.7. The jugular vein is distended and elevated without pulsating. This is usually due to mediastinal lymphadenopathy (*media-sty-nal-limf-adder-nop-path-ee*) secondary to lung carcinoma (*car-sin-owe-ma*). Hepatojugular reflux is negative (because of the obstruction).
5. **Atrial fibrillation.** Here, there is no atrial systole so consequently the jugular venous waveform has no A wave.

How to examine

The vein is usually examined with the patient at 45°. This is because of the following.

1. The normal maximum right atrial pressure is 7 cm water.
2. With the patient sitting straight up, the venous pulsations are normally too deep in the chest to be seen (Fig. 4.13).
3. With the patient lying flat, the vein is always full and there is no visible pulsation.
4. With the patient at 45°, the venous pulsations are normally at the level of the clavicle between the heads of sternocleidomastoid. They may or may not be visible here. In a patient with elevated venous pressure, the pulsation is seen higher up in the neck.

If the jugular venous pressure is extremely elevated, the top of the pulsation may be above the neck and so not visible. In such patients, the internal jugular vein is better observed with the patient sitting up straight.

Initial inspection

See Fig. 4.11.

1. Ensure the patient is at 45°, with head and neck relaxed back against a pillow.
2. Ask the patient to turn their head slightly (perhaps 30°) to the left (keeping the neck relaxed).
3. If lighting is poor, switch on the patient's bedlamp and focus it on the neck.
4. The internal jugular vein is best seen tangentally, so lean slightly across the patient.
5. Inspect between heads of sternocleidomastoid just above the clavicle. This is where the jugular vein may be seen in normal patients.
6. Look slightly higher in the neck along the medial aspect of sternocleidomastoid for a pulsation. If you see a pulsation here, this suggests an increased jugular venous pressure.
7. If none is seen, look also at the earlobe in case this is pulsating.
8. Next assess for hepatojugular reflux (sometimes called abdominojugular reflux). This is helpful in two ways: (1) in deciding if a particular pulsation is venous and (2) in making the diagnosis of right heart failure

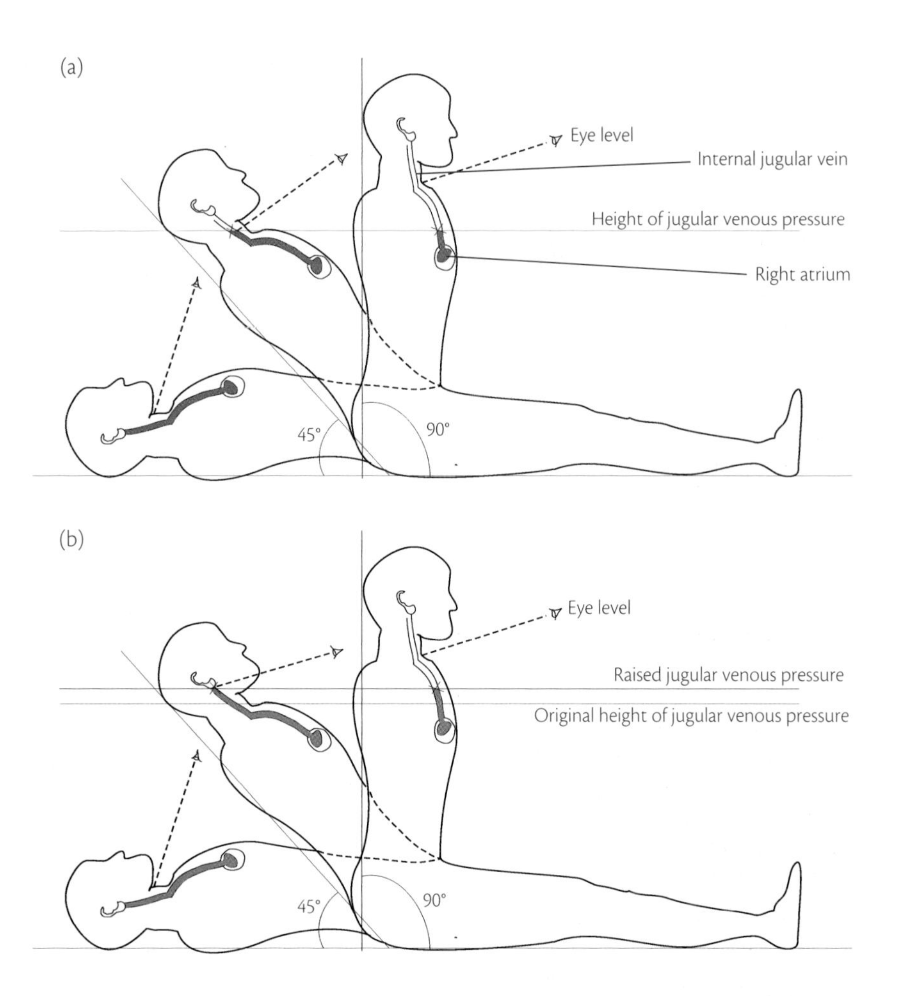

Fig. 4.13 Visibility of the internal jugular vein in different positions. (a) Normal JVP, (b) raised JVP.

On initial inspection, you may seen a pulsation but not be sure whether it is venous or arterial. Pressing on the abdomen increases venous pressure transiently so the internal jugular vein becomes more prominent for a few seconds. This is known as hepatojugular reflux. Usually, the venous pulsation quickly returns to normal (even while pressure is maintained on the abdomen). If it persists at its new level for longer than a few seconds, this is suggestive of right heart failure. Arterial pulsations, on the other hand, are not affected by pressing in the abdomen. The following points should be noted.

1. Patient should stay in the same position with neck relaxed against the pillow and turned to the left.
2. Ask the patient if their 'tummy' is tender, pointing to the right upper quadrant.
3. Ask permission to press on the 'tummy', being especially considerate if the patient admits to having some discomfort. Proceed if permission is given.
4. If you have previously seen what you think is a venous pulsation, you should concentrate on it throughout the procedure. If not, keep focused on the root of the neck (between the heads of sternocleidomastoid just above the clavicle).
5. Press gently in the right upper quadrant of the abdomen for 10 s (Fig. 4.14) and be aware that this may be uncomfortable. If discomfort is a problem, stop.
6. If you have seen a pulsation on initial inspection, check if it alters when you press on the abdomen. If so, it is venous. If not, it is arterial. If venous, decide how high it is above the clavicle. Also, decide if it stays at its new level for more than 5 s. If so, this suggests right heart failure.
7. If you did not see a pulsation on initial inspection, look carefully at the root of the neck. The jugular vein pulsation may just become visible here as you press in the abdomen.

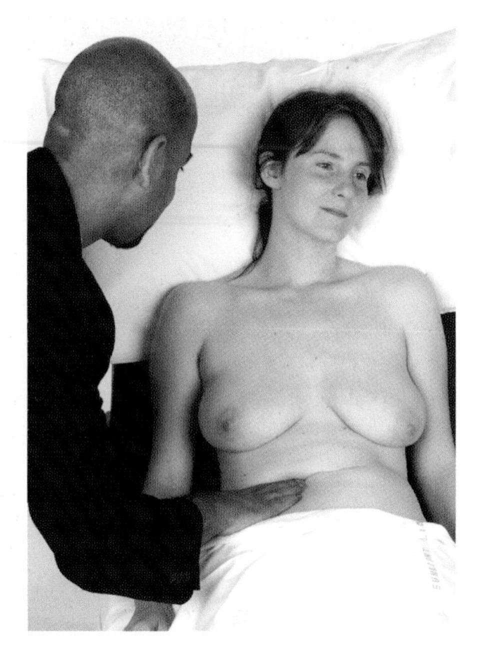

Fig. 4.14 Assessing for hepatojugular reflux.

By the end of this examination you should have decided whether the jugular vein is visible. If it is, you should be able to state whether the pressure is elevated and by how much (in terms of centimetres above the clavicle). In normal patients, the internal jugular vein is often not visible with the patient sitting at 45° and may not even appear when you press on the abdomen. However, seeing it in the root of the neck is reassuring in that it means you have not missed a vein with elevated pressure. See Fig. 4.15.

Inspection of praecordium

11. Take sheet off chest (female patients). Inspect praecordium in general and specifically for scars, cardiac impulse, and any other abnormal pulsations (DF 5/10).

The praecordium

The praecordium is the front of the chest over the heart. Various areas on the praecordium are of particular importance (Fig. 4.17).

1. **Apex/mitral area.** The area around the left fifth intercostal space in the mid-clavicular line is the area where the apex beat (p. 48) is normally felt and mitral valve sounds are best heard. Hence, it is known either as the 'apex' or the 'mitral area'.
2. **Tricuspid area.** The area around the left fourth intercostal space just lateral to the sternum is where tricuspid valve sounds are best heard and is known as the 'tricuspid area'.
3. **Pulmonary area.** The area around the left second intercostal space just lateral to the sternum is where pulmonary valve sounds are best heard and is known as the 'pulmonary area'.

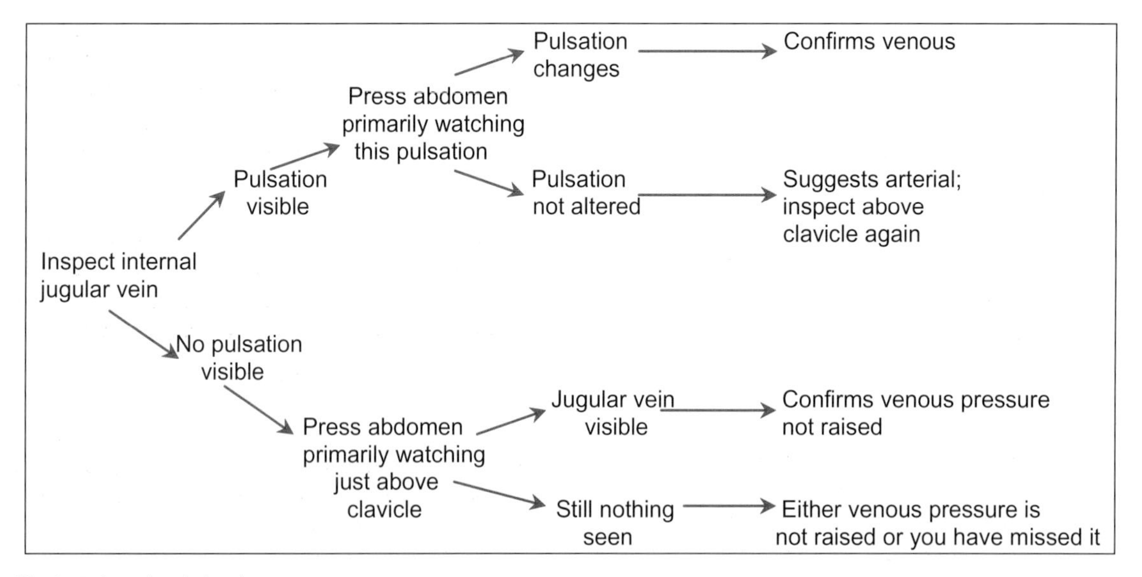

Fig. 4.15 Assessing the jugular venous pressure.

CASE 4.13

Problem. I can't see the internal jugular vein. Why might this be?

Discussion. Of course you may just have missed it but there are other possible reasons.

1. It is not actually visible. Often, the venous pressure is not high enough for the jugular vein to be visible in the neck with the patient lying at 45°.
2. The internal jugular vein cannot be seen if the neck is not relaxed. The main problem with technique is that at various points in the procedure the patient's neck may not be relaxed in the correct position: (1) if the head is not against the pillow at any time, (2) when you ask patient to turn to the left, or (3) when you ask patient about abdominal tenderness and they turn their head to answer you.

A relaxed sternocleidomastoid should just blend into the neck. If the muscle is prominent (Fig. 4.16) it is not relaxed. If the patient is not relaxed, ask them to rest their head back against the pillow and 'sink into the bed'. You may have to say this several times at different stages of the examination (telling patients to relax rarely has the desired effect).

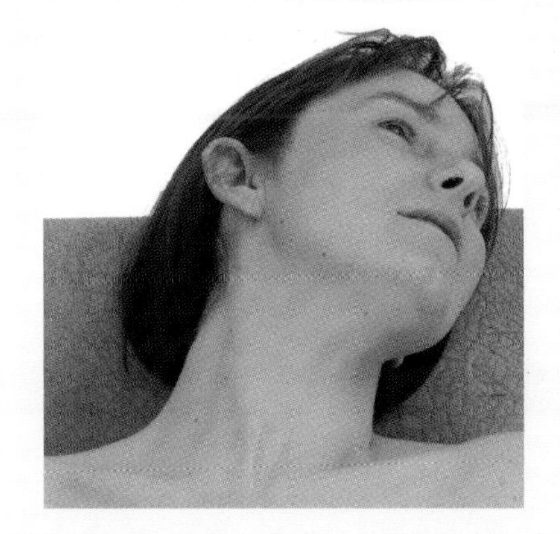

Fig. 4.16 Non-relaxed sternocleidomastoid. Note how clearly visible the muscle is. It should blend into the neck.

4. **Left sternal edge.** The area just to the left of the sternum is known as the 'left sternal edge'—significant because the murmur of aortic regurgitation is best heard here.
5. **Aortic area/base.** The area around the right second intercostal space just lateral to the sternum is

CASE 4.14

Problem. I can't see the deep pulsation you're talking about but I can see the external jugular vein. Is this not just as good?

Discussion. This is a contentious point. The external jugular vein lies lateral to the sternocleidomastoid muscle and is more superficial so it is much easier to see. Traditionally, it is taught that it **should not be used** because it has valves—so its height is an unreliable index of the right atrial pressure. However, it is now accepted that the internal jugular also has valves and these do not cause any problems. It is probably also true that the external jugular is prone to kinking. Experience shows, though, that the internal and external jugulars generally give the same result. So if you cannot see the internal jugular, the external jugular is a reasonable substitute.

CASE 4.15

Problem. The patient can't turn their neck to the left. Should I examine the left internal jugular vein?

Discussion. Yes. However, it is not ideal as veins from the left side of the neck reach the heart by traversing the mediastinum and may be compressed by the aorta, occasionally resulting in distortion of the pressure level.

Tip

Practise with the patient (or your friend) lying at 30°. This makes it easier to see the internal jugular vein in patients with normal right atrial pressure.

CASE 4.16

Problem. I see a pulsation but I'm not sure whether hepatojugular reflux is positive or not.

Discussion. This happens when you're not watching the pulsation before as well as when you press on the abdomen. Always make sure that you are focused on any possible pulsation in the neck **just before** you press in the abdomen. That way, you will be able to follow it clearly and so decide whether hepatojugular reflux is present.

CASE 4.17

Problem. Are there any other ways of assessing whether pulsations in the neck are venous or arterial?

Discussion. There are many ways of distinguishing arterial from venous pulsations. The best is checking for **hepatojugular reflux.** Sometimes, you will still not be sure. A good alternative is to apply pressure in the root of the neck. Gently press between the two heads of sternocleidomastoid just above the clavicle. If the pulsation alters, particularly if it becomes less visible, then it is venous. Other ways are as follows.

1. A very high jugular venous pressure may produce a waggling earlobe. Arterial pulsations do not do this.
2. Venous pulsations, unlike arterial pulsations, vary with posture. Sitting the patient up or lying them flat will alter a venous but not an arterial pulsation.
3. Venous pulsations, unlike arterial pulsations, vary with respiration. This is quite subtle, not least because of movement of the neck during respiration.
4. Venous pulsations are not usually palpable, whereas arterial pulsations are. However, when the venous pressure is very high, the venous pulsation may be palpable.

CASE 4.18

Problem. I've been told to use the manubriosternal angle as the reference point for the jugular venous pressure.

Discussion. Potentially, the manubriosternal angle is a useful reference point (and widely described) because the right atrium is around 5 cm inferior to the manubriosternal angle no matter what angle the patient is lying at. The right atrial pressure is around 7 cm of blood. So normally the internal jugular vein pulsation should be no higher than 2 cm above the manubriosternal angle no matter what position the patient is in. This can be considered unnecessarily complicated. If you see the internal jugular vein around the level of the clavicle with the patient lying at 45°, this is normal. If the pulsation is higher up in the neck, the jugular venous pressure is elevated by that amount.

CASE 4.19

Problem. I can't see the triple waveform and if I'm honest I can't see the double waveform.

Discussion. The triple waveform A, C, and V is not visible. However, with time (a lot of time, perhaps) it is possible to see that the venous pulsation has a double peak. These are the A and V waves. Picking up the giant V wave of tricuspid regurgitation or the cannon A wave of complete heart block can be very difficult—it can be simply seen that the venous pressure is elevated. Similarly, the absent A wave of atrial fibrillation is a tricky sign to identify. If you do see a double pulsation and wish to identify the A and V waves, the heart sounds are useful. The A wave tends to be in time with the first heart sound and the V wave with the second heart sound.

CASE 4.20

Problem. My patient is acutely breathless with an elevated jugular venous pressure but the chest sounds clear and the chest X-ray is normal. What's going on?

Discussion. It is so common for an elevated jugular venous pressure to be due to right heart failure, which in turn is due to left heart failure, that we can sometimes assume this to be the case when the evidence for left heart failure is limited. Beware of such assumptions. Pulmonary embolism is a strong possibility in this patient. This produces right (but not left) heart strain and breathlessness.

Keypoints

- The pressure in the internal jugular vein is a reflection of right atrial pressure.
- It is an important sign because the jugular venous pressure is elevated in right heart failure.
- The internal jugular vein is often not visible.
- To see the internal jugular vein, it is essential that the patient's neck is relaxed.
- Deciding whether a neck pulsation is arterial or venous is never easy; assessing for hepatojugular reflux can be very helpful.

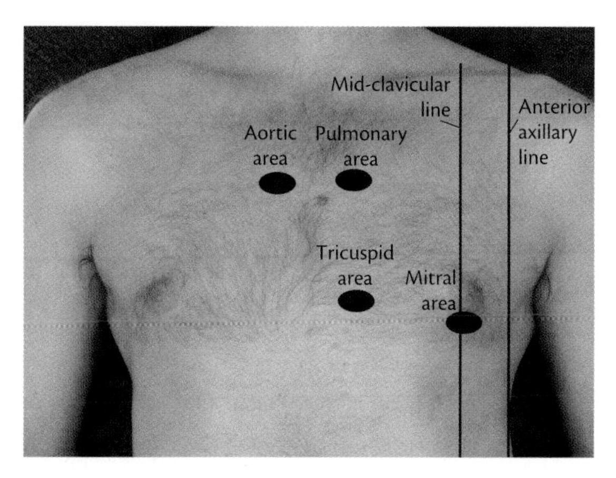

Fig. 4.17 The praecordium.

where aortic valve sounds are best heard and is known as the 'aortic area'. The aortic area may also be referred to as the 'base' or the 'base of the heart'.

The areas do not relate to the surface markings of the appropriate valve because sounds produced by the valves radiate from their point of origin (the surface marking is the point on the skin underneath which the valve is sited). Further important markings are

- the mid-clavicular line
- the anterior axillary line
- the mid-axillary line.

These are imaginary vertical lines usually used to define apex beat position.

What you are looking for on inspection

Scars

The most useful finding on inspection of the praecordium is the presence of a scar, suggesting previous surgery. Scars are of two main types

1. **Mid-line sternotomy (*stern-not-tummy*) scar.** This is a vertical scar over the sternum. The usual reason is coronary artery bypass grafting (commonly known as CABG and pronounced *cabbage*). Aortic and mitral valve replacements also require a mid-line sternotomy scar so such a scar should alert you to the possibility of prosthetic valves.
2. **Left thoracotomy (*thor-ack-cot-tummy*) scar.** Here the scar lies in a diagonal from underneath the left breast to the left axilla. The most common reason is mitral valvotomy surgery. Mitral valvotomy was used in the past as a treatment for mitral stenosis; here an object (dilator) is passed through the narrowed mitral valve to open it up. Patients who have had mitral valvotomy may have signs of mitral regurgitation (which may be caused by the operation) or mitral stenosis (as this tends to recur around 10 years after the operation).

Chest deformity

Sternal depression, scoliosis, and kyphosis may all result in an ejection systolic murmur or a displaced apex beat. So if you find no other cause for these, chest deformities may be the explanation.

Cardiac impulse

This may be seen at the apex—and often is easier to see than to palpate. If it is seen lower or more lateral, it is displaced. For causes of a displaced apex beat, see p. 48.

Pacemaker

A permanent pacemaker may lie under the skin, just inferior to the left clavicle (occasionally on the right).

How to inspect the praecordium

If this is part of a general cardiovascular system examination, you will just have finished assessing the jugular venous pressure. If the patient is female, she may have a sheet covering her chest.

1. At this stage, you should ask the woman's permission to remove the sheet from her chest and if given, then do so.
2. Make a brief (seconds only) general inspection for chest deformity, abnormal pulsations, pacemaker, and scars.
3. Inspect the mid-line for mid-line sternotomy scar—usually easy to see but be careful in men with a lot of chest hair.
4. Now inspect under the left breast for cardiac pulsation and possible left thoracotomy scar.
5. With women, you will usually need to lift the left breast to see this area properly. Ask permission first, 'Do you mind if I lift up your breast?' and if granted, proceed to lift breast with your left hand and inspect (Fig. 4.18).
6. Decide (1) whether you can see the cardiac pulsation and make a subjective decision on its position (this will be quantified when you palpate) and (2) whether there is a left thoracotomy scar; keep the left breast held up so that any skin creases (which may hide the scar—surgeons prided themselves on this) are smoothed out and look very carefully under the breast and in the axilla.

Keypoints

- The aortic area is on the right side of the chest.
- Left thoracotomy scars may be well hidden; you may have to lift the patient's breast to see one. Such a scar should alert you to the possibility of mitral regurgitation and/or stenosis.
- It may be easier to see the cardiac pulsation at the apex than to palpate it.

Palpation of praecordium

12. Palpate at apex for apex beat, assessing position and character (DF 9/10). Palpate for left parasternal impulse (DF 9/10) and aortic and pulmonary thrills (DF 6/10).

Why palpate?

The cardiac impulse

This is a brisk but light movement felt against the hand just after the start of systole, which retracts before the end of systole. Its exact origin is unclear. The apex beat is the cardiac impulse at the most lateral and inferior position at which it can be felt. Normally, the apex beat is felt around the fifth intercostal space in the region of the mid-clavicular line.

Cardiac impulse abnormalities

The cardiac impulse beat may either be displaced or have an abnormal character. A displaced cardiac impulse is not always due to cardiac pathology; pulmonary conditions and skeletal abnormalities may also displace the cardiac impulse. The character of the cardiac impulse is usually only altered in cardiac disease.

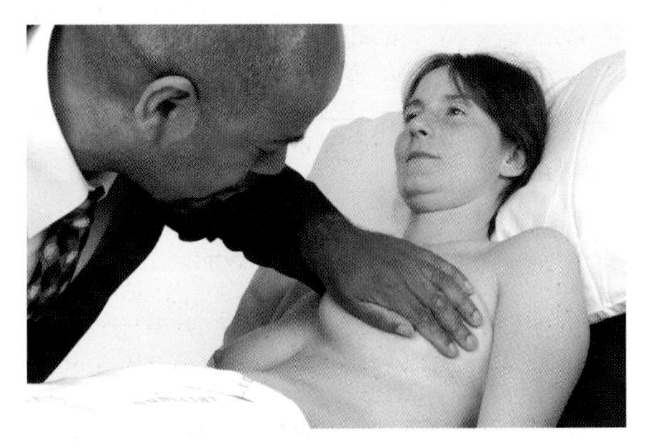

Fig. 4.18 Inspection of the cardiac impulse.

1. In mitral stenosis, the cardiac impulse is tapping in character but not displaced. The tapping character is due to a palpable first heart sound (the first heart sound is the noise made by closure of the mitral and tricuspid valves—p. 50).
2. Aortic stenosis and hypertension both cause obstruction to outflow. This high 'pressure load' causes left ventricular hypertrophy (*high-purr-tra-fee*), which in turn produces a sustained, heaving, minimally displaced (down and out) cardiac impulse.
3. In both mitral regurgitation and aortic regurgitation there is increased filling of the left ventricle to compensate for the retrograde flow associated with these conditions. The resultant 'volume overload' of the left ventricle results in a forceful, thrusting, and displaced (down and out) cardiac impulse. Because there is no obstruction to outflow, the cardiac impulse is not unusually sustained.
4. Left ventricular dilation (as in heart failure) produces a displaced (down and out) cardiac impulse. The cardiac pulsation is diffuse and may be felt from the apex to the left parasternal area.
5. Left ventricular aneurysms produce a dyskinetic (*dis-kye-net-tick*) cardiac impulse—where the impulse appears to have several different components.

Left parasternal impulse

A left parasternal impulse is produced by left atrial hypertrophy (as in mitral stenosis or regurgitation) or right ventricular hypertrophy (which may be secondary to right or left heart disease or lung disease—cor pulmonale).

Thrills

Rarely, murmurs (p. 52) are palpable producing a vibrating sensation a bit like a cat purring. A thrill nearly always indicates a significant lesion. Aortic stenosis, which may produce a thrill in the aortic area, is the only common cause.

How to examine

1. **Palpate the cardiac impulse.** If you have seen a pulsation during inspection, palpate for this first with the index, middle, ring, and little fingers of your right hand. If you did not see anything on inspection, palpate around the fifth intercostal space, in the mid-clavicular line (Fig. 4.19). Always wait at least 10 s before deciding you cannot feel it and try elsewhere.
2. **Find the apex beat.** Once you have found an apical pulsation, feel a little further down and out to see if it is still palpable. Continue until it is no longer

palpable. Go back to the furthest point down and out at which you felt the cardiac impulse. This is the apex beat.

3. **Decide on the character of the cardiac impulse.** While doing this you should also be deciding if the cardiac impulse character is normal or abnormal. If abnormal is it tapping, heaving, or thrusting? Does it last longer than normal (sustained)?
4. **Ascertain apex beat position.** First, decide on how lateral the apex beat is—whether the position you have found coincides with the mid-clavicular line (normal), the anterior axillary line, or the midaxillary line (both displaced). Next decide on the vertical level. This is done (in rather undignified fashion) by 'counting down the ribs'. Keep the fingers of your right hand over the apex. Using your left hand, palpate for the manubriosternal (*man-oo-brio-sternal*) angle. Palpate the intercostal space next to this. This is the second intercostal space. Now, by palpating the ribs, count down the intercostal spaces. When you reach the fifth space palpate laterally along it and so decide if the apex beat coincides with this or another intercostal space. This may feel very clumsy, particularly in women, but keep practising. However, many experienced physicians have made their minds up on the apex beat position before they have counted down the ribs. When you have palpated enough normal apex beats, you will get a feel for when its position is abnormal—without counting down.
5. **Palpate for left parasternal impulse.** Next, place the heel of your hand (fingers pointing upwards) over the praecordium, just to the left of the sternum (Fig. 4.20). Normally, you will feel the movement of respiration. If a left parasternal impulse is present the heel of your hand is lifted with each heartbeat (this is sometimes described as a left parasternal heave).

Tip

A tapping apex beat represents a palpable first heart sound. If you do not hear a loud first heart sound on auscultation, reconsider whether you really felt a tapping apex. Similarly, decisions on whether the cardiac impulse is sustained or whether it is heaving or thrusting are quite subtle. Consider your other signs before deciding on these nuances. Thus, if you have found other signs of aortic regurgitation, you are likely to be correct if you felt cardiac impulse was thrusting and non-sustained.

CASE 4.21

Problem. I can't feel the cardiac impulse. Why might this be?

Discussion. In 50% of patients, the cardiac impulse is not detectable—so don't panic. There are a number of reasons for this (1 and 2 are the most common):

1. **Obesity.** The subcutaneous fat masks the cardiac impulse
2. **Emphysema.** In this condition the lungs overinflate, increasing the barrier between the hand and the heart.
3. **Pericardial effusion.** Fluid in the pericardial sac.
4. **Dextrocardia.** Occasionally the heart develops on the right side of the chest. Suspect this if when auscultating the heart, sounds get louder as you move away from the apex to the left sternal edge.

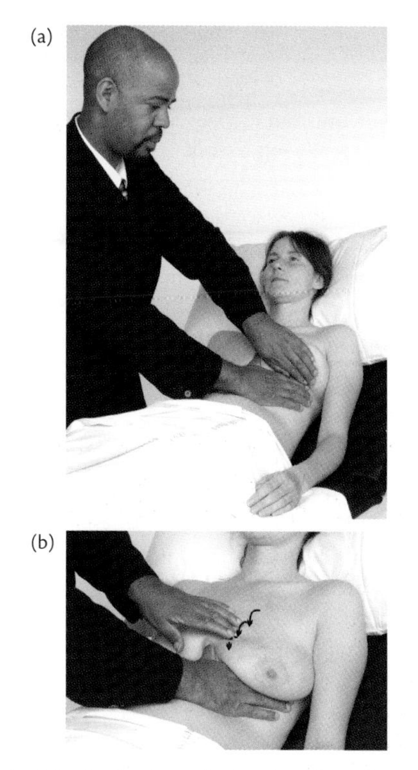

Fig. 4.19 Palpating for the cardiac impulse. (a) Locating the apex beat, (b) counting down the ribs.

Tip

A thrill represents a palpable murmur. If you do not hear a loud murmur on auscultation, reconsider whether you really felt a thrill.

Keypoints

- The apex beat is the cardiac impulse at the most lateral and inferior position at which it can be felt.
- The cardiac impulse is often impalpable.
- You should ascertain apex beat position and character of the cardiac impulse.
- Counting down the ribs may appear clumsy especially in female patients.
- Abnormalities of cardiac impulse character are subtle—only by practising in normal patients will you get a sense of when character is abnormal.
- Right ventricular hypertrophy causes a left parasternal heave.
- Left ventricular hypertrophy causes a sustained, heaving, minimally displaced cardiac pulsation.

6. **Palpate for thrills.** Now, palpate the pulmonary area with the index, middle, and ring fingers of your right hand, then the aortic area in the same way. Any thrill will be felt as a vibration like a cat purring.

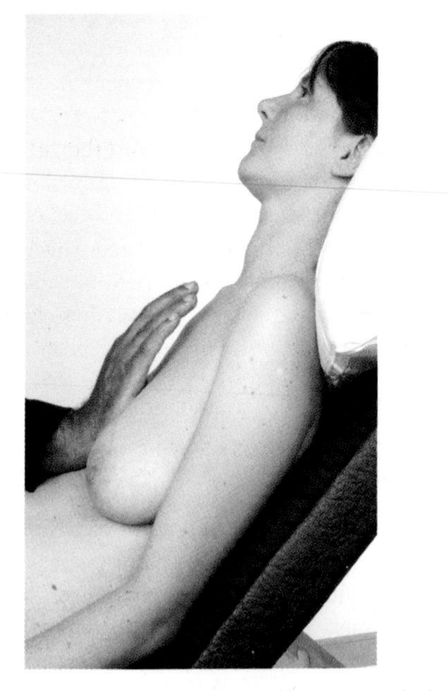

Fig. 4.20 Palpating for a left parasternal heave. Press the heel of your right hand on the chest to the left of the sternum.

Percussion

You may have noticed that percussion has been omitted from this cardiovascular system routine. In the past, percussing out 'cardiac dullness' was used as a method of determining heart size. This was unreliable and has been superseded by the chest X-ray. Hence it is no longer used.

Keypoints

- Do not percuss over the heart.

Auscultation of the heart

13. Auscultate (DF 8/10) while palpating carotid pulse to time any murmur.

Initially, auscultation (*os-cull-tay-shun*) of the heart will seem like a new language. This is not helped by mention of the myriad of rare or trivial abnormalities—split heart sounds and the like—which may be heard on auscultation. However, with practice, auscultation becomes one of the easier parts of clinical examination. In the pages that follow, the most important abnormalities are highlighted. Four areas are discussed:

(1) a description of the normal heart sounds;

(2) a description of various abnormal noises that may occur;

(3) a routine for auscultating the heart;

(4) an action plan on how to decide what you are hearing.

The stethoscope was invented by the French physician Rene Laennac in 1816. Before its introduction, physicians placed their ears directly on the chest to auscultate the heart! Your stethoscope has two settings: a 'bell' and a 'diaphragm' (Fig. 4.21). The bell is better for listening to very-low-pitched sounds. It should be pressed only very lightly on the skin—otherwise it actually acts like a diaphragm. The diaphragm is for listening to higher pitched sounds—though even these are usually quite low pitched.

Normality

There are normally two heart sounds, called the first and second heart sounds. The first heart sound results from the closure of the mitral and tricuspid valves (which happen at about the same time). The second heart sound results from the closure of the aortic and pulmonary valves (which again happen at about the same time).

There are various ways of denoting the heart sounds. The first heart sound may be written HS1, S1, or I. The second heart sound may be written HS2, S2, or II. The time after S1 until S2 is in time with systole. From S2 to S1 is in time with diastole.

Which heart sound is which?

1. The heart sounds come in pairs, with S1 first and S2 second. This is because systole is normally shorter than diastole (Fig. 4.21). During a tachycardia, diastole shortens and it becomes more difficult to detect the pairings.
2. S1 is lower pitched than S2. S1 gives a 'lubb' sound and S2 gives a 'dup' sound: 'lubb–dup'.

Splitting of S2

This is a normal finding. You should understand what it is about but hearing it is difficult and not essential. Both heart sounds result from the shutting of two separate valves. Very rarely—and to the skilled ear only—it may be possible to detect splitting of S1. Splitting of S2, though still a difficult finding, may be easier to hear—especially when the patient is breathing in. Inspiration decreases thoracic pressure and so increases peripheral venous return. The right side of the heart takes longer to fill and thus longer to contract—so that pulmonary valve closure is delayed. Thus in inspiration it may be possible to hear a split S2. This is best heard in the pulmonary area. This 'extra' sound after S2 is sometimes known as P2.

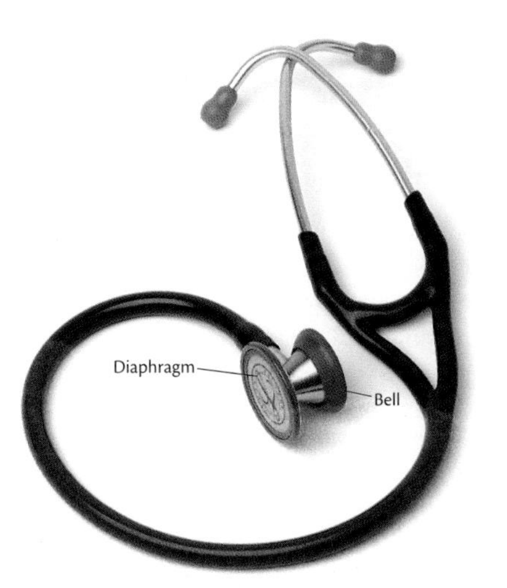

Fig. 4.21 A stethoscope. New stethoscopes have just one ending which functions as either bell or diaphragm depending on pressure applied.

Abnormal ausculatory findings

Altered heart sounds

1. **Loud S1.** Occurs in mitral stenosis. Although the mitral valve is narrowed, when it shuts, it does so suddenly, producing a loud first heart sound. It shuts suddenly because the valve is stiff and does not close at the end of diastole as it should. As the ventricle contracts, the chordae tendinae tense and force it suddenly shut.
2. **Soft S1.** Occurs in mitral regurgitation, because the mitral valve does not close completely.
3. **Soft S2.** Occurs in calcific aortic stenosis because of reduced valve movement.
4. **Wide fixed splitting of S2.** Occurs in atrial septal defect. The left-to-right shunt increases right heart work so right ventricular filling is delayed—resulting in a wide split. It is 'fixed' in that the split does not vary with respiration—unlike the normal splitting of S2. This is because the two atria communicate, equalizing pressure in both throughout respiration.
5. **Prosthetic heart sounds.** Metallic artificial valves produce clicking heart sounds, which are often audible without the stethoscope. Prostheses vary, but metallic mitral valves usually produce a loud S1 and a loud 'opening snap' (which occurs after S2.) Metallic aortic valves usually produce a loud S2 and an 'ejection click' after S1 (as well as an ejection systolic murmur). Artificial tissue valves produce relatively normal heart sounds.

Extra heart sounds

1. **Third heart sound (S3).** This is a low-pitched sound best heard with the bell at the mitral area. It comes just after S2, giving the impression of a double beat S2. The exact mechanism of the third heart sound is unclear. It occurs in the early period of diastole when diastolic filling is most rapid. Two factors seem to be important in its production: unusually rapid diastolic flow and a non-compliant ventricle. S3 is often a normal physiological finding in healthy young people and pregnant women who have a large stroke volume resulting in particularly rapid diastolic flow. The most important pathological cause is left ventricular failure. Here S3 occurs despite a reduced stroke volume. The left ventricle is stiff and in some way this results in S3 at the time of rapid diastolic flow. Other causes include mitral regurgitation and aortic regurgitation—in these, increased stroke volume is the cause.
2. **Fourth heart sound (S4).** This is also a low-pitched sound and like S3 is best heard with the bell at the

mitral area. It occurs just before S1 giving the impression of a double-beat S1. S4 is produced at the time of atrial contraction when a sudden bolus of blood contacts the stiff ventricle. It is never normal—occurring in conditions with a non-compliant ventricle—aortic stenosis, systemic hypertension, congestive cardiac failure, and hypertrophic obstructive cardiomyopathy.

The addition of either S3 or S4 to the normal heart sounds results in a 'triple rhythm'. This is also known as a gallop rhythm if in combination with the tachycardia of heart failure. If both occur together, as in cardiac failure, this may be called a summation gallop. It should be noted that both S3 and S4 are difficult to hear. Research studies have shown that even cardiologists often disagree on their presence.

Additional noises

1. **Opening snap.** Opening of the mitral valve is normally not audible. In mitral stenosis there is elevated left atrial pressure, which causes forceful opening of the mitral valve. This results in a high-pitched 'opening snap' after the second heart sound, best heard at the mitral area or tricuspid area with the diaphragm (as the mitral stenosis progresses and the valve stiffens and calcifies, the opening snap may become quieter and disappear).
2. **Aortic ejection click.** Similarly, opening of the aortic valve is normally not audible. However, if the cusps are abnormal, as occurs in congenital bicuspid aortic stenosis, aortic valve opening may be audible as an 'ejection click' just after the first heart sound; this is best heard in the aortic area. The 'click' precedes the aortic stenosis murmur.
3. **Mid-systolic click.** This occurs in mitral valve prolapse. Mitral valve prolapse involves a 'floppy' mitral valve prolapsing into the atrium during systole. If the prolapse is severe, there is also an element of regurgitation. The 'mid-systolic click' arises at the point when the prolapsing mitral valve leaflet has reached the full extent of its prolapse. Interestingly, a mid-systolic click may also occur in left-sided pneumothorax. The cause is unclear but it may result from contact and separation of the pleural surfaces in synchrony with the heartbeat.

Murmurs

Murmurs result from turbulent flow in the heart. Such turbulent flow may be due to rapid flow in a normal heart (innocent flow murmur) or turbulent flow in an abnormal heart. Murmurs have a blowing quality and are quite prolonged compared to the short-lived banging qualities of heart sounds. Murmurs are normally classified according to their timing in the cardiac cycle, so there are two main categories—systolic and diastolic.

The murmur may be described further by

- its exact timing
- the site at which it is best heard
- where else it radiates to
- any procedures which accentuate it
- its pitch
- its loudness.

Loudness is graded as below:

- grade 1—just audible with patient's breath held
- grade 2—quiet
- grade 3—quite loud
- grade 4—loud enough to have accompanying thrill
- grade 5—very loud
- grade 6—can be heard without a stethoscope.

It is important to point out, though, that the loudness often does not relate to the severity of the lesion. Thus, a small ventricular septal defect (VSD) causes much more turbulence than a large VSD and so produces a much louder sound. Similarly, as aortic stenosis worsens, left ventricular failure develops and cardiac output is reduced. This results in decreased flow across the damaged valve so the murmur gets quieter. However, in mitral and aortic regurgitation, the intensity of the murmur usually increases with the severity of the pathology.

Systolic murmurs are of three main types: pansystolic, ejection systolic, and late systolic. Below, their individual characteristics are discussed, though in practice, distinction can be very difficult.

1. **Pansystolic murmurs.** These are heard throughout systole. They are more or less uniform in intensity throughout systole—thus usually producing a gentle, blowing quality. The most common cause is mitral regurgitation where the mitral valve cannot close fully. It remains open during systole so blood flows backwards across the mitral valve when the left ventricle contracts. The murmur of mitral regurgitation is best heard at the mitral area but may radiate all over the praecordium. It may radiate to the axilla.
2. **Ejection systolic murmurs.** Here the murmur does not start immediately after S1. When it does begin, it builds up intensity before reducing—

described as 'crescendo–decrescendo'. This tends to result in a harsher quality. The most important cause is aortic stenosis. Here, there is turbulent flow across the stenosed aortic valve during left ventricular ejection. Left ventricular ejection starts after the aortic valve opens—just after S1. Thus the murmur does not start immediately after S1. The murmur of aortic stenosis is usually best heard in the aortic area though in patients with calcific aortic stenosis, the murmur may be loudest at the mitral area. Either way, the murmur may be heard all over the praecordium and sometimes radiates to the carotids in the neck. If you hear a murmur-like sound over the carotids but no heart murmur, you should consider a 'carotid bruit' as an alternative. This is a very similar sound but is often caused by narrowing of the carotid artery. Such a narrowing is an important cause of stroke disease. Other common causes of ejection systolic murmurs are innocent flow murmur and aortic sclerosis. Innocent flow murmurs are not pathological. They are due to rapid flow through normal valves and occur especially in children and young adults. They are quiet and often have a musical tone. Aortic sclerosis is a condition seen in older people; the aortic valve is thickened but not stenosed. The murmur is similar to aortic stenosis, but it does not usually radiate to the carotids.

3. **Late systolic murmurs.** These begin late in systole. The most common cause is mitral valve prolapse. If the prolapse is severe, there is also an element of regurgitation, so resulting in a late systolic murmur. Hypertrophic obstructive cardiomyopathy may cause damage to the papillary muscle and consequent mitral regurgitation, resulting in a late systolic murmur.

Diastolic murmurs are of two main types: early and mid-diastolic. Diastolic murmurs are always abnormal.

1. **Early diastolic murmurs.** An early diastolic murmur has a high-pitched quality. It begins loudly and quickly gets quieter. The most common cause is aortic regurgitation. Here, the murmur occurs because of retrograde leakage of blood through the regurgitant aortic valve. The pressure in the aorta is highest at the beginning of diastole and then falls, so resulting in a murmur that is initially loud but then becomes quieter. The murmur of aortic regurgitation is best heard at the left sternal edge with the patient sitting up and breath held in expiration (this is how the aortic valve is brought closest to the stethoscope).
2. **Mid-diastolic murmurs.** A mid-diastolic murmur starts later in diastole. It has a low-pitched 'rumbling' quality and is best heard with the bell. The key cause is mitral stenosis. Blood normally flows across the mitral valve during filling of the left ventricle in diastole. This starts after the mitral valve opens shortly after S2. Thus the turbulent flow of mitral stenosis begins in the middle period of diastole. In theory, when atrial contraction occurs near the end of diastole, flow across the mitral valve will increase, resulting in a louder murmur—so-called 'presystolic accentuation'. Almost always, though, mitral stenosis is associated with atrial fibrillation so there is no atrial contraction—and no presystolic accentuation. The murmur of mitral stenosis is best heard at the mitral area with the patient lying slightly on their left side to bring the mitral valve closest to the stethoscope. It is rare to hear it other than at the mitral area.

Pericardial friction rub

This is a sign of acute pericarditis. It is a scratching sound that may be heard in systole or diastole. It is best heard at the left sternal edge with the patient sitting up and holding their breath in expiration. Like the pain of pericarditis, it may vary from hour to hour. The rub is thought to be due to the inflamed visceral and parietal pericardial sacs rubbing against each another—and so should not occur in the presence of a pericardial effusion. However, one study has shown that a rub is just as likely to occur in the presence of a pericardial effusion.

The auscultation routine

There is no consensus on what constitutes the correct auscultation routine. Any routine should take account of the fact that while a loud sound may be heard all over the praecordium, a quiet sound may be heard only at particular places using particular techniques. The routine on the next page achieves this in a quick but thorough way. Throughout this routine, if you hear what you think are abnormal sounds you should time them by feeling the carotid pulse—which is synchronous with systole.

Tip

Overall auscultation should take no more than 2 min. Spend 40 s on the mitral area and the rest elsewhere.

Tip

Sometimes breath sounds may make it very difficult for you to hear the heart: if need be, ask the patient to hold their breath for a few seconds.

1. Listen over the mitral area with the diaphragm. If you hear a systolic murmur, move the stethoscope to the axilla and listen there too. Systolic murmurs of all types may be heard here, so hearing a murmur in this area does not clinch a diagnosis. However, the pansystolic murmur of mitral regurgitation is usually louder here than in the aortic area. The opposite applies to the ejection systolic murmur of aortic stenosis. The opening snap of mitral stenosis may also be heard here. The pansystolic murmur of mitral regurgitation may radiate into the axilla (ejection systolic murmur does not usually), so if you hear a systolic murmur here, then edge your way with the diaphragm into the axilla, listening to see if it radiates there.
2. Next, ask the patient to roll over slightly on to their left-hand side and listen over the mitral area with the bell at the apex (Fig. 4.23). This is the ideal method for auscultating the low-pitched mid-diastolic murmur of mitral stenosis. S3 and S4 are also best heard here with the bell.
3. Ask the patient to roll back to a straight position. Listen over the tricuspid area with the bell. This is the position for the mid-diastolic murmur of tricuspid stenosis.
4. Listen over the tricuspid area with the diaphragm. This is the best position for the pansystolic murmurs of tricuspid regurgitation, pericardial friction rubs, and innocent flow murmurs. The opening snap of mitral stenosis may also be heard here.
5. Listen over the pulmonary area with the diaphragm (best place for pulmonary murmurs). Note that there is no specific role for listening with the bell at the pulmonary area.
6. Listen over the aortic area with the diaphragm (Fig. 4.24). This is the best place for ejection systolic murmurs of aortic stenosis and aortic sclerosis—although occasionally sometimes these are better heard at the mitral area). Note that there is no specific role for listening with the bell at the aortic area.
7. Listen over the right, then the left carotid with the diaphragm (listening for (1) radiation of a murmur to the carotids, a feature of aortic stenosis (not sclerosis) and (2) carotid bruits).
8. Ask the patient to sit forward, breathe in, breathe out, and then hold their breath (without taking

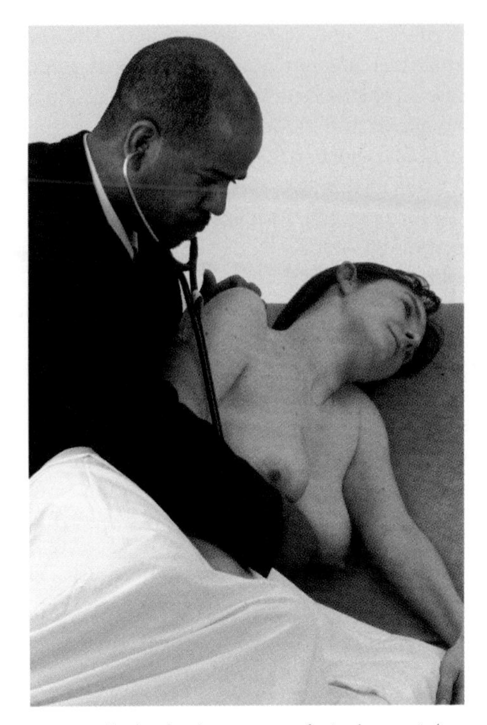

Fig. 4.23 Auscultating for the murmur of mitral stenosis (see text above).

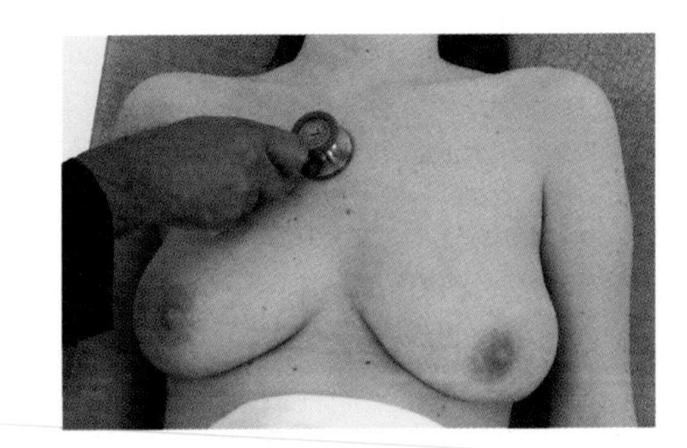

Fig. 4.24 Auscultating over the aortic area with the diaphragm.

Fig. 4.22 The first and second heart sounds.

S1------S2-----------S1-------S2------------S1------S2------------S1-------S2
systole diastole systole diastole systole diastole systole

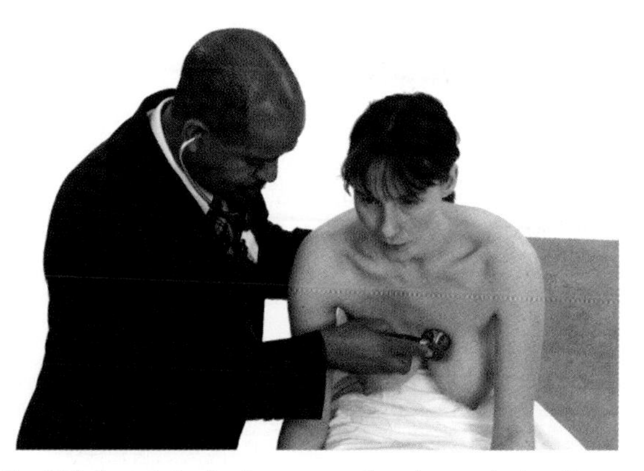

Fig. 4.25 Ausculating for the murmur of aortic regurgitation. Listen with the breath held in expiration.

another breath in) and listen with the diaphragm at the lower left sternal edge (Fig. 4.25). This accentuates the murmur of aortic regurgitation. Let the patient know they can breathe again before moving on.

Tip

Do not listen too long here or the patient will collapse.

9. With patient still sitting up, listen with the diaphragm at the lung bases at the back. Here you are listening for the fine, late inspiratory crackles of left ventricular failure (see p. 106).

Tip

Most valvular lesions can produce murmurs audible all over the praecordium. Thus a murmur at the pulmonary area does not guarantee pulmonary valve pathology. However, if this is the only place it is heard, it makes the pulmonary valve the likely candidate.

An action plan for auscultation

Initially, auscultation may seem like a new language, but do not be put off! Your first priority should be to get to grips with normal heart sounds. Then, learn how to recognize a loud first heart sound and the murmurs of aortic stenosis, aortic regurgitation, mitral stenosis, and mitral regurgitation. Thankfully, these abnormalities, are not only the most important findings, they are also the easiest. Ideally, you should also be able to hear an opening snap and third and fourth heart sounds.

You should have a reasonable stethoscope costing around £40. The £10 stethoscopes are clearly inferior. The £120+ 'cardiology' stethoscopes are only slightly better than the £40 ones—but much more annoying to lose.

Your first test is to get to grips with normality (DF 6/10). There are two normal heart sounds, S1 and S2. These are best heard at the mitral and tricuspid areas with the diaphragm. Note that they may be very quiet, particularly in the aortic and pulmonary areas and particularly in patients with hyperinflated chests, as in emphysema. Furthermore, the heart sounds become quieter with age. To distinguish S1 from S2 remember that because systole is normally shorter than diastole, the heart sounds seem to come in pairs with S1 first and S2 second. Also, S1 is a lower pitched sound—'lubb' than S2—'dupp'.

Having mastered the normal, your next test is to unravel the abnormal.

1. **Detecting an abnormality**. First, you need to hear that something is wrong. How easy this is depends on the actual abnormality:
   - loud or soft S1 or S2 (DF 3/10)
   - extra 'bumps'—S3, S4, opening snap, clicks (DF 8/10)
   - systolic murmur (DF 4/10)
   - diastolic murmur (DF 9/10).

('Bump' is the author's own term, not to be repeated in front of experts.)

Your other physical findings should put you on the alert for particular auscultatory findings. For example, if you have found a collapsing pulse you should listen very carefully for the early diastolic murmur of aortic regurgitation.

2. **If there is an abnormality, take a moment to decide if S1and S2 are normal.** This is normally quite easy (DF 3/10) but may be more difficult if there is a loud murmur.

For each abnormality you must decide 3–6.

3. **Is the abnormality a 'bump' or a murmur? (DF 2/10).** The various 'bumps'—heart sounds, clicks, and snaps—all have a short banging quality, as opposed to the prolonged blowing quality of murmurs, making this an easy decision.
4. **If it is a 'bump', what is it? (DF 6/10).** To decide, you need to make up your mind
   - which area you hear the 'bump'
   - whether it is best heard with the bell or diaphragm

- whether it is high or low pitched
- most importantly, what is its timing in the cycle.

So, having decided on these factors, does your abnormal sound fit with any of the common 'bumps'? (S3—low pitched, heard with bell at the mitral area or left sternal edge, just after S2—making S2 sound like a double beat; S4—low pitched, heard with bell at the mitral area or left sternal edge, just before S1—making S1 sound like a double beat; opening snap—high-pitched, heard with diaphragm at mitral or tricuspid areas, just after S2.)

5. **If it is a murmur, is it systolic or diastolic? (DF 6/10).** Because murmurs can make S1 and S2 difficult to hear, this is best decided by timing the murmur against the carotid pulse (DF 8/10). Less scientific but helpful are the facts that systolic murmurs are much more common and are usually easier to hear than diastolic murmurs and that diastolic murmurs are often heard only when using one specific method.
6. **If it is a diastolic murmur, is it mitral stenosis or aortic regurgitation? (DF 4/10).** There are only two important diastolic murmurs and because one of them, the mid-diastolic murmur of mitral stenosis, is so specific in its site and pitch, it is easy to differentiate this from the other—the early diastolic murmur of aortic regurgitation. The mid-diastolic murmur of mitral stenosis is heard only at the mitral area; it is a low-pitched 'rumbling' sound, best heard with the bell and with the patient lying on their left-hand side. The early diastolic murmur of aortic regurgitation is best heard with the diaphragm at the left sternal edge with the patient sitting up and breath held in expiration. If you hear it in other areas, it will always be audible at the left sternal edge too.
7. **If it is a systolic murmur, what are its characteristics? (DF 9/10)**
    1. Where does it occur in systole? Is it ejection systolic, pansystolic or late systolic? (DF 9/10)
    2. Where on the praecordium is it heard best? (DF 3/10)
    3. Does it radiate? (DF 4/10)
    4. Do any procedures accentuate it?
    5. What is its pitch?
    6. How loud is it?

Tip

'Bumps' and diastolic murmurs are more difficult to hear, but once heard are relatively easy to categorize.

It is usually easy to say where a murmur is best heard and where it radiates to. It is more difficult to decide its exact timing. To ascertain this, you have to decide the following: Is there a gap between S1 and the murmur? Is the murmur uniform or 'crescendo-decrescendo'? Using 1–6, you should be able to describe the murmur.

Tip

Systolic murmurs are easier to hear but harder to describe exactly.

Keypoints

- Practise to get a sense of normality.
- The normal heart sounds come in pairs: S1 and S2.
- Hearing S3 and S4 is tricky.
- Know the basic murmurs: pansystolic murmur in mitral regurgitation; ejection systolic murmur in aortic stenosis; early diastolic murmur in aortic regurgitation; mid-diastolic murmur in mitral stenosis.
- Do not waste time looking for the perfect routine that will satisfy everyone—it does not exist!
- The key to auscultation is timing; this is best done by palpating the carotid pulse, which is in time with systole.
- Your other physical findings prior to auscultation may point towards certain diagnoses, the murmur of which you should listen particularly attentively for.
- Systolic murmurs are easy to hear but it is more difficult to decide exactly which type they are.
- 'Bumps' and diastolic murmurs are more difficult to hear but once heard it is usually quite easy to say which type they are.

8. **Presenting your findings.** Always start by mentioning the heart sounds, whether they are abnormal or normal, and then describe any extra sounds: 'first and second heart sounds are normal, there were no other abnormal sounds' or 'the first heart sound was loud with a normal second heart sound, followed by

an opening snap and there was a quiet, low-pitched, mid-diastolic murmur heard with the bell at the mitral area and with the patient on their left side'.

Peripheral oedema

14. Palpate for ankle or shin oedema over lower anterior tibia (DF 3/10).

See also ankle swelling (p. 29) for definitions and classification.

Why test for ankle oedema in cardiovascular examination?

Peripheral oedema is a common symptom and sign of heart failure, hence its inclusion in the cardiovascular routine. However, it is caused by many other conditions—the most common being postural oedema exacerbated by incompetent venous valves (Table 4.3).

Pathogenesis of peripheral oedema in heart failure

For many years it was thought that increased venous pressure in heart failure caused increased capillary pressure and consequent leakage across the capillary. Thus, it was said that if the jugular venous pressure was not raised, then any oedema present was not cardiac. However, it is now clear that the degree of cardiac oedema does not correlate with the venous pressure: cardiac oedema need not be associated with a raised jugular venous pressure.

Instead, it is fluid overload that is the cause of cardiac oedema—but what causes this? The full answer to this is complex and beyond the scope of this book. However, fluid overload is at least partly related to changes in renal blood flow in cardiac failure, which result in increased renin (*ree-nin*), aldosterone (*al-dough-steer-own*), and vasopressin (*vay-zo-press-in*) production. The consequent sodium and water retention results in fluid overload.

What is pitting oedema?

Oedema caused by fluid with low protein content (as in heart failure) will indent quickly on pressing (within 2–3 s) producing a pit within the subcutaneous tissues—pitting oedema. It is sometimes taught that oedema caused by more proteinaceous fluid as in lymphatic obstruction by a tumour does not indent—non-pitting oedema. However, when such lymphoedema is new, it will usually indent if pressed on for a longer period. As the lymphoedema becomes chronic, it fibroses and hardens and will no longer pit.

How to examine (DF 4/10)

Although usually described as 'ankle' oedema it is actually the shin that is examined. Palpating for oedema may be painful, so be careful and watch the patient's face whilst doing so.

1. Ask permission to examine the patient's legs. You may also have to remove bedclothes to get at the shin.
2. Press your thumb down on the medial aspect of the patient's shin **gently** for 5 s. Watch the patient's face as you press—swollen legs can be tender.
3. Lift your thumb: does the indentation persist (pit) for a few seconds (Fig. 4.26)? If so, there is oedema and it is likely due to low protein fluid. If not, press again for 30 s. Lift your thumb again. Does the indentation now persist? If so, the oedema is likely due to fluid with higher protein content.
4. If oedema is present, you should find the level at which oedema stops. This may be above the knee and the oedema may even progress to the skin of the abdominal wall.

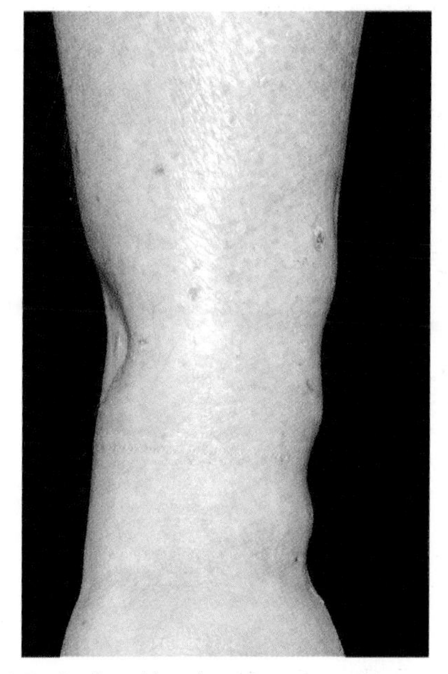

Fig. 4.26 Testing for ankle oedema. Press on medial aspect of lower shin.

CASE 4.22

Problem. My patient is overweight. Could her leg swelling simply be due to fat?

Discussion. Certain factors point towards leg swelling being due to fat: (1) the foot is relatively spared from swelling; (2) the swelling does not pit.

Tip

In a patient known to have heart failure, the degree of oedema gives useful information on the progress of treatment. Thus, in hospitals, patients with peripheral oedema secondary to heart failure often have their weight recorded regularly to monitor progress.

Keypoints

- Ankle oedema is tested for over the shin.
- Ankle oedema is a sign of heart failure but also occurs in many other situations.

Other cardiovascular signs

15. Consider looking for other signs such as radio-femoral delay and pulsatile liver.

As mentioned on p. 33, the cardiovascular system routine is an abbreviation of all possible cardiovascular signs. Some cardiovascular signs normally omitted from the routine are discussed in the next pages.

Blood pressure measurement

The most important of these other cardiovascular signs is blood pressure measurement—and I do not understand why this is not routinely required when examining the cardiovascular system.

What is blood pressure?

Blood pressure is the pressure exerted by the flow of blood in the main arteries. It varies through the cardiac cycle, being highest in systole and lowest in diastole (Fig. 4.1). Until recently blood pressure was usually measured with a machine that used mercury and so it is usually expressed in terms of millimetres of mercury (mm Hg).

The systolic blood pressure is normally given first, followed by the diastolic blood pressure. If a patient has a systolic blood pressure of 120 mm Hg and a diastolic blood pressure of 80 mm Hg, this is written as 120/80 mm Hg and expressed as '120 over 80'. Although expressed as a fraction, the reading is not used as a fraction. The difference between the two (120 - 80 = 40) mm Hg is known as the pulse pressure.

What is a normal blood pressure?

There is no easy answer to this question. What represents low blood pressure (hypotension) for an individual depends on their normal blood pressure. Thus, a blood pressure of 110/70 is hypotensive in a patient with a normal blood pressure of 180/110. However, a systolic blood pressure less than 80 mm Hg is rarely normal and usually indicates serious hypotension.

Hypertension (high blood pressure) is commonly defined as a blood pressure **persistently** greater than 140/90 mm Hg. Hypertension is a diagnosis, therefore, that can only be made after several consultations and blood pressure measurements.

Significance

Blood pressure measurement is an absolutely essential part of examining acutely unwell patients in whom low blood pressure is a critical finding. Hypotension may be caused by many illnesses but the most common are myocardial ischaemia/infarction, sepsis, and hypovolaemia secondary to bleeding. High blood pressure (hypertension) is an important risk factor for ischaemic heart disease and cerebrovascular disease.

The principle of blood pressure measurement

To measure arterial blood pressure directly would require an intra-arterial catheter connected to a pressure-measuring device! A more convenient indirect method makes use of a sphygmomanometer (*sfig-mow-man-om-meter*) (Fig. 4.27). This consists of a tourniquet (*tour-knee-kay*) with an inflatable cuff connected to a balloon (to inflate the tourniquet) and a pressure-measuring device. In the past the pressure was measured using a column of mercury. Because of concern with mercury toxicity, mercury sphygmomanometers are being replaced by aneroid sphygmomanometers.

The tourniquet with inflatable cuff is tied around the upper arm and inflated. Once the pressure in the tourniquet is higher than that in the brachial artery, arterial blood flow is occluded. Then, as the pressure in the cuff is reduced, brachial artery flow returns, but initially this occurs only momentarily at the point at which arterial

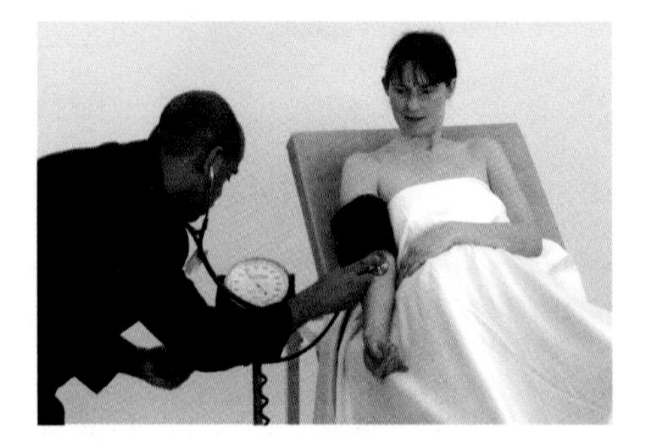

Fig. 4.27 Checking blood pressure by auscultation. Tourniquet inflated, diaphragm over the brachial artery.

blood pressure is at its highest. As the cuff pressure is further reduced, blood flow occurs throughout more and more of the cardiac cycle—until cuff pressure is less than the lowest diastolic pressure and blood flow is continuous throughout the cardiac cycle.

If you auscultate with the stethoscope over the brachial artery during this procedure, you will hear various noises, known as Korotkoff (*core-rot-cough*) sounds (*Nikolai Sergeievichj Korotkoff (1874–1920), Russian surgeon*). These are divided into five phases as the cuff pressure is reduced. In phase I, there is a thudding sound in time with the heartbeat. The thud is due to the short-lived flow of blood at the height of systole. Phase I signifies the systolic blood pressure. As the cuff pressure reduces, the sounds first increase in intensity (phase II), before gradually reducing (phase III) (phases II and III are of no practical significance). When the cuff pressure is less than the diastolic pressure and blood flow occurs throughout the whole cardiac cycle, the sounds quieten quite suddenly (phase IV) before stopping completely (phase V). Sometimes, though, the sounds never stop completely—there is no phase V. There is some debate over whether phase IV or phase V should be used as the diastolic pressure. Although phase IV is a more accurate estimation of diastolic blood pressure, phase V produces more consistent readings when taken by different individuals (less inter-observer variation) and is therefore preferred. If the sounds never stop completely, phase IV is used.

A less accurate method for measuring the systolic blood pressure is to palpate the radial pulse during cuff inflation and deflation. The point at which the pulse disappears and reappears is roughly the systolic pressure (the diastolic pressure cannot be gauged by palpation).

How to measure blood pressure

1. Patient should be relaxed, laid down for 5 min (see Case 4.27 for exception). The patient's arm should be straight, uncovered, and relaxed, either lying on the bed or held by you. It is reasonable to roll the patient's sleeve up but only if this does not impinge on the tourniquet. Otherwise, the shirt sleeve must be removed.
2. Tie the tourniquet around the arm with its lower border 2 cm from the antecubital fossa and with the centre of the inflatable cuff over the brachial artery. There is often an arrow at the centre of the cuff. The brachial artery is positioned roughly a third of the way across the antecubital fossa on the medial side. The cuff should be roughly at the patient's heart level—it usually is.
3. First, check the blood pressure by palpation:
   (1) palpate the radial pulse;
   (2) inflate the cuff by squeezing the balloon—watch the sphygmomanometer dial rising, indicating the cuff pressure;
   (3) feel the point at which the radial pulse disappears—this is the blood pressure by palpation.
4. Now, check blood pressure by auscultation (Fig. 4.27):
   (1) deflate the cuff (to allow the patient's arm to recover);
   (2) then, re-inflate the cuff to a pressure 20 mm Hg higher than the blood pressure by palpation;
   (3) place the diaphragm of the stethoscope on the brachial artery and auscultate;
   (4) now deflate the cuff 5 mm Hg at a time;
   (5) ascertain the points at which you first hear heart sounds (phase I), at which the sounds become muffled (phase IV), and at which the sounds disappear (phase V).
5. The blood pressure is described to the nearest 5 mm Hg as phase I over phase V, such as 120/85 mm Hg—'120 over 85 millimetres of mercury'. Phase IV is used if there is no phase V.

Tip

Measuring blood pressure can hurt especially in frail patients. Do not dither too long deciding exactly what the systolic blood pressure is with the tourniquet at high pressure.

CASE 4.23

Problem. My patient's blood pressure is very high but I'm not sure if the cuff is working properly. He's a very big man.

Discussion. The pressure exerted by the inflatable cuff on the brachial artery depends not only on the amount of air in it but also on the size of the patient's arm. Thus, a normal adult cuff will exert an excessively high pressure on a child's brachial artery, producing an artificially low reading—the converse applies to overweight patients. So there are a variety of cuff sizes to suit different patients—neonate, child, normal adult, and obese adult.

CASE 4.24

Problem. I hear a phase I sound but, on further listening, it disappears. Why might this happen?

Discussion. This may be because the patient is in atrial fibrillation. Here the systolic blood pressure varies with each beat.

CASE 4.25

Problem. I keep hearing a rustling noise, which doesn't seem to relate to the point at which the radial pulse disappears. Why is this?

Discussion. This is likely to be caused by you inadvertently moving your stethoscope. Keep it still!

CASE 4.26

Problem. My patient looks very unwell, the nurses are looking worried, and my blood pressure skills have deserted me. I can't hear the blood pressure. What's going on? What else could I try?

Discussion. The patient's blood pressure is probably very low (less than 80 mm Hg). In such situations, taking the blood pressure is difficult and it is often easier to palpate using the radial pulse than to auscultate.

CASE 4.27

Problem. My patient looks unwell. Can I afford to wait 5 minutes to take their blood pressure (allowing the patient to relax)?

Solution. No, in such a patient your main concern is hypotension. Waiting 5 minutes is only important when assessing for high blood pressure.

Postural blood pressure measurement

Normally, when a person stands up, their blood pressure alters a little: the systolic blood pressure falls by around 3 mm Hg whilst the diastolic blood pressure rises by around 5 mm Hg. A fall in systolic blood pressure greater than 20mm Hg on standing is arbitrarily defined as postural hypotension. Such a blood pressure reduction occurs in 25% of patients over 75 years and is often asymptomatic. However, some patients may be symptomatic, that is, become dizzy on standing. Causes depend on whether this is a recurrent or a one-off phenomenon. Recurrent postural hypotension is most commonly caused by drugs, particularly diuretics (causing chronic hypovolaemia) and vasodilators such as nitrates. Acute postural hypotension has the same causes as hypotension itself.

How to measure

1. Take blood pressure with patient lying down as normal.
2. Reduce cuff pressure to zero, but keep cuff on.
3. Stand the patient up and make sure they are steady.
4. Immediately, re-inflate cuff to 5 mm Hg above the lying systolic pressure and gradually reduce cuff pressure listening for the standing blood pressure.
5. Ask the patient to stay standing and repeat again in 2 min.

Tip

Ask the patient if they felt dizzy when they stood up. In some patients with postural hypotension, the fall in blood pressure is very brief and you may have missed it by the time you get a reading. If the patient admits to transient dizziness on standing it is worth trying again and rechecking lying and standing blood pressures.

Keypoints

- Blood pressure measurement is an absolutely essential part of examining acutely unwell patients.
- The diagnosis of hypertension (high blood pressure) should only be made after a series of blood pressure checks on different days.
- Blood pressure measurement is easy (DF 6/10) in patients with normal or high blood pressure, but difficult (DF 8/10) in those with very low blood pressure (systolic <80).
- Phase IV is a more accurate measure of diastolic pressure but phase V produces more consistent readings when taken by different people.
- Cuff size should vary depending on the individual.

Peripheral pulses

Significance

Both chronic ischaemia due to atherosclerosis (peripheral vascular disease) and acute ischaemia due to thrombosis or embolism are common conditions that need early identification, so it is important that you can palpate the peripheral pulses.

How to examine

Brachial artery (DF 6/10)

1. Use your thumb.
2. Locate the artery in the antecubital fossa about one-third the way across on the medial (ulnar) side — just medial to biceps tendon.

Femoral (fem-uh-ral) artery (DF 7/10—more difficult in overweight patients)

1. The patient should be lying flat or almost flat.
2. Use your index and middle fingers together—pointing upwards and slightly medially.
3. Locate the femoral artery in the groin area, half way between the pubic tubercle and anterior superior iliac (*eye-lee-yak or ill-lee-yak*) crest.

Popliteal (pop-lit-tea-al) artery (DF 9/10)

1. Use both hands; the patient should be lying flat or almost flat.
2. Bend the patient's knee to 120°.
3. Put thumbs on either side of front of knee with fingers in the popliteal fossa palpating for the pulse.

Posterior tibial (tibby-al) artery (DF 6/10)

1. Use your index finger.
2. Inspect for pulsation behind the medial malleolus (it is often visible here).
3. Feel for pulsation behind the medial malleolus.

Dorsalis pedis (door-sallis-pee-diss) artery (DF 9/10)

1. Use index and middle finger.
2. Locate dorsalis pedis, just lateral to the extensor hallucis tendon—about one-third of the way down the dorsum of the foot. Press down against the tarsal bones here (Fig. 4.28).

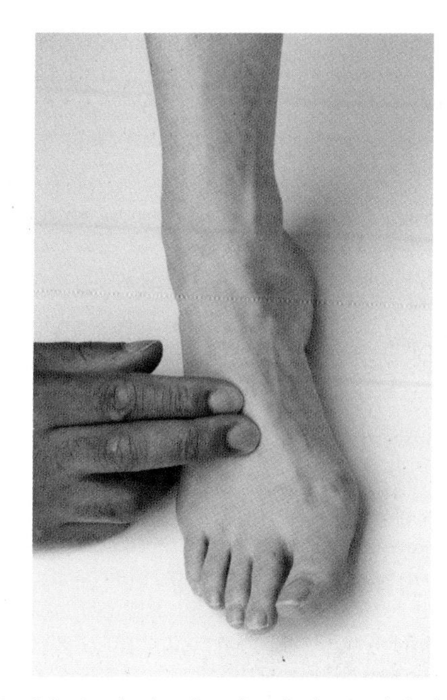

Fig. 4.28 Palpating the dorsalis pedis pulse (see text below).

Radiofemoral delay

(DF 9/10.)

What is it?

This is a subtle sign only rarely seen. The femoral pulse is felt half way between the pubic tubercle and the anterior superior iliac spine. Normally, the radial and femoral pulses coincide in time; if the femoral pulse is delayed and appears to come after the radial pulse, this is 'radiofemoral delay'.

Significance

Radiofemoral delay is a sign of coarctation (*co-ark-tay-shun*) of the aorta (see Fig. 16.58). In this condition there is a stricture in the aortic arch distal to the left subclavian artery, so that blood flow to the arms is good, but flow to the legs is reduced. As well as radiofemoral delay, the femoral pulse is weaker than the radial pulse. Blood pressure is usually elevated. There is often a systolic murmur at the left sternal edge and a continuous (systolic and diastolic) murmur over the scapula.

How to examine

1. The femoral pulse is best located with the patient lying flat.
2. Palpate the right femoral pulse as above (with your right hand.)
3. Now palpate the right radial pulse with your left hand. Decide if the two pulses coincide in time, and if the femoral pulse is weak compared to the radial.

Your teacher may query why you have not included this in the routine. This is a moot point. It can be considered best to exclude it from the routine because it is so rarely present and because it requires poking in the patient's groin early on in the examination (a bit confusing for the patient, who expects you to listen to the heart). It is advised to check it in all patients with hypertension or in any patient in whom other features point to coarctation.

Keypoints

- Radiofemoral delay is a subtle sign.
- It is seen in coarctation of the aorta—and should be checked for in all patients with hypertension.

Sacral oedema

(DF4/10.)

Generalized oedema collects in a site dependent on gravity. Normally, the site is the feet and ankles but in bed-bound patients the oedema collects around the sacrum. If present, sacral oedema is a more useful sign of generalized fluid overload than ankle oedema. This is because there are multiple causes of ankle oedema such as venous damage—whereas sacral oedema has few other causes.

1. Ask permission.
2. Sit patient forward.
3. Press over sacrum for 10 s (be aware of any tenderness).
4. Lift your thumb and observe for any indentation in the skin.

Keypoints

- Sacral oedema may occur in bed-bound patients; when present it is a more specific sign of heart failure than ankle oedema.

Pulsatile liver

This occurs in tricuspid regurgitation. Here, the tricuspid valve cannot shut fully so when the right ventricle contracts, blood refluxes into the superior vena cava into the jugular veins producing the giant V wave. Similarly, blood refluxes into the inferior vena cava and then into the hepatic vein—so causing the liver to pulsate. Also, because it is engorged with blood, the liver is enlarged. The pulsatile liver is examined for in the same way as the liver is normally examined (p. 166).

1. The patient should be lying flat.
2. Palpate superficially over the right upper quadrant for a pulsation.
3. Then, assess for an enlarged liver: perform deep palpation starting in the right iliac fossa, moving superiorly to the right upper quadrant.

Wash your hands

16. Wash your hands.

Once you have finished your examination you must wash your hands. This simple measure will reduce the spread of infections among your patients yet it is so easy to forget when you are learning new techniques or are trying hard to make sense of a case.

Presentation of findings

17. Now say 'I would like to check the blood pressure'. Pause briefly and then present findings.

Having felt for ankle oedema (and checked other signs as appropriate), stand up straight and say 'I would like to check the blood pressure'. The examiner will usually indicate that this is not necessary.

Then, start the presentation. The exact style of presentation depends on your findings. If your findings are compatible with a condition then start off by mentioning it. 'This woman has aortic stenosis as shown by a slow rising pulse, a heaving, sustained, non-displaced apex beat, and an ejection systolic murmur heard throughout the praecordium, loudest at the mitral area, radiating to both carotids. She is comfortable at rest, there is no clubbing or splinter haemorrhages, pulse was 62 per minute and regular, jugular venous pressure was not raised, there were no abnormal heaves or thrills in the praecordium, and heart sounds were normal. There was no evidence of heart failure.'

If your findings are inconclusive, detail them, give a differential diagnosis and if this includes a valvular lesion, suggest an echocardiogram. The following presentation refers to the same patient. 'This woman is comfortable at rest, there is no clubbing or splinter haemorrhages. Pulse was 62 per minute and there wasa regular sinus rhythm with a normal character. Jugular venous pressure was not elevated. There were no heaves or thrills. The apex beat is heaving and non-displaced. There is an ejection systolic murmur radiating to the carotids. The most likely diagnoses are aortic stenosis and aortic sclerosis and I feel an echocardio-

Tip

Do not forget to mention the blood pressure.

gram would be useful to decide.' Here, the student has not identified the slow rising pulse but has made a highly acceptable presentation.

Keypoints

- If you are fairly sure of the diagnosis, mention it early in your presentation.

Cardiovascular diseases and investigations

Echocardiogram (echo)

This is a 'heart scan'. It uses an ultrasound technique. An echo is especially useful for assessing valves and left ventricular systolic function.

Exercise test

This is used to diagnose and assess the severity of coronary artery disease. The patient is exercised, usually on a treadmill. They are monitored for symptoms of angina and ischaemia on the ECG.

Coronary angiogram

A coronary angiogram (*ann-jee-owe-gram*) is used to assess the coronary arteries for evidence of coronary artery disease. A cannula is inserted, usually into the femoral artery and passed to the coronary arteries where dye is released to delineate the arteries.

Cardiac catheter

This involves direct assessment of the heart valves and pressures. Again, a cannula is inserted, usually into the femoral artery and passed to the heart.

Rheumatic fever

This is an acute illness resulting from an immunological reaction to group A β haemolytic streptococcus (also known as *Streptococcus pyogenes* (*pie-oj-en-knees*)). Typically, the patient develops pharyngitis from which they recover. Then, around a month later, the patient develops various problems including fever, sweats, arthritis, and carditis. Although cardiac function is usually normal initially, there is healing with scarring, which may affect the valves. Around 25% of patients suffer long-term damage to their heart valves—the condition is then known as rheumatic heart disease. The mitral valve is most commonly affected (75%), followed by the aortic valve (50%), the tricuspid valve (10%), and the pulmonary valve (2%). Sydenham's chorea (*sid-en-ams-core-ear*) (St Vitus (*vie-tuss*) Dance) is characterized by jerky, purposeless movements. It may occur as part of rheumatic fever or on its own. In either case, it may later result in rheumatic heart disease (*Thomas Sydenham (1642–1689), English physician*).

Infective endocarditis

This is infection of the heart valves or adjacent endocardium—usually resulting in valvular regurgitation. Previously infective endocarditis was divided into subacute bacterial endocarditis and acute bacterial endocarditis but in recent decades the distinction has become blurred. Furthermore, non-bacterial organisms have been implicated. Hence the simple term 'infective endocarditis'. The most common infecting organism is *Streptococcus viridans* (*viri-dans*), which is responsible for around 50% of cases. *Streptococcus viridans* refers to a group of α haemolytic streptococci including *Streptococcus mitis* (*my-tiss*), *Streptococcus sanguis* (*sang-wiss*), *Streptococcus mutans* (*mute-anns*), and *Streptococcus millieri* (*milly-air-ee*).

Keypoints

- Rheumatic fever is an immunological reaction to infection by group A β haemolytic streptococcus (*Streptococcus pyogenes*).
- 25% of patients suffer long-term damage to heart valves.
- Infective endocarditis is a direct infection of the heart—the most common infecting organism is *Streptococcus viridans* (α haemolytic strep).

Mitral stenosis

This is narrowing of the mitral valve.

Cause

Rheumatic heart disease is the only significant cause.

Pathophysiology

Narrowing of the mitral valve results in reduced left ventricular filling during diastole. The normal mitral valve area is 5 cm^2. If this reduces to 2.5 cm^2 or less, symptoms start to occur.

Features

See Fig. 4.29.

How do you measure the severity of mitral stenosis?

1. Severity of symptoms.
2. Length of murmur (reflects degree of left atrial hypertrophy). The longer the murmur, the more severe the stenosis.

3. The time between S2 and opening snap (reflects degree of left atrial hypertrophy). The shorter the time, the more severe the stenosis.
4. Signs of pulmonary hypertension (see Fig. 4.29).
5. Area of valve on echocardiogram. A small area indicates severe stenosis.

Key signs of mitral stenosis

Irregularly irregular pulse, malar flush, tapping cardiac impulse, loud first heart sound, mid-diastolic murmur, opening snap.

Mitral regurgitation

This is where the valve cannot shut completely

Causes

The main causes are rheumatic heart disease, mitral valve prolapse, and 'functional', where left ventricular dilation caused by, say, ischaemic heart disease produces dilation of the valve—the valve itself is not actually abnormal.

Pathophysiology

The mitral valve cannot shut completely so when the left ventricle contracts to eject blood during systole,

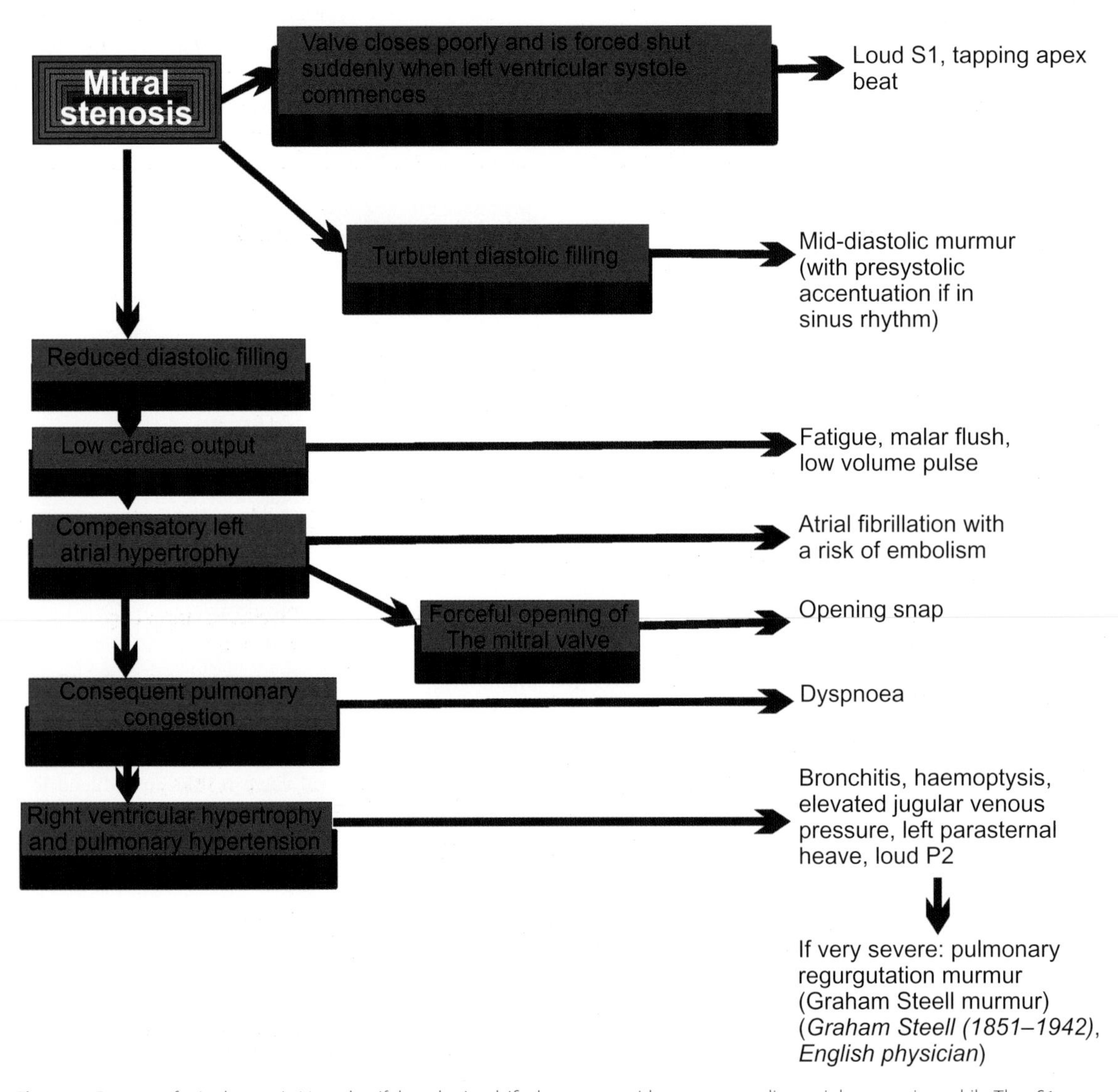

Fig. 4.29 Features of mitral stenosis. Note that if the valve is calcified, as occurs with more severe disease, it becomes immobile. Thus S1 may not be loud and there is no opening snap.

some blood flows backward to the left atrium rather than forward to the tissues.

Features

See Fig. 4.30. Mitral regurgitation may occur acutely as a result of (1) myocardial infarction, producing dysfunction or rupture of papillary muscles or (2) infective endocarditis. When acute, it presents with pulmonary oedema. The left atrium is not dilated.

Key signs of mitral regurgitation

Displaced, thrusting cardiac impulse, soft S1, pansystolic murmur.

Mixed mitral valve disease

Mitral stenosis and mitral regurgitation may co-exist—this is mixed mitral valve disease. It is usually due to rheumatic heart disease but may also result from endocarditis of a stenotic valve. The systolic murmur of mitral regurgitation is easy to hear, the diastolic murmur of stenosis more difficult. It may be possible to say which is more significant using clinical signs. The key to this is the apex beat. If mitral stenosis predominates, this will be tapping and not displaced; if mitral regurgitation predominates, this will be thrusting and displaced. The heart sounds may also be helpful. S1 is soft in mitral regurgitation and loud in mitral stenosis (this is not so clear cut as a calcified stenotic valve does not produce loud S1). Furthermore, S3 may be present in mitral regurgitation but not in mitral stenosis.

Keypoints

- In mixed mitral valve disease, the apex beat and S1 help to decide whether the regurgitation or stenosis is more important.

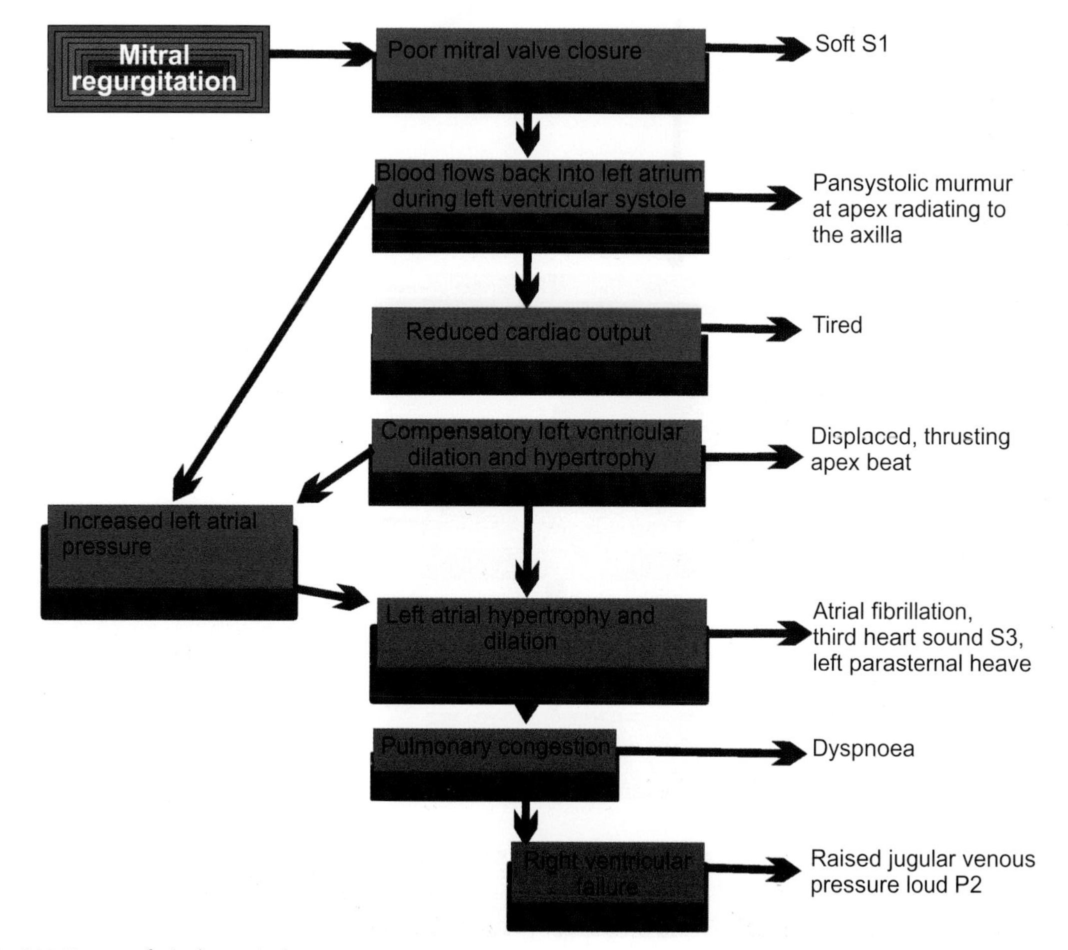

Fig. 4.30 Features of mitral regurgitation.

Tip

S1 should be soft in isolated mitral regurgitation. If it is not or if it is loud, listen carefully for the opening snap and murmur of mitral stenosis.

Aortic stenosis

This is narrowing of the aortic valve. Normal aortic valve area is 2 cm². Narrowing to less than 1 cm² causes significant aortic stenosis.

Causes

Rheumatic, calcific degeneration (elderly), congenital bicuspid valve (presenting in adults), and congenital aortic stenosis (presenting in childhood).

Pathophysiology

Aortic stenosis makes it difficult for the left ventricle to eject blood to the tissues when it contracts.

Features

See Fig. 4.31. The murmur tends to get louder with increasing severity of stenosis, but then becomes quieter

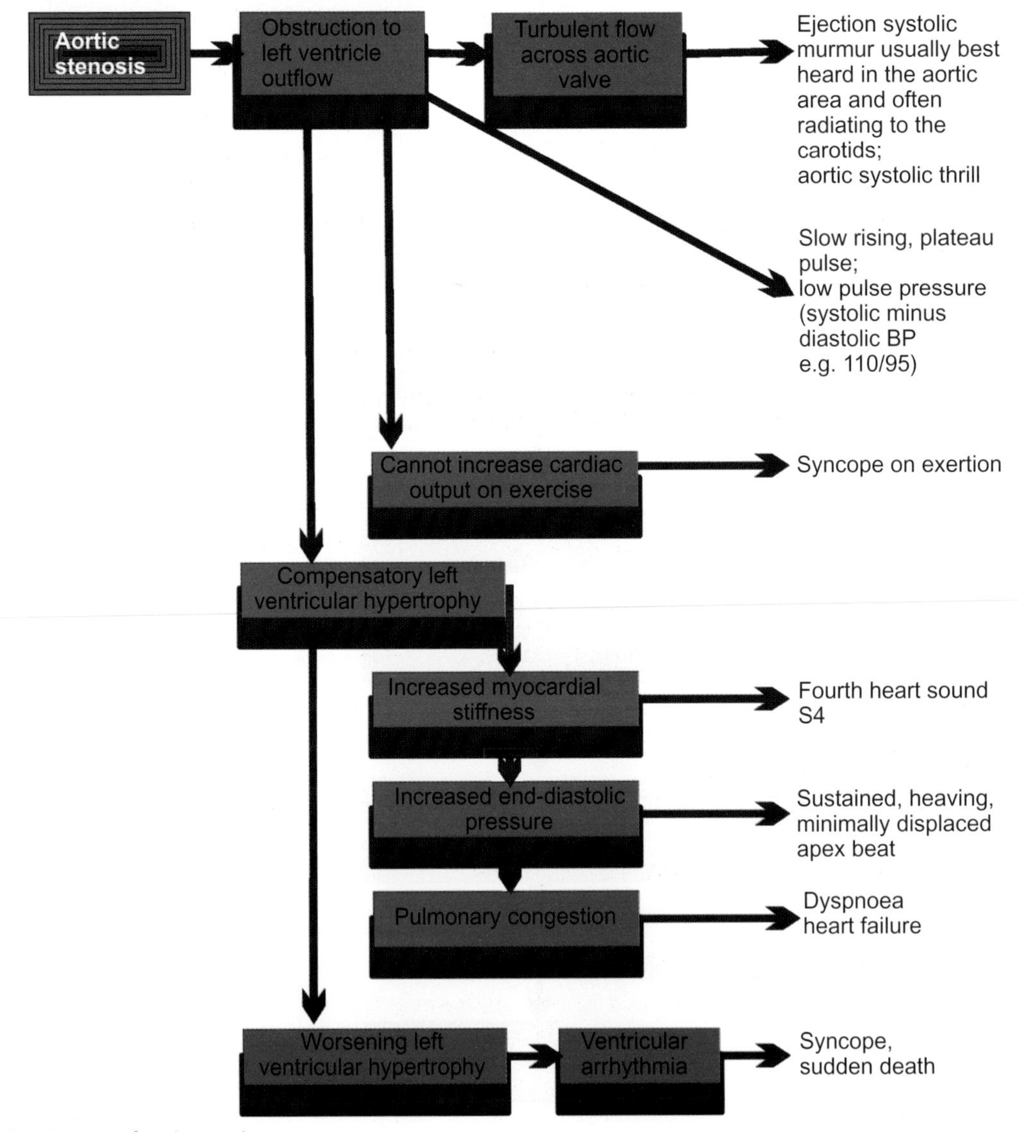

Fig. 4.31 Features of aortic stenosis.

as left ventricular failure supersedes. A thrill—suggesting a loud murmur—indicates quite severe stenosis.

Key signs of aortic stenosis

Pulse character slow rising, sustained, heaving, slightly displaced cardiac impulse, ejection systolic murmur.

Aortic sclerosis

This is a degenerative condition of elderly people. The aortic valve thickens and there is a consequent ejection systolic murmur. Because of this, it can be mixed up with aortic stenosis. However, there are no haemodynamic problems and it is asymptomatic. Signs of aortic sclerosis differ from aortic stenosis in that the pulse character is normal, there is no thrill, and there is only slight radiation to the carotids. However, these signs are not always present in aortic stenosis so in practice, an echocardiogram is often required to differentiate the two.

Aortic regurgitation

This is when the aortic valve cannot shut completely.

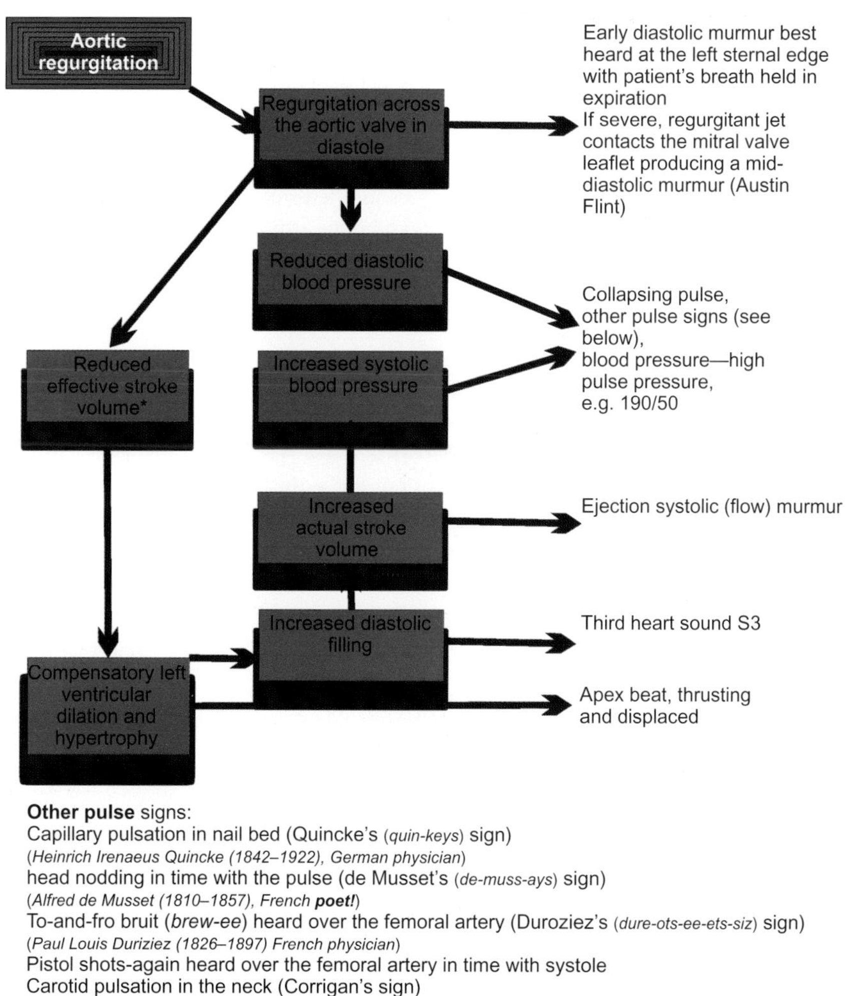

Fig. 4.32 Features of aortic regurgitation. †The actual stroke volume is the volume of blood the left ventricle ejects with each contraction. *The effective stroke volume is the volume of blood that actually reaches the tissues with each contraction. This is the actual stroke volume minus the volume of blood that regurgitates back into the ventricle.

Causes

Congenital or acquired (rheumatic fever, infective endocarditis, trauma, dilation of aorta—syphilis, ankylosing spondylitis, Marfan's, and atherosclerosis).

Pathophysiology

During diastole the pressure in the aorta is much higher than that in the left ventricle. The closed aortic valve prevents blood flowing backwards into the left ventricle. In aortic regurgitation, the aortic valve cannot shut completely so some blood flows back into the left ventricle during diastole.

Features

See Fig. 4.32.

Key signs of aortic regurgitation

Collapsing pulse, thrusting, displaced cardiac impulse, early diastolic murmur.

Mixed aortic valve disease

Aortic stenosis and aortic regurgitation may co-exist—this is mixed aortic valve disease. It is nearly always caused by rheumatic heart disease but may also result from endocarditis affecting a stenotic valve. A characteristic sign of mixed aortic valve disease is a bisfiriens pulse (Fig. 4.9)—this refers to the character of the pulse, which gives an impression of a double pulse. The following features are helpful in deciding clinically whether the stenosis or regurgitation is more important (though echo is best used).

	Aortic regurgitation	Aortic stenosis
Pulse	Collapsing	Slow rising
Pulse pressure	Wide	Narrow
Cardiac impulse	Thrusting, displaced	Heaving, minimal displacement
Systolic murmur	Not loud or harsh	Loud and harsh
Systolic thrill	No	Yes

Note that in a patient with aortic regurgitation, a systolic murmur does not necessarily indicate aortic stenosis. It may simply be a flow murmur.

Heart failure

'Heart failure' is not an ideal term but it is the one that is used. 'Heart weakness' would be more accurate. Avoid using the term 'heart failure' in front of patients—it invariably increases anxiety levels. Heart failure is where the heart cannot maintain adequate cardiac output or does so only by maintaining elevated filling pressure.

Elevated filling pressure

The heart works better (initially at least) when it dilates to increase filling pressure (the Starling mechanism) *(Ernest Henry Starling (1866–1927), English physiologist)*. Thus, one of the first responses of the heart to reduced function is to dilate in order to increase filling pressure and cardiac output.

Classification

There are several different ways of classifying heart failure:

- right or left
- acute or chronic
- high output or low output.

The simplest classification divides heart failure by causes into left-sided heart failure, right-sided heart failure, and non-cardiac heart failure. Table 4.8 is by no means exhaustive, but gives the main causes. The most common type of heart failure is where right and left heart failure co-exist—this is known as congestive heart failure.

Features

In most cases of heart failure, it is the compensatory mechanisms producing increased backward pressures that cause the predominant features. So in left heart failure, pulmonary congestion predominates and in right heart failure it is peripheral tissue congestion that predominates. In Tables 4.9 and 4.10, the features are divided into right and left sided; however, as already mentioned, these most commonly co-exist in congestive heart failure.

Signs of fluid retention

The old idea that fluid retention relates purely to increased venous pressure is losing sway (p. X). It is now thought that it is abnormal renal flow and the consequent compensatory mechanisms that produce fluid retention. All the same signs of fluid retention are common in right heart failure, particularly ankle and sacral oedema. If severe, hepatic congestion producing tender hepatomegaly, ascites, and pleural effusion may also occur.

Investigations

The key signs of heart failure on chest X-ray are enlarged heart (>50% of thoracic diameter), upper lobe venous diversion, lymphatic congestion producing

TABLE 4.8 Causes of heart failure

Left heart failure
Generalized myocardial disease, producing left ventricular systolic dysfunction (due to ischaemic heart disease, alcohol consumption, idiopathic cardiomyopathy*)
Segmental myocardial dysfunction (due to myocardial infarction)
Valvular lesions (such as aortic stenosis and regurgitation, mitral stenosis, and regurgitation)
Hypertension
Right heart failure
Secondary to left heart failure (congestive heart failure)
Segmental myocardial dysfunction (due to right ventricular myocardial infarction)
Valvular lesions (such as tricuspid, pulmonary valve lesions)
Pulmonary vascular hypertension (idiopathic (primary), secondary to lung disease (cor pulmonale) as in chronic obstructive pulmonary disease, secondary to pulmonary emboli)
Non-cardiac (increased demand)
Anaemia
Thyrotoxicosis

* Cardiomyopathy: a disease of the myocardium where no cause is identified.

TABLE 4.9 Features of left heart failure

Produces pulmonary congestion leading to pulmonary oedema	
Symptoms	Breathlessness, orthopnoea, paroxysmal nocturnal dyspnoea
Signs	Tachypnoea, tachycardia (due to increased sympathetic tone), fine late inspiratory basal crepitations (due to pulmonary congestion), third heart sound (poorly compliant left ventricle), fourth heart sound (poorly compliant left ventricle)
If severe, dilation of left ventricle also causes dilation of the mitral valve, which cannot shut completely resulting in mitral regurgitation (known as functional mitral regurgitation). Such mitral regurgitation may produce signs of its own	

TABLE 4.10 Features of right heart failure

Produces peripheral congestion and consequent tiredness, ankle swelling, abdominal discomfort, and anorexia	
Signs	Raised jugular venous pressure, left parasternal heave, right ventricular S3 (poorly compliant right ventricle), ankle or sacral oedema
If severe, signs of 'functional' tricuspid regurgitation may occur because of dilation of right ventricle involving the tricuspid valve.	

Kerley A and more particularly Kerley B lines, and pleural effusion (see Fig. 16.32). For details on chest X-ray, see p. 442. Echocardiography is useful in assessing left ventricular systolic and valvular function. Left ventricular systolic function is probably best assessed subjectively as good, poor, or very poor. However, computer-generated measurements of left ventricular size and the so-called 'ejection fraction' are often preferred—probably because they produce a handy number. Ejection fraction is the proportion of blood in the ventricle that is ejected with each systolic contraction. Normally this is greater than 45%.

Acute heart failure

This may be provoked by acute myocardial ischaemia or infarction, arrhythmias, chest infection, pulmonary emboli, and reduction of therapy for chronic heart failure.

Finals section

In this section, some specific issues dealing with Finals will be discussed. This is not a summary section. For revision, it is suggested that you read the examination summary (p. 33) and the keypoints throughout the chapter and do the questions on p. 72. The emphasis of this section is on the short cases as this format usually causes the most uncertainty and is still used in some UK medical schools and in many worldwide. The Objective Structured Clinical Examination (OSCE) usually has more straightforward and standardized instructions. Despite the different formats the clinical approach remains the same.

The cardiovascular system is at the centre of general medicine. Because of this and because it is well suited to the format of the formal examination routine, the cardiovascular system is the single most important system for medicine short cases. In your Finals examination, it is very likely you will be asked to examine the cardiovascular system. Do well and you will be on your way. **Thus, if you know nothing else, know how to examine the cardiovascular system.**

The most common serious cardiovascular pathology is ischaemic heart disease. However, this does not produce consistent physical signs and so is unsuitable for Finals short cases. Most Finals short cases will be a lesion affecting the heart valves producing a heart murmur. Valvular lesions have become increasingly rare with the reduced incidence and severity of rheumatic fever (p. 63) in the last 30 years. However, they continue to represent a good challenge in tying together more than one abnormal cardiovascular system sign. So medical schools make an effort to recruit patients with valvular lesions for the Finals examination.

Most patients with valvular lesions will have single lesions. You will be a bit unlucky to get mixed valve lesions and very unlucky to get a mixture of aortic and mitral valve problems. If the patient does have multiple valvular lesions, the examiner will not expect you to get the correct answer. So, if there seem to be multiple different contradictory signs, do not panic! As long as you perform a reasonable examination and give a sensible description of what you have found, you will be all right. Common Finals cases are given in Table 4.11.

In day-to-day ward teaching, patients with systolic murmurs with no other accompanying cardiovascular system signs are most common. These may be non-pathological 'innocent' murmurs (p. 52), as occurs in a minority of normal people, or may represent early valvular disease. So, do not be alarmed if you have found no abnormality by the time you reach auscultation (and do not feel the need to invent an abnormality). Common day-to-day cases are given in Table 4.12.

Key diagnostic clues

In day-to-day clinical practice, the key signs are those pointing to arrhythmia or cardiac failure, such as pulse rate and rhythm, blood pressure, jugular venous pressure, and basal lung crepitations. However, as regards short cases—where diagnosis of valvular lesions is most important—it is **carotid pulse character** and **auscultation of the heart** that provide the most important clues.

Key signs of the most important valvular lesions

1. **Mitral stenosis.** Pulse irregularly irregular, malar flush, cardiac impulse tapping, loud first heart sound, mid-diastolic murmur heard, opening snap.

TABLE 4.11 Common Finals cases

Mitral stenosis
Aortic stenosis
Aortic regurgitation
Mitral regurgitation
Mixed mitral valve disease
Mixed aortic valve disease

TABLE 4.12 Common day-to-day cases

Systolic murmur with no other accompanying cardiovascular system signs
Any of the Finals cases
Cardiac failure

2. **Aortic stenosis.** Pulse character slow rising, sustained, heaving, slightly displaced cardiac impulse, ejection systolic murmur heard all over praecordium and radiating into the carotids.
3. **Aortic regurgitation.** Collapsing pulse, thrusting, displaced cardiac impulse, early diastolic murmur best heard at lower left sternal edge with patient sitting forward and breath held in expiration.
4. **Mitral regurgitation.** Displaced, thrusting cardiac impulse, soft S1, pansystolic murmur.
5. **Aortic sclerosis.** Ejection systolic murmur heard all over the praecordium but little radiation to carotids and normal character pulse.

If you know no other facts about the cardiovascular system, you should know those few signs.

Some advice relating to examination problems

General

Do not waste time looking for the cardiovascular system examination routine that will completely satisfy all examiners. It does not exist! Use the one given on p. 33.

The instruction

The examiner will usually ask you to 'examine the cardiovascular system'. Occasionally, they will say instead 'examine the heart'. These both mean the same thing. However, if the examiner gives a more specific instruction, such as 'examine the praecordium' or 'examine the radial pulse and auscultate the heart', you must do just as they request. With such requests, the possibility of confusion here is in how to fit in the 'general look'. This should be done, as always, while preparing the patient for examination.

Moving infirm patients

Always proceed with the aim of carrying out a full examination, asking the patient's permission as you go. If the examiner feels moving such a patient is inappropriate, they will stop you.

Positioning

Even if the patient is already sitting in bed at around 45°, you should alter their position, albeit minimally, to make it clear to the doctor/teacher that you know the patient should be at that angle.

Hands

Tar staining in the short case context is very often a red herring. However, it may be an indicator of ischaemic heart disease, which may produce signs of heart failure

CASE 4.28

Problem. Some examiners may ask you why you have not looked for anaemia or peripheral cyanosis in the hands.

Discussion. The skin creases of the palms may be paler than usual in anaemic patients—but anaemia is better assessed at the conjunctivae (p. 38). Peripheral cyanosis is either a sign of general hypoxia, in which case examination for central cyanosis (p. 90) in the mouth is more appropriate or simply a sign of being cold. Strictly speaking, it may also occur in peripheral arterial problems such as brachial artery blockage, but such a problem would not be the subject of a medical short case. Therefore, these two signs are not routinely included in the cardiovascular system examination.

or cause myocardial infarction complicated by pericarditis or VSD with resultant signs.

Radial pulse

Pulse character (p. 39) is better assessed at the carotid pulse, so although you may get a sense of pulse character at the radial pulse, it is traditional that you do not comment on it. In the short case context, pulse rate and rhythm are often unremarkable. The most important finding is an irregularly irregular pulse, suggesting atrial fibrillation, which may be present in mitral valve disease.

Face

Not all rosy-cheeked patients will have mitral stenosis. All the same, if your short case patient has rosy cheeks always think of a malar flush and be on the alert for mitral stenosis.

Inspecting praecordium

It is often easier to see the cardiac impulse at the apex than feel it so always inspect before palpating.

CASE 4.29

Problem. Whilst inspecting, you may feel an intense urge to get on with the 'real' examination.

Solution. Do not cut short your inspection! Your examiner expects you to be thorough. Look carefully for a left thoracotomy scar—this may involve asking the permission of female patients to lift the breast. If you find a left thoracotomy scar, be thinking of mitral stenosis or mitral regurgitation.

Palpating praecordium

1. Potentially, palpation provides important information about valvular lesions. Unfortunately, though, signs such as the apex beat are not always reliable thus limiting their usefulness. However, the presence of a tapping apex beat, a displaced apex beat, a left parasternal heave, or any thrills are all fairly reliable clinical signs.
2. A tapping cardiac impulse represents a palpable first heart sound. If you do not hear a loud first heart sound, reconsider whether the cardiac impulse really was tapping.
3. A thrill represents a palpable murmur. If you do not hear a loud murmur on auscultation, reconsider whether you really felt a thrill.
4. Decisions on whether the apex beat is sustained or not, heaving, or thrusting are quite subtle. Consider your other signs before deciding. So, if you have found other signs of aortic regurgitation, you are likely to be correct if you felt the apex beat was thrusting and non-sustained.
5. If you have been asked to examine the apex beat only, you should start with inspection of the apex.
6. In many patients the apex beat is not palpable. During the short cases, do not spend longer than 20 s if you cannot find it. Know the causes of an impalpable apex. Although you may well have 'just missed it', you should always say 'the apex beat is impalpable' and then be prepared to answer the question 'Why do you think that is?' with one or all of the reasons given on p. 49.
7. Counting down ribs is cumbersome but expected.

Auscultation

1. You will not be expected to hear every click and squeak; the main thing is that you listen to the different areas of the heart in a professional way.
2. Your cardiovascular system examination prior to auscultation should have given you a good idea what to listen for before starting auscultation. So, if you have seen a malar flush, palpated atrial fibrillation, and a tapping apex beat, you should be listening hard for the mid-diastolic murmur of mitral stenosis.
3. By the time you lift the stethoscope off the patient's chest, you should have decided what you are going to say about the case as a whole. Whilst listening to the chest at the back, you should be thinking as much as listening.

4. Mitral stenosis is one of the most common short cases and you should know it well.
5. The first heart sound should be soft in isolated mitral regurgitation. If it is not or if it is loud, listen carefully for the opening snap and murmur of mitral stenosis.

Other signs

If you feel any other sign might yield useful information, by all means test for it after you have checked for ankle oedema.

Wash your hands

It may not be normal practice to wash your hands prior to presentation at your medical school. For Finals, it is best if you follow the local protocol.

Presentation

Always offer to check the blood pressure. Try to be confident—avoid the words 'seems' or 'might'.

Good luck!

Questions

All answers are in the text. The more stars, the more important it is to know the answer.

1. What are the murmurs of mitral stenosis, mitral regurgitation, aortic stenosis, and aortic regurgitation? *****
2. Give two cardiac causes of clubbing. **
3. What are splinter haemorrhages? *
4. Give two causes of splinter haemorrhages. Are they embolic or vasculitic? *
5. Describe three reasons for an irregularly irregular pulse. ***
6. Give two causes of asymmetrical radial pulses. *
7. What is a collapsing pulse? In which condition does it occur? ***
8. What is radiofemoral delay? Name the condition in which it features. *
9. What are Korotkoff sounds? **
10. What is the significance of phase I, IV, V Korotkoff sounds? ***
11. What is a malar flush and in what does it occur? **
12. Give two signs of hyperlipidaemia. **
13. What is the waveform of the jugular venous pressure? **
14. What are the causes of a raised jugular venous pressure? **
15. Why is the external jugular vein not used? ***
16. How do you differentiate arterial and venous pulsations in the neck? ****
17. What are the reasons for a mid-line sternotomy scar? **
18. What are the reasons for a left thoracotomy scar? **
19. What is the definition of the apex beat? ****
20. What are the reasons for not being able to feel the apex beat? ****
21. What is the left parasternal heave due to? **
22. To what is the first heart sound due? ****
23. What is the reason for the second heart sound? ****
24. What causes the third heart sound? **
25. Name four conditions in which the third heart sound is heard. **
26. What is the fourth heart sound due to? **
27. Give four conditions in which a fourth heart sound is heard. **
28. How is the murmur of aortic regurgitation best heard? ****
29. What is the best way of hearing the murmur of mitral stenosis? ****
30. What causes a pulsatile liver? ***
31. What organism causes rheumatic fever? **
32. What causes mitral stenosis? ****
33. What are the key signs of mitral stenosis? ***
34. Give three causes of mitral regurgitation. **
35. What are the key signs of mitral regurgitation? ***
36. Give three ways of determining the severity of mitral stenosis. **
37. In mixed mitral valve disease, how can you say which lesion predominates clinically? ***
38. Name three causes of aortic stenosis. ***
39. State the key signs of aortic stenosis. ***
40. How do you differentiate between aortic stenosis and sclerosis? ***
41. Give four causes of aortic regurgitation. *
42. What are the key signs of aortic regurgitation? **
43. What are Corrigan's sign and Corrigan's pulse? *

44. What is a bisfiriens pulse? **
45. How do you tell clinically which condition predominates in mixed aortic valve disease? ***
46. What is congestive cardiac failure? ***
47. What are the signs of left heart failure? ****
48. Name the signs of right heart failure. ****

Score. Give 4 marks for 4 stars, 1 for 1 star, and so on. At the end of the third year, you should be scoring 70-plus and by Finals, 90-plus; 110-plus is very good.

Further reading

Anonymous. Abdominojugular test. *Lancet* 1989; **i**:419–20.

Brugada P, Gursey S, Brugada J, Andries E. Investigation of palpitations. *Lancet* 1993; **341**:1254–8.

Cook DJ, Simel DL. The rational clinical examination: does this patient have abnormal jugular venous pressure? *Journal of the American Medical Association* 1996; **275**:630–4.

Davison R, Cannon R. Estimation of central venous pressure by examination of jugular veins. *American Heart Journal* 1974; **87**:279–82.

Desjardins VA, Enriquez-Sareno M, Tajik AJ, Bailey KR, Seward JB. Intensity of murmurs correlates with severity of valvular regurgitation. *American Journal of Medicine* 1996; **100**:149–56.

Fisher J. Jugular venous valves and physical signs. *Chest* 1984; **85**:685–6.

Hope RA, Longmore JM, Hodgetts TJ, Remrakha PS. *Oxford handbook of clinical medicine.* 3rd edn. Oxford: Oxford University Press; 1995.

Ishmail AA, Wing S, Ferguson J, Hutchinson TA, Magder S, Flegel KM. Inter-observer agreement by auscultation in the presence of a third heart sound in patients with congestive heart failure. *Chest* 1987; **91**:870–3.

Jordan MD, Taylor CR, Nyhuis AW, Tavel ME. Audibility of the fourth heart sound. Relationships to the presence of disease and examiner experience. *Archives of Internal Medicine* 1987; **147**:721–6.

Markiewicz W, Brik A, Brook G. Pericardial rub in pericardial effusion lack of correlation with amount of fluid. *Chest* 1980;**77**:643–6.

McGee S, Abernethy WB, Simel DL. Is this patient hypovolaemic? *Journal of the American Medical Association* 1999; **281**:1022–9.

O'Brien E. Ave atque vale: the centenary of clinical sphygmomanometry. *Lancet* 1996; **348**:1569–70.

Sever P, Beevers G, Bulpit C, Lever A, Ramsay L, Reid J, *et al.* Management guidelines in essential hypertension: report of the second working party of the British Hypertension Society. *British Medical Journal* 1993; **306**:983–7.

Sheth TN. The relationship of conjunctival pallor to the presence of anaemia. *Journal of General Internal Medicine* 1997; **12**:102–6.

Slater EE, DeSanctis RW. The clinical recognition of dissecting aortic aneurysm. *American Journal of Medicine* 1976; **60**:625–33.

Spitell PC, Spittell JA, Joyce JW, Tajik AJ, Edwards WD, Schaff HV, *et al.* Clinical features and differential diagnosis of aortic dissection: experience with 236 cases (1980 through 1990). *Mayo Clinic Proceedings* 1993; **68**:642–51.

Young JB, Will EJ, Mulley GP. Splinter haemorrhages: facts and fiction. *Journal of the Royal College of Physicians of London* 1988; **22**:240–3.

CHAPTER 5

Respiratory system

Chapter contents

Introduction

Chest disease is a common cause of morbidity and mortality in Western countries. Episodes of illness associated with acute increases in breathlessness are one of the commonest causes of hospital admission while lung cancer remains the number one killer of all cancers.

In this chapter, you will learn what questions to ask patients with respiratory diseases and how to examine the respiratory system.

Symptoms

The key symptoms of the respiratory system are cough, phlegm, haemoptysis (*he-mop-ta-sis*), wheeze, breathlessness, and chest pain. Breathlessness and chest pain have been dealt with in the cardiovascular chapter so they will not be discussed in any detail.

Cough

It is normal for the respiratory mucosa to produce a small amount of secretions. These are removed by mucociliary (*mew-co-silla-ree*) action. When there is an abnormal amount of secretions or other foreign material, the normal mucociliary action is unable to cope and a cough is used to remove the material. Involuntary coughing always indicates an abnormality but the causes form a wide spectrum from minor, transient problems to serious, life-threatening disease.

When a patient complains of cough, the first question to ask about is duration. Cough may be categorized (crudely, agreed) according to duration: less than 2 months is acute and more than 2 months is chronic. The two categories have different patterns of causation.

Acute cough

Causes

1. Infection affecting any part of the respiratory tree—nasopharyngitis (*nay-so-fa-rinj-eye-tiss*) to laryngotracheobronchitis (*la-ring-owe-tray-key-owe-bronk-eye-tiss*) to pneumonia.
2. Allergic reactions.
3. Reaction to irritant.
4. Any of the causes of chronic cough at their onset.

How to decide what the cause is

1. **Infections.** Associated fever and chills; sputum, often but not necessarily mucopurulent (thick yellow or green); hoarseness if laryngitis; pain related to affected site—throat pain for pharyngitis or laryngitis, chest pain with tracheitis.
2. **Allergic.** Associated sneezing; watery secretions.
3. **Reaction to irritant.** Recent inhalation of irritant; no sputum.

As regards infections, it is very difficult to distinguish viral from bacterial infections clinically. Two points may help.

1. Viral infections, particularly the common cold, are much more common.
2. Streptococcal pneumonia tends to produce respiratory symptoms, especially pain, early on in its course—within hours of the onset of fever and chills—whereas viral pneumonias tend to have a prodrome of general symptoms before the more obvious respiratory symptoms develop.

Chronic cough

Causes

See Table 5.1. Note that several important causes (postnasal drip, gastrooesophageal reflux disease, and angiotensin-converting enzyme (ACE) inhibitors) are not chest diseases.

How to decide what the cause is

See Table 5.2. Ask about

(1) timing—?nocturnal, ?morning;

(2) exacerbating—?exercise ?cold weather ?meals;

(3) sputum;

TABLE 5.1 Causes of chronic cough

Common
Post-nasal drip*
Asthma
Gastro-oesophageal reflux disease†
Chronic obstructive pulmonary disease
Smokers' cough (due to chronic irritation)
Less common
Bronchiectasis
Lung cancer
Tuberculosis
Angiotensin-converting enzyme inhibitor
Heart failure

* Post-nasal drip is due to pathology in the nasal mucosa or sinuses. It has multiple causes including allergic reactions and irritant reactions and it may be post-infective.

† Gastrooesophageal reflux disease: it is now well recognized that acid refluxing into the larynx may cause a chronic cough.

TABLE 5.2 Analysis of causes of chronic cough

	Timing of cough	Exacerbating	Sputum	Associated symptoms	Other factors
Post-nasal drip	Worst first thing in the morning		Yes		
Asthma	During the night	Exercise, cold weather	No	Paroxysmal breathlessness	
Gastrooesophageal reflux disease		Meals	No	Heartburn	
COPD	On first going to bed and first thing in the morning but not much during the night		Often*	Chronic breathlessness	Usually smoker or ex-smoker
Smokers' cough	As for COPD		As for COPD		Smoker or ex-smoker
Bronchiectasis		Postural changes	Copious, may be blood streaked		
Angiotensin-converting enzyme inhibitor			No		May develop any time in the first year of treatment
Heart failure	During the night		May be frothy, sometimes bloody		
Lung cancer			Initially dry, later purulent sputum due to secondary infection or bloody sputum may develop†	Anorexia,weight loss	Usually smoker or ex-smoker
Tuberculosis			May be bloody	Anorexia, weight loss, night sweats	

COPD, chronic obstructive pulmonary disease.

* Chronic bronchitis is defined as cough productive of sputum on most days of 3 months in 2 consecutive years.

† A rare form of lung cancer—broncho-alveolar carcinoma—may cause production of copious amounts of watery sputum.

(4) associated symptoms—breathlessness, heartburn, weight loss, anorexia, and night sweats;

(5) smoking;

(6) recent ACE inhibitors.

CASE 5.1

Problem. What cough features point towards lung cancer?

Discussion. While lung cancer is a rare cause of chronic cough, the serious nature of the diagnosis means that the cough of lung cancer warrants particular attention. The difficulty is that there are no clear characteristic features. Initially, the cough can be mild and the characteristic blood-stained sputum may not be present. The associated symptoms mentioned in Table 5.2 may also be absent. The diagnosis should be borne in mind in patients presenting with a new, **persistent** cough or in patients with a chronic cough who present with a change in cough pattern. All such patients should have a chest X-ray performed. If normal this makes the diagnosis of lung cancer unlikely. However, even if the X-ray is normal, the presence of weight loss, anorexia, or haemoptysis necessitates referral to a respiratory expert for consideration of bronchoscopy. If the patient is or has been a smoker, the index of suspicion should be higher.

Keypoints

- Cough may be classified according to duration: less than 2 months is acute and more than 2 months is chronic.
- If less than 2 months, think of infections (usually upper respiratory) and allergies.
- If more than 2 months, think more of intrinsic lung disease but also consider sinonasal, gastrointestinal, and cardiac problems.
- In patients with chronic cough ask about timing, exacerbating factors, sputum, associated symptoms, and smoking.
- Do not forget to ask about ACE inhibitors.

TABLE 5.3 Causes of sputum production

Acute
Infection affecting any part of the respiratory tree – nasopharyngitis to laryngotracheobronchitis to pneumonia
Chronic
Common
Post-nasal drip
COPD
Less common
Bronchiectasis (*bron-key-eck-ta-sis*)
Lung cancer
Tuberculosis
Heart failure

COPD, chronic obstructive pulmonary disease.

Sputum

Sputum production accompanying cough is a feature of many conditions (Table 5.3). Sometimes sputum has a particular character that points to certain conditions:

(1) **foul smelling and tasting**—anaerobic infections;

(2) **copious and mucopurulent**—bronchiectasis;

(3) **foamy and pink tinged**—pulmonary oedema;

(4) **rusty**—pneumococcal pneumonia;

(5) **copious, frothy, and saliva like**—bronchoalveolar carcinoma;

(6) **bloody**—see haemoptysis.

Sputum can be divided into serous (runny, clear), mucoid (viscous, clear), and mucopurulent or purulent (viscous, yellow/green). This classification can provide limited assistance in guiding antibiotic treatment. While mucoid or mucopurulent sputum may be either viral or bacterial, serous sputum is rarely bacterial.

Keypoints

- Acute onset mucoid or mucopurulent sputum may be either viral or bacterial; serous sputum is rarely bacterial.

Haemoptysis

Haemoptysis is the coughing up of blood or blood-tinged sputum. It has multiple causes, the most important of which are detailed in Table 5.4. In Hippocrates'

TABLE 5.4 Causes of haemoptysis

Common
Lung cancer
Bronchiectasis
Acute or chronic bronchitis
Pulmonary infarction
Less common
Tuberculosis
Lung abscess
Heart failure
Bleeding diatheses (*die-ath-ee-seize*)* and anti-coagulation

* Bleeding diatheses are conditions such as haemophilia where patients have a propensity to bleed.

day (Hippocrates c.460–370 BC, Ancient Greek physician, often called 'father of medicine'), the chief cause was tuberculosis. While tuberculosis remains an important cause of haemoptysis, bronchitis, bronchiectasis, and lung cancer are now the most common causes.

Causes

The commonest causes of haemoptysis are bronchitis, bronchiectasis, and lung cancer. The following are helpful in making the diagnosis.

1. Heart failure may cause frothy, pink sputum.
2. Large quantities (>200 ml) of haemoptysis occur more typically with tuberculosis, pulmonary infarction, bronchiectasis, and bleeding diatheses.
3. The colour of the blood does not usually help. Generally bright red blood represents fresh bleeding whereas darker blood is caused by blood that has oozed from the bleeding site and has had time to be metabolized before being coughed up.

So clinical evaluation of haemoptysis mainly relies on

(1) assessing other symptoms or signs that might suggest other causes;

(2) identifying causes needing urgent treatment;

(3) evaluating patients for lung cancer.

Assessing other symptoms or signs that might suggest the other causes

See p. 115 for lung cancer, p. 117 for bronchiectasis, p. 116 for acute bronchitis, p. 117 for chronic bronchitis, p. 118 for pulmonary infarction, p. 116 for tuberculosis, p. 116 for lung abscess, and p. 68 for heart failure. As regards bleeding diatheses and anti-coagulation, heparin or warfarin therapy, bleeding from other sites including purpura and bruises, or profuse bleeding should prompt you to do a clotting screen.

Identifying causes requiring urgent treatment

Certain conditions require urgent action.

1. If there is any suggestion of pulmonary embolism, anti-coagulation should be initiated and investigations such as a 'spiral' computed tomography (CT) lung scan arranged.
2. If there is evidence of infection, antibiotics should be started.
3. If heart failure appears a possibility, diuretics should be commenced.

Evaluating patients for lung cancer

Having carried out this initial assessment, there will be a group of patients with unexplained haemoptysis. Many of these will eventually be shown to have bronchitis or bleeding from the nasopharynx. However, a significant minority will be due to lung cancer. All patients with unexplained haemoptysis should have a chest X-ray, chest CT, and bronchoscopy as necessary to exclude lung cancer.

Tip

Haemoptysis due to chronic bronchitis normally settles down within a couple of days. If it persists longer, think of lung cancer. If the cause is lung cancer, the haemoptysis is often preceded by weight loss.

CASE 5.2

Problem. My patient has chronic bronchitis. Four months ago, they had a small amount of haemoptysis. Chest X-ray, CT scan, and bronchoscopy at that time were clear. Now, the patient has had another bout of haemoptysis. Do we need to do the tests all over again?

Discussion. Patients with chronic bronchitis are prone to recurrent bouts of haemoptyses. Clearly, common sense is needed when considering investigation. So, provided the amount of haemoptysis is similar, there are no new symptoms such as weight loss, and the tests were recent, it is reasonable not to repeat them.

CASE 5.3

Problem. My patient isn't sure whether they vomited or coughed up the blood. Do I have to investigate for both?

Discussion. You will usually be able to differentiate the two with a careful history going through the circumstances of the blood production. Failing this a short period of inpatient observation may reveal the source. Occasionally it will remain unclear whether the blood was coughed up or vomited. In such circumstances, you will need to consider gastroscopy as well as the respiratory tests.

Keypoints

- Bronchitis, bronchiectasis, and lung cancer are the commonest causes.
- Always consider causes needing urgent intervention such as pulmonary embolism, infection. and heart failure.
- All patients with unexplained haemoptysis should have a chest x-ray, chest CT, and bronchoscopy as necessary to exclude lung cancer.

Wheeze

When patients complain of wheeze, the first thing to do is establish what exactly they mean by this. Wheeze should have a musical quality to it—more than just noisy breathing—and is usually more prominent in expiration. Wheeze nearly always suggests small airways obstruction as in asthma or chronic obstructive pulmonary disease (COPD). In patients with asthma, they will sometimes notice that the wheeze is increased during exercise or in cold weather.

There are a couple of other causes of wheeze.

1. Occasionally wheeze is a feature of pulmonary oedema.
2. Rarely the inspiratory noise of stridor (*stry-door*) may be mistaken for a wheeze. However it lacks the musical quality of a wheeze. See p. 83.

Keypoints

- Wheeze should have a musical quality and is usually more prominent in expiration.
- Wheeze usually suggests asthma or COPD
- However, do not automatically assume wheeze is due to small airways obstruction: always consider the possibility of pulmonary oedema or stridor.

Other issues to discuss in the respiratory history

Many respiratory conditions have their roots in (1) exposure to noxious substances, (2) previous illnesses or treatments, or (3) contact with other people or animals. Thus, when a patient complains of respiratory symptoms, you need to broaden your enquiry.

Exposure to noxious substances

Smoking history

This is the most important, being a powerful risk factor for COPD and lung cancer; 90% of lung cancers are thought to be due to smoking. You need to get a clear history: roughly how many cigarettes are smoked, how long the patient has smoked, and when they stopped if relevant. When asked 'Do you smoke?', patients are inclined to answer 'no', carelessly omitting the fact that they stopped the previous day. Always ask, 'Did you ever smoke?', 'When did you stop?', 'How many did you smoke—2 per day, 20 per day, 60 per day?' If the patient smoked a pipe, try to get them to quantify tobacco use in ounces per week.

CASE 5.4

Problem. I've heard smoking quantified in terms of pack years. What does this mean?

Discussion. You may find it helpful to quantify the tobacco exposure in terms of 'pack years'. So a patient who smoked 10 a day (half a pack) for 30 years has smoked $0.5 \times 30 = 15$ pack years. A patient who has smoked 40 a day for 15 years has smoked 30 pack years.

Occupational exposure

Always ask patients about current or previous exposures to dusts, fumes, and chemicals at work. The substances that can cause respiratory problems are many, ranging from mouldy hay (farmers' lung) to titanium. If the patient is currently working in such an atmosphere, try to establish if symptoms are worse when at work and better when on holiday. In the UK, you should specifically enquire about coal and asbestos and enquire about any noxious substances produced locally.

1. Coal can cause a form of lung fibrosis—coal-miners' pneumoconiosis (see Fig. 16.37).
2. Asbestos also causes fibrosis (asbestosis) and is also a risk factor for lung cancer and mesothelioma (*meso-thee-lee-owe-ma*) (see Fig. 16.29).

Previous illnesses or treatments

1. Measles and whooping cough in childhood are risk factors for bronchiectasis.

2. Rheumatoid arthritis may be complicated by lung fibrosis.
3. Amiodarone—a cardiac drug—can cause fibrosis.
4. Another cardiac medication - β-blockers - can worsen airways obstruction.

Contact with other humans or animals

If tuberculosis is a possibility always enquire about family contacts. Ask specifically about foreign travel—many UK patients have their origins in India and Pakistan and may contract tuberculosis when they visit their relatives in Asia.

Animals may cause respiratory disease in two ways:

(1) by passing on infection;

(2) through hypersensitvity reactions.

So in patients with pneumonia, always enquire about exposure to birds. Any species of bird can transmit chlamydia psittaci (*cla-mid-ia-sit-ak-eye*). This may cause psittacosis (*sit-ak-owe-sis*), which is a form of pneumonia. Psittacosis responds better to tetracyclines than penicillins. Your suspicions should be particularly aroused if the patient's parrot, budgie, or canary died recently after a brief illness. In patients with chronic breathlessness, enquire about exposure to pigeons. This can result in a hypersensitivity pneumonitis—pigeon-fanciers' lung. Pets, particularly cats and dogs can exacerbate asthma.

Keypoints

- Virtually any substance that can be inhaled can cause respiratory problems.
- Take a detailed smoking history.
- If you are considering tuberculosis, always ask about family contacts and foreign travel.
- If you are considering pneumonia, always ask about birds as psittacosis is managed differently.

The importance of examining the respiratory system

As in many other branches of medicine, modern investigations have reduced reliance on respiratory system examination findings. Tests such as the chest X-ray, lung function tests, and increasingly sophisticated scanning techniques provide much useful information about respiratory disease. Examination is far from being infallible and small pulmonary lesions may not produce any abnormal clinical signs.

That said, examination of the respiratory system remains a very important part of the doctor's assessment of chest problems. In the acutely unwell patient, examination findings may often yield very important and immediate information with regards to the severity and the source of the illness. Furthermore, in patients complaining of long-term breathlessness or symptoms suggestive of malignancy, examination findings are often extremely helpful in analysing the cause of the patient's problem. Examination involves assessing not just the chest but also looking at other areas, particularly the hands, pulses, and face to glean further information as to the cause and severity of chest symptoms. While the scope of respiratory examination is far reaching, there are some general themes, which recur over and over again.

1. Signs pointing towards malignancy.
2. Signs of unilateral pleural effusion (fluid collection), raising the possibility of malignancy, infection, or more rarely autoimmune disease.
3. Signs of unilateral consolidation (solidification), usually suggesting infection but occasionally being due to immune or toxic effects.

Less common but important are the following.

1. Signs of unilateral lung collapse, raising the possibility of malignancy or alternatively a mucus plug in either an asthmatic patient or post-operatively.
2. Signs of lung fibrosis.

Respiratory system examination summary

This summary contains many terms that you will not understand on first reading. These terms are explained in the next section 'Respiratory examination in detail'.

1. Introduce yourself to the patient and ask for permission to examine.
2. Ask the patient to get on to the bed (if not already on the bed). You may need to help! Ask the patient to remove all garments covering chest and arms. For female patients, ensure a chaperone is present and offer to cover the chest with a sheet or towel. Arrange the patient so that their chest is at 45° to the horizontal.
3. While doing 1 and 2, be having a general look and listen.
4. Inspect both hands for clubbing (DF8/10), peripheral cyanosis (*sigh-a-no-sis*), tremor, muscle wasting, and tar staining.

5. Palpate right radial pulse for pulse rate (DF 3/10) and rhythm (DF 6/10) and consider if bounding (DF 6/10). Then, check respiratory rate (DF 4/10).
6. Check for flapping tremor (DF 8/10).
7. Inspect face for swelling (DF 8/10), eyes for Horner's (DF 7/10), and underneath tongue for cyanosis (DF 9/10).
8. Inspect right internal jugular vein for jugular venous pressure (DF 9/10). Check for hepatojugular reflux (DF 8/10).
9. Inspect front of chest from end of bed, assessing breathing pattern (DF 4/10), chest shape (DF 4/10), and movement (DF 8/10).
10. Inspect front of chest and neck close up (DF 5/10).
11. Palpate trachea (DF 9/10).
12. Palpate the praecordium for apex beat position (DF 9/10), axillary lymph nodes (DF 8/10), and if suspected, tender areas (DF 8/10) and subcutaneous emphysema (DF 1/10).
13. Palpate for chest expansion anteriorly, comparing both sides (DF 9/10).
14. Percuss front of chest and in the axillae, comparing the two sides (DF 9/10).
15. Assess tactile vocal fremitus (*frem-it-us*) at the front of the chest and in the axillae, comparing the two sides (DF 9/10).
16. Auscultate over the front of the chest and in the axillae, comparing the two sides (DF 8/10).
17. Assess vocal resonance at the front of the chest and in the axillae, comparing the two sides (DF 9/10).
18. Change the patient's position to facilitate examination of the neck and the back of the chest (DF 6/10).
19. Examine the neck for enlarged lymph nodes (DF 8/ 10).
20. Inspect the back of chest assessing movement (DF 8/10), chest shape (DF 4/10), and other visible abnormalities (DF 4/10).
21. If appropriate, palpate the posterior aspect of the chest for possible rib fractures (DF 8/10).
22. Palpate for chest expansion posteriorly, comparing both sides (DF 8/10).
23. Percuss the back of chest comparing the two sides (DF 9/10).
24. Assess tactile vocal fremitus over the posterior aspect of the chest, comparing the two sides (DF 9/10).
25. Auscultate over the back of the chest, comparing the two sides (DF 8/10).
26. Assess vocal resonance over the back of the chest and in the axillae, comparing the two sides (DF 9/10).
27. Look for other signs such as whispering pectoriloquy or peripheral oedema if appropriate.
28. Wash your hands.
29. Pause briefly and then present findings.

Respiratory system examination in detail

Getting started

1. Introduce yourself to the patient and ask for permission to examine.

Put out your hand to shake the patient's hand. Say something like 'Hello, I'm Friedrich Wegener, a third-year medical exchange student. Do you mind if I examine your chest and hands?' Don't just say 'chest'! The patient will wonder what you are up to when you start looking at his hands!

2. Ask the patient to get on to the bed (if not already on the bed). You may need to help! Ask the patient to remove all garments covering chest and arms. For female patients, ensure a chaperone is present and offer to cover the chest with a sheet or towel. Arrange the patient so that their chest is at 45° to the horizontal.

If the patient is unable to get on to the bed himself, offer your assistance and if necessary ask for help from the nurses. The respiratory system can only be examined properly with the patient's chest bare. Students, quite understandably, are often unsure if this is appropriate, particularly for women patients. Such doubt can create a confidence problem—not a good thing at this early stage of the examination. For a man, simply say something like 'It's best if I examine you with your chest bare. Could you take off your shirt and vest, please.' For a woman, say something like 'Ideally, it's best if I examine you with your chest bare. Is that all right? I can cover up your chest with a sheet for part of the examination.' Give the patient good opportunity to refuse. If she refuses, do not take this as a slight—just get on with the examination as best you can. If she's happy to undress, give her time to do so. Then, if requested, cover the chest up with a sheet or towel until you get to the examination of the chest itself. And remember, for a male doctor, a woman—medical student or nurse—should be present to act as a chaperone.

The best position for examining the respiratory system is not universally agreed. The two main options are sitting upright or lying at 45° as for the cardiovascular system. It is suggested that the examination is started with the patient at 45° as this is comfortable for most patients and good for examining the jugular venous pulse. Later in the examination, the patient can sit forward so that the back of the chest can be examined (p. 108). However, if the patient is very breathless, they may be more comfortable sitting fully upright either in a chair or with their feet over the side of the bed from the start.

CASE 5.5

Problem. My patient is very breathless needing to sit up. Do I insist on him lying at 45°?

Discussion. Definitely not. Common sense must prevail—examine the patient sitting up.

3. While doing 1 and 2, be having a general look and listen.

Consider respiratory effort and pattern, stridor and hoarseness, cyanosis, nebulizer, oxygen, and sputum pot. See p. 15 for details on 'general look'.

Moderate or severe respiratory distress may be suggested by (1) noisy or laboured breathing, which may be brought on or worsened by the effort of undressing and positioning, (2) a need to sit upright, or (3) the presence of an oxygen mask or a nebulizer machine (Fig. 5.1) by the bed. A nebulizer machine is used to supply high-dose bronchodilators and normally implies either asthma or COPD.

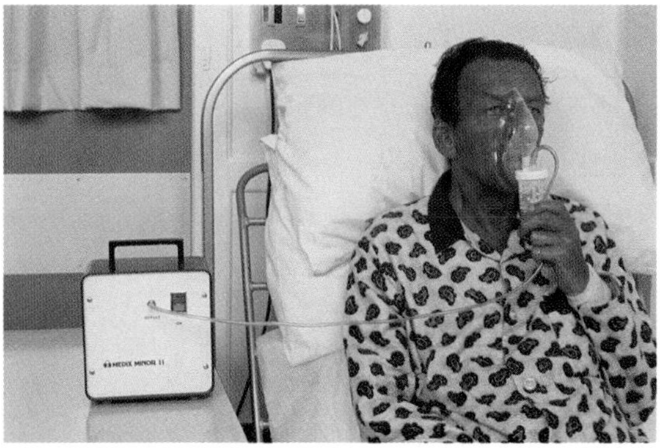

Fig. 5.1 Using a nebulizer machine.

TABLE 5.5 Causes of stridor

Sudden
Inhaled foreign body
Anaphylactic reaction
Gradual
Tumours of pharynx, larynx, or trachea
External compression of the trachea by enlarged lymph nodes or goitre

A rasping noise prominent in inspiration is suggestive of 'stridor'. This implies obstruction of the upper airways (Table 5.5) and requires expert attention. If the onset is sudden, immediate action is required to relieve the obstruction. Although rare, stridor is a particularly important sign because the standard basic respiratory tests—chest X-ray, blood gases, and spirometry—will rarely identify this as the source of breathing difficulties.

The patient may sound hoarse. This is most commonly due to laryngitis but there are more serious causes: (1) lung cancer causing laryngeal nerve palsy (p. 115) or (2) laryngeal cancer.

If you see a sputum pot by the bed, open it up and have a look. Large volumes of yellow/green sputum suggest bronchiectasis, foul-smelling sputum may point to an anaerobic lung abscess, and blood in the sputum (haemoptysis) needs to be thoroughly evaluated (p. 78).

CASE 5.6

Problem. The patient is using a nebulizer, which is making considerable noise during your examination.

Discussion. Like any other complicated task, a physical examination is best performed with the minimum of distractions. As a doctor you will have to decide for yourself whether the potential longer-term benefit from a clearer analysis of symptoms and signs outweighs the immediate benefit to the patient of the nebulizer. As a student, you need to ask the patient's doctor or simply wait till the nebulizer treatment is finished—it usually takes around 10 min.

Hands

4. Inspect both hands for clubbing (DF8/10), peripheral cyanosis, tremor, muscle wasting, and tar staining.

Clubbing

What is it?

Clubbing is a painless enlargement of connective tissue in the terminal phalanges of the digits. When severe, the ends of the digits look like clubs (Fig. 5.2). It is usually symmetrical and affects fingers more than toes. Clubbing was first described by Hippocrates and the term 'hippocratic fingers' is occasionally used. Initially, the soft tissue swelling causes tenseness within the skin and alters the 'nailbed angle'. What is the nailbed angle? The contour of the fingernail and the skin on the back of the finger do not run seamlessly together. The nailbed angle is the angle formed at the junction between the skin of the finger and the nail (Fig. 5.3).

When the soft tissue of the terminal phalanx enlarges, it pushes the nail upwards and the nailbed angle is gradually lost. At this stage clubbing is present (even if the fingers do not look like clubs). Later the nail becomes increasingly curved, especially in the long axis until finally swelling of the terminal phalanx leads to the classical appearance of the fingers, which resemble clubs (Fig. 5.2).

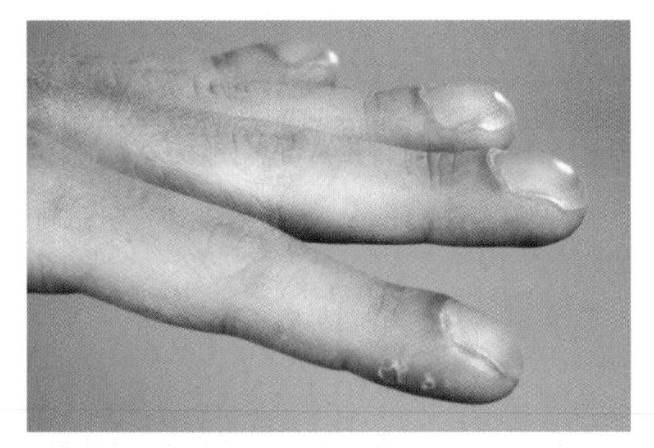

Fig. 5.2 Severe clubbing.

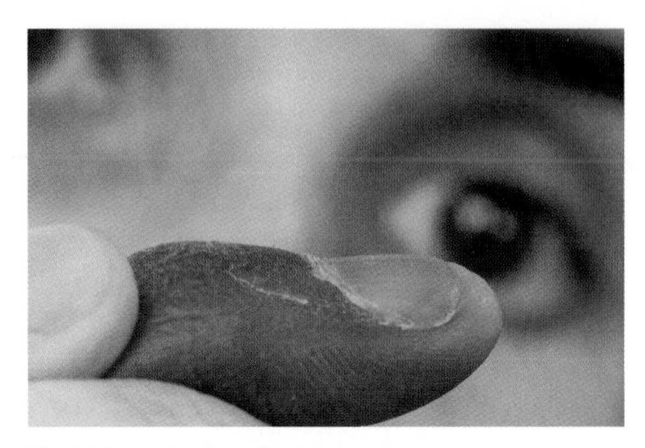

Fig. 5.4 Inspecting the nailbed angle.

Significance

Clubbing is associated with a variety of diseases (Table 5.6), most of them respiratory in origin. It is not associated with asthma or COPD. Table 5.6 does not give the full story. Whilst it is true to say that patients with cyanotic congenital heart disease with clubbing are uncommon, 95% of patients with cyanotic congenital heart disease will have clubbing compared to 75% of patients with idiopathic pulmonary fibrosis, 30% of patients with bronchiectasis, and 25% of patients with lung cancer.

How does clubbing happen?

This question remains unanswered. The theory currently most favoured implicates megakaryocytes (*mega-carry-owe-sites*). Normally megakaryocytes (the precursors of platelets) are trapped in the pulmonary capillaries

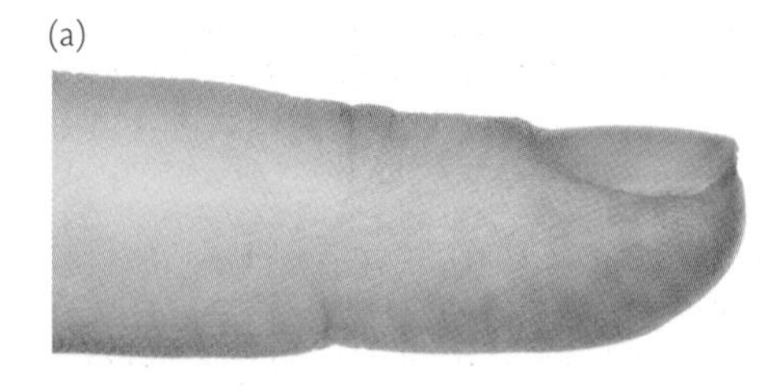

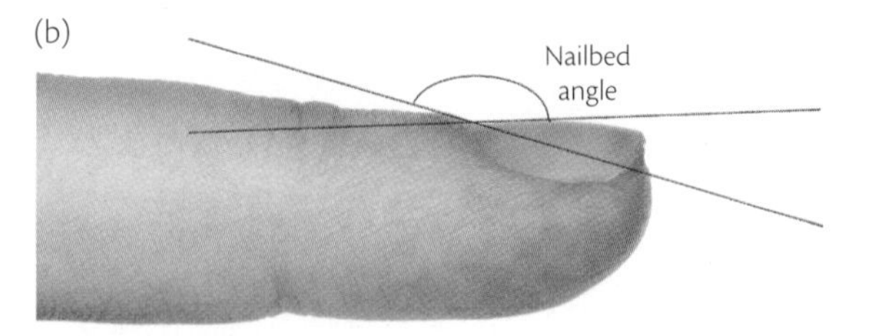

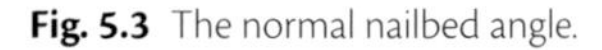

Fig. 5.3 The normal nailbed angle.

TABLE 5.6 Causes of clubbing

Common	
Bronchiectasis	
Lung cancer	
Idiopathic pulmonary fibrosis	
Rare	
Respiratory	Lung abscess, empyema, asbestosis, mesothelioma
Cardiac	Congenital heart disease with right-to-left shunt, infective endocarditis
Gastrointestinal	Cirrhosis, inflammatory bowel disease, coeliac disease
Others	Thyrotoxicosis, familial, pregnancy

and do not appear in the systemic circulation. In the presence of lung disease, damage to the pulmonary capillaries results in megakaryocytes gaining access to the systemic circulation. They are then trapped in the capillaries of the fingers where they release growth factors into the surrounding tissue. This theory is supported by the fact that patients suffering from congenital heart disease with right to left shunt (bypassing pulmonary capillaries) are highly likely to have clubbing.

How to examine

1. Say to the patient, 'Do you mind if I examine your hands and fingers?'
2. Lift the patient's right hand up a few inches.
3. Bend down so that your eyes are at the same level as the patient's hand and look at the patient's fingers from the side (Fig. 5.4).
4. Focus on one finger, the right middle is best, and look at the nailbed angle.
5. Decide if the angle is lost or preserved.
6. Next, examine other fingers on the right hand and then the left hand.

Hypertrophic pulmonary osteoarthropathy

What is it?

This is rare. It is an inflammation of the periosteum (*perry-os-tea-um*) at the ends of long bones and may cause tenderness and swelling over the fingers and wrists. It has been described as a late manifestation of clubbing though this is probably not true: it may occur without clubbing and has different causes (80% associated with lung cancer, 10% with mesothelioma) implying a different pathological process altogether.

While examining for clubbing, other clinical features may provide clues to respiratory disease.

1. Fine tremor may be a side-effect of bronchodilator therapy for COPD or asthma.
2. Wasting of intrinsic muscles of the hand (T1 distribution) may be due to brachial plexus damage caused by an apical lung cancer.
3. A bluish discoloration of the fingers may be part of a central cyanosis (p. 90).
4. The yellowish tinge of tar staining on the fingers suggests smoking-related disease such as lung cancer or COPD. The degree of staining does not predict the amount of tobacco smoked.

Radial pulse, respiratory rate, and flap

5. Palpate right radial pulse for pulse rate (DF 3/10) and rhythm (DF 6/10) and consider if bounding (DF 6/10). Then, check respiratory rate (DF 4/10).

CASE 5.7

Problem. I think the nailbed angle is lost but the patient's fingers don't look clubbed.

Discussion. This is the most common appearance of clubbing (Fig. 5.4). The club-like appearance is a late development. It can be difficult to be sure and this is one reason to look at several fingers on both hands—the loss of angle tends to vary a little from finger to finger so you may see a clearer example on another finger. It's also worth knowing that in Coury's original paper describing 350 cases of clubbing, 20% are classified as borderline or possible clubbing—so clearly, it is not always easy.

CASE 5.8

Problem. The patient's fingers look clubbed but there is no loss of nailbed angle.

Discussion. This appearance is thought to be normal. If the angle is not lost it's not clubbing. Soft tissue swelling sufficient to make fingers look clubbed should be more than sufficient to obliterate the nailbed angle.

CASE 5.9

Problem. I find the nailbed angle technique difficult. Are there any other ways of examining for clubbing?

Discussion. The nailbed angle technique may seem difficult initially but it is the most reliable. However, there are a couple of other techniques.

The first method is based on the fact that the increased soft tissue in the terminal digit makes it more fluctuant—and involves assessing the fluctuancy of the nailbed (Fig. 5.5).

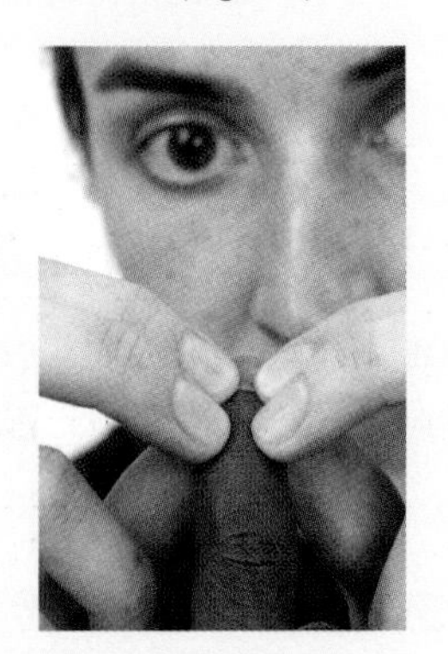

Fig. 5.5 Assessing nailbed fluctuancy.

1. Take the patient's right middle finger.
2. Position both your thumbs underneath the pulp of the finger.
3. Hold the proximal interphalangeal joint steady with the tips of your middle fingers.
4. Now palpate the nail with the tips of your index fingers.
5. Normally, there should only be very slight fluctuation. With clubbing, the nailbed may feel very spongy. This distinction between normal and abnormal fluctuation is very tricky and not one I have found convincing.

The second method was first proposed by *Leo Schamroth (1924–1988, South African cardiologist)*, who developed clubbing himself while suffering from endocarditis. Schamroth's sign is based on the finding that if a normal person places the terminal phalanges of corresponding fingers of both hands back to back, it produces a small diamond shaped aperture between both nail beds. When clubbing is present, this window is abolished. I like this method although it is not well studied.

Keypoints

- Clubbing is a painless enlargement of connective tissue in the terminal phalanges of the digits.
- Clubbing is a clue to many illnesses, the most common being idiopathic pulmonary fibrosis, lung cancer, and bronchiectasis.
- Clubbing is not associated with COPD.
- Clubbing is best examined by assessing for loss of the nailbed angle.

Pulse rate and rhythm

Significance

The pulse rate and rhythm may be altered in respiratory disease.

1. Chest infections or pneumonias may cause a tachycardia or may be complicated by atrial fibrillation (irregularly irregular pulse, see p. 36, or atrial flutter with 2:1 block (Case 5.10).
2. In the context of an asthma attack, a pulse rate >110/min indicates a severe attack. On the other hand, bradycardia in the asthmatic patient may be an indicator of life-threatening cardiac insufficiency in asthma.
3. A large-volume 'bounding' pulse may be a sign of carbon dioxide retention suggesting respiratory failure.

How to examine

Palpation of the right radial pulse is described on p. 35. In the respiratory system, the aim is to assess rate and rhythm and consider whether the pulse is large volume ('bounding').

CASE 5.10

Problem. My patient has symptoms of a chest infection and is somewhat breathless but otherwise comfortable. I'm worried, though, because their pulse is 150/min and regular, suggesting a worrying development.

Discussion. You're quite right to be worried. Normally a tachycardia of this degree suggests your patient is approaching a critical juncture. However, your observation that the patient looks well suggests this is much more likely to be atrial flutter with 2:1 block (p. 417).

CASE 5.11

Problem. My friend is a keen sportsman but suffers with asthma. I've checked his pulse and it's bradycardic (50/min). Does this mean his asthma is badly controlled even though he's well and not breathless?

Discussion. When evaluating the pulse in the respiratory system, it should be used in the context of the patient's condition. This man simply has a resting bradycardia because he is physically fit.

CASE 5.12

Problem. I was seeing a patient with severe asthma today and the consultant asked me if there was evidence of pulsus paradoxus. What's that?

Discussion. This is a difficult sign to elicit and as a result is rarely performed. Normally, the blood pressure falls slightly during inspiration. With pulsus paradoxus this is exaggerated and systolic blood pressure falls by more than 10 mm Hg. It may occur in severe acute asthma, constrictive pericarditis, or cardiac tamponade. It can normally only be elicited by sphygmomanometry but in tamponade, it may be possible to palpate a reduced radial pulse volume on inspiration.

Respiratory rate

What is the respiratory rate?

The respiratory rate is the number of breaths per minute.

What is the normal rate?

There is some disagreement over the normal rate. A rate around 14 breaths per minute is commonly quoted. However, at least one study (see 'Further reading') suggests that the normal rate averages 20 breaths per minute with a normal range of 16–25 per minute. The author's experience is that the normal respiratory rate averages around 18 per minute.

What is abnormal?

Clearly, given the lack of clarity over what the normal rate is, it is a little difficult to say what is abnormal. However, it is generally agreed that the respiratory rate increases (tachypnoea) (*tack-kip-knee-a*) in patients with chest conditions such as pneumonia, pleurisy, and asthma/COPD. It may also be increased in patients with fever of any source or anxiety.

British Thoracic Society guidelines use respiratory rate as an important indicator of severity in patients with acute asthma. In such patients, a respiratory rate >25/min indicates that the attack is severe. In patients with community-acquired pneumonia, a respiratory rate >30/min has been shown to be one of the three key indicators (along with blood urea >7 mmol/l and diastolic blood pressure <60 mm Hg) that predict a worse outcome. The respiratory rate is reduced (bradypnoea) in cases of opiate overdose or neurological conditions such as stroke or raised intracranial pressure. In such circumstances, there may also be Cheyne–Stokes (*chain-stokes*) breathing (p. 92).

How to examine

The respiratory rate is one of the few signs that can be altered voluntarily. If patients realize you are watching their chest closely, they find it very difficult to ignore and tend to breathe self-consciously. Thus a little duplicity is required.

1. Having assessed the patient's pulse, continue to give the impression that you are examining it.
2. While doing this, inspect the patient's breaths in and out and count them over 30 s (10 s is too short).

6. Check for flapping tremor (DF 8/10).

What is a flapping tremor?

This is an irregular, coarse, jerky movement of the wrist.

Significance

In the context of respiratory disease this is a sign of carbon dioxide retention due to respiratory failure (usually in COPD, see p. 117). It is said to indicate the patient is in a critical condition, but this is unreliable. It can occasionally be present in mild illness and is often absent in

Keypoints

- Check pulse rate and rhythm and consider whether it is bounding in nature.
- In the context of an asthma attack, a pulse rate >110/min indicates a severe attack.
- Continue to palpate the pulse while checking the respiratory rate.
- The respiratory rate needs to be measured over at least 30 s.
- Respiratory rate >30/min in the context of community-acquired pneumonia suggests severe pneumonia.
- In the context of an asthma attack, a respiratory rate >25/min indicates a severe attack.

severe illness. It may also be found in liver failure or kidney failure.

How to examine

1. The tremor may be difficult to observe at rest. It is maximized by getting the patient to hold their arms outstretched, with wrists cocked and fingers spread slightly whilst showing them what you mean (Fig. 5.6). It may be easier to demonstrate the position you want for your patient.
2. Look for a coarse, irregular flapping movement at the wrists. Make sure you observe for at least 15 s before deciding that a flapping tremor is absent.

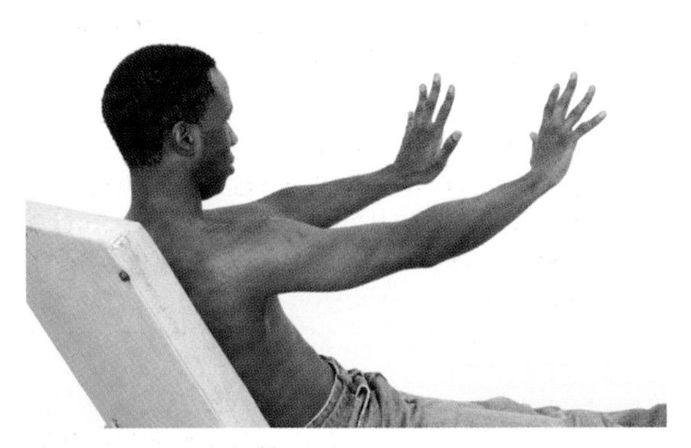

Fig. 5.6 Assessing for flap.

CASE 5.13

Problem. I've tried to test for flapping tremor but the patient won't co-operate.

Discussion. Carbon dioxide retention also causes drowsiness and confusion so testing for a flap can be difficult. Make sure you demonstrate clearly to your patient what you mean. Sometimes, the patient simply cannot co-operate. If so, think about performing a blood gas to resolve the issue.

CASE 5.14

Problem. The patient seems shaky but is it a flap?

Discussion. A flapping tremor means what it says—a flap. It is quite different from the tremor due to β-agonist treatment seen in many patients being treated for respiratory disease.

Keypoints

- A flapping tremor may be a sign of respiratory failure (but unreliable).
- Show the patient what to do.
- A flapping tremor is also found in liver failure and rarely kidney failure.

Face, eyes, and tongue

7. Inspect face for swelling (DF 8/10), eyes for Horner's (DF 7/10), and underneath tongue for cyanosis (DF 9/10).

Facial swelling

Significance

Lung cancer may cause blockage of the superior vena cava either by direct tumour invasion or by thrombosis. This is known as superior vena caval (SVC) obstruction (Fig. 5.7). The SVC receives blood from the head, neck, and arms. When the SVC is blocked, the head and neck veins become engorged and there is a loss of the normal jugular pulsations (that is, a raised non-pulsatile jugular venous pressure (JVP)). The face and neck also become oedematous but the arms tend to be less swollen as they are able to use an alternative collateral circulation involving the inferior vena cava. There may be visible distended veins on the chest wall providing this collateral circulation from the arms.

How to examine

1. Briefly look at the face. Is the face abnormally swollen? Is it plethoric or cyanosed?
2. If you think the face might be swollen, then look at external jugular vein (p. 45). Is it distended and is it

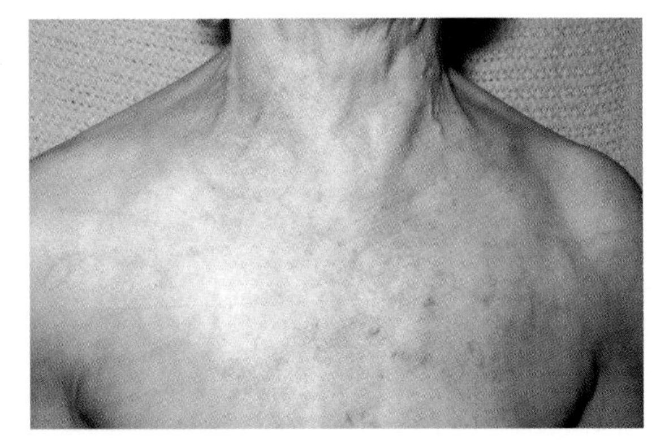

Fig. 5.7 Superior vena caval obstruction.

CASE 5.15

Problem. The patient's face is a bit puffy but he's a bit overweight so maybe that's the cause.

Discussion. SVC obstruction is rare and most 'swollen' faces will be due to fatty tissue. What is important is that any sort of facial swelling prompts you to briefly check the external jugular and chest wall veins for evidence of SVC obstruction. If you don't think of it, you won't find it.

pulsating? Look at the chest wall. Are there distended veins?

The combination of a swollen face with a distended non-pulsatile external jugular vein suggests SVC obstruction and prominent chest wall veins lend support to the diagnosis.

Horner's syndrome (Johann Horner (1831–1886), Swiss ophthalmogist)

What is it?

This is a syndrome characterized by a small pupil (miosis) accompanied by drooping of the eyelid (partial ptosis) on the same side with reduced sweating (anhidrosis) on the same side of the face.

How does it happen?

Horner's syndrome is caused by damage to the sympathetic nerves to the eye and face. The sympathetic pathway to the eye takes a roundabout route:

1. First-order neurones travel from the hypothalamus to the spinal cord between levels C8 and T2.
2. Second-order neurones pass from the spinal cord over the apex of the lung and then up along the carotid artery to the superior cervical ganglion.
3. Third-order neurones emerge from the superior cervical ganglion and then diverge into two separate pathways, one going via the cavernous sinus to the eye—where it innervates the pupillary muscle and the eyelid—the other travelling alongside the external carotid artery to innervate the facial sweat glands.

Significance

A lung tumour situated in the apex of the lung may damage second-order neurones causing Horner's. Other causes are listed in Table 5.7.

How to examine

See Chapter 11.

TABLE 5.7 Causes of Horner's

First-order neurone damage	Stroke
Second-order neurone damage	Lung tumour—usually squamous cell, thyroid tumour, neck or chest trauma
Third-order neurone damage	Skull fracture, cavernous sinus thrombosis

CASE 5.16

Problem. I'm sure I've been told that there's a fourth feature of Horner's, that is, the eye looks to be more sunken within the orbit (enophthalmos). Why haven't you mentioned this?

Discussion. Enophthalmos is often described as a feature of Horner's. It's difficult to be sure if the eye is truly indrawn or whether the ptosis simply makes it look indrawn. Either way, I don't think it helps very much in deciding whether Horner's is present.

CASE 5.17

Problem. The patient appears to have Horner's but when I shine a light into the pupil it constricts normally. Should this happen?

Discussion. The size of the pupil depends on the relative influence of the sympathetic nerves (which dilate) and parasympathetic nerves (which constrict). In Horner's, the parasympathetic nerves are undamaged so pupillary constriction to light still occurs.

CASE 5.18

Problem. I've noticed that patients' pupils are often slightly different in size but there doesn't seem to be ptosis. Any advice?

Discussion. In normal individuals, the pupils are often slightly different in size. The difference is usually less than 1 mm in contrast to the size difference in patients with Horner's where it is usually more than 1 mm.

Cyanosis

What is it?

Haemoglobin that has not been oxygenated (deoxygenated haemoglobin) gives blood a blue colour. Cyanosis is a bluish discoloration of the skin and mucous membranes due to excess deoxygenated haemoglobin (usually >2.5 g/100 ml). Cyanosis may be peripheral or central. In peripheral cyanosis, only the blood supply to the extremities such as the fingers is reduced. Because of the reduced blood flow, the tissues remove more oxygen from the blood so resulting in an increase in deoxygenated haemoglobin and hence a blue discoloration. In central cyanosis, all arterial blood is poorly oxygenated, so even tissues such as the tongue, with a good blood supply, go blue. Cyanosis is a crude estimate of arterial oxygenation and doctors vary greatly in their ability to pick out this subtle hue.

CASE 5.19

Problem. Surely you're making things over-complicated by talking about deoxygenated haemoglobin. Is cyanosis not simply a sign of hypoxia?

Discussion. True, hypoxia and cyanosis go together. But there is another important variable—the haemoglobin level. In a patient with a haemoglobin of 16 g/100 ml, oxygen saturation needs to fall to 85% (PO_2 7kPa) to produce deoxygenated haemoglobin greater than 2.5 g/100 ml (and so cyanosis). In an anaemic patient with a haemoglobin of 6 g/100 ml, oxygen saturation needs to be 60% (PO_2 is 4 kPa) for enough deoxygenated haemoglobin to be present to produce cyanosis. Either way, though, it is quite clear that patients need to be severely hypoxic before cyanosis is visible.

CASE 5.20

Problem. Is deoxygenated haemoglobin the only substance that makes the skin go blue?

Discussion. Blue discoloured skin may also occur in certain conditions characterized by abnormal haemoglobin such as methaemoglobinaemia. Methaemoglobin has a bluish colour. It is the same as haemoglobin except that the iron ion is in the ferric (3+) form rather than the ferrous (2+) form. There is normally a small component of methaemoglobin in the blood but enzyme deficiencies can result in increased levels especially in the presence of certain drugs (methaemoglobinaemia). In contrast to hypoxic cyanosis, oxygen treatment has no effect on the skin colour and the PO_2 is not reduced.

Significance

Any condition that reduces oxygen levels may cause cyanosis. Cyanosis may come on suddenly in patients with chest infections, pneumonia, or pulmonary emboli. Patients with chronic lung disease such as COPD or pulmonary fibrosis are particularly prone to develop cyanosis when such acute problems develop. Some patients with severe COPD or more rarely fibrosis may have chronic cyanosis. Pulmonary oedema due to cardiac pathology may also cause cyanosis.

How to look for central cyanosis

It is blood in the superficial venules and capillaries that give the skin and mucous membranes their colour. Cyanosis is best seen where the epidermis is thin and these subepidermal blood vessels predominate—places such as lips, nose, ears, and oral mucous membranes. However it is usual to evaluate cyanosis by inspecting the mucous membranes under the tongue because unlike the other extremities above, it is not affected by peripheral cyanosis.

1. Ask the patient to put out their tongue and inspect underneath the tongue.
2. Do not expect a bright blue discoloration; cyanosis has more of a purplish hue.

Keypoints

- SVC obstruction may occur in patients with lung cancer.
- When examining the respiratory system, stop for a second to think whether the face is swollen.
- Horner's is characterized by miosis, partial ptosis, and anhidrosis of the same side of the face.
- Horner's is due to damage of the sympathetic nerve supply to the eye and face.
- Cyanosis is due to an excess of deoxygenated haemoglobin.
- Cyanosis can provide a crude estimate of arterial oxygenation.
- Cyanosis usually represents severe hypoxia.
- The blue hue of cyanosis can be difficult to spot.
- Cyanosis occurs very late in anaemic patients (and early in polycythaemic patients).

Jugular venous pressure

8. Inspect right internal jugular vein for jugular venous pressure (DF 9/10). Check for hepatojugular reflux (DF 8/10).

Why examine?

Advanced pulmonary disease may cause right heart failure (cor pulmonale) (*cor-pull-ma-nail-ee* or *cor pull-ma-narly*) and hence an elevated JVP. Two mechanisms are thought to be responsible for the right heart failure: (1) alveolar hypoxia or arterial hypoxaemia causing vasoconstriction and hence pulmonary hypertension and (2) lung disease causing direct damage to the pulmonary vessels so increasing vascular resistance. The JVP may also be elevated but non-pulsatile in SVC obstruction (see p. 88).

How to examine

See Chapter 4, p. 42.

Inspection of praecordium including chest expansion

The chest itself

It is now time to move on to examination of the chest itself. First, the front of the chest and the axillae are assessed. The examination is carried out in a sequence of inspection, palpation, percussion, tactile vocal fremitus (TVF), and auscultation, comparing the right and left sides. Then the back of the chest is examined in the same way. It is helpful to know the surface markings of the lobes of the lungs (Fig. 5.8) so that you can correlate signs with lung anatomy. If right middle lobe pathology is present, you might expect to detect abnormal signs

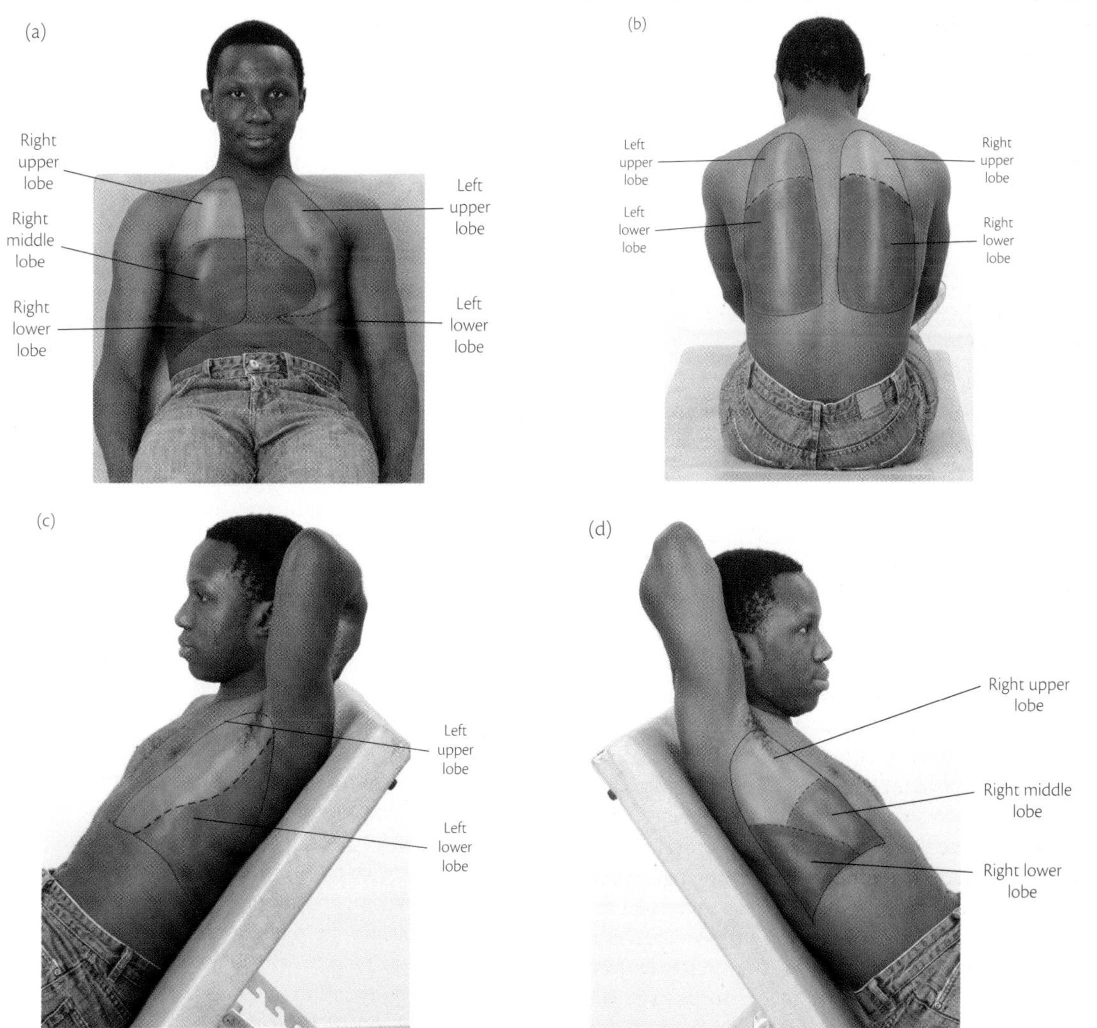

Fig. 5.8 Surface markings of the lung lobes: (a) anterior view, (b) posterior view, (c) left lateral view, and (d) right lateral view.

Keypoints

- In the absence of cardiac failure, an elevated JVP in the context of respiratory disease suggests cor pulmonale.
- Cor pulmonale indicates advanced respiratory disease.

over the lower part of the right chest at the front and over the right axilla inferiorly and anteriorly but would not expect to detect any abnormality over the back. Disease in the upper lobes produces signs mainly in the upper chest at the front and back of the chest: sometimes signs may be found in the axillae. Disease in the lower lobes produces signs mainly over the lower back of the chest, sometimes in the axilla, and less often over the front of the chest.

9. Inspect front of chest from end of bed, assessing breathing pattern (DF 4/10), chest shape (DF 4/10), and movement (DF 8/10).

The aim now is to take a concentrated look at the overall chest shape as well as the breathing pattern and chest movement. These features are best assessed by stepping back a little and viewing the chest from the end of the bed.

Breathing pattern

1. **Pursed lips.** Patients with COPD sometimes purse their lips when they breathe out. This happens particularly during exacerbations. In such patients, there is good evidence that this improves ventilation and oxygenation.
2. **Accessory muscle use.** Normally, the diaphragm is the only muscle that plays a part in breathing—and even then, it is only involved in inspiration; expiration is a passive process. However, in patients with respiratory muscle fatigue or COPD, particularly during an exacerbation, additional muscles may become involved. To aid inspiration, the sternocleidomastoids (*stern-owe-clyde-owe-mast-oids*) (anterior superficial neck muscles), the scalene (*scay-lean*) muscles (deep neck muscles), and the trapezius (posterior neck and back muscles) lift the rib cage. Expiration may be supplemented by the external oblique muscles (anterolateral abdominal muscles).
3. **Leaning forward with hands on knees.** Patients with exacerbations of COPD often adopt this position
4. **Cheyne–Stokes (or 'periodic') breathing.** Here patients' breaths become gradually deeper and deeper and then more and more shallow. As the breathing becomes more and more shallow, it slows down and there may be apnoeic pauses for several seconds before the cycle resumes. Cheyne–Stokes breathing (*John Cheyne (1777–1836), Scottish physician and William Stokes (1804–1878), Irish physician*) may occur in patients with heart failure or in patients with a reduced level of consciousness due to neurological causes such as opiate overdose, stroke, or head injury.
5. **Fast, deep breathing.** Usually, when patients are breathless, their respiration is fast but shallow. Sometimes, though, you may notice that the patient is breathing not just fast but also deep. This suggests hyperventilation. Hyperventilation is said to occur when the rate of ventilation is excessive for the level of carbon dioxide. Therefore it can only be properly diagnosed by finding a low carbon dioxide level in blood gases. Various conditions may cause hyperventilation: hypoxia, heart failure, asthma, fever, pain, and anxiety to name a few. Hyperventilation causes a metabolic alkalosis. This in turn reduces the level of ionized calcium in the blood. The resultant hypocalcaemia may be symptomatic with tingling of the fingers or around the mouth. Hyperventilation may be a compensatory response to metabolic acidosis as occurs in diabetic ketoacidosis and renal failure—in which case it is known as Kussmaul's (*kus-malls*) breathing (*Adolf Kussmaul (1822–1902), German physician*). Here, there is no alkalosis and so no hypocalcaemia or tingling.

CASE 5.21

Problem. I've heard doctors talking about lung zones. What's the difference between zones and lobes?

Discussion. Lung zone is a term best reserved for analysis of chest X-rays. When a lung abnormality appears on a standard chest X-ray, it is often difficult to say which lobe it is in based on the chest X-ray alone. Thus a shadow in the middle of the left lung on the X-ray may represent pathology either in the left upper or lower lobes. Which lobe the lesion is in depends on how close to the front or the back of the chest the lesion is—and this is information the chest X-ray doesn't provide. Thus, when assessing chest X-rays, it is more logical to divide the lungs into thirds (zones—upper, middle, and lower) to describe the radiological situation of any lung abnormality.

Chest appearance

'Barrel chest'. Normally, the lateral diameter of the chest is greater than the anterior-posterior (A–P) diameter (4:3 approximately). In patients with barrel chest, the A–P diameter is increased so that the proportion approaches 1:1. Barrel chest is a feature of COPD and is thought to be due to the accessory muscles pulling the ribs upwards. The presence of barrel chest usually suggests quite advanced COPD, though the degree of chest deformity is not a reliable indicator of disease severity.

1. **Other abnormalities of chest shape.** The chest shape may be deformed in various ways although these are becoming less common (see Table 5.8):
   (1) if the patient's sternum is depressed (pectus excavatum) (*peck-tus-ex-ca-vay-tum*), this puts them at risk of breathing difficulties;
   (2) a prominent sternum (pectus carinatum) (*peck-tus-carry-nar-tum*) suggests the patient may have suffered from chest disease in childhood;
   (3) a severely deformed spine (kyphoscoliosis) puts patients at considerably increased risk of breathing difficulties in later life;
   (4) a severe deformity of one side of the chest raises the possibility of a thoracoplasty for tuberculosis in the past.

Other features you may observe from the end of the bed

1. **Chest drains for pneumothorax (*new-mow-thor-axe*) (p. 119) or pleural effusion (p. 113).** For a pneumothorax, the chest drain is normally inserted in the front of the chest (second intercostal space in the mid-clavicular line) or in the axilla, whereas for a pleural effusion, the drain is usually inserted posteriorly. Thus a tube coming out of the front of the chest or armpit suggests recent pneumothorax whereas a tube coming out of the back suggests recent pleural effusion.
2. **A general swelling of the neck and supraclavicular regions.** This may be due to air in the subcutaneous tissues (subcutaneous emphysema). It is usually diagnosed much more easily on palpation (p. 97). It is a complication that can follow the insertion of a chest drain for a pneumothorax. Some air escapes through the hole created in the chest wall tissues rather than through the tube and tracks upwards resulting in swelling of the neck. This looks worse than it is. Subcutaneous emphysema may also be a result of air in the mediastinum (pneumomediastinum), the discussion of which is beyond the scope of this book.

TABLE 5.8 Chest deformities

Funnel chest (pectus excavatum)	
What is it?	A depressed sternum
How does it happen?	It is congenital; usually idiopathic but may be associated with connective tissue disorders such as Marfan's (*ma-fans*) syndrome
Effects	Cosmetic; effects on lung function usually minor but in some cases, it may cause breathlessness.
Pigeon chest (pectus carinatum)	
What is it?	A prominent sternum
How does it happen?	Develops in childhood in patients with rickets or severe chest disease. In those with chest disease, it is thought to be due to repeated strong contractions of the diaphragm while the ribcage is still pliable
Effects	Cosmetic; little additional effect on lung function beyond the causative condition
Kyphoscoliosis	
What is it?	Spinal deformity resulting in increased A–P curvature (kyphosis) and lateral curvature (scoliosis) of the spine. It affects 1 in 1000 people with 1 in 10 000 affected severely. The patient's posture may look abnormal
How does it happen?	Mostly idiopathic, first noticed in childhood, but may be due to bone or connective tissue disease affecting the spine (osteoporosis, Ehlers–Danlos (*er-luz-dan-loss*) syndrome)
Effects	Cosmetic; may have quite severe effects on lung capacity resulting in breathlessness presenting in middle age
Thoracoplasty	
What is it?	Thoracoplasty was an operation used in the past to treat tuberculosis. It involved removing several ribs and so can result in the treated side of the chest looking very deformed
Effects	Reduces lung capacity, which becomes more important with advancing years resulting in an increased propensity to breathing difficulties

3. **Evidence of previous radiotherapy.** Sharply demarcated patches of erythematous or thickened skin raise the possibility of cancer, particularly lung cancer and lymphoma.
4. **Prominent chest wall veins.** These suggest SVC obstruction (p. 88).

Chest movement

Why examine?

Many chest conditions reduce chest movement. Most diseases are bilateral and so result in reduced chest movement on both sides. However, some important conditions (consolidation, effusion, collapse, fibrosis, and pneumothorax) may affect just one lung so resulting in reduced movement on that side. The consequent asymmetry of movement makes detection easier. Both inspection and palpation (p. 97) are used to assess chest movement.

How to examine

1. Walk confidently to the end of the bed.
2. Explain to the patient 'I now want to have a thorough look at your chest.' For female patients, if appropriate add, 'Could you please remove the towel?'
3. Stand and look carefully at the patient's chest.
4. Certain abnormalities will be obvious such as pursed lip breathing, the presence of a chest drain, a depressed or prominent sternum, kyphoscoliosis, or previous thoracoplasty.
5. Go through a checklist in your mind.
    1. Is the patient's breathing pattern normal? If not, decide what is abnormal. Is the patient's breathing becoming deeper and deeper before ceasing for a period (suggesting Cheyne–Stokes respiration)?
    2. Are they using their accessory muscles? Sometimes, pursed lip breathing and accessory muscle usage will go together.
    3. Is the chest shape normal? If not, does the chest look barrel shaped?
    4. Are there prominent chest wall veins (suggesting SVC obstruction)?
5. Look at the neck. Is there swelling of the neck (suggesting subcutaneous emphysema)?
6. Next, ask the patient to take a deep breath in and then out through their mouth. Show the patient what you want them to do: 'Please take a deep breath in and out ... like this.'
7. As the patient breathes, watch the chest carefully and concentrate on whether one side is moving more than the other. Force yourself to decide whether both sides move equally or if there is a difference.
8. Then, ask the patient to repeat their deep breath in and out. If your opinion remains unchanged, this part of the examination is complete. If not, ask the patient to breathe in and out again until your findings are consistent.

CASE 5.22

Problem. I can't decide if my patient has asymmetrical chest movement and now he says he's dizzy.

Discussion. You have to be a little careful during the chest examination not to make your patient hyperventilate. Over-breathing can result in tingling, dizziness, and even collapse. I suggest a maximum of four deep breaths in and out at any one point in the examination.

Keypoints

- Chest shape and movement are best assessed by standing at the foot of the bed.
- Accessory muscle use and pursed lip breathing suggest a deterioration in chest condition, most commonly an exacerbation of COPD.
- Barrel chest is a sign of COPD.
- Inspection of chest movement is a useful way of detecting unilateral chest pathology.
- When inspecting chest movement, demonstrate to the patient how you would like them to breathe.

10. Inspect front of chest and neck close up (DF 5/10).

Why examine?

Having taken a look at the chest from the distance it is now time to look more closely at the chest. The aim is to (1) examine more closely any abnormalities seen from the end of the bed and (2) identify smaller pathology not easily visible from the end of the bed.

How to examine

1. Go back to the left-hand side of the patient's bed.
2. If there were any possible radiotherapy patches, inspect for small tattoo marks, which are often over the irradiated skin.
3. Inspect for prominent chest wall veins suggesting SVC obstruction.
4. Look for a chest drain scar over the second intercostal spaces in the mid-clavicular line.

CASE 5.23

Problem. On close inspection of the chest I've noticed a long vertical scar over the front of the sternum. Does this give a clue to respiratory disease?

Discussion. Big scars on the front of the chest usually represent cardiac operations. See p. 47 for more information.

5. Ask the patient to lift up their right arm and look in the axilla for a chest drain scar—in the fourth, fifth, or sixth intercostal spaces in the mid-axillary line. Do the same for the left axilla.

Palpation of trachea and praecordium

11. Palpate trachea (DF 9/10).

The trachea can normally be felt in the neck. It lies in the mid-line between the suprasternal notch and the cricoid (*cry-coid*) cartilage.

Why examine?

Examination of the trachea is somewhat uncomfortable for the patient but it is important to do it because displacement of the trachea to one side is an important sign. The trachea may be pulled to the side by unilateral upper lobe fibrosis or collapse. Upper lobe fibrosis usually suggests tuberculosis in the past. Lung cancer causing blockage of a main bronchus is usually responsible for upper lobe collapse. Furthermore, if the lung cancer has been treated surgically by removal of lung (pneumonectomy), the trachea will be pulled to that side. Rarely, the trachea may also be displaced by a tension pneumothorax or by a large pleural effusion—both of which push the trachea towards the opposite side.

How to examine

1. Keep the patient positioned at 45° with their neck relaxed against the pillow.
2. Say to the patient something like, 'I need to feel your windpipe. It's a little uncomfortable but I'll try to be gentle.'
3. Then, using your right middle finger, gently palpate the patient's neck about 2 cm superior to the suprasternal notch in the mid-line (Fig. 5.9).
4. You will feel a resistance there. If you move your finger 0.5 cm to the right or left, the resistance is more difficult to palpate. This resistance is the trachea.
5. Palpate the space either side to get a feel for whether the trachea is central.

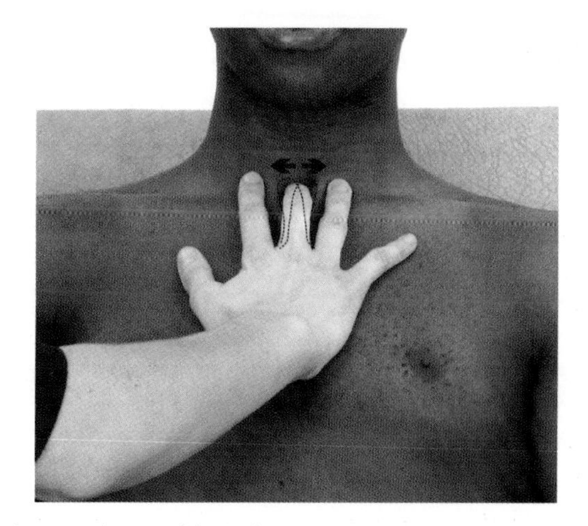

Fig. 5.9 Palpation of the trachea.

6. Decide whether the trachea central or is it displaced to one side.

12. Palpate the praecordium for apex beat position (DF 9/10), axillary lymph nodes (DF 8/10), and if suspected, tender areas (DF 8/10) and subcutaneous emphysema (DF 1/10).

Tip

Practise palpation of the trachea on your (consenting) friends; patients will not thank you for poking around unnecessarily in their necks.

CASE 5.24

Problem. I thought I had had got the hang of finding the trachea but I'm having great difficulty palpating this patient's.

Discussion. The usual reason for increased difficulty is excess adipose tissue in patients who are overweight—this can make it very difficult to identify the trachea.

CASE 5.25

Problem. The patient's trachea seems to be slightly deviated to the right but when I've examined the chest I've found nothing (collapse, fibrosis, and so on) to suggest a cause.

Discussion. Very slight deviation to the right can be a normal variant.

CASE 5.26

Problem. I've heard of a sign called 'tracheal tug'. What's this?

Discussion. Tracheal tug is said to be a sign of COPD. I have never found it helpful. It is said that in COPD, if you palpate the trachea during inspiration, it seems to move downwards—tracheal tug.

Keypoints

- Examining the trachea is somewhat uncomfortable for the patient—be gentle.
- Tracheal deviation usually suggests unilateral upper lobe pathology.

Why examine?

Palpation of the praecordium often provides only limited information about the respiratory system—but occasionally there may be positive findings.

1. **Rib fracture.** The presence of an exquisitely tender area on the chest may suggest a rib fracture. This may be associated with a grinding/crunching sensation called crepitus (*crep-it-us*) where the broken ends of bone rub against each other. Rib fractures are usually due to trauma and may be complicated by a pneumothorax or haemothorax. Rarely this may be a pathological fracture where secondary spread of a cancer to the bones may cause the ribs to break from trivial trauma.
2. **Subcutaneous emphysema.** General swelling of the upper chest and neck may suggest subcutaneous emphysema (p. 93). When palpated this produces a very characteristic crackling sensation under the hand.
3. **Apex beat.** The apex beat (p. 48) is defined as the most lateral and inferior position at which the cardiac impulse is felt. Its normal position is the fifth intercostal interspace in the mid-clavicular line. The apex beat position may give a clue to unilateral lower lung lobe pathology in the same way that the tracheal position gives clues to upper lobe pathology. Thus right lower lobe collapse (often due to lung cancer) or fibrosis (often after pneumonia) may result in slight movement of the apex beat to the right so it is felt more medially than the mid-clavicular line. Left lower lobe collapse or fibrosis may cause the apex beat to be displaced laterally. As with the trachea, a large pleural effusion or a tension pneumothorax will push the apex beat away from the side of the pathology.
4. **Axillary lymph nodes.** The lymphatic drainage of the lung is primarily through the neck nodes so lymph nodes are discussed in more detail on p. 110. The axillary nodes drain the breasts and the pleurae. In normal patients, it is often possible to palpate small axillary lymph nodes (<0.5 cm). A large (>1 cm) lump is nearly always pathological. If it is hard, this is suspicious of breast cancer—or rarely mesothelioma. If firm rather than hard, any of the causes of generalized lymph node enlargement detailed on p. 110 may be responsible.

How to examine?

See Fig 5.10.

1. Ask the patient, 'Is the front of your chest painful or tender?'
2. If the answer is 'yes', ask for permission to examine: 'Do you mind if I examine the painful or tender areas?' If permission is granted gently palpate the painful spots. Can you elicit tenderness? Is the painful or tender spot within a hard bony area suggesting rib injury?
3. If you have previously observed chest or neck swelling suggestive of subcutaneous emphysemas, gently palpate the area. If subcutaneous emphyse-

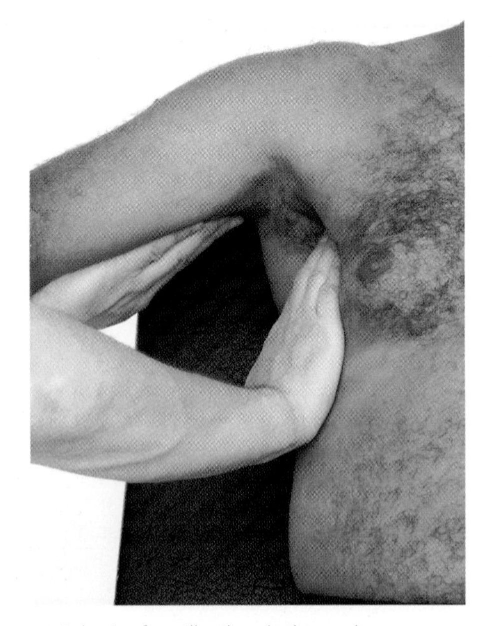

Fig. 5.10 Palpating for axillary lymphadenopathy.

ma is present you will feel a crackling sensation under the hand.

4. Palpate the apex beat position as per p. 48.
5. To examine for axillary lymph nodes, the patient needs to abduct their arms: 'Please lift your right arm out to the side ... Do you mind if I check in your armpit for glands?'
6. If the muscles and tendons around the axilla are tense, it is very difficult to palpate nodes so take the weight of the patient's right arm by holding it at the elbow with your left arm (to allow the shoulder muscles to relax) (Fig. 5.10).
7. Using the palmar aspect of the fingers of your right hand, palpate in sequence the medial, anterior, lateral, posterior, and apical aspects of the axilla. Do you feel any rounded masses?
8. If so, palpate these specifically with the tips of your fingers to get a clearer idea of size and consistency.
9. Then, do the same for the left axilla—this time using your right arm to support the patient's arm and your left hand to palpate for nodes.

Tip

Avoid wiggling your fingers in the patient's armpit; this is tickling!

CASE 5.27

Problem. I can't palpate the apex beat. Why might this be?

Discussion. The apex beat is impalpable in around 50% of patients (p. 49). One common cause relating to the respiratory system is hyperinflation of the lung associated with COPD.

CASE 5.28

Problem. The apex beat is displaced laterally. But on further examination I've found nothing such as left lower lobe collapse or fibrosis or right pleural effusion to suggest a cause. Why might this be?

Discussion. The apex beat is primarily a sign of cardiac disease and displacement of the apex is usually due to cardiac pathology—so it's usual not to find any explanatory respiratory pathology to explain a change in its position.

CASE 5.29

Problem. When examining the cardiovascular system, I've been taught to assess the apex beat character. Is this useful in the respiratory system?

Discussion. No, respiratory disease does not affect the character of the apex beat.

CASE 5.30

Problem. When examining the axilla for nodes, I tend to feel prominent areas but they don't feel like nodes.

Discussion. The tendons in the axilla, especially if they are tense, may feel hard and lumpy and may mimic nodes—but if you palpate carefully you will note that they have a linear character rather than the lumpiness of a node.

Keypoints

- Apex beat displacement may suggest unilateral lower lobe pathology.
- To examine for axillary lymph nodes, make sure the muscles and tendons are as relaxed as possible.

The remainder of the chest examination is dominated by a sequence of testing for expansion, percussion, tactile vocal fremitus (TVF), auscultation, and vocal resonance (VR). This is done first over the front of the chest and the axillae and then over the back. As the principles are the same front and back, each technique will be described in one section rather than in separate sections for front and back.

Palpation of chest expansion

13. Palpate for chest expansion anteriorly, comparing both sides (DF 9/10).

Why examine

Palpating for chest expansion is a comparative technique. The aim is to compare the two sides and detect any reduction in expansion on one side. Unilateral reduction in expansion at the front of the chest may be due to pathology of any lobe. Unilateral reduction in expansion low down the chest posteriorly suggests lower lobe pathology. The lower lobe is the most common site for important pulmonary conditions such as consolidation, effusion, fibrosis, and collapse. Unilateral reduction in expansion high up the chest posteriorly suggests upper lobe pathology.

Front of the chest

How to examine

1. Your examination of the praecordium should have identified any areas of tenderness—be careful of these.
2. Ask the patient to breathe in and then out and to hold their breath in expiration (so that the subsequent expansion will be maximal).
3. Then, having warned the patient, place your hands firmly on the chest wall with fingers gripping their sides (the lower ribcage).
4. Bring your thumbs together to meet in the mid-line around the inferior part of the sternum but not touching the chest (Fig. 5.11a). Exactly where you grip the patient's side will vary according to the patient's size but essentially you grip in the position that allows you to bring you thumbs together to meet in the mid-line.
5. Ask the patient to take a deep breath in and watch your thumbs (Fig. 5.11b). If one thumb moves less than the other, this indicates reduced expansion on that side.

Back of the chest

How to examine

First concentrate on the lower lobes. The same procedure is followed as for the front of the chest, this time with the doctor standing behind the patient.

1. Ask the patient to breathe in and then out and to hold their breath in expiration.
2. To assess lower lobes,
   (1) place your hands firmly on the chest wall with fingers gripping their sides (the lower ribcage) and bring your thumbs together to meet in the mid-line around the lower thoracic spine but not touching the chest (Fig. 5.12);
   (2) ask the patient to take a deep breath in and watch your thumbs, assessing if one thumb moves less than the other—indicating reduced expansion on that side.
3. To assess upper lobes,
   (1) do the same again this time higher up with thumbs meeting around T3 level.

(a)

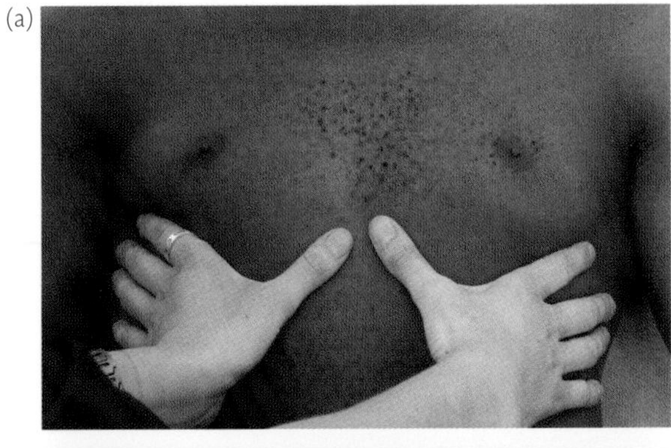

(b)

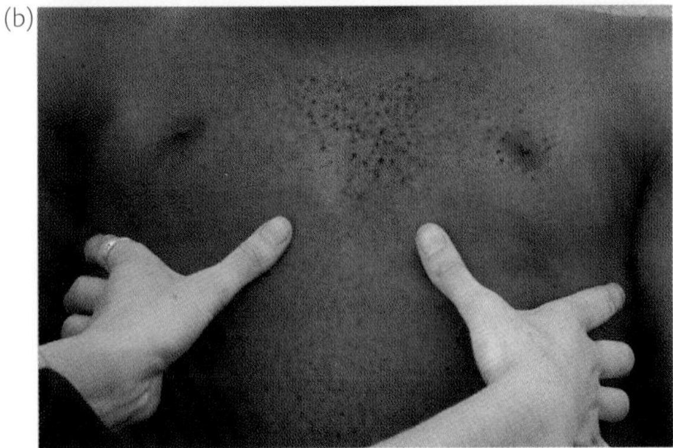

Fig. 5.11 Palpation of chest expansion anteriorly.

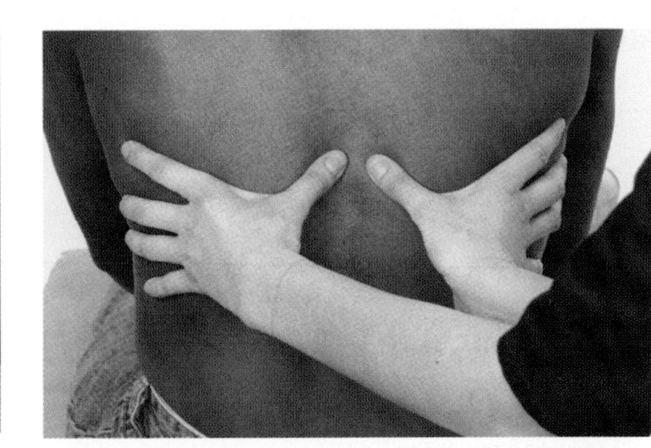

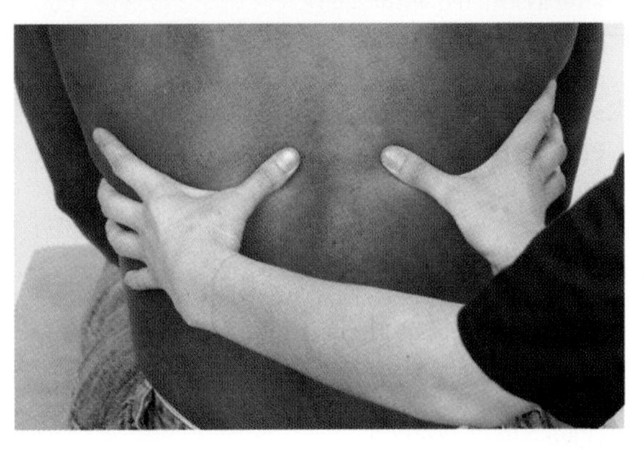

Fig. 5.12 Palpation of chest expansion posteriorly—lower lobes.

CASE 5.31

Problem. I've checked expansion but wasn't sure if the two sides were equal. When I tried again, it didn't seem to work very well.

Discussion. When repeating expansion, the temptation is just to ask the patient to breathe in again and see what happens to your thumbs. This never works—your thumbs will be separated by this stage. You have to release your grip and start again.

CASE 5.32

Problem. When testing for expansion at the front, do my hands go over or under the breasts?

Discussion. Under. You may have to lift the patient's left breast up with your left hand (ask permission) so that you can grip the left ribcage properly with your right hand. Then, slide your left hand under the patient's right breast so that you can grip the right ribcage and bring your thumbs together in the mid-line.

CASE 5.33

Problem. Is there any benefit in measuring actual chest expansion overall (as opposed to simply comparing the two sides)?

Discussion. This is not recommended as a routine test, but chest expansion overall can be measured.

1. Wrap a tape measure around the patient's chest (under each axillae).
2. Ask the patient to breathe out and hold it.
3. Tighten the tape measure round the chest and measure.
4. Loosen your grip.
5. Ask the patient to breathe in and hold it.
6. Tighten the tape measure again and measure.

The difference between the two measurements is the patient's chest expansion. Normally, this is >5 cm. A measure <2 cm is clearly abnormal and indicative of lung or chest wall disease. However, this measure does not correlate well with lung capacity.

CASE 5.34

Problem. I've noticed senior doctors sometimes lean over from the front to examine expansion at the back of the chest. Is this a better way?

Discussion. This method involves the same principle, that is, grip at the sides and compare how much the thumbs move in the centre. Some doctors find this more cumbersome and the line of sight can make it difficult to compare the movement of both sides of the chest satisfactorily.

CASE 5.35

Problem. I feel a little awkward when leaning across to examine expansion at the back of the chest. Is it alright to sit down on the bed behind the patient whilst checking expansion?

Discussion. This can be more comfortable for the examiner but it can also be more awkward. However, it is not unreasonable to sit down to check expansion posteriorly if you personally find it more comfortable.

CASE 5.36

Problem. Both inspection from the end of the bed (p. 94) and palpation are used to assess chest movement—which is better?

Discussion. This is a matter of personal preference. Some doctors find inspection from the end of the bed more informative but others prefer the palpation method. So experiment and find out what suits you.

Keypoints

- The main aim is to compare the two sides.
- Grip the patient's ribcage with your fingers and bring your thumbs together in the mid-line.
- Reduced expansion on one side of the chest anteriorly may be due to pathology in any lung lobe.
- Reduced expansion on one side of the **lower** chest posteriorly suggests either pathology overlying the lower lobe (such as effusion) or pathology within the lower lobe (such as fibrosis, collapse, or consolidation).

Chest percussion

14. Percuss front of chest and in the axillae, comparing the two sides (DF 9/10).

Chest percussion is one of the great arts of medicine. It requires considerable practice to achieve proficiency but once mastered provides useful clues to chest disease. Percussion was first described in 1761 by *Josef Leopold Auenbrugger (1722–1809, Austrian physician)*. As with many great discoveries, Auenbrugger's ideas were pretty much ignored for 50 years, until they were adopted by *Rene Laennac (1781–1826, French physician, the inventor of the stethoscope)* and colleagues. At that time, percussion was a major diagnostic advance because it provided the first way to distinguish between pleural effusions and consolidations. Since the discovery of X-rays in 1895, percussion's importance has somewhat diminished but it remains an extremely useful tool for evaluating chest diseases when they first present.

How to examine: basic technique

There are two different techniques—a normal technique for percussing over the chest wall in general and a modified technique for over the clavicle.

Percussion over the chest wall

See Fig. 5.13.

1. Place your left hand palm down on the chest wall.
2. Align your fingers with the ribs so that your middle finger is between ribs.
3. Spread your fingers slightly apart (Fig. 5.13a).
4. Press your left middle finger firmly against the chest wall.
5. Now, hold your right hand extended at the wrist with the middle metacarpophalangeal (MCP) joint slightly flexed, so that the distal phalanx is roughly at right angles to the hand.

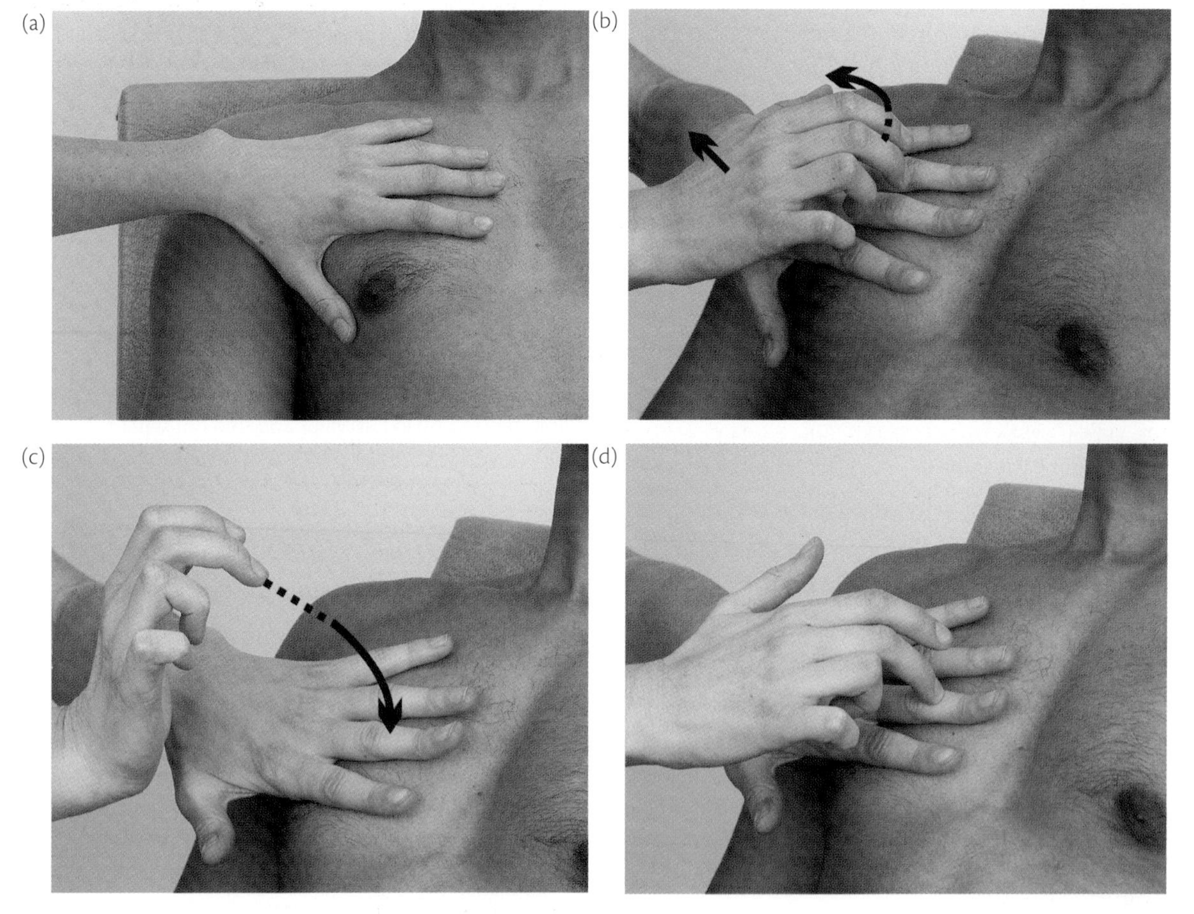

Fig. 5.13 Percussion over the chest wall

6. Now hyperextend the wrist further in preparation to strike your left middle finger (Fig. 5.13b).
7. Then, briskly flex the wrist and use the pad of your right middle finger to strike the dorsum of the middle phalanx of the left middle finger (Fig. 5.13c).
8. Remove the percussing finger immediately (Fig. 5.13d).
9. With the same motion of the right hand, strike the left middle finger for a second time, again removing the percussing finger quickly (this second strike is non-essential and merely provides confirmation of your first attempt; if you are confident striking once, this is acceptable).
10. Whilst doing 7., listen to noise made and sense the feeling of the two fingers meeting—the percussion note is both heard and felt.

Tip

Make sure the left middle finger is placed firmly against the chest wall. Lifting it even slightly makes the percussion note much duller.

Tip

Keep the fingernail of your right middle finger very short.

Percussion over the clavicle

For percussing the clavicle, only the right hand is used. The same technique is applied except that the pad of the right middle finger strikes the clavicle directly rather than the left middle finger. This can be painful for the patient, so be gentle.

How to examine: normality

The aim of chest percussion is to compare the right and left sides of the chest. There are three normal percussion sounds/sensations, which you can check on yourself using the chest wall two-hand technique:

Tip

Practice is essential to achieve the consistent action and force required. Percussion particularly in the learning stages can be awkward (and uncomfortable at the clavicles) so it is helpful if students practise on each other first.

Tip

Initially your percussion action may be feeble and you will have to devote time to producing a stronger strike. However, as you improve, it can be easy to get carried away and use too much force—avoid this. The aim is to produce a consistent, audible note without hurting the patient.

(1) dull—occurs over solid organs such as the liver;

(2) resonant—occurs over the lung;

(3) tympanic—occurs over the abdomen.

The resonance over the lung is present to approximately the sixth rib anteriorly, the eighth rib in the axilla, and the tenth rib posteriorly. There is usually a dull area over the liver and heart anteriorly.

Why examine?

The percussion note is altered if lung tissue becomes airless, as in consolidation or collapse, or if lung tissue is pushed away from the chest wall by fluid, air, or pleural thickening (Table 5.9). Pleural effusion, consolidation, and lung collapse commonly produce signs over the lower lobes. It should be noted that the percussion note is normal in many patients with important lung disease (notably lung cancer) and can also be normal in minor degrees of the conditions in Table 5.9.

How to examine: a system

Front of the chest and axillae

The patient should remain at 45°, supported by pillows.

1. First, percuss the patient's right clavicle over its medial third (only the medial third overlies lung tissue).
2. Next percuss the left clavicle using the same force, comparing the noise and the sensation—is one side duller than the other?
3. Now percuss the chest wall anteriorly: upper right, upper left, middle right, middle left, lower right, lower left always using the same force and comparing the sides as you go. In women patients, their

TABLE 5.9 Types of abnormal percussion

Pleural effusion	Very (stony) dull
Consolidation	Dull
Collapse	Dull
Pneumothorax	Hyper-resonant

breasts may make the percussion note dull and percussion more difficult.

4. Ask the patient to abduct their right arm and then percuss the right upper axilla and compare with the left upper axilla; next percuss the right and then left lower axillae.
5. If at any point you think there might be a difference but are unsure, repeat the percussion in that area.

Tip

With the axilla it is perfectly acceptable to percuss down each intercostal space on one side before comparing it with the other axilla. This avoids the need to abduct each arm with consecutive percussion.

Back of the chest

1. The patient should be sitting up (p. 109) and percussion performed with the doctor standing slightly behind him (Fig. 5.14).
2. Percuss the chest wall posteriorly: upper right, upper left, middle right, middle left, lower right, lower left, always using the same force and comparing the sides as you go.

Tactile vocal fremitus

15. Assess tactile vocal fremitus at the front of the chest and in the axillae, comparing the two sides (DF 9/10).

Traditionally, medical examination is performed according to a sequence: inspection, palpation, percussion, and expansion—so strictly speaking TVF would be done before percussion. However, TVF is most effective at evaluating areas that have been found to be dull to percussion—in particular differentiating between effusion and consolidation. Therefore, although a form of palpation, the author's view is that TVF is best done following percussion.

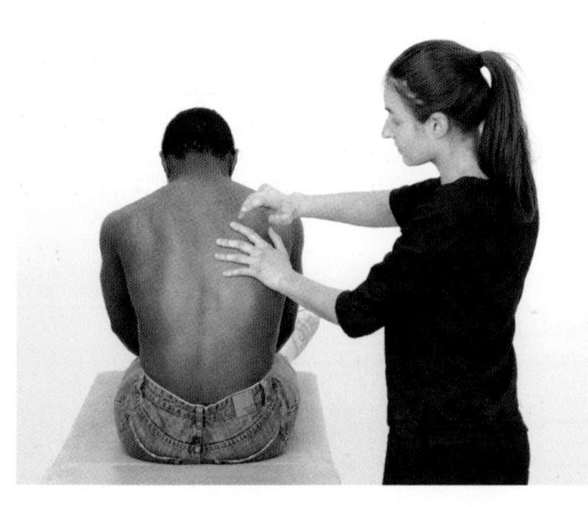

Fig. 5.14 Percussion of the posterior chest.

CASE 5.37

Problem. The patient seems perfectly well but there seems to be a large area of dullness over the left side of the chest at the front.

Discussion. This is the patient's heart and so is completely normal. Normal cardiac dullness does make comparison of the percussion note on the front of the chest difficult. However, if the right side of the chest is duller than the left, this does suggest pathology.

CASE 5.38

Problem. The right lung seems dull to percussion yet it appears to be expanding better than the left. Can you explain why?

Discussion. We tend to automatically assume that the side with the dull percussion note contains the pathology. This is usually but not always true. It is the lung that is not expanding that **is** always the one with the pathology. The likelihood is that this patient has a pneumothorax—so rather than the right chest being dull, the left chest is hyper-resonant making the right side appear dull.

CASE 5.39

Problem. I'm a bit disappointed. I found no abnormality on percussion but the chest X-ray shows large bilateral pleural effusions. Yet, I thought I percussed the patient's chest fairly competently.

Discussion. Percussion is essentially a comparative technique, which relies on you identifying differences between the two sides. When there is bilateral pathology, this difference is abolished, making detection of any abnormality more difficult. As you become more familiar with the percussion technique, you will start to get a sense of dullness even when it occurs bilaterally. However even in the most experienced hands errors can still be made.

CASE 5.40

Problem. So consolidation produces a dull note, pleural effusions are stony dull. Am I really supposed to be able to tell the difference?

Discussion. You're right, it isn't easy. But the differentiation between effusion and consolidation was one of percussion's original benefits. Nowadays, TVF, VR, and the breath sounds provide supplementary information to help distinguish between effusions and consolidation clinically.

Keypoints

- Use one hand when percussing over the clavicle, two hands elsewhere.
- Make sure the left middle finger is placed firmly against the chest wall.
- The percussion note is both heard and felt.
- The aim is to compare the right and left sides of the chest using consistent force to produce an audible note without hurting the patient.
- The dull side is usually the abnormal side (the exception is pneumothorax).
- Pleural effusion produces a very (stony) dull note, consolidation and collapse produce a dull note, whilst pneumothorax produces a hyperresonant note.
- The percussion note can be normal in many patients with serious lung disease.
- Cardiac dullness makes useful comparisons of percussion note at the front of the chest difficult.

Why examine?

Low-frequency vibrations (100–200 Hz) can be detected at the chest wall by a palpating hand. Most speech contains low-frequency harmonics (<300 Hz) so when we speak, low-frequency vibrations are transmitted through the lungs to the chest wall and can be detected by the palpating hand as TVF. The degree of TVF is affected by the thickness of the chest wall—being reduced in overweight patients. It is easier to detect TVF in men than in women because the vibrations created by their deeper (lower frequency) voices are easier to palpate and are better transmitted through normal lung. When assessing TVF, the aim is to detect differences between the two sides: consolidation increases transmission of speech vibrations so TVF is increased, whereas effusion, collapse and pneumothorax result in reduced transmission and TVF.

How to examine

You should already have established if there are any tender areas—if so you may need to modify your examination to avoid these areas.

Front of the chest and axillae

1. **Assess TVF at the apices**
   1. The vibrations over the clavicle are used to assess apical TVF.
   2. Place the ulnar border of your right hand on the patient's right clavicle.
   3. Ask the patient to say 'ninety-nine'. Whilst they are speaking, concentrate on the vibration transmitted to your right hand.
   4. Next, place the ulnar border of your right hand on the patient's left clavicle, ask the patient to say 'ninety-nine', and again assess the vibration transmitted to your right hand. Is the vibration the same on both sides? It should be.
   5. If you are not sure, recheck.
2. **Assess TVF of the upper lobes**
   1. Place the flat of your right hand over the top of the right side of the patient's chest.
   2. Ask the patient to say 'ninety-nine', concentrating on the vibration transmitted to your right hand.
   3. Do the same on the patient's left side and consider if the two sides are equal.
   4. If you are not sure, recheck.
3. **Assess TVF of lateral aspects of the lungs**
   1. Ask the patient to abduct their right arm: 'Please lift your right arm out to the side ... Do you mind if I feel in your armpit (again).'
   2. Place the flat of your right hand on the medial aspect of the patient's right axilla.
   3. Ask the patient to say 'ninety-nine', concentrating on the vibration transmitted to your hand.
   4. Do the same for the left axilla, again comparing the two sides.

Back of the chest

You should be standing behind the patient.

1. **Assess TVF of the upper lobes**

Place the flat of your right hand over the top of the right side of the patient's chest and repeat as for the front, comparing both sides

CASE 5.41

Problem. I find it easier to use my left hand when detecting TVF over the right side of the patient's chest—is that alright?

Discussion. There are no hard and fast rules. Use whichever hand gives you the most consistent results. The advantage of using the right hand (or left hand) throughout is that the same hand is sensing the vibration consistently. However, using the right hand throughout does result in a slightly awkward asymmetry in the way your hand contacts the patient's chest. Using your left hand on the patient's right side and your right hand on the patient's left side avoids this asymmetry. Another option is to use both hands together. This can be more difficult and a little embarrassing when examining women.

CASE 5.42

Problem. Why don't you assess TVF on the lower chest anteriorly?

Discussion. The heart causes a normal asymmetry in TVF between the right and left lower chest so there is little value in comparing TVF there.

CASE 5.43

Problem. Can I ask the patient to use phrases other than 'ninety-nine'?

Discussion. TVF was first demonstrated by German physicians who used 'neunzig und neun'. The English translation 'ninety-nine' conveniently produces the same resonances. There's little reason why ninety-nine is better than other phrases sometimes used, such as 'one-hundred-and-one', 'one, two, three', or 'one, one, one'.

CASE 5.44

Problem. What happens if the patient changes the volume of their voice as they repeat 'ninety-nine'?

Discussion. The louder the patient's voice, the greater the TVF. If the patient varies the volume, explain to them that they need to keep the volume even and try again.

Keypoints

- TVF is most effective at evaluating areas that have been found to be dull to percussion.
- Consolidation increases TVF.
- Effusion, collapse, and pneumothorax reduce TVF.
- Assess TVF at apices, upper chest, and axillae anteriorly and over the upper and lower lobes posteriorly.

2. Assess TVF of lower lobes

Place the flat of your right hand over the lower aspect of the right side of the patient's chest and repeat as above, comparing both sides

Chest auscultation

16. Auscultate over the front of the chest and in the axillae, comparing the two sides (DF 8/10).

Like chest percussion, auscultation of the chest remains one of the great arts of medicine.

How to examine: basic technique

Chest auscultation is performed with the stethoscope (p. 50, CVS). There is no consensus on whether the bell or the diaphragm should be used. The case for the bell is strong: in theory it should be better for hearing breath sounds as these are mostly low pitched; skin or hairs being stretched under the diaphragm may create unwanted artefacts. However, these issues seem to be of little practical importance and it is common practice to auscultate using the diaphragm apart from the lung apices where good contact with the diaphragm is difficult and the bell is used.

(1) Place the diaphragm on the chest wall.

(2) Ask the patient to breathe in and out through their mouth deeply and quite fast—respiratory rate about 30 breaths per minute.

(3) Listen to the sounds generated.

Bear in mind that too much deep breathing may make the patient dizzy or even collapse (hyperventilation).

Tip

It may be helpful to spend a few seconds showing the patient how to breathe in the manner that you wish.

> **Tip**
>
> It may be best to keep saying 'In ... out ... in ... out ...' so that the patient is continually prompted.

How to examine: normality

The normal breath sounds over the chest wall are called 'vesicular' (*vee-sick-you-lar*). The quality of these sounds is soft. The French physician and inventor of the stethoscope, Rene Laennac (1781–1826) compared them to leaves gently rustling. Their origin is not completely understood. The inspiratory sound is thought to be due to air turbulence within the small airways and alveoli (*al-vee-owe-lie*). Thus, the intensity of the sound gradually increases through inspiration as more and more air reaches the alveoli. The initial part of the expiratory sound is initially due to air flowing out of the alveoli. Once these have emptied, the sound heard originates in the large airways —further away from the stethoscope—so that the noise becomes quieter in the second half of expiration, fading away to become inaudible.

Why examine: abnormalities

Two types of abnormality may occur: abnormal breath sounds and added sounds.

Abnormal breath sounds

As most of the sound produced in normal breath sounds originates in the small airways and alveoli, diseases that damage these may alter the breath sounds.

1. Small airway and alveolar damage is most severe when areas of the lung become consolidated, collapsed, or fibrosed. In such conditions, the breath sounds do not have the soft rustling component produced by turbulence within the alveoli. Instead, noises from the larger airways predominate producing a harsher sound—known as 'bronchial breath sounds' (DF 9/10). In bronchial breathing, the sounds gradually increase through inspiration but stop near the end of inspiration (when air would normally be flowing round the alveoli) and restart after a gap when air flows back through the larger airways during expiration. The expiratory sounds tend to be louder and longer than the inspiratory sounds. Detecting such areas of bronchial breathing can be surprisingly difficult (DF 9/10). However, in the case of consolidated lung, the solidified lung conducts sounds very well so that the bronchial breathing is easier to identify. The features of bronchial breathing are compared with those of vesicular breathing in Table 5.10.
2. If just some of the alveoli are damaged, again through consolidation, collapse, or fibrosis, the normal vesicular lung sounds may be reduced in intensity. This may also happen in COPD or asthma. A similar reduction in intensity may also occur where fluid (pleural effusion) or air (pneumothorax) have pushed the alveoli away from the chest wall (and consequently, the stethoscope).
3. The expiratory component of the breath sounds may be prolonged in airways obstruction—as air takes longer to leave the alveoli.

Occasionally, in very thin patients, the vesicular breath sounds are louder than normal.

> **Tip**
>
> Because bronchial breath sounds are harsher and tend to sound louder than vesicular sounds, there is a tendency to overdiagnose any loud breath sounds as bronchial sounds. Before diagnosing bronchial breath sounds make sure that the expiratory sound is louder and longer than the inspiratory sound and that there is a gap between inspiration and expiration.

TABLE 5.10 A comparison of bronchial and vesicular breath sounds

	Vesicular	**Bronchial**
Quality	Soft, rustling	Harsh, blowing
Inspiratory sound: origin	Small airways and alveoli	Large airways
Expiratory sound: origin	Alveoli and small airways, then large airways	Large airways
Louder component	Inspiratory	Expiratory
Longer component	Inspiratory	Expiratory
Gap	Between expiration and inspiration	Between inspiration and expiration

Tip

Sounds similar to but louder than bronchial breathing can be heard over the trachea normally. Listen to your own breath sounds over your chest and trachea and compare what you hear.

CASE 5.45

Problem. I'm listening over the upper chest anteriorly and it's difficult to say if the breath sounds are bronchial or vesicular. Can you explain why?

Discussion. Over certain parts of the chest wall overlying the large airways, sounds from these airways dominate so that the normal breath sounds are not vesicular. Over the manubrium, the breath sounds may be bronchial. Close to the manubrium, over the first and second intercostal spaces, the breath sounds may be 'bronchovesicular'. Broncho'vesicular sounds are half way between vesicular and bronchial sounds with inspiration and expiration of similar length and intensity and only a short gap between the two.

Added sounds

There are three types of added sounds (also known as 'adventitial' (*ad-vent-tish-al*) sounds): crackles (DF 5/10), wheeze (DF 2/10), and friction rub (DF 9/10).

1. **Crackles.** Sometimes referred to as crepitations (*crep-it-ay-shuns*) ('creps') or rales (*rahls*), these are short crackly sounds similar to that heard when pulling apart strips of Velcro. They are predominantly (90%) inspiratory. In the past, it was thought that crackles were always due to air bubbling through fluid within the small airways and alveoli. Whilst this is clearly the case for patients with left ventricular failure, it does not explain the marked crackles often heard in pulmonary fibrosis. In such patients, the crackles are thought to be due to changes in gas pressure causing sudden opening of small airways that had collapsed during the previous expiration. Crackles in different conditions have different origins and characteristics (Table 5.11). While crackles may occur in all these conditions, they are not always present, especially early in the disease process. Crackles can be described as fine, medium, or coarse. Fine crackles tend to be high pitched, scratchy sounds like rubbing your hair between your fingers or opening Velcro. Coarse crackles are lower pitch, wet bubbly noises, and medium crackles are in between the two. You will pick these sounds up with experience.
2. **Wheeze.** Also known as rhonchi (*ronk-eye*), wheeze is a continuous whistling sound due to the vibration of opposing walls of narrowed airways as air passes through them. The term used to be restricted to the noise that could **only** be heard with the unaided ear. However the sound is similar when heard with the stethoscope and hence the term wheeze has been adopted to embrace all such noises (doctors will often talk of 'wheezes heard on auscultation' to avoid confusion with its traditional definition). They are usually due to small airway obstruction as in COPD or asthma. In such cases the following should be noted.

TABLE 5.11 Features of crackles

	Origin: site	Origin: pathology	Timing	Character	Coughing effects
Fibrosis	Alveoli	Pressure effects	Inspiratory (throughout inspiration or second half)	Fine	No
Chronic obstructive pulmonary disease	Small airways	Pressure effects	Early inspiration	Medium	No
Left ventricular failure	Alveoli	Fluid	Inspiratory (throughout inspiration or second half)	Medium (variable)	No
Bronchiectasis	Alveoli	Fluid and pressure effects	Inspiratory (throughout inspiration or second half)	Coarse	Reduces, sometimes completely
Resolving pneumonia	Alveoli	Fluid and pressure effects	Inspiratory (throughout inspiration or second half)	Coarse	Reduces, sometimes completely

1. Wheezes are either confined to expiration (40% of patients) or heard throughout inspiration and expiration (60% of patients).
2. The pitch and duration of the wheeze is related to the degree of obstruction (and not its loudness). With severe asthma, so little air moves through the airways that the chest is effectively silent. The wheeze of asthma tends to be of higher pitch than that of COPD.
3. The wheezes are widespread throughout the lungs and tend to have variable pitch (polyphonic) (polly-fon-ic).

There are other causes of wheeze. Heart failure may cause wheeze due to associated bronchospasm. The old-fashioned term 'cardiac asthma' sums this up succinctly. Features tend to be similar to asthma or COPD with polyphonic wheezes, either confined to expiration or heard throughout inspiration and expiration. An obstructing lesion within a lung due to a tumour or a foreign body produces wheezes with similar features except that they are monophonic (the same pitch) and localized to one area of the lung. An obstruction proximal to the extra-thoracic trachea produces a monophonic rhonchus, which is confined to inspiration and is louder over the neck than over the chest (stridor).

3. **Friction rub.** Also known as a pleural rub, this is a grating sound like creaking leather due to rough thickened, pleural surfaces rubbing together as the lungs expand and contract. Such pleural inflammation may be due to pneumonia, pulmonary infarction, or occasionally malignancy. In contrast to crackles, a friction rub tends to predominate in expiration and around two-thirds are confined to expiration. The patient usually complains of pain in the area when it is known as pleurisy. You have to be very thorough and patient to hear a rub as it may be very localized.

How to examine: a system

Front of the chest and axillae

1. Place the diaphragm of your stethoscope over the patient's chest starting just below the right clavicle.
2. Ask the patient to breathe in deep and fast through the mouth. Demonstrate this to the patient.
3. After each breath move your stethoscope to the next site, comparing both sides. You may need to encourage the patient to keep breathing by saying 'In ... out ... in ... out ...'.
4. Decide on the intensity and character of the breath sounds and the presence or absence of added sounds as you go.
5. If you suspect an abnormality, listen longer in that area and confirm whether this is true; if so determine its nature (abnormalities may be quite localized so the abnormal sounds are heard only over a small area).
6. Finally, use your bell to listen to the right and left apices in turn.

Back of the chest

1. Stand behind the patient.
2. Use the diaphragm.
3. Auscultate over the chest: upper right, upper left, middle right, middle left, lower right, lower left.

Vocal resonance

17. Assess vocal resonance at the front of the chest and in the axillae, comparing the two sides (DF 9/10).

Why examine?

This is a very similar test to TVF (p. 102) and indeed Cases 5.42, 5.43, and 5.44 apply equally to VR. Normally, if you listen over a patient's chest with a stethoscope while they speak, you will hear muffled indistinct sounds. This is known as vocal resonance (VR). The sounds seem to come from the chest piece of

> **Tip**
>
> If the patient has severe pain on inspiration (as in pleurisy), it is kinder to reduce the auscultation procedure and rely on X-ray investigation.

> **Tip**
>
> Keep away from the mid-line where the breath sounds may tend to be dominated by upper airways noise.

> **CASE 5.46**
>
> **Problem.** I've heard a crackling sound but I'm not sure if it's a friction rub or crackles.
>
> **Discussion.** The following points may be helpful: (1) crackles tend to be more prominent in inspiration whereas a rub is usually more prominent in expiration; (2) crackles may be altered by coughing whereas a rub never is; (3) pain over the area on inspiration or on coughing makes a rub more likely.

Keypoints

- Normal vesicular breath sounds originate primarily from small airways or alveoli.
- Vesicular breath sounds have a rustling quality, the inspiratory component predominates, and there is a gap between expiration and inspiration.
- Breath sounds are reduced in intensity in many common conditions such as COPD and asthma, as well as pulmonary fibrosis, pleural effusion, pneumothorax, and lung collapse.
- Bronchial breathing occurs when the small airways or alveoli have been damaged. They are best heard in consolidation but also occur in lung collapse or fibrosis.
- Bronchial breath sounds are harsh and blowing, the expiratory component predominates, and there is a gap between inspiration and expiration.
- Crackles are due to air bubbling through fluid or pressure effects in damaged small airways or alveoli.
- Wheezes are due to small airways narrowing.
- The pitch and duration (but not loudness) of wheezes correlate with the severity of obstruction.
- When auscultating, compare both sides as you go for the intensity of breath sounds and to ascertain whether they are bronchial or vesicular and note any added sounds.
- If you think there may be an abnormality, listen longer, confirm its presence, then determine its nature.

the stethoscope. Normal lung conducts lower frequency sounds better so VR is greater in men than in women. As for TVF, the degree of VR is also affected by the thickness of the chest wall and so is reduced in overweight patients.

Abnormalities

1. Over an area of consolidation, sound transmission is increased. Words appear more resonant (though not necessarily intelligible) through the stethoscope and appear to be generated closer to the earpiece.
2. Effusion, collapse, and pneumothorax result in reduced transmission and VR.

When assessing VR, the aim is to detect differences between the two sides.

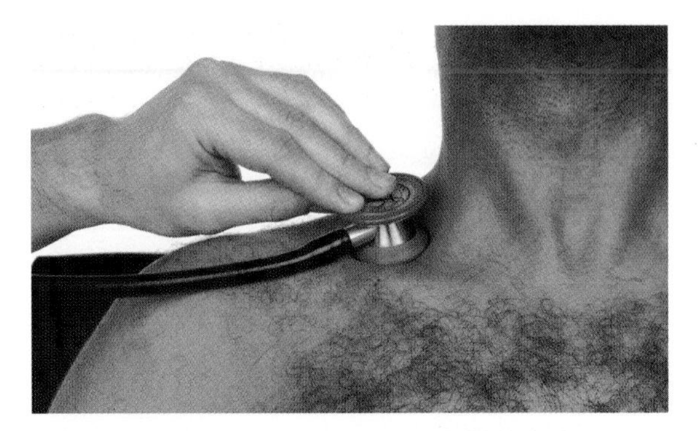

Fig. 5.15 Assessing vocal resonance over the apices.

How to examine

Front of the chest and axillae

1. **Assess VR at the apices**
   1. Place the bell of the stethoscope over the patient's right supraclavicular fossa (Fig. 5.15).
   2. Ask the patient to say 'ninety-nine'.
   3. Whilst they're speaking, concentrate on the sound coming through the stethoscope. Next, place the bell of the stethoscope over the patient's left supraclavicular fossa.
   4. Ask the patient to say 'ninety-nine' and again assess the sound coming through the stethoscope.
   5. Is the sound the same on both sides—they should be?
   6. If you are not sure recheck.
2. **Assess VR of the upper lobes**
   1. Place the diaphragm of the stethoscope over the top of the right side of the patient's chest.
   2. Ask the patient to say 'ninety-nine', concentrating on the sound transmitted through the stethoscope.
   3. Do the same on the patient's left side and consider if the two sides are equal.
   4. If you are not sure recheck.
3. **Assess VR of the lateral aspects of lungs**
   1. Ask the patient to abduct their right arm: 'Please lift your right arm out to the side ... Do you mind if I listen in your armpit.'
   2. Place the diaphragm of the stethoscope on the medial aspect of the patient's right axilla.
   3. Ask the patient to say 'ninety-nine', concentrating on the sound transmitted through the stethoscope.
   4. Do the same for the left axilla, again comparing the two sides.

Back of the chest

1. Stand behind the patient.
2. Use the diaphragm.

CASE 5.47

Problem. Which is better, TVF or VR? Do I really need to do both?

Discussion. There is no definite answer. They are both testing the same thing—sound transmission through the lungs. TVF is more cumbersome but does have an advantage in that you can more readily notice any variations in the patient's voice intensity that may be producing bogus results. The author finds both tests difficult but useful so prefers to do both using them to confirm or refute findings suspected with the other. Thus, if an area where TVF is suspected to be increased is found but this is not certain, it is useful to be able to test VR over that area: if TVF was truly abnormal, VR should be too. However, if you are very confident in your TVF findings, it is not unreasonable to omit VR (or vice versa).

Keypoints

- VR tests the same phenomenon as TVF.
- Consolidation increases VR; effusion, collapse, and pneumothorax reduce it.
- Assess VR at apices, upper chest, and axillae anteriorly and over the upper, middle, and lower chest posteriorly.

3. Assess vocal resonance over the chest: upper right, upper left, middle right, middle left, lower right, lower left.

Sitting forward

18. Change the patient's position to facilitate examination of the neck and the back of the chest (DF 6/10).

Now it is time to get the patient to sit forward. This allows examination of the neck and the posterior aspect of the chest. Examination of the anterior aspect of the chest and axillae has allowed a thorough examination over the upper and middle lobes of the lungs, but only a minor portion of the lower lobes. Examination of the back of the chest is particularly important as it allows the evaluation of the lower lobes (Fig. 5.8) where many pulmonary conditions tend to be prominent. The upper third of the posterior aspect of the chest overlies the upper lung lobes whilst the lower two-thirds overlies the lower lobes.

CASE 5.48

Problem. The patient can't sit forward.

Discussion. Common sense is necessary. Depending on the patient's condition various solutions are possible.

1. If the patient is slightly weak, help the patient to sit forward and then stabilize in the above position.
2. If the patient is moderately weak, help the patient to sit over the side of the bed leaning on a table.
3. If the patient is severely weak, it may not be appropriate to sit the patient up and you may have to confine yourself to auscultating from the front over posterior aspect of the axilla.

When patients are weak, you may need to abbreviate the subsequent examination to the most useful tests: percussion and auscultation at the bases of the lungs.

Keypoints

1. Examination of the back of the chest allows thorough evaluation of the lower lobes of the lungs.
2. Make sure the patient is comfortable.
3. You may need to adopt a different position and approach if the patient is weak.

How?

1. Ask the patient to sit forward. The ideal position is arms crossed—so that the scapulae are rotated laterally. However, patients may have difficulty maintaining this position. A more comfortable alternative is for the patient to sit with their hands on their knees.
2. Explain that you now wish to examine their neck and the back of their chest.
3. Remove pillows and let down the headrest of the bed to allow easy access to the patient's back.
4. If need be, ask the patient to shuffle down the bed to give you more room behind him.
5. Check that the patient is comfortable—they will need to stay in this position for a few minutes.

Palpation for lymph nodes in neck

19. Examine the neck for enlarged lymph nodes (DF 8/10).

Why examine?

Enlarged lymph nodes at any site may be due to either generalized or local disease (Table 5.12). When lung disease spreads via the lymphatics, it tends to involve the nodes of the neck particularly the supraclavicular nodes. Thus, enlarged nodes in the neck may be an important sign of lung disease. About one in five patients with lung cancer have enlarged lymph nodes in the neck. The nodes tend to be hard. They may be very small initially but later may fuse together to form a mass that is fixed to structures underneath. The nodes tend to develop in the supraclavicular area especially deep between the sternal and clavicular heads of sternocleidomastoid. Other common causes of enlarged lymph nodes in the supraclavicular region are lymphoma, tuberculosis, and sarcoidosis. In these cases, the enlarged nodes are firm, rubbery (not hard), and discrete and do not attach to underlying structures. The exception is advanced tuberculosis, which can produce matted nodes that fuse together. Rarely, enlarged supraclavicular nodes are due to other cancers, such as those affecting the head or neck. Cancer affecting the stomach or pancreas may cause an enlarged node in the left supraclavicular region, known as Virchow's node (*Rudolf Virchow (1821–1902), German pathologist and politician*). Higher up the neck, enlarged nodes are most commonly due to local infections particularly throat infections, which usually produce tender, enlarged submandibular nodes.

How to examine

Also see Chapter 12. As for the axillary nodes, it is important for the muscles to be as relaxed as possible to facilitate palpation of any neck nodes. Also, it is better (less painful) if in general you use the flats of the palmar aspects of your fingers and only use the tips of your fingers where necessary to get a better feel.

1. Stand behind the patient.
2. Ask the patient to flex their head slightly (so that the neck muscles are relaxed).
3. If you palpate any lumps, ascertain their approximate size, consistency (firm or hard), whether they are discrete or fused together, and whether they are attached to underlying structures.
4. Supraclavicular
    1. Using your index, middle, and ring fingers together, gently palpate both supraclavicular fossae (Fig. 5.16).
    2. Use the tips of your index fingers to palpate the space between the two heads of sternocleidomastoid (Fig. 5.17).

TABLE 5.12 Causes of enlarged lymph nodes

Generalized	
Malignant	Lymphoma, acute and chronic lymphatic leukaemia
Viral	Infectious mononucleosis, cytomegalovius, human immunodeficiency virus
Bacterial	Tuberculosis, syphilis, brucellosis
Toxoplasmosis	
Sarcoidosis	
Local	
Acute or chronic infection	
Metastatic cancer	

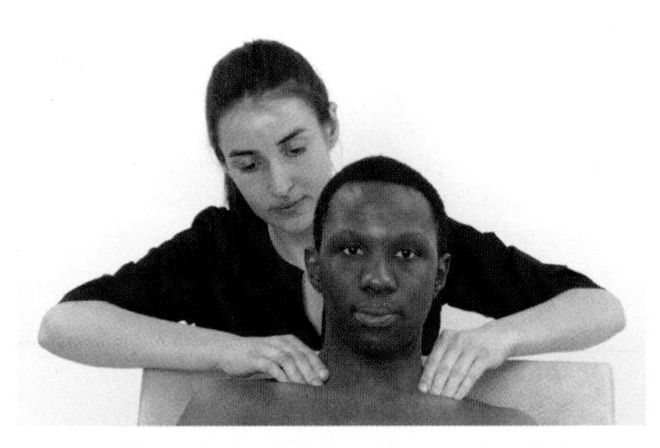

Fig. 5.16 Palpating for lymph nodes in the supraclavicular fossae.

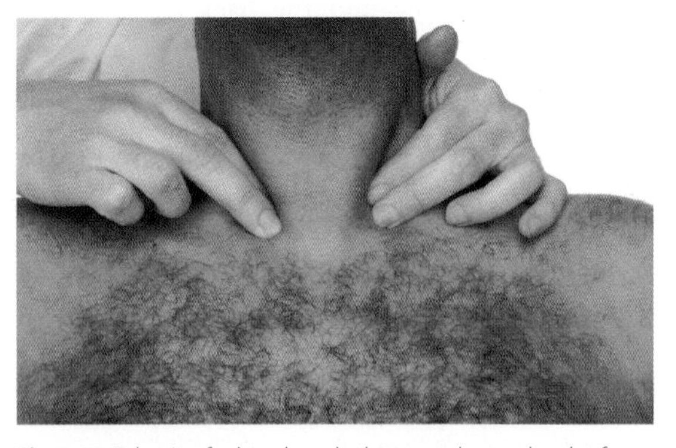

Fig. 5.17 Palpating for lymph nodes between the two heads of sternocleidomastoid.

3. Sternocleidomastoids
    1. It is best to examine the two sides separately—avoiding potential bilateral palpation of the carotid sinus, which may cause fainting.
    2. Use your right index, middle, and ring fingers together to slowly palpate up the right sternocleidomastoid to the angle of the jaw.
    3. Use your left hand to do the same on the patient's left side.
4. Submandibular
    1. Here, you really have to use the tips of your fingers. Use index, middle, and ring fingers together to palpate both sides simultaneously.
    2. Palpate under the angle the jaw.
    3. Work your way forward on both sides to meet at the chin.

Keypoints

- When lung disease spreads via the lymphatics, it may involve the nodes of the neck.
- Lung cancer tends to produce hard nodes, which may fuse together to form a mass fixed to structures underneath.
- Nodes due to lung cancer usually develop in the superclavicular area especially deep between the sternal and clavicular heads of sternocleidomastoid.
- Other causes of enlarged lymph nodes tend to result in firm, rubbery, discrete nodes, which do not fix to underlying structures.
- To examine for lymph nodes, make sure the muscles and tendons are as relaxed as possible.

Posterior chest inspection and palpation

20. Inspect the back of chest assessing movement (DF 8/10), chest shape (DF 4/10), and other visible abnormalities (DF 4/10).

See also inspection of front of chest (p. 91).

Why examine?

The aim is to examine for abnormalities of the back of the chest including:

(1) kyphoscoliosis (see p. 93);

(2) thoracotomy scar—operations on the lungs especially for lung cancer often require a long, diagonal incision usually near the base of one lung;

(3) chest drains (p. 93), indicating pleural effusion;

(4) sequelae of investigation or treatment of pleural effusions (large bandage or 0.5–1 cm scar indicating recent chest drain, 1mm mark or small plaster indicating recent pleural aspiration).

How to examine

1. Stand behind the patient and inspect the back of the chest.
2. Certain abnormalities will be obvious such as kyphoscoliosis, thoracotomy scar, or a plaster over a chest drain or aspirate site.
3. Inspect carefully for marks at the base of the lungs suggesting recent chest drain or aspiration.
4. Next, ask the patient to take a deep breath in and then out through their mouth.
5. As the patient breathes, watch the chest carefully and concentrate on whether one side is moving more than the other—assymetrical expansion suggests unilateral disease.
6. Then, ask the patient to repeat their deep breath in and out. If your opinion remains unchanged, this part of the examination is complete. If you are unsure get your patient to continue breathing until you are.

Keypoints

- The principles are the same as for the front of the chest
- Look carefully for thoracotomy scars and sequelae of pleural effusions.

21. If appropriate, palpate the posterior aspect of the chest for possible rib fractures (DF 8/10).

See also palpation of the praecordium re: rib fractures (p. 96).

How to examine

1. Ask the patient 'Is the back of your chest painful or tender?'
2. If the answer is 'yes', ask for permission to examine: 'Do you mind if I examine the painful or tender spots?'
3. If your patient consents, gently palpate the painful area. Can you elicit tenderness? Is the painful or tender spot within a hard bony area suggesting rib injury or tumour?

22. Palpate for chest expansion posteriorly, comparing both sides (DF 8/10).

See 'Palpation of chest expansion' (p. 97).

23. Percuss the back of chest, comparing the two sides (DF 9/10).

See 'Chest percussion' (p. 100).

24. Assess tactile vocal fremitus over the posterior aspect of the chest, comparing the two sides (DF 9/10).

See 'Tactile vocal fremitus' (p. 102).

25. Auscultate over the back of the chest, comparing the two sides (DF 8/10).

See 'Chest auscultation' (p. 104).

26. Assess vocal resonance over the back of the chest and in the axillae, comparing the two sides (DF 7/10).

See 'Vocal resonance' (p. 107).

Other respiratory signs

27. Look for other signs such as whispering pectoriloquy or peripheral oedema if appropriate.

As mentioned on p. 15 (Case 3.7), the respiratory routine is an abbreviation of all possible respiratory signs. Some respiratory signs normally omitted from the routine are discussed in the next pages.

Whispering pectoriloquy

(DF 8/10.) This is a very similar test to VR. Instead of the patient saying 'ninety-nine', they whisper the words. Compared to normal speech, whispering produces higher frequency sounds (well over 400 Hz). Normally, whispered words are muffled when auscultated with the stethoscope and are not often heard. Consolidated lung conducts high frequencies even better than low frequencies so that in some cases of consolidation the whisper is heard well: this is whispering pectoriloquy. Whispering pectoriloquy can sometimes be heard at the top of large pleural effusions where some collapse or consolidated lung may be found.

Keypoints

- Whispering adds confirmatory evidence in the presence of increased VR.
- Whispering pectoriloquy can sometimes be heard at the top of large pleural effusions if there is consolidation above the effusion.

Various

Peripheral oedema

Peripheral oedema has many causes (see p. 30). However, if combined with an elevated JVP in a respiratory context it may indicate cor pulmonale. Cor pulmonale occurs when respiratory disease causes chronic hypoxia, which in turn results in pulmonary hypertension and right heart failure. Cor pulmonale indicates that the respiratory system is under considerable strain and as such represents a serious development in a patient with respiratory disease. So you should always check for peripheral oedema if you have found an elevated JVP suggesting cor pulmonale or if there are signs of chronic chest disease such as COPD or fibrosis.

Tip

Beware the trap of assuming all patients with respiratory disease with a raised JVP and peripheral oedema have cor pulmonale. As ischaemic heart disease is also common, your patient may have COPD and concurrent congestive heart failure.

Temperature

Fever (pyrexia) is defined as a temperature higher than the 99th percentile of temperature found in normal individuals. In healthy people between the ages of 18 and 40 years, this has been found to be an oral temperature >37.2°C in the morning and an oral temperature >37.7°C in the evening. The different cut-offs in morning and evening reflect the diurnal variation in temperature (mean temperature is 36.4°C in the morning and 36.9°C in the evening). Chest infections commonly (though not always) produce a pyrexia.

Sputum pot

If the patient has symptoms or signs suggestive of infection, you should ask if there is a sputum pot and if so request to inspect the sputum (p. 78). Yellow/green sputum will point you towards an infection. Copious amounts produced in one day should make you consider bronchiectasis. Also look out for signs of blood. Although blood can be found in infections, it does raise the spectre of cancer or tuberculosis. Your suspicions may deepen if other worrying symptoms such as weight loss or a persistent hoarse voice are present.

Wash your hands

28. Wash your hands.

Do not forget this important infection control measure!

Presentation of findings

29. Pause briefly and then present findings.

The aim is to describe your findings emphasizing any abnormality. Because you will have examined so many different areas, it is reasonable to omit certain signs if normal. However, certain findings must always be commented on whether normal or abnormal:

(1) general appearance;

(2) presence or absence of cyanosis;

(3) presence or absence of clubbing;

(4) pulse rate;

(5) respiratory rate;

(6) signs of carbon dioxide retention;

(7) signs of cor pulmonale;

(8) tracheal position;

(9) chest expansion, percussion, TVF, breath sounds (bronchial or vesicular, added sounds), and VR.

As regards carbon dioxide retention, a flapping tremor or bounding pulse need not be specifically mentioned if not present. Similarly if there is no evidence of elevated JVP or peripheral oedema, these need not be specifically mentioned. When describing expansion, percussion, TVF, breath sounds, and VR, it is not necessary to detail your findings over each area of the lungs. It is more important to emphasize any abnormal findings. An example might be as follows. 'This woman looks generally well and is not cyanosed. However, she is tachycardic with a pulse rate of 110/min though has a normal respiratory rate at 14/min. She shows no signs of cor pulmonale or carbon dioxide retention. The trachea is not deviated. Percussion note, TVF, and VR are normal over most of the chest with vesicular breath sounds. However, expansion is reduced on the right side and there is an area of dullness over the right lower lobe with bronchial breath sounds and increased TVF and VR. There are no added sounds. This is consistent with an area of consolidation in the right lower lobe.'

Notice that many features that were examined for have not been mentioned, such as the face, eyes, tremor, and tar staining.

CASE 5.49

Problem. My findings don't add up. I think I heard bronchial breathing at the right base but found no other abnormality on auscultation or percussion and no change in TVF or VR.

Discussion. You must have got something wrong. The findings should add up. If there really is bronchial breathing, there should be other signs of lung consolidation, collapse, or fibrosis. Check again. The other possibility is that the breath sounds are really vesicular (normal).

Keypoints

- Emphasize any abnormality.
- If your findings don't add up, think again.

Respiratory diseases and investigations

See Table 5.13.

Pleural effusion

Pleural effusion refers to abnormal fluid in the pleural space. What is the pleural space? The visceral pleura is closely applied to the underlying parietal pleura, which in turn is adherent to the thoracic wall. The pleural space is the potential space between the visceral and parietal pleurae. This space is normally filled by a thin layer of lubricating fluid, which ensures friction-free movement of the pleural surfaces.

Causes

There are multiple causes of pleural effusion (Table 5.14). These are usefully categorized into transudates and exudates according to the protein content of the fluid. For this reason it is common to evaluate pleural effusions by aspirating a small amount of pleural fluid through a needle. The most important part of the diagnostic evaluation is to decide whether there is evidence of malignancy.

In general, transudates are bilateral though they may occasionally be unilateral (in which case they are usually right sided). Exudates are usually unilateral, though in the case of collagen vascular disease can be bilateral. Pulmonary emboli without infarction causes a transudate; if infarction is present, the fluid is an exudate.

Symptom

Breathlessness.

Signs

1. Expansion is reduced.
2. Percussion is very (stony) dull
3. VR and TVF are reduced.
4. Breath sounds are vesicular but of reduced intensity (often absent).
5. If the effusion is large the trachea and apex beat may be displaced away from it.

TABLE 5.13 A summary of clinical signs associated with important clinical conditions

Clinical condition	Position of trachea	Expansion	Percussion	Vocal resonance and tactile vocal fremitus	Whispering pectoriliquy	Auscultation
Normal	Central	Symmetrical	Resonant	Normal	Absent	Vesicular
Consolidation	Central	Decreased	Dull	Increased	May be present	Breath sounds bronchial with coarse crackles
Lobar collapse	Towards the lesion*	Decreased	Normal or dull	Decreased	May be present	Decreased breath sounds, may be bronchial breathing
Unilateral fibrosis	Towards the lesion*	Decreased on side of fibrosis	Normal	Increased	Absent	Fine crackles. Breath sounds usually vesicular but may be bronchial if fibrosis severe
Interstitial lung fibrosis	Central	Symmetrically decreased	Resonant	Increased	Absent	Fine crackles. Breath sounds usually vesicular but may be bronchial if fibrosis severe
Pleural effusion	Away from the fluid*	Decreased	Very (stony) dull	Decreased	Absent but may be present above a large effusion	Breath sounds vesicular but decreased
Pneumothorax	Central	Decreased	Hyper-resonant	Decreased	Absent	Breath sounds vesicular but reduced
Tension pneumothorax	Away from the pneumo-thorax*	Decreased	Hyper-resonant	Decreased	Absent	Absent breath sounds (may hear breath sounds from opposite lung)
Asthma or chronic obstructive pulmonary disease	Central	Symmetrically decreased	Resonant	Normal	Absent	Breath sounds vesicular with prolonged expiration and wheeze (either inspiratory and expiratory or both). Sometimes coarse crackles with added infection

* Any condition with the potential to shift the trachea (and hence the mediastinum) will only achieve this if it is of sufficient magnitude. Minor examples of these conditions will not cause a mediastinal shift.

Other types of fluid

The term 'pleural effusion' is usually reserved for serous fluid (though it may be blood stained) within the pleural space. Other types of fluid are given specific names:

(1) **haemothorax**—blood in the pleural space;

(2) **chylothorax**—chyle in the pleural space;

(3) **empyema**—pus in the pleural space.

Lung consolidation

Consolidation is where an area of lung is filled with fluid or solid matter. This classically occurs in infective pneumonia but may also be a feature of pulmonary haemorrhage or pneumonitis (lung inflammation due to non-infective causes such as drugs and auto-immune reactions). In the latter conditions, the consolidation is usually patchy and the signs variable. It is in infective pneumonia that enough lung is consolidated to give the classical signs of consolidation.

1. Expansion is reduced.
2. Percussion is dull.
3. VR and TVF are increased.
4. Breath sounds are bronchial breathing.

Lung collapse

If a bronchus is blocked off, the air in the part of the lung distal to the blockage is gradually reabsorbed leaving a portion of collapsed lung.

TABLE 5.14 Causes of pleural effusion

Transudate (protein content <30g/l)
Heart failure***
Hypoalbuminaemia due to chronic liver failure** or nephrotic syndrome*
Meig's syndrome (associated with an ovarian fibroma)* (Joe Vincent Meig (1892–1913), professor of gynaecology)
Pulmonary emboli**
Hypoalbuminaemia of other causes

Exudate (protein content > 30g / litre)
Pneumonia***
Tuberculosis**
Tumour (effusion may be bloody)—bronchial carcinoma**, breast cancer*, lymphoma **, mesothelioma*
Collagen vascular disease (rheumatoid arthritis* and systemic lupus erythematosus*)
Pulmonary infarction (may be bloody)**
Asbestos exposure*
Abdominal pathology (subphrenic abscess, pancreatitis)**

Ranging from * (uncommon) to *** (common).

Causes

1. **Pathology within the lumen.** Secretions—postoperative, asthma, cystic fibrosis, foreign body (classically a peanut).
2. **Pathology in the wall.** Bronchial carcinoma.
3. **Pathology compressing the wall from outside.** Enlarged lymph nodes usually due to bronchial carcinoma or lymphoma.

Symptom

Breathlessness.

Signs (may be minimal)

1. Expansion is reduced.
2. Percussion is dull.
3. VR and TVF are reduced.
4. Breath sounds are usually vesicular but of reduced intensity; there may be an area of bronchial breathing.
5. If the area of collapsed lung is large, the trachea (especially with upper lobe collapse) or the apex beat (especially with lower lobe collapse) may be displaced towards it.

Lung cancer

Lung cancer, variously known as cancer of the bronchus, lung carcinoma, or bronchial carcinoma, continues to be the commonest cause of cancer death in the UK. The major risk factor is smoking though one form of lung cancer (adenocarcinoma) appears not to be smoking related. Lung cancer may present with no symptoms or signs (when it has been identified by chance on a chest X-ray) otherwise it can cause a variety of symptoms and signs. Some of the more common features are described here.

1. Local damage within the lung, producing
   (1) cough, haemoptysis, breathlessness, chest pain, and wheeze (symptoms);
   (2) inspiratory wheezes, signs of lung collapse or pleural effusion, and clubbing (signs).
2. Direct spread within the thorax,
   (1) affecting the recurrent laryngeal nerve causing hoarseness;
   (2) affecting the sympathetic nerve chain causing Horner's syndrome;
   (3) affecting the phrenic nerve causing paralysis of the diaphragm (the paralysed diaphragm elevates, pushing the lung upwards; thus the part of the chest wall that normally overlies the lower lung overlies solid tissue such as liver instead (producing signs similar to a pleural effusion);
   (4) invading the superior vena cava causing SVC obstruction.
3. Metastatic spread to
   (1) supraclavicular lymph nodes;
   (2) liver producing hepatomegaly;
   (3) bones producing tender spots and pathological fractures;
   (4) brain with signs of hemiparesis.
4. Non-metastatic extra-pulmonary manifestations:
   (1) anorexia, weight loss, and fever;
   (2) hypercalcaemia;
   (3) neuropathy;
   (4) hypertrophic pulmonary osteoarthropathy;
   (5) myasthenia-like syndrome.

Mesothelioma

Mesothelioma is a malignant tumour of the pleura due to previous asbestos exposure. It is much less common than bronchial carcinoma.

Symptoms

1. Pain (sometimes but not usually pleuritic).
2. Breathlessness.

3. Tiredness.
4. Weight loss.

Signs

1. Clubbing.
2. Hypertrophic pulmonary osteoarthropathy.
3. Signs of a pleural effusion.
4. Enlarged supraclavicular or axillary lymph nodes.

Lung infections

Various infections may occur.

1. **Tracheitis.** Affects the trachea; usually viral; causes chest pain, cough, and sputum; no specific lung signs.
2. **Bronchitis.** Affects the main bronchi; usually viral; causes chest pain, cough, and sputum; no specific lung signs.
3. **Infective exacerbation of COPD.** Affects small bronchioles; usually due to viral infection, haemophilus influenzae, or streptococcus pneumoniae (pneumococcus); causes increased breathlessness, chest pain, increased cough and sputum, and wheeze; signs of carbon dioxide retention (flapping tremor, bounding pulse) may occur; lung signs—reduced intensity of breath sounds and increased wheezes; chest X-ray shows no new changes.
4. **Bronchopneumonia.** Affects the lung parenchyma (mainly alveoli) in a patchy fashion; usually caused by bacteria of low virulence such as haemophilus influenzae; causes breathlessness, chest pain, cough, and sputum; lung signs—crackles; chest X-ray shows patchy shadowing.
5. **Lobar pneumonia.** Affects the lung parenchyma such that whole areas of lung are solidified due to the inflammation; usually due to more virulent organisms such as pneumococcus; causes breathlessness, chest pain, cough, and sputum; lung signs—signs of consolidation (see p. 114), may sometimes be complicated by pleural effusion (see p. 113) or empyema (see below) producing mixed signs; as the consolidation resolves crackles develop; chest X-ray shows a distinct area of shadowing (Fig. 16.25).
6. **Pleurisy.** Affects the pleurae; usually a consequence of lobar pneumonia; causes pleuritic chest pain and pleural rub.
7. **Lung abscess.** Occurs when there is a localized collection of pus within the lung; may complicate pneumonia (especially that due to staphylococcus or klebsiella), aspiration of food into the lung, or bronchial obstruction by a foreign body; causes production of large amounts of foul-smelling sputum; produces clubbing and signs of consolidation or crackles; chest X-ray shows one distinct area of shadowing, typically with a fluid level within it (see Fig. 16.31) (lung abscess can be multiple).
8. **Empyema.** Occurs when there is a localized collection of pus within the pleural space; may complicate pneumonia but may also follow a subphrenic abscess or penetrating chest wound including surgery; produces clubbing and signs consistent with a pleural effusion; chest X-ray shows pleural effusion.
9. **Tuberculosis.** The tubercle bacillus deserves particular mention. Its various stages can cause lung collapse, fibrosis, consolidation, and effusion or empyema. Clubbing is not a feature of tuberculosis.

There are a few points to add.

1. Strictly speaking, tracheitis, bronchitis, pneumonia, and pleurisy are all defined as inflammation of the specific part of the respiratory tract. So they may result from physical, chemical, or allergic processes as well as infections. In the case of pneumonia, it is common parlance to use the term 'pneumonia' purely for infective processes. The term 'pneumonitis' is commonly used to describe non-infective processes.
2. All these conditions may produce generalized symptoms and signs such as fever, lethargy, anorexia, weight loss, and sweats. The severity of these systemic symptoms (and the disease in general) tends to be greater for bacteria than viruses, for distal disease (such as pneumonia) than proximal disease (such as tracheitis), and where there are collections of pus as in empyema or lung abscess.
3. The term 'chest infection' is often used. This is a vague, poorly defined term usually used to describe lung infections that do not produce shadowing on the X-ray, such as tracheitis, bronchitis, and infective exacerbations of COPD.
4. Bronchiectasis is a condition which results in dilated bronchi and is often a sequela of childhood infections. It is characterized by regular production of large amounts of purulent sputum. There may be associated breathlessness. Signs include clubbing and coarse crackles.

Small airways obstruction

There are two conditions characterized by small airways obstruction—asthma and COPD. Small airways obstruction primarily causes difficulty with expiration.

Asthma

Asthma is a clinical syndrome of unknown aetiology characterized by three components.

1. Recurrent episodes of small airways obstruction that resolve spontaneously or with treatment.
2. Airway hyper-responsiveness. This is an exaggerated tendency to bronchoconstrict to stimuli that have little effect on normal individuals.
3. Inflammation of the airways.

Asthma can be a life-threatening condition and is a common cause of hospital admission. The characteristic symptoms are breathlessness and wheeze. On examination, the characteristic findings are increased respiratory rate and heart rate and on auscultation reduced breath sound intensity with prolonged expiration and expiratory wheezes (though there may also be inspiratory wheezes). The British Thoracic Society have produced guidelines that use clinical features to recognize severe or life-threatening attacks.

Severe acute asthma is indicated by the presence of **any** of the following:

(1) unable to complete sentences because of breathlessness;

(2) respiratory rate ≥25 breaths/min;

(3) heart rate persistently ≥110 beats/min;

(4) peak expiratory flow rate (PEFR) <40% of normal;

(5) a drop in systolic blood pressure on inspiration ≥10 mm Hg (pulsus paradoxus).

A life-threatening attack of asthma is indicated by the presence of **any** of the following:

(1) silent chest on auscultation;

(2) cyanosis;

(3) bradycardia;

(4) exhaustion, confusion, and unconsciousness.

Chronic obstructive pulmonary disease

Chronic obstructive pulmonary disease is characterized by airway obstruction due to chronic bronchitis or emphysema. This obstruction may vary but never returns to normal: there is an irreversible component. Chronic bronchitis is defined as the presence of cough productive of sputum on most days of at least 3 months of at least 2 successive years. The diagnosis of emphysema is pathological: destruction of air spaces distal to the terminal bronchioles due to destruction of their walls (mostly alveolar destruction). Both emphysema and chronic bronchitis are usually due to tobacco consumption and tend to occur together.

Effects

The characteristic symptoms of COPD are cough, sputum, breathlessness, and wheeze. Examination may reveal the following:

(1) increased antero-posterior chest diameter (barrel chest);

(2) pursed lips breathing;

(3) use of accessory muscles of respiration;

(4) reduced expansion bilaterally;

(5) percussion note may be a little hyperresonant;

(6) VR and TVF may be reduced bilaterally;

(7) breath sounds are vesicular, but of reduced intensity, prolonged expiration, wheezes that may be confined to expiration or occur both in inspiration and expiration and crackles;

(8) as the disease progresses, chronic hypoxia may produce cyanosis and signs of cor pulmonale (elevated JVP, ankle oedema, and right ventricular heave).

There are three points to add.

1. Many patients have combinations of asthma and COPD where there is some reversibility. It may be difficult to say which is the more important component in such cases. Table 5.15 gives some differences, albeit stereotypical, which may help to decide which is more important.
2. β_2-agonist drugs such as salbutamol are one of the mainstays of treatment for both asthma and COPD

TABLE 5.15 Asthma compared with chronic obstructive pulmonary disease

	Asthma	Chronic obstructive pulmonary disease
Age group	Young	Old
Smoker for more than 10 years	No	Yes
Breathless between attacks	No	Yes

TABLE 5.16 Causes of pulmonary fibrosis

Causes
Auto-immune
Idiopathic (= cryptogenic) pulmonary fibrosis (L)
Scleroderma (L)
Sarcoidosis (U)
Rheumatoid arthritis (L)
Inhalation of irritants
Asbestosis (L)
Coal-miners' pneumoconioisis (U)
Silicosis (U)
Extrinsic allergic alveolitis (U)
Drugs (amiodarone, methotrexate) (L)
Post infection or tuberculosis (U)

U, predisposition to upper lobes; L, predisposition to lower lobes.

treatment. They themselves may produce clinical signs, for example, tremor and tachycardia.

3. Clubbing is not a feature of COPD.

Pulmonary fibrosis

Fibrosis of lung tissue is the reaction of the lung tissue to a variety of insults (Table 5.16). Different conditions tend to affect different parts of the lung to greater or lesser extents. Fibrosis can also be localized or generalized in distribution. Localized fibrosis may be caused by infection especially tuberculosis, infarction, or previous radiotherapy. Generalized fibrosis may be caused by the inhalation of irritants, auto-immune disorders, or drugs. An immune response leads to a diffuse infiltrate in the lungs, which can lead to thickening and fibrosis around alveolar walls (called fibrosing alveolitis). The fibrosing alveolitis is called idiopathic or cryptogenic when the cause cannot be identified. More recently different histopathological groups have been identified with different natural histories and therefore prognoses. The term 'idiopathic interstitial pneumonia' has become the all-embracing term for these different groups and idiopathic fibrosing alveolitis has become one of the sub-groups (and is also known as usual interstitial fibrosis) (see Fig. 5.18). Whatever the cause, pulmonary fibrosis tends to cause breathlessness and a dry cough. The main signs are clubbing and crackles over the affected lobes. Breath sounds are usually vesicular but if the fibrosis is severe may be bronchial. Clubbing is a particular feature of idiopathic pulmonary fibrosis and asbestosis. It is rare in scleroderma, silicosis, sarcoidosis, tuberculosis, and in drug-induced fibrosis.

Pulmonary embolism

This is where part of the pulmonary arterial circulation is blocked off by a thrombus that originated from the venous system. It is sometimes complicated by pulmonary infarction (where a portion of lung tissue infarcts).

Effects

The effects depend on size of thrombus, whether the embolism is persistent, and whether it causes pulmonary infarction:

(1) **small embolism, one-off**—no clinical features;

(2) **small emboli due to persistent embolism (chronic thrombo-embolic disease)**—breathlessness and signs of pulmonary hypertension—elevated jugular venous pulse, right ventricular heave, and tricuspid regurgitation murmur;

(3) **medium embolism, no infarction**—breathlessness and tachypnoea;

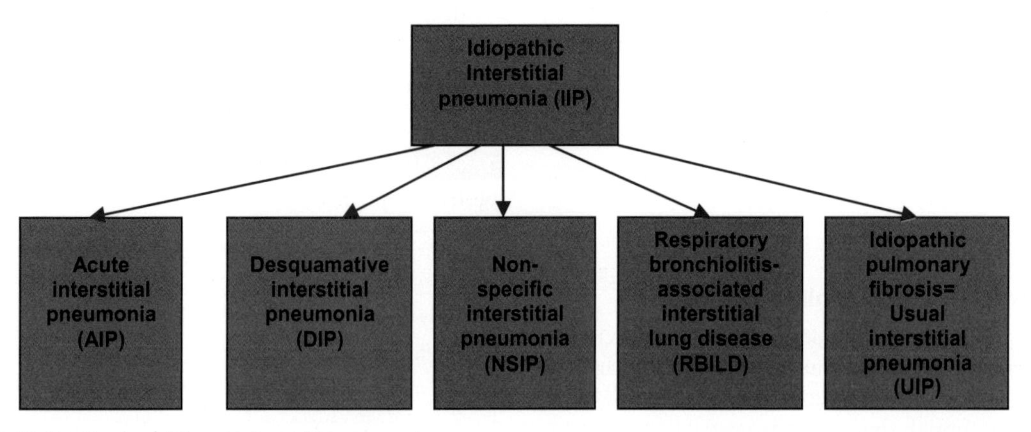

Fig. 5.18 Classification of idiopathic interstitial pneumonia.

(4) **medium embolism with associated pulmonary infarction**—breathlessness, pleuritic chest pain, tachypnoea, pleural rub, and pleural effusion;

(5) **major embolism**—breathlessness, central chest pain, hypotension, cyanosis, elevated jugular venous pulse, and sudden death.

The clinical features of pulmonary embolism are neither sensitive nor specific in making the diagnosis.

1. The diagnosis is best confirmed with a 'spiral' CT lung scan (or isotope ventilation/perfusion scan). However, because of the potential seriousness of the diagnosis, anti-coagulant treatment should be started as soon as the diagnosis is suspected—do not wait for the scan result.
2. Patients with medium embolism and no infarction produce very non-specific clinical features. So always consider pulmonary embolism in patients with unexplained breathlessness.

> **Tip**
>
> Always check the legs for signs of a deep venous thrombosis: unilateral leg swelling, stiffness of the calf muscles, increased warmth of the affected side, and tenderness between the heads of the gastrocnemius muscle. Such signs are present in around one-third of pulmonary embolism patients.

Pneumothorax

Pneumothorax refers to air in the pleural space. A pneumothorax occurs when damage to the lung causes air to leak from the lung, through the visceral pleura into the pleural space. Such damage may occur either spontaneously or less commonly following trauma (see Table 5.17).

TABLE 5.17 Causes of pneumothorax

Spontaneous
Any lung disease, especially emphysema
Subpleural bleb, usually in young adults (mostly men) with otherwise normal lungs
Trauma
Iatrogenic, following pleural aspiration or central line insertion
Chest wall injury

Effects

The presence of air in the pleural space abolishes the negative pressure within the space, which provides the suction force that maintains the inflation of the lungs.

Symptoms

The air within the pleural space may cause pleuritic pain while the lung collapse causes breathlessness.

Signs

1. Expansion is reduced.
2. Percussion is hyper-resonant.
3. VR and TVF are reduced.
4. Breath sounds are vesicular but reduced.

Tension pneumothorax

In this condition, air in the pleural space accumulates creating sufficient pressure to force the mediastinum and its contents to away from the side of the pneumothorax. This is a dangerous development (see below).

Causes

In most cases of pneumothorax, the leak closes off as the lung deflates. In the case of a tension pneumothorax, the opening from the lung into the pleural space not only persists but acts as a valve so that air enters the pleural space in inspiration but cannot exit on expiration. Tension pneumothorax usually follows trauma and only rarely occurs spontaneously.

Effects

This is an emergency situation. As the pressure in the pleural space builds up, not only does the lung collapse, but the mediastinum is pushed further towards the opposite side until venous return to the heart is reduced with a consequent reduction in cardiac output.

Symptoms

1. Pleuritic pain.
2. Severe breathlessness.

Signs

1. Expansion is minimal.
2. Percussion is hyper-resonant.
3. VR and TVF are absent.
4. Breath sounds are absent.
5. Often accompanied by hypotension, cyanosis, and tachypnoea. There may be signs of mediastinal

displacement with the trachea and apex beat shifted away from the affected side.

Spirometry

The spirometer is a machine that measures the volume of air blown into it.

There are two key measurements:

1. **Forced vital capacity (FVC).** This is the volume of air expelled by a maximal expiration—from an initial position of full inspiration.
2. **Forced expiratory volume over 1 s (FEV1).** This is the volume of air expelled in the first second, again from an initial position of full inspiration.

The ratio of FEV1/FVC is usually calculated. This is normally around 70% (somewhat higher in young people). In small airways obstruction, both the FEV1 and FVC are reduced but the FEV1 disproportionately so—so that the FEV1/FVC ratio is reduced. In pulmonary fibrosis, again both FEV1 and FVC are reduced but the FVC disproportionately more so—so that the FEV1/FVC is increased.

Peak expiratory flow rate

The PEFR is the maximal rate of flow of expired air. The measurement is obtained using a peak expiratory flow meter (Fig. 5.19). As in spirometry, the patient should start after taking a full inspiration. However, rather than a prolonged expiration, the aim is to blow as hard as possible into the meter. The meter measures this maximal flow rate. The PEFR is reduced in small airways obstruction and as such is commonly used to monitor asthma control.

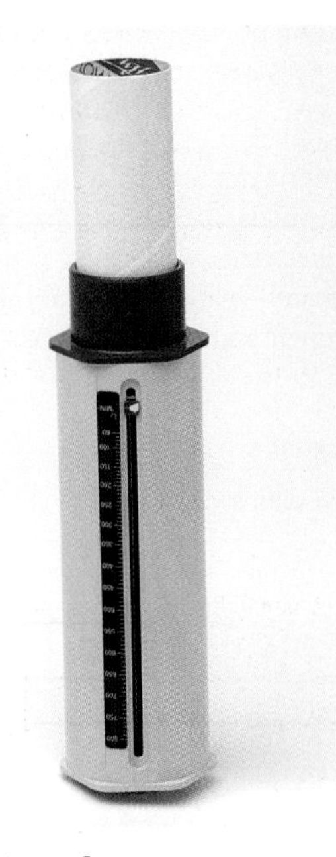

Fig. 5.19 A peak expiratory flow meter.

Bronchoscopy

This is where a fibre optic instrument (similar but smaller to that used in gastroscopy, see p. 180) is passed into the bronchial tree to inspect it for pathology. Only proximal lesions close to the bronchial tree are usually suitable for this procedure (peripheral lesions are best investigated using CT scanning with or without fine needle biopsy). As well as observing lesions there is also the facility to biopsy specimens for histological analysis, aspirate fluid for culture and cytology, and sometimes remove mucus plugs or other thickened secretions that can cause respiratory embarrassment.

Finals section

In this section, some specific issues dealing with Finals will be discussed. This is not a summary section. For revision, I suggest you read the keypoints throughout the chapter and the examination summary (p. 81) and do the questions on pp. 122–3.

In exams, the examiners need patients with consistent signs. Thus, patients with pulmonary fibrosis and bronchiectasis are common Finals diagnoses whereas in day-to-day practice, students will more often be tested on patients with pleural effusions and consolidation (see Tables 5.18 and 5.19). The latter is particularly uncommon in examinations, as pneumonia is an unpredictable illness the signs of which usually resolve in a matter of weeks with treatment.

TABLE 5.18 Common Finals cases

Pulmonary fibrosis
Bronchiectasis
Pleural effusion

TABLE 5.19 Common day-to-day cases

Asthma or chronic obstructive pulmonary disease
Pleural effusion
Consolidation
Pulmonary fibrosis
Bronchiectasis

Key diagnostic clues

In day-to-day medicine, the key signs are those pointing to severity of asthma or COPD such as pulse and respiratory rate and any added auscultatory sounds. However, as regards Finals, the key signs are clubbing, expansion (as measured by both inspection and palpation), and percussion or auscultation especially at the bases of the lungs posteriorly.

Key signs for Finals

1. **Pulmonary fibrosis.** Clubbing, fine crackles at bases of lungs bilaterally posteriorly.
2. **Bronchiectasis.** Clubbing, coarse crackles at bases of lungs bilaterally posteriorly.
3. **Pleural effusion.** On affected side—expansion reduced, very (stony) dull to percussion, reduced breath sound intensity, reduced TVF and VR, trachea may be deviated away from affected side
4. **Consolidation.** On affected side—expansion reduced, dull to percussion, bronchial breathing, increased TVF and VR.

Some advice relating to examination problems now follows.

Some advice relating to examination problems

General

Do not waste time looking for the respiratory system examination routine that will completely satisfy all examiners. It does not exist! Use the one given on p. 81.

The instruction

The examiner will usually ask you to 'examine the respiratory system'. Occasionally, they will say 'examine the chest'. These both mean the same thing. However, if the examiner is more specific, such as 'auscultate at the bases', you must do just as they request. With such requests, the possibility of confusion here is in how to fit in the 'general look'. This should be done, as always, while preparing the patient for examination.

Moving infirm patients

Always proceed with the aim of carrying out the full examination requested asking the patient's permission as you go. If the examiner feels moving such a patient is inappropriate, they will stop you.

Positioning

Even if the patient is already sitting in bed at around 45°, you should alter their position, albeit minimally, to make it clear to the examiner that you know the patient should be at that angle.

Hands

Clubbing is the key sign. You need to make a clear decision on its absence or presence. Clubbing is much more common in examination patients so if you think it is present, you are probably correct. Try not to spend longer than 30 s.

Face

With respect to Horner's, it can be very easy to over-diagnose anhidrosis and ptosis. The clearest sign in Horner's is the miosis; if this is not present it would be unwise to diagnose Horner's. SVC obstruction, is very easy to overlook; just make sure you consider it as a possibility before moving on.

Neck

While the JVP can be an important sign in the respiratory system, it is nowhere near as fundamental as it is in the cardiovascular system. If you cannot see it, do not spend ages analysing why. Simply consider it not elevated.

Inspect front of chest from end of bed

This is the best way of identifying unilateral disease. Pleural effusion, pneumothorax, and consolidation all cause a reduction in expansion on the affected side—so concentrate. Three breaths in and out is enough: more than this is unlikely to enlighten you further but may cause the patient to become light-headed.

Palpate apex beat

As for the JVP, the apex beat is a sign that can be difficult to assess whilst not adding much information to the respiratory examination. It is often impalpable as in COPD and even if you do suspect that it is not in the normal position, there are lots of cardiac reasons to explain this. So, if you cannot feel the apex beat, move on quickly. If you think the apex beat is in an abnormal position it would be unusual to find a respiratory cause to explain this.

Percussion, tactile vocal fremitus, breath sounds, and vocal resonance

It is clearly important to examine over the whole of the chest. However, you will need to combine brevity with thoroughness.

Percussion

Practise percussion as much as possible (perhaps more than other signs) because your technique will be seen as an indicator of how much time you have spent with patients. Even if you get the case wrong, the examiner cannot fail to be impressed if your percussion technique is slick

Tactile vocal fremitus and vocal resonance

Stick to 'ninety-nine'. You do not want to stand out (other than for your expertise).

Examination of the front of the chest as a whole

In the examination setting, common cases such as pulmonary fibrosis, bronchiectasis, and pleural effusion may produce little in the way of signs on the front of the chest. So if you have not found any abnormality by the time you begin examination of the back of the chest, do not worry. It is the bases posteriorly that usually hold the answer.

Axillae

The axillae should be examined whilst examining the front of the chest. Sometimes, you will realize that in the heat of the moment, you have forgotten to do this. If this is the case, it is quite reasonable to examine the axilla from behind.

Putting the signs together

The signs should make sense. If you find an area of dullness, the breath sounds should also be altered (reduced in pleural effusion or bronchial in consolidation) as should the TVF and VR (reduced in pleural effusion and increased in consolidation). It is reasonable to perhaps expect that one or two of the five key features (expansion, percussion, TVF, breath sounds, and VR) do not quite add up, but to find one isolated abnormality is very unlikely. Clubbing combined with crackles has three key causes (Table 5.20).

TABLE 5.20 Causes of clubbing and bilateral basal crackles

Idiopathic pulmonary fibrosis
Bronchiectasis
Asbestosis

Washing hands

See p. 72.

Presentation

Vocal resonance at the back is the last part of the examination of the chest itself. Whilst doing this, formulate your thoughts as to what you have found overall.

Good luck!

Questions

The more stars, the more important it is to know the answer.

1. Give three causes of chronic cough not due to chest disease. *
2. Does the cough of lung cancer have clear characteristic features? *
3. What might foul-smelling sputum be indicative of? *
4. What is the nailbed angle? *
5. What are the three commonest causes of clubbing? ****
6. Name another six causes of clubbing. **
7. Why does clubbing occur? *
8. What is hypertrophic pulmonary osteoarthropathy? *
9. Give two features that suggest that an acute asthma attack is severe. **
10. What are the three key features of Horner's syndrome? **
11. Give four causes of haemoptysis. ****
12. What circumstances would require urgent action in a case of haemoptysis? ****
13. What is pigeon fancier's lung? **
14. What is a flapping tremor and what is its possible significance in respiratory cases? ***
15. Give three causes of Horner's syndrome. ***
16. What is the difference between a lung lobe and zone? *
17. Give three causes of tracheal deviation. *
18. If one side of the chest is duller than the other, it is usually that side that is abnormal. What is the exception to this rule? **
19. What is the tobacco exposure in pack years for a patient who has smoked 40 cigarettes per day for 30 years? *
20. What conditions can be associated with asbestos exposure? **
21. What respiratory infection would you suspect if a patient's pet bird had recently died following an illness? **
22. Give one cause of increased tactile vocal fremitus and three causes of reduced tactile vocal fremitus. **
23. Describe the difference between bronchial and vesicular breath sounds. ****
24. Give two mechanisms by which crackles occur. *
25. What two features of wheezes correlate with the severity of obstruction? **
26. Which lymph node site does lung cancer usually spread to? **

27. Which lymph node site does breast cancer usually spread to? **
28. What are the two main categories of pleural effusion? ****
29. Give 10 causes of pleural effusion. ****
30. What is Schamroth's sign? **
31. What is Cheyne-Stokes respiration? Name two associations. **
32. How is cyanosis produced? ***
33. What is methaemaglobinaemia? **
34. Give four physical signs of superior vena caval obstruction. ****
35. Compare percussion note, breath sounds, and tactile vocal fremitus in lung consolidation, lung collapse, and pleural effusion. ****
36. What is Cor pulmonale? ***
37. What is Kussmaul's respiration? ***
38. What are the accessory muscles of breathing? *
39. What happens to the FEV1/FVC in small airways obstruction and pulmonary fibrosis? **
40. What examination features would you expect with a left-sided pneumothorax? ****
41. What is surgical emphysema? **
42. What is pectus excavatum? *
43. What is pectus carinatum? *
44. Describe the characteristics of bronchial breathing. In which conditions might you encounter it? ****
45. When might you hear a pleural rub? **
46. What is whispering pectoriloquy and when might you encounter it? ***

Score. Give 4 marks for 4 stars, 1 for 1 star, and so on. At the end of the third year, you should be scoring 60-plus and by Finals, 80-plus; 90-plus is very good.

Further reading

British Thoracic Society. Community acquired pneumonia in adults in British hospitals in 1982–1983: a survey of aetiology, mortality, prognostic factors and outcome. *Quarterly Journal of Medicine* 1987; **62**:195–220.

British Thoracic Society. Guidelines for the management of asthma in adults: II—acute severe asthma. *British Medical Journal* 1990; **301**:797–800.

Buller AJ, Dornhorst AC. The physics of some pulmonary signs. *Lancet* 1956; **ii**:649–51.

Coury C. Hippocratic fingers and hypertrophic osteoarthropathy. A study of 350 cases. *British Journal of Diseases of the Chest* 1960; **54**:202–9.

Currie GP, Gray RD, Mc Kay J. Chronic cough. *British Medical Journal* 2003; **326**:261.

Hirschberg B, Biran I, Glazer M, Kramer MR. Hemoptysis: etiology, evaluation and outcome in a tertiary referral hospital. *Chest* 1997; **112**:440–4.

Hooker EA, O'Brien DJ, Danzi DF, Barefoot JAC, Brown JE. Respiratory rates in emergency department patients. *The Journal of Emergency Medicine* 1989; **7**:129–32.

Irwin RS, Curley FJ, French CL. Chronic cough. The spectrum and frequency of causes, key components of the diagnostic evaluation, and outcome of specific therapy. *American Review of Respiratory Disease* 1990; **141**:640–7.

Mackowiak PA, Wasserman SS, Levine MM. A critical appraisal of 96.8° F, the upper limit of the normal body temperature, and other legacies of Carl Reinhold August Wunderlich. *Journal of the American Medical Association* 1992; **268**:1578–80.

Martin JF, Kristensen SD. Finger clubbing. *Lancet* 1991; **338**:947.

Murphy RLH, Holford SK, Knowler WC. Visual lung-sound characterisation by time-expanded wave-form analysis. *New England Journal of Medicine* 1977; **296**:968–71.

CHAPTER 6

Abdominal system

Chapter contents

Introduction

The abdominal system includes the gastrointestinal tract from mouth to anus and the organs within the abdominal cavity. It is important because the abdomen is affected by several common (and some potentially serious) diseases, for example, peptic ulcer, gastro-oesophageal reflux disease, irritable bowel syndrome, inflammatory bowel disease, and cancer. Also, diseases from other systems may cause abdominal symptoms—diarrhoea, constipation, vomiting, weight loss, and so on. In this chapter, you will learn what to ask patients with abdominal diseases and how to examine the abdominal system.

Symptoms

There are many diseases that affect the gastrointestinal tract. To be able to diagnose these conditions you will need to learn about them and how they present. Although this chapter will concentrate on common symptoms that affect the abdomen, it must be remembered that no one symptom is diagnostic. What you will learn to do is ask about a range of symptoms and the responses you get from your patients will help to build a picture of the disease, that with practice, will help guide you to a diagnosis.

Abdominal pain

Abdominal pain (particularly of the upper abdomen) is a common complaint. Pain in the epigastric region can often be mistaken for retrosternal pain and vice versa, leading to problems with diagnosis (see Case 4.1).

The approach to abdominal pain is similar to that of pain anywhere else in the body. However your questions will be modified to reflect this area of enquiry. Common causes of abdominal pain are given in Table 6.1.

1. **Oesophagitis.** Inflammation of the oesophagus caused by the reflux of gastric acid back into the oesophagus.
2. **Gastro-oesophageal reflux disease**. This is also due to reflux of gastric acid back into the oesophagus but many patients do not exhibit the inflammatory changes of the oesophagus despite having similar symptoms.
3. **Gastritis.** Inflammation of the stomach mucosa (*mew-cose-a*), which can be due to bile reflux, *Helicobacter pylori* infection, non-steroidal anti-inflammatory drugs (NSAIDs), or an autoimmune cause (pernicious anaemia).
4. **Peptic ulcer.** This is simply a deficit in the mucosa of the stomach or duodenum that penetrates the muscularis mucosae (*musk-you-lar-iss-mew-cose-a*) layer.
5. **Gallstones.** These are precipitates of cholesterol or bile pigments, which can occur in the gallbladder or bile ducts. The majority are asymptomatic but they can cause abdominal pain if they impact in a biliary duct, or jaundice (*jawn-dis*) if they lodge in the common bile duct. Stones in the ducts or gallbladder can act as a source of infection and cause ascending cholangitis (*coal-ann-jite-iss*) or cholecystitis (*coal-ee-sis-tight-iss*) respectively.
6. **Pancreatitis.** Inflammation of the pancreas, which can occur acutely or chronically. Alcohol and gallstones are major factors in causing pancreatitis.
7. **Kidney stones.** These can be made of a number of materials, for example, calcium oxalate. If they block a ureter they can cause severe pain, termed renal colic.
8. **Constipation**. Definitions vary but a useful one is a bowel frequency of less that three per week or having to strain for more than a quarter of the time during defaecation (usually because of hard stools).
9. **Diverticulitis diverticulae** (*die-ver-tick-you-lee*). In the context of the large bowel, these are outpouchings of the bowel due to an increased pressure within the lumen. They are common and asymp-

Tip

If there is any doubt that you could be dealing with a myocardial infarction arrange an electrocardiogram.

TABLE 6.1 Common causes of abdominal pain

Oesophagus	Oesophagitis, gastro-oesophageal reflux disease
Stomach/duodenum	Gastritis, peptic ulcer
Hepatobiliary tract	Biliary colic, cholecystitis
Pancreas	Pancreatitis
Kidneys	Renal colic
Large bowel	Constipation, diverticulitis, irritable bowel syndrome
Appendix	Appendicitis
No cause found	

tomatic in a large number of Western adults. However if a diverticulum becomes inflamed it can become painful and is called diverticulitis.

10. **Irritable bowel syndrome.** This is a condition that can exhibit a range of symptoms including constipation, diarrhoea, and abdominal pain. However there is no obvious organic cause and all gastrointestinal investigations including colonic biopsies are normal. It is more common in Western society and particularly in people with anxiety or depression. One theory suggests that certain individuals are simply hypersensitive to normal gastrointestinal functions.
11. **Appendicitis.** Inflammation of the appendix. The most common predisposing cause is a faecolith within the lumen of the appendix.

What to ask

This can be broken down into two sections: (1) questions about the pain itself and (2) questions about potential causes of the pain.

Questions about the pain itself

Begin with an open question, 'Tell me about the pain?' but as with chest pain, you need to establish certain key facts.

1. Was this a single bout of pain or were there several bouts?
2. Where was the pain? This is an important question, as the site of pain can give a clue to which organ is affected. Also ask about radiation (spread) of pain, that is, through to the back (pancreatitis?) or around to the scapula (biliary colic?).
3. What kind (character) of pain is it? Pain is always difficult to describe so give options, that is, knife like, burning, or aching. One particular character you should look for is the **colicky** pain. This is a squeezing pain that builds up and then eases off and usually comes in waves. This sort of pain indicates a blockage in a duct or hollow organ and represents the body's attempt to overcome the blockade
4. Onset? Was this a gradual build-up or was the pain severe at the start?
5. Did anything bring it on? Ask specifically about certain foods, for example, gallstone disease exacerbated by fatty foods, peptic ulcer by spicy foods, or oesophagitis by hot tea.
6. Did anything make it better? Ask about effect of treatments, for example, relief with antacids or milk for oesophagitis or peptic ulcer.
7. How long did it last? You need an answer in seconds, minutes, hours, and so on. Reassure the patient that you only need an estimate and give options: 'Did it last seconds only, 5 minutes, about 12 hours?'

Try to get some indication of the severity of the pain. With acute abdominal pain the pain can be very severe. The pain of renal colic is so intense that the patient will roll around in agony. The pain of a perforated peptic ulcer is so bad that the patient dare not move. In each case there may be pallor and sweating.

The answers to the previous questions will offer some signposts to the cause of pain. The descriptions of pain for each condition detailed below will add further clues. Also see Table 6.2 to review the causes of acute and chronic abdominal pain.

1. Oesophagitis tends to result in a pain that is retrosternal and burning, is made worse by citrus fruits and spicy foods, and is eased by milk and antacids. It may last from a few minutes to several hours. It tends to be recurrent. It may occasionally be relieved by glycerine trinitrate (GTN), where this reduces oesophageal spasm through its muscle relaxant properties.
2. Peptic ulcer pain is usually located in the epigastrium (*epi-gas-tri-um*) and is burning or gnawing in nature. It is said that the pain of gastric ulcer comes on after a meal while that of a duodenal ulcer is relieved following a meal. However this distinction is not often true and is unhelpful. Sometimes the pain of duodenal ulcer can wake a patient from sleep. Often the pain is so localized that the patient can put a finger on where it is. One complication of a peptic ulcer is perforation leading to peritonitis. When this occurs the pain is severe and the patient can only lie still.
3. Gallstones, when they obstruct a duct or the outlet to the gallbladder, cause biliary colic. The pain is experienced in the epigastrium or right upper quadrant and often radiates around to the back under the scapula. It occurs suddenly and builds up to a severe pitch lasting for several hours. The pain is severe and the patient usually rolls around in agony. Although the pain is labelled as colic the pain rarely fluctuates.
4. Pancreatitis, when acute, can also cause severe pain in the epigastrium, which often radiates through to the back. It needs to be considered in any diagnosis of acute abdominal pain. The pain of chronic pancreatitis is usually less intense if experienced at all.
5. Renal stones can cause renal colic if they get stuck in the renal pelvis or the ureters. The pain is felt in the loins and is severe enough to cause the patient

to roll around in agony also. The pain can radiate down the abdomen and can be felt in the testes in the male or labia in the female.

6. Constipation may cause pain but usually in the elderly patient. The pain can be dull or sharp and may be constant or colicky. It tends to be diffuse and the patient has some difficulty pointing to a specific area. The pain may also move site (the elderly patient can sometimes be accused of being confused or lying because their story changes).
7. Diverticulitis can cause pain, which can be severe and acute in onset. It may originate in the centre of the abdomen before localizing in the left iliac fossa (or be felt in the left iliac fossa immediately). The pain can behave like the mirror image of appendicitis (see below) and is sometimes called left-sided appendicitis.
8. Irritable bowel syndrome can cause a variety of painful experiences. The pain can be dull, sharp, or burning in nature and can affect any part of the abdomen. The pain however is rarely severe.
9. Appendicitis, during a classical attack, causes colicky, central abdominal pain before localizing to the right iliac fossa. However the appendix can occasionally lie in different positions within the abdomen and can lead to the pain localizing in more unusual places (which may lead to a delay in diagnosis).

Questions about the potential causes of the pain

You should always ask about the other abdominal symptoms—has the patient had nausea, vomiting, or a change in bowel habit? When did they last open their bowels? If it is longer than 48 h (and unusual for them) the patient may have developed intestinal obstruction (especially if they are unable to pass wind (flatus) as well). With any luck, your previous questions will have given you some idea of what the diagnosis is, so obtain further information about what you think are the likely causes. Ask about **associated symptoms** and **risk factors** relevant to the condition(s) you suspect.

1. **Oesophageal pain**. Associated symptoms—nausea, vomiting, abdominal pain. Risk factors—smoking, alcohol.
2. **Peptic ulcer**. Associated symptoms—anorexia, nausea, vomiting, belching, waterbrash. Risk factors—*Helicobactor pylori* (*heli-co-back-ter-pie-lorry*) infection, NSAIDs, smoking, alcohol.
3. **Gallstones**. Associated symptoms—anorexia, nausea, vomiting belching, jaundice, fever (with cholecystitis or chalangitis). Risk factors—high cholesterol, age >40 years, female sex.
4. **Pancreatitis**. Associated symptoms—anorexia, nausea, vomiting, fever, hypotension, weight loss (chronic pancreatitis). Risk factors—gallstones, alcohol, viral infections, drugs, for example, steroids.
5. **Renal stones**. Anorexia, nausea, vomiting, urinary frequency, haematuria (*he-mat-you-rear* or *he-mat-chew-rear*). Risk factors—dehydration, immobility, hypercalcaemia (*high-per-cal-see-mia*), stagnant or infected urine, hyperuricaemia, for example, after chemotherapy.
6. **Constipation**. Associated symptoms—anorexia, nausea, vomiting, flatulence, spurious diarrhoea (see p. 141). Risk factors—dehydration, lack of dietary fibre, drugs.
7. **Diverticulitis**. Associated symptoms—anorexia, nausea, vomiting, diarrhoea or constipation, bleeding per rectum (PR), fever. Risk factors—poor dietary fibre, increasing age.
8. **Irritable bowel syndrome**. Associated symptoms—nausea, constipation or diarrhoea, belching, heartburn, flatulence. Risk factors—anxiety, depression.
9. **Appendicitis**. Associated symptoms—anorexia, nausea, vomiting, urinary frequency, constipation or diarrhoea. Risk factors—poor dietary fibre.

You may have noticed that the associated features of many of the acute causes of abdominal pain are very similar. In fact, many of the causes of an '*acute abdomen*' can be difficult to distinguish on history alone and you will have to consider them all in your differential diagnosis. An acute abdomen is an emergency and needs to be recognized. The crucial decision when dealing with one, is whether urgent surgery is needed. This is one instance when clinical examination is more important than the history. If during your examination you find signs of peritonitis, for example, abdominal rigidity, guarding, or rebound tenderness (see p. 161), you need to refer your patient to the surgeons immediately.

I have not mentioned less common causes of abdominal pain, such as bowel obstruction, mesenteric (*me-sent-eric* or *mez-ent-eric*) ischaemia, diabetic ketoacidosis (*key-toe-acid-owe-sis*), acute intermittent porphyria (*pour-firi-a*), and hypercalcaemia. These are described briefly at the end of this chapter.

Anorexia, weight loss, and weight gain

Anorexia

Anorexia means a loss of appetite. Most of us have experienced temporary anorexia, say after a short illness, or if we find a fly in our soup. However a loss of appetite is only important if it is prolonged and associated with significant weight loss. Care must be taken not to take anorexia at face value. Dig a little deeper. Sometimes there are other symptoms that put your patient off eating, for example, vomiting, difficulty swallowing (dysphagia) (*dis-fage-a*), or loss of taste (ageusia) (*ay-goo-zia*), yet your patient may report all these as simply being off their food.

Weight loss

Weight loss is an important symptom that can be difficult to evaluate. It needs to be assessed in two stages: (1) verify weight loss (and define amount and time scale) and (2) search for a cause.

Verify weight loss. Unfortunately the degree to which a patient complains about weight loss does not always correlate with the true amount lost. Some may complain bitterly that they have lost weight but a flick through their notes (if available) may show that their weight is unaltered say after a year. Others may seem unconcerned but on further questioning will have lost gross amounts of weight. Therefore you must be diligent and try to confirm the presence of true weight loss. Some patients will be pretty accurate, for example, 'I have lost a stone in 2 months.' If they cannot be precise try asking questions that might imply significant weight loss, for example, 'Are your clothes loose and ill fitting these days?' or 'Do you have to tighten your belt a further notch or two?' If your patient remains vague and looks well nourished, you may have to take their story with a pinch of salt. In this situation I would simply record their weight and do some baseline blood tests, for example, full blood count (FBC), urea and electrolytes (U&Es), liver function tests, and thyroid function tests.

Search for a cause. If you are convinced that there is weight loss, you must search for a cause. The first question you should ask is about food intake. Some weight loss may be deliberate in the case of dieting. Otherwise anorexia may herald a wide range of diseases. Less obvious causes of anorexia include depression. You may suspect this from the patient's demeanour (hunched posture, lack of eye contact, and so on) Sometimes it is less apparent and you need to ask about key symptoms: 'Do you have trouble sleeping?', 'Do you wake up early in the morning and have difficulty getting back to sleep?', 'Do you sleep excessively?', 'Have you lost interest in your work or hobbies?' Another condition that can be hard to spot is anorexia nervosa. You need to have an index of suspicion especially if you are dealing with a young girl with weight loss. It is a sign of the times that girls afflicted with anorexia are getting even younger and that boys are also being affected. Sometimes weight loss may occur despite a normal or increased appetite. This can occur in thyrotoxicosis (an overactive thyroid), diabetes mellitus, or some malignant conditions. Also ask about night sweats. What you are looking for are episodes that lead to drenching of their nightclothes or bed sheets. This symptom together with weight loss may be due to tuberculosis or lymphoma (*lim-foam-a*). Any further questions will depend on any further symptoms volunteered by your patient., for example, an elderly patient with alternating diarrhoea and constipation may suggest cancer of the colon and you should ask further gastrointestinal questions about bleeding PR, abdominal pain, tenesmus (*ten-ez-muss*) (a feeling that defaecation is incomplete), and so on. An intolerance to a warm environment and irritability may suggest hyperthyroidism and you should ask about diarrhoea, excessive sweating, tremor, lack of periods in a woman (amenorrhea) (*ay-men-owe-rear*), or eye problems (Grave's disease). If no symptoms are forthcoming, you will have to screen the patient by asking questions from all of the systems review and seeing if any clues occur.

Weight gain

People do not often complain of weight gain. Some patients with depression, rather than lose their appetite, eat excessively for comfort and put on weight. Another important cause of weight gain is an underactive thyroid (hypothyroidism). Other symptoms include intolerance of a cold environment, constipation, dry skin, and heavy periods in women (menorrhagia) (*men-owe-rage-ia*). Rarely a lesion of the hypothalamus or pituitary can lead to hypopituitarism (*high-poe-pit-you-it-are-izm*) and sufferers may have an increased appetite and weight gain. If weight gain is rapid this may be due to fluid retention. This could be due to congestive cardiac failure or ascites (*a-sigh-tease*) (see later) or drugs such as non-steroidal pain-killers or steroids (steroids also stimulate appetite).

Keypoints

- Verify if weight loss has actually taken place.
- Weight loss despite a good appetite suggests thyrotoxicosis (or malignancy).
- Ask about night sweats, which might indicate tuberculosis or lymphoma.
- Weight gain may be due to fluid retention (as well as fat).

Heartburn

Heartburn is a common symptom and most of us will have experienced it at some point in our lives. It is a retrosternal burning pain, which can sometimes radiate into the neck. In most cases this is due to gastro-oesophageal reflux, or peptic ulcer disease. However occasionally it is due to cardiac ischaemia or even infarction. With hospital patients, the proportion of people with a cardiac cause for heartburn is likely to be a lot higher than in the community. If patients say they have heartburn, get them to describe it, so you know you are both on the same wavelength. Also ask for accompanying symptoms, for example, nausea or fluid rising into the mouth (waterbrash). Heartburn aggravated by spicy or citrus foods, or by lying flat, suggests a gastrointestinal origin. If the pain is relieved within half an hour by antacids, or within days by a proton pump inhibitor (a powerful acid suppressant), for example, omeprazole, then this will strengthen the hypothesis that the heartburn is of gastrointestinal origin. Always check to make sure that heartburn is not related to exertion (that is, anginal in nature). If there are any doubts, perform an electrocardiogram (ECG).

Keypoints

- Make sure you and your patient understand what is meant by 'heartburn'.
- Ask about other gastrointestinal symptoms particularly those related to gastro-oesophageal reflux and peptic ulcer.
- Always give a thought to cardiac disease.

Dyspepsia

What is it?

This is an elusive term because it can mean different things to different doctors, for example, some use it to describe indigestion. Perhaps an easy way of describing dyspepsia (*dis-pepsi-a*) is that it is a collection of symptoms including epigastric pain, heartburn, nausea, upper abdominal bloating, and belching. Therefore dyspepsia is not a precise entity. Luckily you will not meet many patients who will complain they have dyspepsia. It is a term used predominantly by doctors. I find it a vague and unhelpful term. If I hear a patient has dyspepsia, all I can deduce is that they have some upper gastrointestinal pathology and nothing more. I prefer to concentrate on the individual symptoms such as heartburn or epigastric pain and investigate these accordingly. Peptic ulcers are a common cause of dyspepsia and because of this a distinction is sometimes made between this (as a cause) and non-ulcer dyspepsia. A patient must be investigated (usually by endoscopy) and have a peptic ulcer excluded before being categorized as having non-ulcer dyspepsia. The final thing to say is that you should always be alert to malignant conditions that can masquerade as dyspepsia. Danger signs include anorexia, weight loss, dysphagia, vomiting, haematemesis (*he-mat-emma-sis*), and constant abdominal pain. If a patient has these signs they should be thoroughly investigated.

Keypoints

- Dyspepsia is a collection of symptoms including epigastric pain, heartburn, bloating, belching, and nausea.
- The distinction is usually made between ulcer dyspepsia (a common and important cause) and non-ulcer dyspepsia.
- Beware of dyspeptic patients with anorexia, dysphagia, vomiting, haematemesis, constant abdominal pain, and weight loss. These need further investigation.

Dysphagia

What is dysphagia?

Dysphagia means difficulty in swallowing. The problem usually resides in the oesphagus but you have to ask specific questions to exclude other causes that can affect swallowing. Other factors include (1) local factors in the mouth, (2) pain on swallowing (odynophagia) (*owe-die-no-fay-jah*), and (3) globus hystericus (*glow-bus-hysteric-us*).

1. Local factors in the mouth include aphthous (*apf-thus*) ulcers, herpes simplex, and candida, which may cause pain when chewing food. This pain may be sufficient to put the person off eating. A lack of dentures can prevent a patient from chewing food sufficiently to be able to swallow anything other than a soft or pureed diet.
2. Pain on swallowing may be caused by tonsillitis or pharyngitis or by inflammation of the oesophagus itself, for example, by candidal infection. The patient will experience a raw, painful sensation as food is swallowed and this is usually enough to put the patient off their food.
3. Globus hystericus is a terrible name for this condition. The 'hystericus' label conveys the impression

of some screaming, out-of-control patient, who is frankly mad. This is a recognized condition that affects anxious people who complain that they have a lump in their throat usually at the level of the larynx. This sensation may be intermittent but the crucial thing is that the patient is still able to swallow normally despite its presence.

In **all** these cases the normal function of the oesophagus is retained. To exclude the above ask if there is pain in the mouth or the throat on swallowing. Check elderly patients for dentures and ask if they fit well. The small number of patients with globus hystericus will normally volunteer this symptom. The term globus pharyngeus is being increasingly used.

TABLE 6.2 Causes of acute and chronic pain in the abdomen

Organ	Acute	Chronic
Oesophagus		Oesophagitis, gastro-oesophageal reflux disease
Stomach/duodenum	Perforated peptic ulcer, peptic ulcer	Peptic ulcer
Biliary tract	Biliary colic, cholecystitis	Cholecystitis
Kidneys	Renal colic	
Pancreas	Pancreatitis	Pancreatitis
Large bowel	Diverticulitis	Diverticulitis, irritable bowel syndrome

TABLE 6.3 Causes of dysphagia

Mechanical
Stricture
Carcinoma
*Brown-Kelly Paterson/Plummer Vinson syndrome

Neurological
Stroke
Motor neurone disease
Multiple sclerosis
Parkinson's disease
Achalasia (*ay-ka-lazier*) of the oesophagus

* *Adam Brown-Kelly (1865–1941), Scottish ear, nose, and throat surgeon, Donald Ross Paterson (1863–1939), Scottish ear, nose, and throat surgeon, H. S. Plummer (1874–1936), American physician, and P. P. Vinson (1890–1959), American physician,* all described oesophageal stricture associated with iron deficiency anaemia.

The causes of dysphagia can be divided into mechanical and neurological causes (see Table 6.3). With mechanical causes a physical barrier to the passage occurs because of narrowing of the lumen. The dysphagia usually worsens in a progressive fashion, starting with difficulties with large boluses of food, then smaller pieces, until even liquids and the patient's own saliva cannot be swallowed in extreme cases. With neurological causes the normally coordinated contractions of the oesophagus are impaired. Patients tend to have difficulties swallowing liquids more than solids. Sometimes they may experience nasal regurgitation of fluids. With some neurological causes of dysphagia, the swallowing problem is just part of a bulbar or pseudobulbar palsy (a lower motor neurone lesion or upper motor lesion of the IX, X, and XII cranial nerves respectively). They may also experience difficulties in the articulation of their speech (dysarthria) (*dis-are-thria*) or in the power of their speech (dysphonia) (*dis-phoney-a*) and you should be alert to this when you are listening to your patient.

In all cases of dysphagia, it is possible for regurgitation of food to occur. Sometimes your patient will mistakenly call this vomiting. The key feature here is the absence of retching and usually undigested food is brought back. Of more concern is that regurgitation can occur while the patient is asleep and can lead to aspiration of contents into the respiratory tract.

CASE 6.1

Problem. A 65-year-old man is admitted with a pneumonia. He has a 2-year history of Parkinson's disease and is on treatment to control his symptoms. He is an ex-smoker of 20 cigarettes per day for 40 years. He claims he has never had a bad chest until recently but he admits this is his third attack of pneumonia in the last 6 months. What is happening?

Discussion. To have three attacks of pneumonia in such a short time should ring alarm bells. You should be considering what could be predisposing your patient to repeated attacks of pneumonia. An ex-smoker may have developed lung cancer and this needs excluding. However a patient with Parkinson's disease is at risk of aspiration pneumonia. Silent aspiration of food, particularly at night, can easily be missed. If you suspect this, a speech therapy assessment will be of great value. A therapist may identify problems with swallowing and can offer strategies that may help with dysphagia and reduce the risk of aspiration.

Keypoints

- Exclude local problems in the mouth or pain on swallowing before labelling a symptom as dysphagia.
- Dysphagia may be due to mechanical obstruction or neurological diseases.
- Mechanical causes of dysphagia usually lead to progressive problems with solids greater than liquids.
- Neurological causes of dysphagia usually lead to problems with liquids greater than solids.
- Dysphagia may lead to aspiration pneumonia.

Nausea and vomiting

Everyone at some stage in their lives will have experienced nausea and vomiting, whether through a bout of food poisoning, travel sickness, the fear of medical exams, or the alcoholic celebrations (or consolation) following an examination. There are many causes of nausea and vomiting and it is easier to consider them in broad categories. Here, vomiting will be concentrated upon, as this is the more serious symptom of the two. See Table 6.4.

What to ask

Questions can be divided into (1) questions about the vomiting itself and (2) questions about the potential cause of vomiting.

Questions about the vomiting itself

Don't spend too much time finding out details about the vomit. Vomiting is a non-specific marker of disease and it is ultimately the cause you are most interested in. Nonetheless, there are certain important features you need to look into.

1. Is it acute or chronic?
2. Is there nausea or retching preceding the vomit? Effortless vomiting may in fact be regurgitation and suggest oesophageal pathology.
3. How much did they vomit? You only need a rough guide. Give suggestions such as an eggcupful, a cupful, a bucketful.
4. What is in the vomit? Was it undigested food (for example, from a pharyngeal pouch)? Was it digested food (large quantities vomited in a projectile fashion may be pyloric stenosis)? Was it dark and did it smell faeculant (this could indicate a bowel obstruction)?
5. Does it contain blood? Or did it contain elements that resembled coffee grounds (this is called haematemesis, see later).

Questions about the potential cause of vomiting

As the causes of vomiting are so great it will provide a significant challenge to your history taking skills. Sometimes your patient will help narrow your focus straight away by telling you about associated features unprompted. Otherwise you will need to be methodical and patient in your hunt for clues.

1. Start by asking if there are any precipitating factors. Can they pinpoint the start of vomiting to eating suspect food? This usually occurs at social gatherings or at restaurants where food may be insufficiently prepared. The time to vomit following consumption of contaminated food can be as little as 6 h with toxin-forming organisms, for example, *Bacillus cereus* (*ba-sill-us-serious*) to 12–24 h for other organisms, for example, salmonella.
2. Pain is another important feature to ask about. Severe pain anywhere in the body can cause nausea and vomiting. Ask specifically about chest pain, which could signify a myocardial infarction (MI) or epigastric pain, which could be due to a range of abdominal pathologies, for example, peptic ulcer, pancreatitis, and cholecystitis, not to mention MI again. Colicky abdominal pain with faeculant vomiting could indicate intestinal obstruction.
3. From this point it is recommended that a review of gastrointestinal symptoms such as heartburn, dysphagia, and bowel habit be performed.

TABLE 6.4 Causes of vomiting

Gastrointestinal
Peptic ulcer
Pancreatitis
Cholecystitis
Bowel obstruction
Non-gastrointestinal
Psychogenic (*sigh-co-jennik*)
Sepsis
Severe pain, e.g. myocardial infarction, aortic dissection
Endocrine, e.g. diabetes, Addison's disease, hyperparathyroidism
Central nervous system, e.g. meningitis, space-occupying lesion
Drugs, e.g. opiates, non-steroidals, digoxin, cytotoxic drugs

4. Do not forget to check the past medical history for significant events such as previous operations (which can cause adhesions in the abdomen leading to bowel obstruction).
5. Check for diabetes, renal problems, liver problems, and so on.
6. A drug history is mandatory. Just about any drug can cause nausea and vomiting, whether in normal dosage, for example, antibiotics, cytotoxic (*sigh-toe-toxic*) drugs, and non-steroidal medication or in overdosage. Some drugs have a narrow therapeutic index, that is, the dose range that produces a beneficial effect is small and any further increase in dose can lead to toxic side-effects. Drugs in this category include digoxin (*di-jox-in*), aminophylline (*am-in-off-i-lin*), and phenytoin (*fen-it-toe-in*). Alcohol should be asked about because it can cause vomiting following a binge or through chronic damage to other organs, particularly the liver.
7. If no clear signposts have emerged with these questions then you will have to slowly review all the other non-gastrointestinal systems looking for clues. Do not discount the effect of emotions and be prepared to ask tactfully about stresses in a patient's life, for example, exams or bullying at work.

CASE 6.2

Problem. A 72-year-old woman who is a type 2 diabetic is admitted to your ward. She has vomited four times at home and now looks clammy and unwell. How do you assess this woman?

Discussion. This woman is unwell and you need to get answers fast. You must modify your history taking to reflect the urgency of the situation. Your first steps will include a cursory examination of your patient and the instigation of some preliminary investigations; all this must be done while taking a focused history. Ask the nursing staff to do some preliminary observations, for example, pulse, blood pressure, and temperature (this was 58/min, 80/40, and 36.8°C in this case). Insert a venflon and withdraw blood for analysis (at least an FBC, U&Es, and random blood sugar (RBS)) and ask for an ECG and chest X-ray. Any patient with low blood pressure who looks clammy and unwell should initially trigger three important groups of causes in your mind: cardiac, sepsis, and haemorrhage. Ask if there is any pain anywhere, particularly the chest or epigastrium. Is there any breathlessness (could suggest pulmonary embolism or pneumonia)? Is there any blood in the vomit (suggesting gastrointestinal haemorrhage as a cause)? Have they passed any black, tarry motions (melaena) (again suggesting haemorrhage)? Have they felt cold and shivery then hot with bouts of uncontrollable shaking (rigors) (which may indicate underlying sepsis)? If these questions are negative then you need to ask detailed questions from your systems review. Record your clerking while you wait for the results of your investigations to percolate back to you.

This patient had no pain but was later found to have an inferior MI. This case also demonstrates the 'silent MI' and you need to be aware of such cases, particularly when you deal with high-risk patients like those who are elderly or have diabetes.

Keypoints

- There are a large number of causes of nausea and vomiting.
- Severe pain and vomiting suggests a serious underlying condition.
- Give a thought to food poisoning.
- Always ask about travel.
- Ask if there is blood in the vomit.
- Always ask about drug treatment.

Haematemesis and melaena

What are they?

Haematemesis and melaena (*muh-leaner*) are important symptoms, which should be taken seriously. The causes of these symptoms are given in Table 6.5.

Haematemesis

This is the vomiting of blood. This can be bright red blood from a fresh bleeding site or if the blood has been in the stomach for long enough, it is transformed by the stomach acid into a coffee-ground appearance.

TABLE 6.5 Causes of haematemesis and melaena

Oesophagus	Stomach	Duodenum
Severe oesophagitis	Gastric ulcer	Duodenal ulcer
Mallory–Weiss tear	Gastric erosions	Duodenitis
Oesophageal varices	Gastic varices	
Oesophageal cancer	Gastric cancer	

Melaena

This is the faecal output from the anus following a bleed from the upper gastrointestinal tract. The stools look black and tarry and can occur because of bleeding anywhere from the oesophagus down to the right side of the colon. In general the bleeding has to be slow enough to allow the blood time to be chemically altered during its transit through the bowel.

What to ask

Haematemesis

The questions follow a similar pattern to ordinary vomiting with some critical differences. You need to ask (1) questions about the haematemesis and (2) questions about the potential causes of the haematemesis.

There are four questions you need to ask about haematemesis: What is the appearance? Is the patient haemodynamically stable? Is there nausea or retching? How much did they vomit?

1. The appearance of the vomit is all important in the diagnosis of haematemesis. Bright red blood is usually easy to spot but dark vomit can be misleading because not all dark vomit is coffee ground in nature. It is also worth a quick question to see if any port, red wine, or blackcurrant beverages have been drunk beforehand, as this can be mistaken for haematemesis if vomited up.
2. The next question to ask is whether the patient is haemodynamically stable or hypovolaemic (*high-poe-vol-ee-mick*). If blood loss is severe enough, the patient will complain of dizziness particularly on standing (see haematemesis). Your questions should be supplemented by a quick visual inspection and examination of the patient. Look and see if they are pale and clammy. Check the pulse for a tachycardia (>100 is serious) and the blood pressure, looking for hypotension (systolic <100 mm Hg). If these signs are positive you have an emergency on your hands and you need to resuscitate and investigate your patient urgently. Other symptoms that might be experienced include palpitations, angina, and dyspnoea.
3. Ask if there was any nausea or retching beforehand. The crucial observation is the timing of blood with the vomiting episodes. If a person has retched repeatedly before blood finally appears, this suggests a Mallory–Weiss (*mal-lorry-vice*) tear of the oesophagus (*George Kenneth Mallory (born 1900), American pathologist, Soma Weiss (1898–1942), American physician*). Blood or coffee grounds found early in the vomit suggest another pathology, for example, peptic ulcer. Effortless vomiting of large amounts of bright red blood (often by the bucketload) suggests bleeding oesophageal varices (*va-ri-seize*). This is an emergency and suspect this in a patient who is known to have varices, is an alcoholic, or has chronic liver disease.
4. Ask how much blood they vomited, for example, eggcupful, cupful, or bucketful.

The causes of haematemesis are more limited compared with those of vomiting.

1. Ask about repeated retching, which could signify a Mallory–Weiss tear.
2. Ask about pain, which may suggest peptic ulcer disease, gastritis, or duodenitis (*duo-de-night-iss*). It must be noted that these conditions can present with haematemesis without pain.
3. Check the past medical history. Some patients will be well known and may be alcoholics or have chronic liver disease. Alarm bells should ring if these patients are admitted with haematemesis and oesophageal varices or ulcers should be on the top of your list. There may be times when people known to have oesophageal varices are admitted with haematemesis. These people can bleed from lesions other than their varices and the cause of bleeding should always be looked for with an urgent gastroscopy.
4. Check for other gastrointestinal symptoms, particularly danger symptoms such as anorexia, dysphagia, or weight loss, which may signify underlying malignancy.
5. Ask about medication, for example, aspirin, NSAIDs, warfarin (*war-fa-rin*), and steroids. NSAIDs are a potent cause of gastric erosions and ulceration. Their use is widespread particularly amongst the elderly population. Do not just accept standard medications. Ask about 'over-the-counter' preparations that can be bought from the local chemist as some of these may contain aspirin or non-steroidal anti-inflammatory elements. Warfarin does not cause bleeding but it can cause significant bleeding from minor lesions or exacerbate a major bleed. I have also included steroids in this list because in the past many doctors have believed they also cause ulcers. However research has shown that this is not the case. However if they are combined with NSAIDs they markedly increase the risk of bleeding.
6. Always ask about alcohol and the amount of units that are drunk in a week.

Melaena

The appearance of melaena is unmistakable. The only time there may be confusion is with a patient taking iron or bismuth compounds where the stools may also appear black (they usually lack the tarry consistency!). Also beware that patients on iron can still have melaena, so do not accept that black stools are solely due to iron until you have fully assessed the patient. All the causes of haematemesis can lead to melaena if sufficient blood passes through the bowel, therefore the questions you ask to define the causes of haematemesis are relevant for melaena alone. In addition, lesions in the right side of the colon, for example, cancer of the caecum (*see-cum*), can cause melaena and therefore questions relevant to the large bowel should also be asked, for example, change in bowel habit, tenesmus abdominal pain, and weight loss.

Keypoints

- Haematemesis: confirm that haematemesis has taken place, for example, bright red blood or coffee-ground vomit.
- Repeated retching or vomiting before blood appears suggest a Mallory–Weiss tear.
- Melaena: confirm that melaena has taken place, that is, black stools are not due to iron or bismuth ingestion.
- Melaena is due to bleeding in the upper gastrointestinal tract (or right-sided colonic lesions).
- Both: ascertain whether the patient is haemodynamically stable (pulse <100/min, blood pressure >100 systolic).
- Is the patient on NSAIDs or warfarin?
- Always ask about alcohol consumption.

Bleeding per rectum

Bleeding can occur in two forms: (1) melaena (which has already been described) and (2) frank bleeding. The most common source of bright red bleeding is the anorectal region, although sources in the sigmoid and descending colon can also be responsible. The further proximally you go in the bowel the longer the blood takes to work its way to the anus and the darker it will look. The exception to this is torrential bleeding from an upper gastrointestinal source, where the blood can rush through the bowel and manifest as bright red bleeding. In these cases the patient is usually ill with a tachycardia and low blood pressure and will need urgent intervention. See Table 6.6 for causes of bleeding PR.

TABLE 6.6 Causes of bleeding per rectum

Anus/rectum	Colon	Upper gastro-intestinal tract
Haemarrhoids	Ulcerative colitis	Torrential bleed
Anal fissure	Crohn's colitis	
Carcinoma of rectum	Ischaemic colitis, carcinoma of colon, polyps, angiodysplasia (*an-ji-owe-dis-play-zia*)	

What to ask

The first question to ask is whether the patient is haemodynamically stable or hypovolaemic. If blood loss is severe enough the patient will complain of dizziness particularly on standing (see haematemesis). Your questions should be supplemented by a quick visual inspection and examination of the patient. Look and see if they are pale and clammy. Check the pulse for a tachycardia (>100 is serious) and the blood pressure, looking for hypotension (systolic <100 mm Hg). If these signs are positive you have an emergency on your hands and you need to resuscitate and investigate your patient urgently.

If the situation is not life threatening you can take a more measured history. As the most common causes of bleeding PR are due to ano-rectal pathology, this is a good place to start.

1. Ask if the blood is bright red or dark red. The more proximal the bleeding lesion is in the bowel, the darker red it will be.
2. Ask if the blood is mixed in with the motion. You will have to ask supplementary questions here because most people will finish in the toilet and will see a mixture of blood and faeces and claim that the blood is mixed in. Therefore ask if any blood dripped in the toilet bowl after they finished defaecation and if any blood was wiped off with the toilet paper. If the answer to both is yes, the likelihood is that you are dealing with haemorrhoids or occasionally an anal fissure.
3. Now ask about pain on defaecation. If it is painless when a motion is passed, the diagnosis is likely to be to be haemorrhoids. If it is painful, then an anal fissure is more likely (usually after constipation

with the passage of hard faeces). Before accepting that rectal bleeding is due to haemorrhoids ask about other abdominal symptoms. More than one cause of bleeding PR can co-exist and you may still have to investigate the large bowel even if you do demonstrate haemorrhoids or a fissure. If there are no other bowel symptoms you can be confident that bleeding PR is a local ano-rectal problem and you can spare your patient needless investigations.

4. Ask about diarrhoea and constipation. Profuse diarrhoea may suggest inflammatory bowel disease, for example, ulcerative colitis (*ulcer-at-ive-coal-eye-tiss*) or Crohn's (*crones*) disease and constipation could herald an anal fissure (*Burrill Bernard Crohn (1884–1983), American physician*).
5. Ask if there is any mucus passed as this also suggests an inflammatory cause of diarrhoea and bleeding PR.
6. Do not forget to ask about recent travel because some infective conditions can cause rectal bleeding, for example, shigella (*shig-ella*) or amoebic (*am-ee-bic*) dysentery or schistosomiasis (*shis-toe-so-my-a-sis*).
7. Abdominal pain may be a feature of a number of conditions. Ask about the nature of the pain, particularly if it is colicky and note its site, radiation, and relation to defaecation; for example, pain with ulcerative colitis may be colicky or cramp like prior to defaecation and is relieved by the act.
8. Finally in some cases the blood loss may be chronic and occult and the patient may present to you with symptoms of anaemia, for example, dyspnoea, dizziness, or angina.

Jaundice

Jaundice is another challenge to your history taking skills. There are many causes of jaundice and to help you understand these there is a section explaining the physiology of jaundice near the end of this chapter (see p. 177). The key to learning about jaundice is the liver because this is the focal point of bilirubin (*billy-rue-bin*) metabolism.

What is it?

Jaundice is the yellow discoloration of the skin and sclerae due to the deposition of the bile pigment bilirubin. Some old-fashioned textbooks call this icterus (*ick-ter-us*). Bilirubin is the breakdown product of haemoglobin and is modified in the liver (conjugated) before being excreted in the bile.

CASE 6.3

Problem. A 56-year-old man is admitted unconscious into casualty and you shadow the resident medical officer (RMO) as they assess the patient. The only history available is that he had been complaining about indigestion on and off for a month. He is normally fit and well except for hypertension, for which he takes atenolol (50 mg). He is pale and clammy, his pulse is 60/min, his blood pressure is 100/70, and he is apyrexial. The RMO suspects that the patient has had an inferior MI leading to bradycardia and collapse; however the ECG only shows left ventricular hypertrophy with lateral ischaemia. The RMO now considers performing a head computed tomography scan to find out why the patient is unconscious. Can you save them from making a mistake?

Discussion. The RMO's working diagnosis is a good one. The month's history of indigestion could have been unstable angina leading up to an inferior infarct, which can affect the conduction system of the heart and cause bradycardias and even complete heart block. Do not be put off a diagnosis of an infarct because of a normal ECG; if necessary repeat one a few hours later and follow up with cardiac enzymes as changes may develop later. Your priority in this case is to first check that the patient is breathing and that their airway is patent. A venflon should be inserted for venous access and blood sent for analysis. An ECG and later a portable chest X-ray will be of value.

In this case however there are a number of catches. The first is that the patient's blood pressure of 100/70 might be dismissed as normal. However as a hypertensive individual, his blood pressure might normally run at a higher level, for example, 190/110 and this new blood pressure could represent a significant drop. Another catch is that he is on a β-blocker, atenolol, which slows the pulse and can mask a tachycardia. Therefore you must be aware of these pitfalls. Re-evaluate the clues again. He is pale and clammy suggesting that his circulation is under stress. Sepsis has not been demonstrated and a cardiac cause is still possible if not proven. Remember this patient has complained of indigestion and it is possible that they may have a peptic ulcer. It can bleed without obvious haematemesis and therefore if you suspect this as a

(*continued*)

CASE 6.3 (continued)

possibility then you should perform a PR examination. In this case a PR examination revealed melaena and the cause of his collapse became clear. He was resuscitated with fluids with further blood sent for cross-matching and once stable he was sent for urgent endoscopy, which revealed a bleeding gastric ulcer, which was injected.

Keypoints

- Bleeding PR can be in the form of bright red or dark red blood or melaena.
- Bright red or dark red blood suggests a lower gastrointestinal source of bleeding.
- Is the patient haemodynamically stable?
- Always ask about diarrhoea or constipation.
- Painless bleeding following defaecation with blood on the toilet paper suggests haemorrhoids (but you must still rule out other causes).

Causes

See Table 6.7. As the liver is the key organ in bilirubin metabolism it is useful to divide the causes into pre-hepatic, hepatic, and post-hepatic causes. Sometimes you may read about a different classification of jaundice into **hepatitic** and **cholestatic** causes. Hepatitic causes simply mean those agents that damage the liver cells, interfering with their functions (including bilirubin metabolism). Cholestatic causes are those that obstruct the normal flow of bile into the small intestine and these are subdivided into intrahepatic cholestasis (*coal-ee-stay-sis*), where the disturbance occurs in the intrahepatic bile ducts and canaliculi (*can-a-lick-you-lie*) and the intrahepatic ducts and extrahepatic cholestasis, where the disturbance is in the extrahepatic ducts, for example, the common bile duct. This distinction between hepatitic and cholestatic causes is somewhat artificial because elements of both may co-exist in the same patient; for example, viral hepatitis or cirrhosis (*si-roe-sis*) may include damage to the liver cells as well as some intrahepatic cholestasis.

TABLE 6.7 Causes of jaundice

Pre-hepatic	Hepatic	Post-hepatic
Haemolytic anaemia, e.g. auto-immune hereditary spherocytosis	Hepatitis, e.g. viral hepatitis A, B, or C	Gallstones in common bile duct
	Leptospirosis	Bile duct stricture
	Hydatid disease	Cholangiocarcinoma
	Drugs, e.g. halothane	Chronic pancreatitis
	Autoimmune, e.g. primary biliary cirrhosis	Cancer head of pancreas
	Alcohol	Sclerosing cholangitis
	Malignancy, especially at porta hepatis (*porter-hepat-iss*)	

What to ask

1. Ask how long the patient has had jaundice.
2. Also ask about the colour of their stools and urine. In obstructive causes of jaundice, bilirubin in the bile does not reach the intestine where it contributes to the colour of the stools. Instead the faeces are a pale, clay colour. The excess bilirubin is excreted in the urine giving it a dark colour.
3. Also ask about itching. Bilirubin deposited in the skin is an irritant and can cause itching (the mechanism is not known).
4. Ask about pain. The pain of biliary colic may suggest gallstones. Dull pain in the epigastrium or right hypochondrium (*high-poe-con-dree-um*) may be due to hepatitis. Painless, progressive jaundice is supposed to be the hallmark of carcinoma (*car-sin-owe-ma*) of the head of the pancreas, although other conditions can sometimes mimic this.
5. Ask about fever. Sweating and rigors may suggest ascending cholangitis, a condition where infection occurs in the bile ducts (usually with a gallstone as a source) and ascends up the biliary tree. The triad of jaundice, pain, and fever is known as Charcot's (*shark-owes*) triad.
6. Also ask about travel. This usually means travel abroad where your patient may pick up exotic infections. Hepatitis A is common in certain areas and can be acquired through seafood. Don't forget about journeys closer to home, for example, hydatid (*high-dat-id*) disease can be picked up in Wales (if you spend your time amongst the sheep!).
7. Occupation should be noted as certain jobs may occasionally put a person at risk of jaundice:

sewage workers—leptospirosis (*lept-owe-spy-roe-sis*); sheep farmers—hydatid disease; doctors and nurses—hepatitis B and C.

8. Review the patient's past medical history as this may be packed full of useful information. Relevant questions include past blood transfusions (hepatitis B and C) although the risks with modern screening techniques should be miniscule these days. Ask about previous operations particularly around the biliary tree, which could lead to bile duct stricture. Ask if they have had jaundice before and medical conditions such as autoimmune disease, for example, systemic lupus erythmatosis (SLE), which may be associated with an autoimmune hepatitis or inflammatory bowel disease, which can lead to sclerosing cholangitis.
9. Always ask about drugs. Many drugs can cause jaundice through a variety of mechanisms (usually liver cell damage). As the list is so large it is always worth consulting the *British national formulary* (*BNF*), the drugs 'bible' for doctors, nurses, and pharmacists, if you are unsure of a particular drug.
10. Do not forget to ask about alcohol, which can lead to chronic liver disease.
11. Enquire about a family history. Some haemolytic diseases may be inherited, for example, hereditary spherocytosis (*sphere-owe-site-owe-sis*)—autosomal dominant.
12. Take a social history. You will need to be tactful with your enquiries here. You will be asking about high-risk activities that can lead to viral infections and you will have to probe gently into the patient's sexual activities. Some people may be affronted by your questions and others may respond with nervous silence. All will feel some measure of embarassment. So just explain calmly why you need to ask these questions beforehand and reassure them that their answers will be confidential. Questions to ask include a history of intravenous drug abuse and unprotected sex with multiple partners, particularly amongst homosexuals or bisexual people. All these activities increase the risk of infection with hepatitis B and C and human immune-deficiency virus.
13. Finally do not forget your systems review (especially if the cause is still not clear) because multi-system diseases, for example, autoimmune diseases, can affect any organ and malignancy in just about any system can lead to metastases in the liver.

Keypoints

- Ask about pale stools and dark urine (suggest an obstructive jaundice).
- Ask if there is pain associated with the jaundice.
- Is itching or fever associated?
- Ask about travel and previous blood transfusions.
- Ask tactfully about certain lifestyles, for example, homosexuality or drug abuse.

Bowel habit

It seems there is no aspect of a person's life that cannot be probed by a doctor and their bowels are no exception. Questions about bowel habit are a real test of your ability to control the consultation. The British (of yesteryear) are obsessed with their bowels. The patient who is virtually mute whilst talking about their heart attack may suddenly come alive when you ask them about their bowels.

Constipation

What is it?

Many people have their own idea of what constitutes constipation and therefore you must be clear that you and the patient are on the same wavelength. A useful definition of constipation is a bowel frequency of less than three times per week or where the patient has to strain for at least a quarter of the time during defaecation. See Table 6.8 for causes of constipation.

What to ask

1. The important question is to ask how long the patient has suffered with constipation. Somebody with symptoms for more than a year is unlikely to

TABLE 6.8 Causes of constipation

Idiopathic
Diet
Drugs, e.g. opiates, anti-cholinergics
Cancer of the colon/rectum
Diverticular disease
Acute bowel obstruction
Spinal cord disease
Parkinson's syndrome
Hypothyroidism
Hypercalcaemia

have sinister pathology. If they have had constipation all their life then the constipation is likely to be idiopathic or just a normal variant. It might be worth asking why they have complained if they have tolerated the symptoms for so long. Sometimes patients develop painful anal fissures or they may be worried about the possibility of cancer.

2. Ask about the patient's diet. Find out what they eat in a typical day. It is amazing how little some people eat, or the lack of fibre in their diet. Adequate fluid (at least 1.5 l) is required along with exercise to maintain a regular bowel habit. Simple advice regarding adequate fibre, fluid, and exercise may be all that is required. It may also be worth checking a calcium level and carrying out thyroid function tests to rule out hypercalcaemia and hypothyroidism.

3. Also check the patient's occupation. Some jobs might not allow for a regular bowel habit, for example, lorry drivers or salesmen and these people often get used to 'hanging on' until a more appropriate moment.

4. Anyone who has recently developed constipation or is alternating between diarrhoea and constipation requires further investigation. The diagnosis to worry about is cancer of the bowel, although diverticular disease and inflammatory bowel disease can present this way.

5. A patient presenting with absolute constipation (even to flatus) together with colicky abdominal pain and faeculant vomiting should make you think of acute bowel obstruction.

6. Do not forget to ask about other abdominal symptoms such as vomiting, pain, and indigestion. One further symptom you may not have heard of is tenesmus. It is a sensation of incomplete evacuation following defaecation and often leads to the patient returning to the toilet repeatedly. This may be due to an obstructive lesion such as carcinoma of the rectum but may be experienced in other diseases such as inflammatory bowel disease.

7. Constipation may be a feature of other disease even if it is not the presenting complaint. Enquiring about this symptom can be an opportunity for you to improve the patient's quality of life by tackling the constipation. In cases of spinal injury, stroke, Parkinson's syndrome, and so on, be aware of the possibility of constipation and always ask about it because although it has a low priority amongst health care workers it has the ability to cause great misery.

8. Never forget about the role of medication in causing constipation; ask for details. Common culprits include the opiates (*owe-pee-ates*), anti-cholinergics (*anti-coal-in-err-jicks*) (including classes of drugs with anti-cholinergic side effects, for example, anti-depressants or oxybutinin (*ox-ee-beauty-nin*) for incontinence), and aluminium-containing antacids, for example, aludrox or algicon. Be especially sensitive to patients undergoing palliative care who may be on large doses of opiate analgesia. Even now doctors outside palliative care still forget to write patients up for laxatives even though it is inevitable their patients will become constipated.

Diarrhoea

What is it?

Diarrhoea is a condition that all of us will have experienced, yet it is difficult to define. We all recognize at one extreme, loose watery stools being passed up to 10 times per day as obvious diarrhoea, yet normal stools being passed more than five times a day could be diarrhoea according to some definitions. Some institutions have used the passage of 250 g per day of stool weight as a quantitative expression of diarrhoea. Although useful in a research setting, this definition has no practical value to a general practitioner faced with a patient in their surgery. The author's view is that if you are dealing with a patient with loose, watery stools, you are dealing with diarrhoea. You will have to make your own judgement on more borderline cases where there may just be a small increase in the frequency of bowel action or 'the motion is not quite as solid as it usually is.'

Causes

The causes of diarrhoea are great in number and here only some broad categories along with some examples will be given.

What to ask

1. The first fact you need to establish is whether you dealing with diarrhoea. Ask what the stool looks like, whether it is formed, semi-solid, or watery? You also need to know the approximate frequency of the bowel action: two times per day, six times per day, 15 times per day, and so on. Most people (understandably) do not scrutinize their stools in great detail and may be unable to give an accurate account of what they produce. If their diarrhoea is continuing, it may be helpful if they keep a 'diarrhoea diary,' charting the appearance and frequency of their bowel action.

2. Ask if the diarrhoea is acute or chronic. Diarrhoea is usually regarded as chronic if it lasts longer than 3 weeks. This is important because acute causes are usually short lived by definition and are predominantly infective.
3. Ask about recent attendances to parties, restaurants, or food outlets of dubious reputation. This may point to food poisoning as a cause of the diarrhoea. Although most causes of food poisoning are over within a week, some cases can last for several weeks, for example, campylobacter (*camp-ee-low-back-ter*), so an infective cause is still worth looking for in an apparently chronic case of diarrhoea.
4. Ask about recent travels abroad. The causes of diarrhoea contracted abroad are many and some of them have notable names such as 'Montezuma's revenge' or 'Delhi belly'.
5. You will need to find out more detail about the diarrhoea. Ask if there is any blood mixed in with the motion, which might suggest an infective colitis, diverticular disease, inflammatory bowel disease, or malignancy.
6. Ask about associated mucus, which can also be found in inflammatory conditions.
7. Find out if the stools are loose, pale, and bulky and float in the toilet bowl. Are they difficult to flush away? This form of diarrhoea is called steatorrhea (*stee-at-owe-rear*) and is caused by malabsorption. Malabsorption can occur for a number of reasons, that is, small bowel mucosal disease, for example, coeliac (*seal-ee-yak*) disease or pancreatic disease, where the nutrients in the small intestine cannot be absorbed. The high fat content in the stool gives it a loose, bulky quality that makes it difficult to flush away. It is also important to realize that malabsorption can occur in the presence of normal-looking stools and you should still be suspicious if the clinical picture and blood tests suggest this.
8. Check the patient's occupation. This is probably more important for counselling rather than for a clue to a cause. People with infectious diarrhoea who work in 'sensitive' jobs such as cooks, food preparers, teachers, doctors, or nurses should not work until they are no longer a risk.
9. Do not forget to ask about drugs. Many drugs can cause diarrhoea and it is worth checking any medication you are unsure of in the *BNF*. A common cause of diarrhoea is the broad-spectrum antibiotics. If taken for long enough, the antibiotics kill off the useful commensal organisms in the gut allowing more resistant pathogens such as *Clostridium deficile* (*clos-trid-iium-de-fitch-ee-lee* or *de-fe-seal*) to thrive, causing diarrhoea and in severe cases 'pseudomembranous' (*sue-dough-mem-bren-us*) colitis. Also ask about the use of laxatives especially in older patients. In the past a regular bowel habit was deemed essential and everything from prune juice to laxatives were used to achieve this aim. Many older people omit this aspect of the history when they complain of diarrhoea.
10. Other drugs that commonly cause diarrhoea are given in Table 6.9.
11. If you still have no clear idea as to the cause of diarrhoea then you will have to review all the systems. Pay particular attention to conditions, for example, hyperthyroidism (diarrhoea, normal appetite, weight loss, and intolerance to warm

Tip

If a nurse informs you a patient has diarrhoea (particularly someone who was previously constipated), quickly check the drug chart and see if they are still on laxatives because doctors and nurses are notorious for not reviewing medication (particularly bowel medication and night sedation).

TABLE 6.9 Causes of diarrhoea

Diet	Curry, malnutrition
Stress	Tests/examinations, irritable bowel syndrome
Infection	Viral gastroenteritis, food poisoning, 'traveller's diarrhoea', dysentery
Chronic inflammation	Ulcerative colitis, Crohn's disease, ischaemic colitis, radiation colitis,
Endocrine	Hyperthyroidism, carcinoid syndrome, Zollinger–Ellison syndrome*
Malabsorption	Small bowel mucosal disease, e.g. coeliac disease, bacterial overgrowth, surgery, e.g. ileal resection
Pancreatic disease	
Drugs	Laxative abuse, antibiotics, digoxin, theophylline, magnesium compounds
Spurious diarrhoea	

* Robert Milton Zollinger (1903–1992), US surgeon, Edwin Homer Ellison (1918–1970) US surgeon.

environments), carcinoid (*car-sin-oid*) syndrome (diarrhoea, wheezing, and facial flushing), and Zollinger–Ellison syndrome (diarrhoea and recurrent peptic ulcers).

12. One final point to make is that paradoxically, patients with constipation can present with diarrhoea, faecal soiling of underwear, or faecal incontinence. This is called spurious diarrhoea. How liquid stools are formed around impacted stools is not known but the situation has to be explained carefully, or your patient will think you are crazy prescribing laxatives for diarrhoea.

Keypoints

- Constipation: there are a number of causes of constipation.
- Check diet for adequate fibre and adequate fluid intake.
- Always check a drug history.
- Diarrhoea: there are a large number of causes of diarrhoea.
- Give a thought to food poisoning.
- Always check a travel history.
- Pale, bulky stools that are difficult to flush (steatorrhoea) suggest fat malabsorption.
- Always check the drug history.
- In the elderly patient do not forget spurious diarrhoea.

TABLE 6.10 Causes of urinary frequency

Causes
Fluid intake
Increased
Decreased
Alcohol ingestion
Kidney disease
Diabetes mellitus
Diabetes insipidus
Psychogenic polydipsia
Prostatic disease
Detrusor instability
Drugs, e.g. diuretics (*die-you-ret-ticks*)

Genitourinary system

This section will concentrate on urinary tract symptoms and sexual history taking will not be covered. There are a number of symptoms you need to know.

Dysuria

What is it?

Dysuria (*dis-you-ria*) is pain on passing urine. It is often described as burning or scalding in nature and usually indicates a lower urinary tract infection.

What to ask

Ask if there is burning or stinging when passing water. Look out for smart replies such as, 'I'll check the next time I drive past the river.'

Frequency

What is it?

As the name suggests this is where people pass urine many times during the day. It is difficult to define a point when going to the toilet becomes pathological because of the renal response to a wide range of fluid intakes. Nevertheless if a patient is going to the toilet so often that it affects their life it deserves to be investigated. See Table 6.10 for causes of frequency.

What to ask

1. Try to get some idea of how often the patient is going to the toilet; 'lots' or 'a million times' is inadequate. Ask whether it is two times per day, five times per day, 10 times per day, and so on. Or ask if it is frequent what the average interval between passing urine is, for example, 10 min, 30 min, 1 h, and so on. Also try to get an idea of the amount of urine they are passing. Small volumes passed frequently might suggest prostatic disease, while large amounts might suggest diabetes mellitus or diabetes insipidus or psychogenic polydipsia.
2. Ask how much fluid they drink in a day. A person drinking gallons of fluid is likely to pass a lot of urine, for example, in psychogenic polydipsia (a condition where the patient always feels thirsty and drinks continually). Paradoxically, too little fluid (<1 l) may lead to frequency because concentrated urine in the bladder is an irritant. Try to gauge the amounts by cupfuls or glasses of drink, for example, a cup of tea or coffee = 150 ml, a mug of tea or coffee = 250 ml, and a glass of drink = 250 ml.
3. This form of questioning is fairly crude and the majority of people cannot give accurate estimations of what they drink and pee. A useful thing to do is to give a diary and a measuring jug so that they can

chart their fluid intake and output over a 3-day period (please do not get them to measure their fluid intake and urine output from the same jug).

4. Ask about past attacks of cystitis or kidney infections (which may cause kidney damage).
5. Ask about drugs, particularly diuretics. Most people are acutely aware of the relationship of their frequency and their diuretics (although some still neglect to mention that they are on them). When they are reminded, you will soon learn how they plan trips to town, for example, via a succession of toilets (most simply do not take the tablet).

Oliguria

What is it?

Oliguria *(ollig-you-ria)* means a low urine output. Very few people will complain of a low urine output. This tends to be a medical observation. People who are dehydrated will become oliguric because their kidneys will decrease the excretion of water to conserve the body's supply. Oliguria can also be a sign of renal failure. The rule of thumb is that your patient should produce at least 20 ml of urine per hour (if your patient is at risk of renal failure they will probably be catheterized to help measure the urine output accurately). Sometimes kidney failure may occur with a normal urine output and therefore the quality of urine produced must always be analysed. This is done by looking at the electrolytes in the urine and by comparing the concentration of urea and creatinine with the plasma urea and creatinine. The urine of a normal person will have its urea and creatinine concentrated at least twenty times that of the plasma concentration. The urine of a person in renal failure may almost be at the same concentration as plasma.

Anuria

What is it?

Anuria *(a-new-ria)* means no urine output at all. Even in established renal failure there is usually some urine produced and therefore you must consider an obstruction to the flow of urine. Such a person will need an emergency abdominal ultrasound to try and pinpoint a cause of obstruction or to rule it out.

Urgency

What is it?

This is the desperate need to micturate as soon as the desire is experienced. All the causes of frequency can cause urgency.

What to ask

'When you get the sensation to pee do you have to go to the toilet there and then or can you hold on?'

Incontinence

What is it?

One definition of incontinence is where there is the involuntary loss of urine, which can be objectively demonstrated and is a social or hygienic problem. As the definition of incontinence infers, it is a difficult and embarrassing symptom to cope with and patients often attempt to hide it. You should always ask about this in a tactful and sensitive manner and reassure your patient that there is a lot that can be done to improve the condition.

See Table 6.11 for causes of incontinence. The top two causes are **urge** and **stress** (the two can co-exist). All the causes of urgency can lead to incontinence if the patient is not quick enough getting to the toilet. An overactive bladder (detrusor *(de-true-za)* instability) is the greatest cause of urge incontinence (the detrusor is the bladder muscle). It can develop for no obvious reason or it can be secondary to bladder outflow obstruction. Stress incontinence is commoner in women because of childbirth and the potential damage to the pelvic floor musculature. Typically the patient leaks a small amount of urine, if they cough, sneeze, stand, lift, or exercise. All these activities raise the intra-abdominal pressure, which is also experienced within the bladder. Leakage occurs when the bladder pressure exceeds the pressure exerted by the urinary sphincter. Sometimes the environment is less than optimal for a patient to maintain continence, for example, a urine bottle is placed on the hemiplegic side of a stroke patient, or the toilet is too far away for a patient with Parkinson's disease to reach in time.

Overflow incontinence is a paradox (similar to spurious diarrhoea), in that the fundamental problem is retention of urine. For reasons that are not understood, the patient may pass small amounts of urine at times or may just become incontinent. An examination of the

TABLE 6.11 Causes of incontinence
Urge
Stress
Overflow
Environmental
Giggle
Continuous

abdomen will reveal an enlarged bladder (or you can confirm it with a bladder scanner, a portable ultrasound machine).

What to ask?

Before launching into questions about incontinence it is best if you prepare your patient. Say, 'I am sorry but I have to ask you some personal questions. They are designed to help find out what the problem is and hopefully to help you. Everything you tell me will be kept confidential.'

1. Ask about urgency as before but follow up the question with 'Do you find there are times you do not make it to the toilet and wet yourself?'
2. Ask 'Do you wet yourself if you cough, sneeze, stand, exercise, or lift heavy objects?' (stress incontinence).
3. Ask about fluid intake.
4. Ask about caffeine intake and the amount of tea and coffee drunk in a day (caffeine is a weak diuretic).
5. Ask about medications. Diuretics on their own may be enough to cause incontinence or can make an existing problem worse. Anti-cholinergics can cause urinary retention and may cause overflow incontinence.
6. Check to see if the patient has recently developed constipation because this can also cause urinary retention.
7. Ask about childbirth in women. You need to know how many children they have had. Were they all vaginal deliveries? Find out what size they were if possible and more importantly were instruments involved, for example, forceps (stress incontinence).
8. Ask about previous surgery. Women may have had previous surgery for incontinence, for example, bladder repair. Men may have had previous prostate surgery and their prostatic symptoms may have returned. Occasionally a small proportion of men, following a transurethral prostatectomy, may develop true stress incontinence as a result of damage to the internal urethral sphincter.
9. Find out whether they suffer with diabetes mellitus, kidney, or bladder problems.
10. On rare occasions young girls may become incontinent when they laugh or giggle (giggle incontinence).

Haematuria

What is it?

Haematuria is the passing of blood in the urine. If it is visible it is termed macroscopic haematuria, if it is detected by a dipstick test of the urine it is termed microscopic haematuria. This is an important symptom and needs prompt investigation. See Table 6.12 for causes of haematuria.

TABLE 6.12 Causes of haematuria

Kidney	Tumours, infection, infarction, stones, trauma, nephritis
Ureter	Stones, tumour
Bladder	Tumour, infection
Prostate	Benign prostatic hypertrophy, cancer of the prostate
Urethra	Trauma

What to ask

1. The first thing to do is to establish if haematuria has truly taken place. There are occasions where what you ingest can colour your urine red. The culprits include beetroot, tablets such as rifampicin (*riff-am-pi-sin*) (red-man syndrome), and laxatives such as codanthrusate or codanthromer (these have been withdrawn) and phenolphthalein (*feen-ol-fthalen*), so ask about these.
2. Ask about pain. Colicky pain in the loin radiating to the groin may suggest renal or ureteric stones. Painless haematuria should make you think about malignancy in the urinary tract, for example, kidney or bladder.
3. Ask about recent trauma. Any blow to the loin may damage the kidney. The urethra can be damaged in a road traffic accident or in an 'astride' injury where a person falls astride a bar or beam. Trauma may occur due to instrumentation of the urethra, for example, catheterization. Some confused patients with a catheter *in situ* may tug at it and cause haematuria.
4. Ask about other urinary symptoms, for example, dysuria and frequency may suggest a urinary tract infection or frequency and nocturia may suggest prostatic disease in a man.
5. Check to see if the patient is on warfarin (or has any other bleeding tendency). This may exacerbate any bleeding problem even from a minor source.

Abdominal system examination summary

1. Introduce yourself to the patient and ask for permission to examine.

CASE 6.4

Problem. A 56-year-old man was admitted with haematuria to undergo cystoscopy (*sis-toss-cup-ee*) (use of an instrument to inspect the urethra and bladder). He has passed haematuria on two occasions, which alarmed him. You ask questions about his problem. He tells you he has daytime frequency where he passes only tiny volumes with urgency. He also gets up on average three times per night to pass urine. In addition he noticed that it took a while before he could start urinating, despite having the urge and when he did the stream was poor. Sometimes he thought he had finished but he had to return minutes later to urinate again. What is the diagnosis?

Discussion. Any cause of painless haematuria must make you think of malignancy and that is the reason for this man's admission, so that he can have his bladder inspected by cystoscopy among other investigations. However he describes symptoms that suggest another diagnosis. His difficulty initiating micturition (hesitancy), his poor stream, and having to return to urinate again all suggest bladder outflow obstruction. In a middle-aged man, the likeliest cause is benign prostatic hypertrophy (BPH). A rectal examination demonstrated an enlarged prostate that felt clinically benign. However before BPH can be accepted as the cause of the haematuria, the investigations need to be completed to ensure that malignancy is not responsible.

Keypoints

- Dysuria usually suggests a lower urinary tract infection.
- Urinary incontinence is an embarrassing symptom and its cause should be searched for tactfully.
- For most urinary symptoms it is wise to check the drug history.
- Anuria should trigger a search for any obstruction to the flow of urine.

2. Ask the patient to get on to bed (if not already on the bed). You may need to help!
3. Ask the patient to strip to their underwear.
4. Lie the patient flat on one pillow (if they are elderly or have a kyphosis (*kye-foe-sis*) two pillows may be needed).
5. Whilst doing 1–4, have a 'general look'. Discomfort? Is the abdomen distended? Is there evidence of jaundice, wasting of muscles, scratch marks, and so on?
6. Inspect both hands for signs of chronic liver disease (DF 6/10), for example, clubbing, leuconychia (*loo-co-nick-ia*), koilonychia (*coil-o-nick-ia*), palmar erythema, Dupuytren's (*dew-pit-runs*) contracture, spider naevi (*knee-vie*) (make sure you blanch these), and purpura (*purr-pew-ra*).
7. Look for a flapping tremor (DF 8/10) only if you suspect liver failure (jaundice, spider naevi, and so on). Ask the patient to extend their arms and cock their wrists back.
8. Inspect the face for xanthelasmata (DF 2/10), spider naevi (DF 6/10), and other telangiectasia (DF 9/10); inspect the eyes for jaundice (DF 7/10); and inspect the conjunctivae for anaemia (DF 8/10).
9. Inspect the lips for pigmentation or telangiectasia (*tee-lan-jeck-tay-sia*) (DF 9/10).
10. Examine the oral cavity (DF 8/10). Inspect for telangiectasia, pigmentation, dentition, ulcers, angular stomatitis (*stow-ma-tight-iss*), and candidiasis (*can-did-eye-a-sis*). Also examine the tongue and tonsils and check for odours.
11. Palpate the neck for cervical lymph nodes (DF 6/10), particularly the left supraclavicular region.
12. Inspect the chest for further spider naevi (DF 8/10), gynaecomastia (DF 7/10), and loss of axillary hair in men (DF 6/10).
13. Observe the abdomen for distention, herniae, scars, striae (*stry-ee*), pulsations, peristalsis, and distended veins (DF 8/10).
14. Ask the patient if they have any tender areas before commencing light palpation. Palpate the abdomen lightly, mapping any areas of tenderness and note any masses (DF 4/10). Watch the patient's face for signs of pain!
15. Palpate more deeply and assess any masses felt in more detail (DF 7/10).
16. Palpate specifically for enlarged organs: liver—commence in the right iliac fossa and move upwards towards the right costal margin while

getting the patient to take deep breaths; spleen—commence in the right iliac fossa and move upwards towards the left costal margin while getting the patient to take deep breaths; kidneys—commence in the flanks and 'bimanually ballot' them.

17. Percuss over any masses or organs felt. Check for ascites. If the percussion note is dull in the flanks, go on to demonstrate shifting dullness (DF 7/10) or a fluid thrill (DF 6/10).
18. Auscultate for bowel sounds (DF 8/10) (and for bruits and rubs if necessary) (DF 9/10).
19. Examine the groins for lymphadenopathy and herniae (ask the patient to cough) (DF 8/10).
20. Wash your hands.
21. Now say, 'I would like to examine the external genitalia and perform a rectal examination.' Present findings.

Abdominal system examination in detail

Getting started

1. Introduce yourself to the patient and ask for permission to examine.

Put out your hand to shake the patient's hand. Say something like, 'Hello I'm Berkeley Moynihan, a third-year student. Do you mind if I examine your tummy and hands?'(some people do not understand 'abdomen' and 'belly' sounds a bit rough).

2. Ask the patient to get on to bed (if not already on the bed). You may need to help!

Usually this will be no problem, but if the patient is unable to get on to the bed, offer your assistance. If lifting is required ask a friendly nurse who will show you how to lift properly.

> **Tip**
>
> For women in nightgowns, it is helpful if they gather the nightgown above their waist before getting on the bed. Once on the bed it is a simple matter to slip it over their heads. Otherwise they end up sitting on them and have to go through some undignified wriggling to inch the garment from under their bottoms.

3. Ask the patient to strip to their underwear.

Traditionally it is said that the abdominal examination should be performed with the patient exposed 'from nipples to knees'. Mercifully, these days the patient's dignity can be maintained by covering the groin with a sheet (until this area is examined in detail). Also women patients can be examined with their bra on. There is very little that can be missed under a bra in the abdominal examination. However you must scan very carefully around the chest so as not to miss telangiectasia. These are dilated capillaries or small arterioles that look like thin red streaks or blobs. If you press on them, they disappear or 'blanch' to give it the correct medical term. This is because blood is forced out of the vessels and once the pressure is released the vessel refills and reddens again).

4. Lie the patient flat on one pillow (if they are elderly or have a kyphosis two pillows may be needed).

The abdominal system is examined with the patient lying flat on one pillow. Sometimes people with a kyphosis, usually elderly people, have difficulty lying flat because of the curvature of their spine. In these cases use two pillows to maintain their comfort. Occasionally you may get a person who has orthopnea who becomes breathless when they lie flat. Try and get them as flat as their breathing will allow but sometimes you may be forced to examine them practically upright. **In all cases the patient must be comfortable** (see Fig. 6.1).

5. Whilst doing 1–4, have a 'general look'. Discomfort? Is the abdomen distended? Is there evidence of jaundice, wasting of muscles, scratch marks, and so on?

See p. 15 for more details on 'general look'. Patient distress suggests severe illness. A venflon could suggest

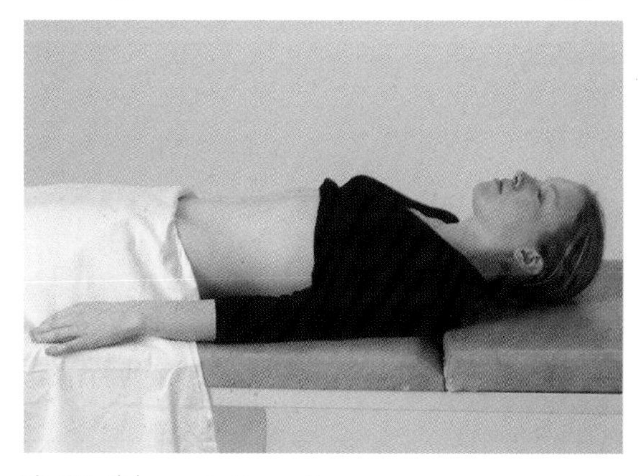

Fig. 6.1 Abdo examination position.

severe pain requiring analgesia, for example, acute pancreatitis or an infection requiring antibiotics and fluids, such as acute cholecystitis (an infection of the gallbladder). A yellow appearance of the skin could suggest jaundice and a distended abdomen could represent ascites. Also check to see if there is general muscle wasting or scratch marks.

Hands

6. Inspect both hands for signs of chronic liver disease (DF 6/10), for example, clubbing, leuconychia, koilonychia, palmar erythema, Dupuytren's contracture, spider naevi (make sure you blanch these), and purpura.

Chronic liver disease is, by definition, liver disease that has lasted longer than 6 months. There are a number of causes of which alcohol is the most common. What you are looking for are signs associated with a malfunctioning liver, including some which reflect the body's attempt to compensate. In addition some signs may be caused by malnutrition, particularly in alcoholic liver disease where a normal diet may be replaced by alcohol. These patients can show signs of anaemia and vitamin deficiency also. There are many signs to look out for. Each individual sign on its own is not diagnostic of liver disease and may have other causes. However the more signs you see in one patient, the greater the likelihood that you are dealing with chronic liver disease.

Clubbing

Clubbing (DF 8/10) is mainly seen in respiratory disease and therefore is discussed in detail on p. 84. It is seen occasionally in abdominal disease, particularly in cirrhosis of the liver. It can also occur in diseases such as ulcerative colitis, Crohn's disease, and coeliac disease.

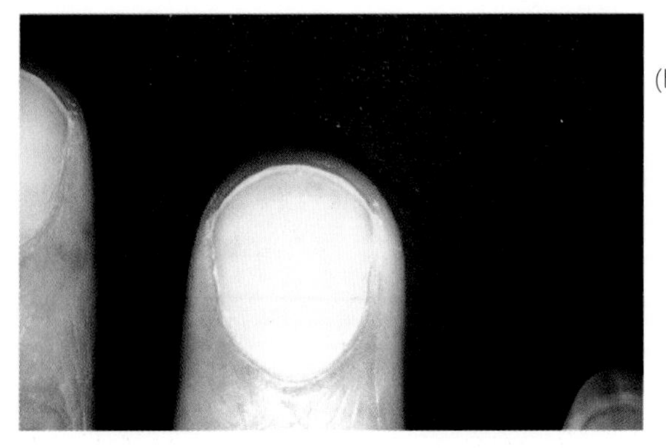

Fig. 6.2 Leuconychia.

Leuconychia

(DF 5/10.) See Fig. 6.2.

What is it?

White nails (compare with your own fingernails to help make the diagnosis).

Causes

Cirrhosis of the liver and nephrotic (*nef-rot-tick*) syndrome.

Significance

White nails are a marker for conditions causing low albumen.

Koilonychia

(DF 8/10.) See Fig. 6.3.

What is it?

Koilonychia is a 'spoon-shaped' depression of the nail plate. In the early stages the convex curvature of the nail is lost as it becomes flattened. Later the nail edges curl up leaving a depression in the centre 'like a spoon'. In advanced cases it is said you can hold a drop of water in the central depression.

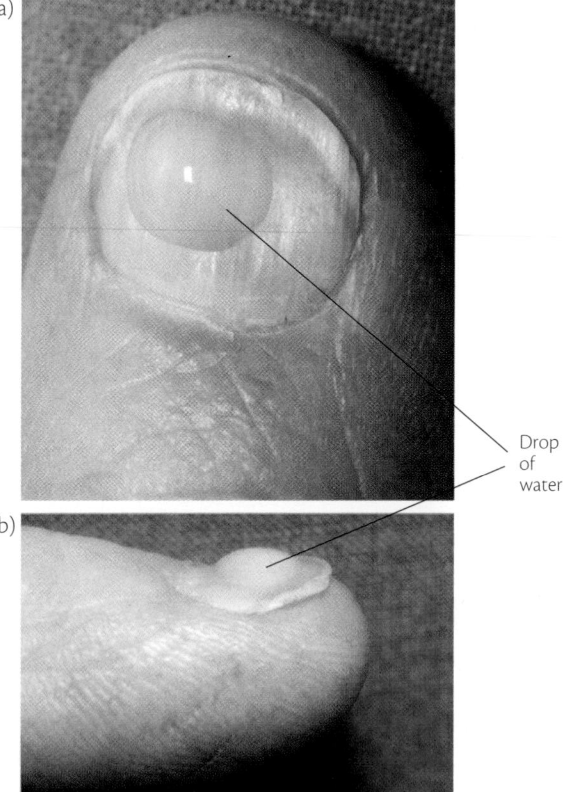

Fig. 6.3 Koilonychia. Note the spoon-shaped nail is able to hold a drop of water.

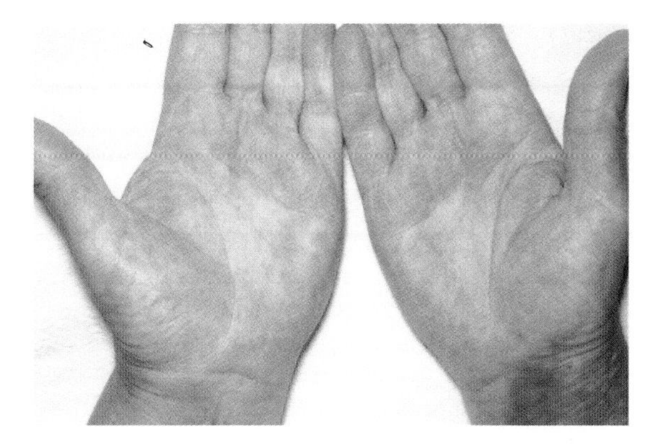

Fig. 6.4 Palmar erythema.

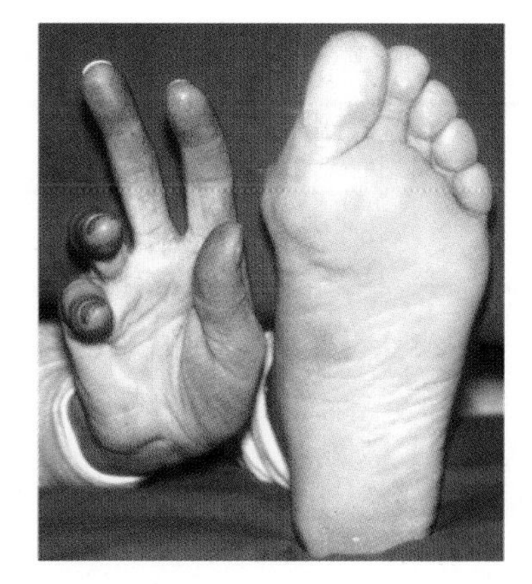

Fig. 6.5 Dupuytren's contracture.

Causes

Chronic anaemia and rarely, exposure to strong detergents.

Significance

This indicates a chronic anaemia (most commonly due to iron deficiency). This finding should prompt a search for a cause of the anaemia.

Palmar erythema

(DF 5/10.) See Fig. 6.4.

What is it?

It is a redness of the palms. The redness is concentrated on the thenar (*th-ee-nar*) eminence (the muscular mound beneath the thumb), the hypothenar eminence (the muscular mound beneath the little finger), and the pulps of the fingers, with the centre of the palm being spared. This can be subtle and easily missed. It is always worth comparing with your own palms to appreciate the difference (unless you have palmar erythema too!)

Causes

Chronic liver disease, pregnancy, the contraceptive pill, and rheumatoid arthritis.

Significance

In the cases of chronic liver disease, the contraceptive pill, and pregnancy, the palmar erythema is due to increased levels of circulating oestrogens. In chronic liver disease (especially due to alcohol), there is gonadal atrophy and depressed testosterone production. A larger proportion of this testosterone is rapidly metabolized to oestrodiol (*east-roe-dial*).

Dupuytren's contracture

(DF 9/10.) See Fig. 6.5. Dupuytren's contracture is named after *Baron Guillaume Dupuytren (1777–1835), French surgeon.*

What is it?

This is the thickening and contracture of the palmar aponeurosis, a fibrous sheet that protects the tendons of the hand. It divides at the bottom of the fingers and attaches to the base of the proximal phalanges. The thickening usually occurs at the root of the ring finger causing it to curl in towards the palm. Later the little finger is also affected. Early cases can be easily missed. If you look carefully at the palm especially in the region of the fourth and fifth fingers you can often see vertical furrows due to the thickening. Running your fingers over this region is also a good way of making the diagnosis. In advanced cases you might get a clue when you shake the patient's hand. They may tickle or scratch your palm with their flexed ring finger. So if you think that you are examining a mason with a funny handshake, make a quick visual check because it might just be a Dupuytren's contracture.

Causes

Alcoholism, chronic liver disease, diabetes mellitus, and heavy manual labour.

Significance

In advanced cases, the hand is unsightly and the contracture interferes with the function of the hand. The condition can be helped by an operation, which can be performed under local anaesthetic.

Spider naevi

(DF 6/10.) See Fig. 6.6.

What are they?

These are telangiectasia with a specific appearance. They consist of a central arteriole with tiny vessels radiating from it like 'spider legs'. This central arteriole feeds the spider legs with blood. You must demonstrate this by **blanching** it. Press on the central blob and very

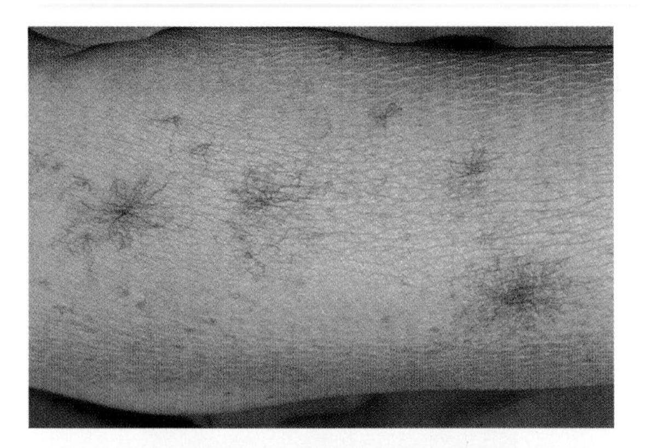

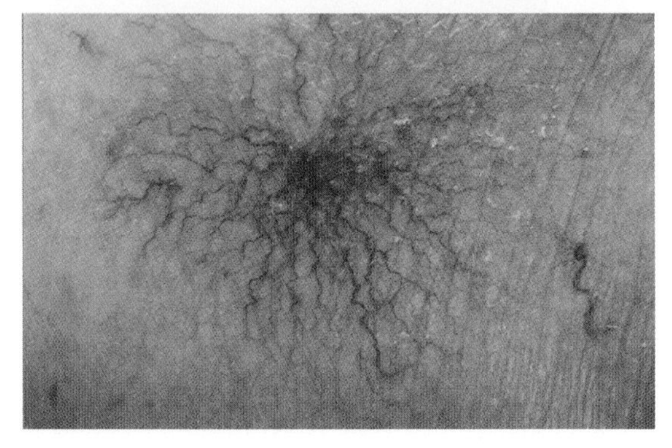

Fig. 6.6 Spider naevi.

quickly remove your finger. If you are quick enough, you should see the blood rush back and the red spider legs reappear.

Causes

Chronic liver disease, pregnancy, and thyrotoxicosis; They can also be a normal finding.

Significance

One or two spider naevi can be found in normal people, in pregnancy, and in thyrotoxicosis. However, if more than five spider naevi are found then it is likely that you are dealing with chronic liver disease (especially if there are other supporting features).

Purpura

(DF 2/10.) See Fig. 6.7.

What is it?

This is due to spontaneous bleeding into the skin. If the bleeding is localized to blobs less than 3 mm across they are called petechiae (*pet-ee-key-eye*). Very large areas of bleeding are called ecchymoses (*eck-ee-moe-seize*).

Causes

See Table 6.13.

> **CASE 6.5**
>
> **Problem.** In casualty you see a 32-year-old woman with abdominal swelling and colicky lower abdominal pain. You also notice five spider naevi on her upper body and palmar erythema. What is the diagnosis?
>
> **Discussion.** This woman is pregnant until proven otherwise. She is of reproductive age and both spider naevi and palmar erythema can be found in pregnancy. Her abdominal swelling is due to the foetus and you need to establish the duration of the pregnancy. Colicky abdominal pain is a concern. If she is near term this could represent the beginnings of labour but the fact that she has presented to casualty rather than labour ward suggests a serious complication and she needs to be seen by an obstetrician without delay.

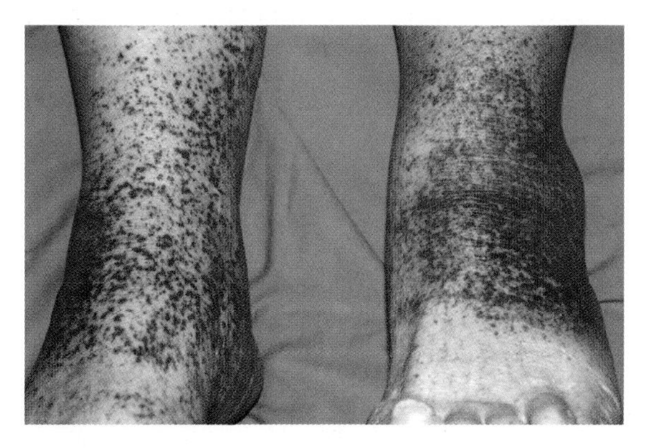

Fig. 6.7 Purpura. Drug-induced purpura affecting the legs.

TABLE 6.13 Causes of purpura

Abnormal blood vessels
Steroid induced
Old age (senile purpura)
Abnormal platelets
Idiopathic thrombocytopenic (*throm-bo-sigh-toe-pee-nick*) purpura (translated this means bleeding due to low platelet count of unknown cause)
Malignant infiltration of the bone marrow, e.g. leukaemia, myeloma, secondary deposits
Abnormal clotting factors
Haemophilia (deficiency of Factor VIII)
Anti-coagulation therapy, e.g. warfarin

Significance

In the case of chronic liver disease, bleeding may be caused because of a deficiency of clotting factors (II, VII, IX, and X).

Flapping tremor

7. Look for a flapping tremor only if you suspect liver failure (jaundice, spider naevi, and so on). Ask the patient to extend their arms and cock their wrists back.

In some textbooks a flapping tremor is called asterixis (*ass-stir-ix-iss*). It is elicited in the same manner as the flapping tremor associated with carbon dioxide retention in respiratory failure (see Fig. 5.5). Sometimes people call it a 'liver flap' to qualify the cause of the tremor.

CASE 6.6

Problem. Your senior house officer is bleeped to see a case urgently in casualty. The patient was originally referred to the surgeons with abdominal pain but the registrar decided there was nothing surgical going on. He is a 17-year-old man who looks very ill. You hear that he has complained of abdominal pain and headache all day. He has stayed in his bedroom with the curtains shut and his mother had became worried when he had started vomiting. In the last 30 min he had developed a purply-blue rash on his abdomen, arms, and legs. What is the diagnosis?

Discussion. You must always be on your guard when people tell you a patient is 'medical', 'surgical', 'cardiac', and so on. Diseases do not respect our boundaries and can often mimic each other, for example, indigestion and cardiac pain. This case illustrates how focusing on the wrong symptom can throw the unsuspecting clinician. This is in fact a case of meningococcal (*men-in-go-cock-al*) meningitis. He had a headache, fever, and probably photophobia (*foe-toe-foe-bee-a*) (an aversion to light) leading him to keep his curtains drawn. Young people can also get abdominal pain (especially babies and children) together with nausea and vomiting. The dangerous aspect of this case is the development of a rash. It does not blanch and is purpuric in nature. This marks the onset of meningococcal septicaemia, a very grave complication. This is a medical emergency and this patient needs intravenous antibiotics, as well as fluids and high-dependency care at the minimum.

Keypoints

- Spider naevi are telangiectasia and should blanch with pressure.
- Purpura is bleeding into the skin and lesions do not blanch with pressure.
- Dupuytren's contracture usually starts with thickening (of the palmar aponeurosis) around the ring finger. Eventually this leads to the ring finger curling in towards the palm.
- Koilonychia should always prompt you to confirm anaemia and to search for a cause.
- There are many signs of chronic liver disease. No one sign is diagnostic (jaundice is the most specific of these) but the more signs you see in one patient the greater the likelihood of chronic liver disease.

Only look for it if you suspect liver failure (you may have spotted jaundice, spider naevi, or other signs described earlier). Get the patient to extend their arms, cock their wrists back, and spread their fingers. If liver failure is present the hands should start flapping rhythmically. In fact it is more of a flapping twitch than a tremor, with the twitching directed down towards the floor. There are other signs of liver failure to look out for. The patient may be confused and drowsy. In the context of liver failure this is called hepatic encephalopathy (*en-keff-a-lop-pathy*). One feature is the inability to reproduce a five-pointed star, which is termed constructional apraxia (*ay-pracks-ya*). Although an interesting sign, in practice it is more important to gauge the conscious level along with liver function tests and other blood measurements in the assessment of such a patient. In addition, patients have a characteristic odour on their breath (hepatic fetor (*feet-or*)), which is described as sweet and musty. You will only really appreciate this when you meet a patient with this problem.

Beware! In some patients with a very acute presentation of liver failure, for example, paracetamol overdose, the pace of liver damage can be so overwhelming that none of the above signs will have time to develop.

Face, eyes, and lips

8. Inspect the face for xanthelasmata (DF 2/10), spider naevi (DF 6/10), and other telangiectasia (DF 9/10); inspect the eyes for jaundice (DF 7/10); and inspect the conjunctivae for anaemia (DF 8/10).

Keypoints

- A flapping tremor is a marker of liver failure.
- Only look for a flapping tremor if you suspect liver failure.
- A flapping tremor can also be found in respiratory failure.
- In rapidly progressive cases of liver failure a flapping tremor (and other signs) may not develop.

Xanthelasma

See Fig. 6.8. These are little yellowish papules (fatty deposits) around the eye that signify hyperlipidaemia. In the context of an abdominal examination they suggest prolonged cholestasis (obstruction of bile drainage). The likeliest cause is primary biliary cirrhosis.

Spider naevi

See previous discussion.

Other telangiectasia

A different form of telangiectasia can be found in hereditary haemorrhagic telangiectasia (HHT), also known as (Osler–Weber–Rondu syndrome (*William Osler (1849–1919), Canadian physician, Fredrick Parkes Weber (1863–1962), English physician, Henri-Jules Louis Rendu (1842–1902), French Physician*). These look like different sized red blebs, which can be seen on the face, the lips, the buccal mucosa, and both sides of the tongue (make sure you look at the underside of the tongue!). Although rare, the importance of this condition lies in the fact that these telangiectasia can be found elsewhere, in the nose, gut, and lungs. They are prone to bleeding and cause epistaxis (*epi-stacks-sis*), gastrointestinal bleeding, and haemoptysis (*he-mop-ta-sis*) respectively. See Fig. 14.18.

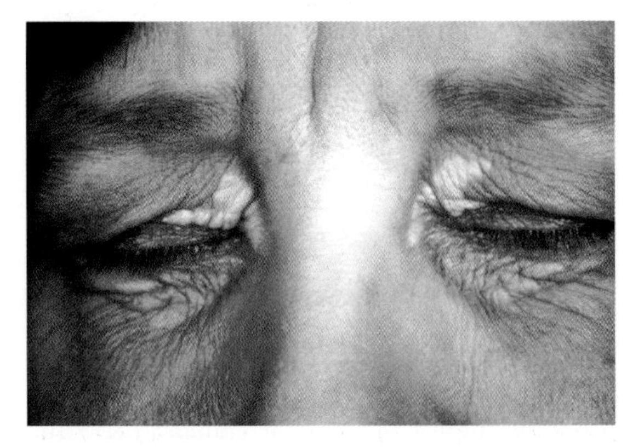

Fig. 6.8 Xanthelasma.

CASE 6.7

Problem. You see a 45-year-old woman who has an iron deficiency anaemia and difficulty swallowing. She has a thin, drawn face and you notice telangiectasia on her face that do not look like spider naevi. Your consultant asks you for a diagnosis and off the top of your head you say HHT. Your consultant says you are wrong. Why?

Discussion. It is likely that your consultant will be impressed by your answer. It is a good attempt because HHT can cause bleeding, leading to an iron-deficiency anaemia and you could make a case for chronic iron deficiency ultimately leading to an oesophageal web and causing dysphagia. However you need to examine your patient a little more closely. Blanch the lesions to prove they are telangiectasia and then look at their distribution. Always look at the lips and in the mouth. In this case there are none on the lips or in the mouth although the lesions do blanch. This is not HHT. Therefore look at your patient again. Her face is thin and drawn, the nose almost beak like with wrinkles and furrows around the nose and mouth. Her skin looks waxy and her fingers are thin and tapering in appearance. Now feel the fingers and notice the hard nodules. These are areas of calcinosis (*cal-sin-owe-sis*). The diagnosis here is systemic sclerosis. This is a condition of unknown cause where skin production (and other organs) is affected leading to thickened, shiny inelastic skin. One variant of systemic sclerosis is called the CREST syndrome (this is an abbreviation of **c**alcinosis, **r**aynaud's phenomenon, **o**esophageal dysmotility, **s**clerodactyly, **t**elangiectasia). Calcinosis is the process of calcium deposition (which is visible in the skin). Raynaud's phenomenon is a vascular condition of the hands and feet leading to arterial spasm in the cold giving the extremities a white appearance. They turn blue and then red as the extremeties slowly warm up. Oesophageal dysmotility leads to dysphagia in 30% of cases. Sclerodactyly is the name given to the thin tapering fingers. Telangiectasia completes the syndrome. Iron deficiency can occur and renal failure is one of its serious complications.

Jaundice

See Fig. 6.9. The best place to check for jaundice is the sclera of the eyes. You may have already noticed yellow skin with your 'general look' but this can be mislead-

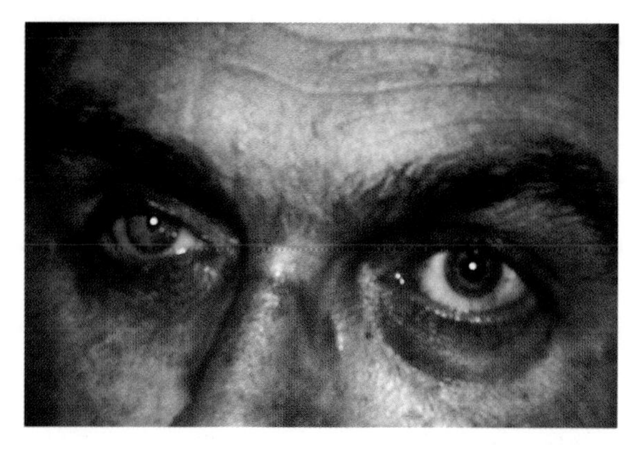

Fig. 6.9 Jaundice. Note the prosthetic eye on the right is unaffected.

CASE 6.8

Problem. You are on a ward round and you see an elderly patient who has yellow skin. She has coarse, thinning hair and looks apathetic. Your consultant asks you the diagnosis and your hurried reply is 'jaundice'. The consultant shakes their head. Why are you wrong?

Discussion. Try not to be hurried into an answer and remember that jaundice is a sign and not a diagnosis. So take your time and be methodical. It is to your credit that you have noticed yellow skin but now check the sclerae. It is white and so this is not jaundice. Review your patient again. The coarse, thinning hair and apathetic expression suggest hypothyroidism (myxoedema). Her skin is dry and yellow and her tongue looks large (it is said that you lose the outer third of your eyebrows but this is not a good sign). Now look for slow relaxing ankle reflexes (other reflexes can be slow relaxing too) and check her memory with an abbreviated mental test score (AMTS) examination. The yellow tinge to her skin is due to hypercarotinaemia (*high-per-carrot-in-ee-mia*), a build-up of carotene in the blood. Carotene is a precursor of vitamin A and is found in abundance in carrots. In myxoedema the body's metabolism slows down because of an underactive thyroid and the conversion of carotene to vitamin A is reduced. In long-standing cases the build-up of carotene leads to its deposition in the skin and to the yellow appearance. This colour disappears, as do all the other fetures of hypothyroidism, with thyroxine treatment. Other causes of a yellow skin include race (oriental races), uraemia, and pernicious anaemia. You need to confirm the presence of jaundice by observing yellow sclera.

How to examine

Ask the patient's permission: 'Can I gently pull down your eyelid?' When you pull down the lower eyelid ask the patient to look down and observe the sclera.

Anaemia

Significance

Anaemia may be the result of blood loss due to a number of causes in the gastrointestinal tract. This loss can be obvious and spectacular as in bleeding oesophageal varices or insidious and occult from a colonic polyp. Anaemia can also be due to malabsorption of iron, folate, and vitamin B12 because of a variety of diseases or can simply reflect an inadequate dietary intake through illness, alcoholism, depression, and so on. Chronic anaemia can also cause signs that you should search for if you find pale conjunctivae. These include koilonychia, angular stomatitis (painful cracks in the corners of the mouth), and atrophic glossitis (*gloss-eye-tiss*) (a smooth, painful tongue). Rarely, iron deficiency anaemia can lead to an oesophageal web, which can cause dysphagia (see p. 130).

How to examine

While you are checking for jaundice, scan down and look between the eyeball and the margin of the eyelid that you are pulling. This aspect of the conjunctiva is usually pink. If it is pale this suggests anaemia. Do not worry if you are never sure. Keep practising seeing normal as well as abnormal conjunctivae and remember, this is a crude test and even experienced physicians are often wrong.

9. Inspect the lips for pigmentation or telangiectasia (DF 9/10).

Pigmentation of lips

Brown freckly pigmentation around the mouth and lips may herald a rare condition called Peutz–Jehger's (*perts-yay-gers*) syndrome (*Johannes Laurentius Augustinus Peutz (1886–1957), Dutch physician, Harold Joseph Jehgers (1904–1990), American physician*). This is associated with polyps in the bowel, which can cause bleeding or bowel obstruction (see Fig. 14.9).

Telangiectasia of lips

Telangiectasia here would be very suggestive of HHT.

Oral cavity

10. Examine the oral cavity (DF 8/10). Inspect for telangiectasia, pigmentation, dentition, ulcers, angular stomatitis, and candidiasis. Also examine the tongue and tonsils and check for odours.

Keypoints

- Always inspect the sclerae to confirm the presence of jaundice clinically.
- Make sure that you check the conjunctivae for pallor and remember that this is a crude clinical test for anaemia.
- Telangiectasia or pigmentation around the lips and in the mouth may be markers of rare but important clinical syndromes (HHT and Peutz-Jehger's respectively).

Important clues can be gained from inspecting the mouth, so you must not be tempted to skimp on this part of the examination. Make sure that you illuminate the inside of the mouth well with a torch.

Telangiectasia

(DF 9/10.) Lesions here may be further confirmation of HHT.

Pigmentation

(DF 9/10.) Brown freckly pigmentation could be further proof of Peutz-Jehger's syndrome (see Fig. 14.19). More diffuse pigmentation could represent Addison's disease (*Thomas Addison (1793 - 1860), English physician*), an endocrine disorder that can present with anorexia, vomiting, and diarrhoea (see Figs 14.12–14.14).

Dentition

(DF 4/10.) Quickly examine the teeth and gums. Poor dentition and inflamed gums (gingivitis (*gin-ji-vie-tiss*)) may be markers of self-neglect. Elderly patients may have ill-fitting dentures, which can prevent them eating properly.

Ulcers

(DF 8/10.) Ulcers can have a variety of causes. One common form of recurrent ulceration is the aphthous ulcer (Fig. 6.10). They may be small or can be over 1 cm in diameter and can be sufficiently painful to deter the patient from eating. They have a yellow base with a surrounding rim of erythema. Some people with aphthous ulcers may have an increased risk of having ulcerative colitis. Patients with severe neutropenia (*new-trow-pee-nia*) (a decrease in a subset of white cells that normally fight infection) may develop similar looking ulcers in the mouth and oropharynx. Herpetic ulcers are also recurrent and tend to occur in painful crops in and around the mouth. A painless ulcer should give cause for concern, as this may be the beginning of a squamous (*squay-muss*) cell carcinoma. Any patient complaining of a long-standing ulcer or swelling in the mouth that is not healing or is increasing in size should have it biopsied to rule out cancer.

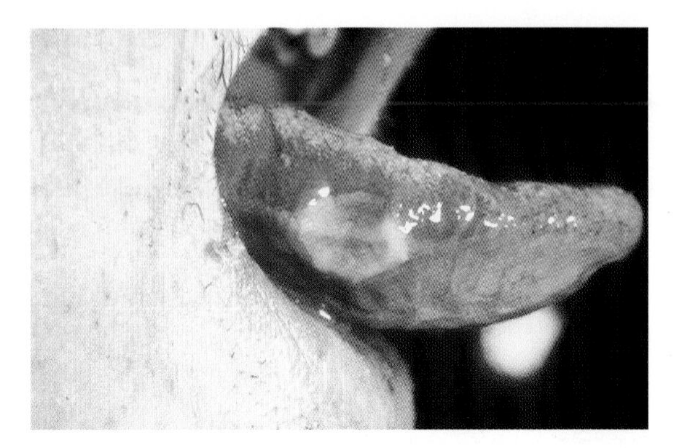

Fig. 6.10 Aphthous ulcer.

Angular stomatitis

(DF 2/10.) Do not forget to look at the corner of the mouth. Painful cracks in the corner suggest angular stomatitis. This may be due to candidal infection, chronic anaemia, or rarely vitamin deficiencies. See Fig. 6.11.

Candidiasis

(DF 8/10.)

What is it?

It is important to recognize the presence of candida (thrush). It is a fungal infection that can cause a sore mouth. In some cases, particularly in those who have a depressed immunity the candida can spread into the oesophagus and cause a painful dysphagia. It can manifest in different forms.

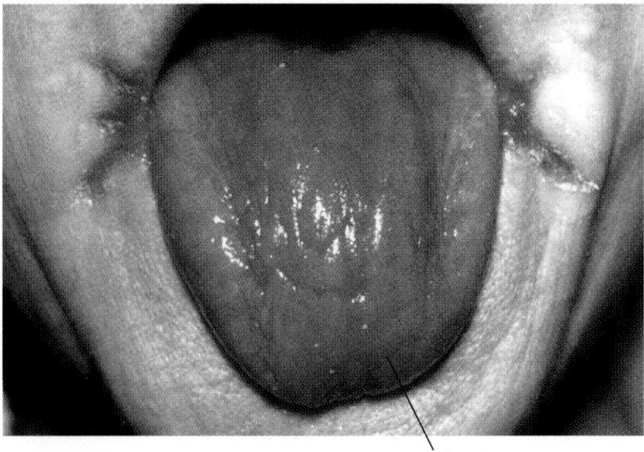

Fig. 6.11 Angular stomatitis. The patient also has a smooth fissured tongue indicative of a glossitis. The common causal feature is iron deficiency.

Causes

Trauma, moist areas, antibiotic therapy, diabetes mellitus, steroid therapy (oral and inhaled), and other forms of immunosuppression.

How to examine

Look for whitish plaques in the oral cavity. Occasionally patients who have drunk some milk may leave some residue that resembles candida. You should scrape the plaque away with a spatula to reveal reddened mucosa (if you are unsure you could send the scrapings to microbiology to identify). If you cannot remove the plaque after a number of attempts, you may be dealing with leukoplakia (*loo-co-play-kia*), a pre-malignant condition (a biopsy is required). A more difficult form of candidiasis to spot is a red inflamed mucosa, which may be erosive (particularly in denture wearers).

Tongue

(DF 7/10.) It is hard to miss the tongue during an inspection of the mouth but it is easy to miss vital clues without careful scrutiny. A furred tongue is supposed to signify illness or a fever but may be found in perfectly healthy people. In some patients, particularly after antibiotic therapy, this furring may be black in colour. This is a benign condition due to overgrowth of the papillae of the tongue together with infection due to *Candida nigricans* (*nigh-gri-cans*). You can reassure the patient that there is no serious disease but it can be a difficult condition to treat. A wasted tongue should signal a neurological cause (see p. 315). You should look for fasiculations (*fa-sick-you-lay-shuns*) (motor neurone disease) and observe the tongue movements for any lesion of the hypoglossal nerve. A large tongue is not always immediately obvious (unless very large). Possible causes include hypothyroidism (the commonest), acromegaly (*ack-crow-meg-alley*), and primary amyloidosis (*am-ee-lloyd-owe-sis*) (see Fig. 6.12).

CASE 6.9

Problem. You examine the oral cavity of a 28-year-old woman who is known to have asthma and who complains of a sore mouth. Inside her mouth you notice white plaques, which you scrape away to reveal underlying red raw areas. What is the cause?

Discussion. The simple answer is candidiasis but you must not be satisfied with this. You must ask yourself a further question. Why should an otherwise fit woman have oral candidiasis? If not due to local causes such as dentures or poor oral hygiene, is there the suggestion of debilitation, malnutrition, or immunosuppression? In this case the key is that she is an asthmatic and likely to be using a steroid inhaler. This can lead to local candidiasis especially if the inhaler technique is poor. She will need treatment with nystatin together with a check of her inhaler technique. If this is poor she needs re-educating on how to use her inhaler. If she still has difficulties she can use a spacer device, which removes the need for her to co-ordinate her breathing with the manipulations of her inhaler. It is also useful for the patient to gargle with water after using her inhalers.

Tonsils

(DF 8/10.) Now you need to view the tonsils. Get your patient to say 'Aaaah!' Quickly watch the central uvula (*you-view-la*), which should elevate in the mid-line. Then look down and to each side and inspect each tonsil. Are they obviously enlarged? Is there pus on them? Very rarely they may be involved in a lymphoma.

Odour

(DF 9/10.) The appreciation of smell on the breath is rarely ever taught because it is a difficult area to describe. Yet important information may be conveyed to your nose. Certain conditions have a characteristic odour, for example, the sweet musty smell of hepatic failure or the sickly sweet, acetone smell of diabetic ketoacidosis. The only real way of learning these smells is to find actual cases during your clinical attachment and memorize them (the odours are unmistakable). Alcohol on the breath is one smell that most medical students are acquainted with and is an important factor in many medical diseases. Foul-smelling breath (halitosis) may be due

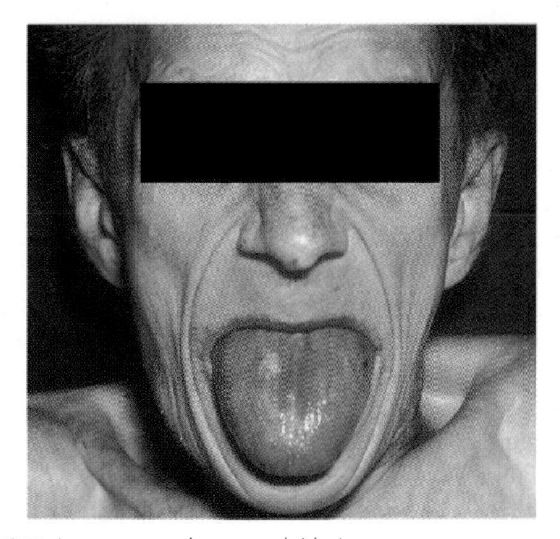

Fig. 6.12 Large tongue due to amyloidosis.

to poor dental hygiene, pathology of the nasopharynx, or bronchiectasis, or it may have no discernible cause.

Other

(DF 9/10.) Although beyond the scope of this chapter it is important to recognize that skin disease may also involve the oral mucosa. Sometimes this can be crucial in supporting a diagnosis, for example, lichen planus (*like-en-plane-us*) or pemphigus vulgaris (*pem-fig-us-vul-gar-iss*).

Keypoints

- Inspection of the oral cavity is very important and must be done with adequate illumination.
- Local disease may cause pain and interfere with nutrition especially in vulnerable people, for example, candida or ulcers.
- Signs of general disease can be found in the mouth, for example, pigmentation in Addison's disease.
- Pay close attention to the tongue and assess its colour, size, and coating (and its neurology also, see later).
- Signs of skin disease may be found in the mouth and may aid in their diagnoses, for example, lichen planus or pemphigus vulgaris.

Palpation of the neck

11. Palpate the neck for cervical lymph nodes (DF 6/10), particularly the left supraclavicular region.

When palpating the neck during an abdominal examination, pay particular attention to the left supraclavicular fossa. An enlarged lymph node here may be caused by spread from a gastrointestinal cancer, especially gastric cancer. This node is often called Virchow's (*ver-koffs*) node and is sometimes referred to as Troisier's (*twa-zee-ers*) sign. This node is preferentially involved because the lymph drains directly from the gut to this area. This area is readily felt with the fingertips with the patient lying flat. However, if you are palpating the rest of the cervical region, you must be aware that more traditional teachers believe that you can only examine this region properly from behind the patient as in the respiratory examination (see p. 110). *Rudolph Ludwig-Karl Virchow (1821–1902), German pathologist, Charles Emile Troisier (1844–1919), French pathologist.*

Keypoints

- The left supraclavicular node is the preferential drainage site for gastrointestinal organs.
- A malignant swelling of the left supraclavicular node is called Troisier's Sign or Virchow's node.

Inspection of the chest

12. Inspect the chest for further spider naevi (DF 8/10), gynaecomastia (DF 7/10), and loss of axillary hair in men (DF 6/10).

Spider naevi

Inspect and blanch as before.

Gynaecomastia

What is it?

Gynaecomastia is the enlargement of the breast tissue in men. See Fig. 6.13.

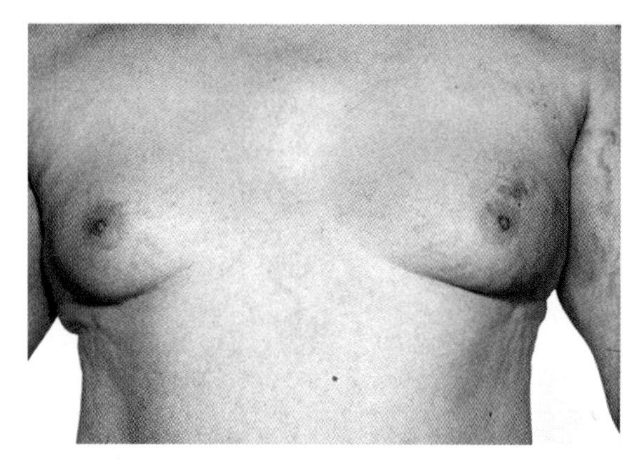

Fig. 6.13 Gynaecomastia.

TABLE 6.14 Causes of gynaecomastia

Puberty
Thyrotoxicosis
Chronic liver disease
Klinefelter's (*kline-felt-hers*) syndrome
Testicular disease/tumours
Pituitary disease
Hypothalamic disease
Drugs

* Harry Fitch Klinefelter (1912–?), US physician: described the syndrome of feminization as result of multiple X chromosomes linked with a solitary Y chromosome.

Significance

In the context of an abdominal examination, it usually occurs in chronic liver disease. Increased circulating oestrogens and decreased testosterone production lead to feminization in men. Other signs to look out for include loss of axillary hair and a female distribution of pubic hair.

Causes

See Table 6.14.

CASE 6.10

Problem. You see a 62-year-old man whom you just got permission to examine. As he undresses you notice he has a distended abdomen and what look like a pair of breasts. You examine him thoroughly but cannot find any other features of chronic liver disease. You find an enlarged regular liver, confirm gynaecomastia by palpation, elicit shifting dullness, and demonstrate pitting oedema of the legs and ankles. As you conclude your examination you notice your patient seems more breathless than before. Does your patient have chronic liver disease?

Discussion. It is possible. You do not always need to have all the classical signs such as leuconychia and spider naevi present (although their presence makes clinical diagnosis easier). However there is a further clue here. You have examined the patient flat and as you finished your patient was noticeably more breathless. This suggests orthopnea. Your patient in fact has congestive cardiac failure with an enlarged liver due to congestion, together with orthopnea and peripheral oedema. Cardiac failure can be severe enough to be accompanied by ascites. The only thing that cannot be explained so far is the gynaecomastia. However if you look at his treatment chart you will see that the patient is on frusemide, spironolactone, and digoxin amongst others. Spironolactone can cause gynaecomastia and digoxin can occasionally. It must be pointed out that spironolactone is rarely used for heart failure treatment with the advent of better drugs (particularly angiotensin-converting enzyme inhibitors) although it is still used in the medical treatment of ascites (note that spironolactone may be making a comeback in heart failure with the advent of new trial results). In the past congestive cardiac failure could be severe and prolonged enough to interfere with the liver function markedly and lead to a situation called cardiac cirrhosis.

How to examine

Checking for gynaecomastia in the thin or cachexic man is relatively simple. In the obese man it can be much more difficult to tell whether enlarged breasts are due to gynaecomastia or simply adipose tissue. Do not be satisfied simply looking at them, you must also palpate them to check if glandular tissue is present. This too is not as easy as it sounds, so do not be put off if you are still unsure. Often, the patient is distressed about it and this can provide a vital clue.

Loss of axillary hair

Another potential sign of increased oestrogen production in men with chronic liver disease.

Other drugs causing gynaecomastia are shown in Table 6.15.

Inspection of the abdomen

13. Observe the abdomen for distention, herniae, scars, striae, pulsations, peristalsis, and distended veins (DF 8/10).

It seems that you have examined everything **but** the abdomen up to this point. As you get confident and slick you will find that it can take you less than a minute to get to this stage. But be patient! You still

TABLE 6.15 Other drugs causing gynaecomastia

Cimetidine (*sigh-met-a-dean*)
Digoxin
Cytotoxic drugs
Methyldopa (*me-thile-dough-per*)
Anti-androgens, e.g. cyproterone (*sigh-pro-ter-own*) acetate*
Oestrogens*
Gonadorelin (*go-nad-owe-rel-in*) analogue*

* These drugs are used in the treatment of prostate cancer. In addition, oestrogens may be administered to men who are preparing to become women as part of gender reassignment.

Keypoints

- If you suspect gynaecomastia always palpate the breast tissue.
- Gynaecomastia has many causes including drugs.
- If you diagnose gynaecomastia look for other effects of feminization, that is, female distribution of pubic hair and testicular atrophy.

should not lay a hand on your patient. You need to focus your inspection on the abdomen itself and note any features. To help with your presentation the abdomen is divided into nine regions by a number of imaginary lines. A simpler version, dividing the abdomen into four quadrants is also acceptable. Any abnormal findings should be mapped to any one of the nine regions (or four quadrants), for example, a 5 × 5 cm mass in the epigastrium or a scar in the left lower quadrant (see Figs 6.14 and 6.15). At this point it is useful to stand at the foot of the bed and observe the abdomen. Check to see that it is roughly symmetrical and if it moves gently outwards with inspiration. If the patient has peritonitis and abdominal rigidity, there may be no visible movement with respiration.

Abdominal distention

(DF 2/10.) There is a range of normal appearances of the abdomen, ranging from the concave abdomen (scaphoid) (*scay-foid*) of the thin person (viewed from the side) to the more generous protuberance of the obese person. You will get a feel for these differences the more patients you examine. Any abdomen that appears swollen requires an explanation. A useful way of remembering the five causes of generalized abdominal distention is 'the five Fs': fat, foetus, fluid, flatus, and faeces. The first two are usually easy to identify. You will instinctively recognize the fatty abdomen of the obese patient and most women will tell you that they are pregnant (although you still hear stories of some women who are unaware of their pregnancy). The other three need further examination to distinguish between them. Sometimes you may notice more localized distention. The swollen area may give you a clue to the cause. If you have a good working knowledge of the anatomy of the abdomen you can make an educated guess, for example, a distended epigastrium could be due to gastric cancer, an enlarged left lobe of the liver, or a pancreatic cyst or pseudocyst. Or a distended hypogastrium (supra-pubic region) could indicate urine retention in an enlarged bladder or an ovarian cyst.

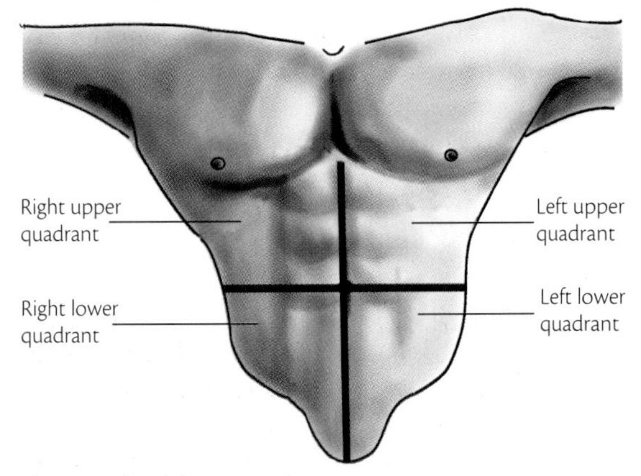

Fig. 6.14 The abdomen quadrants.

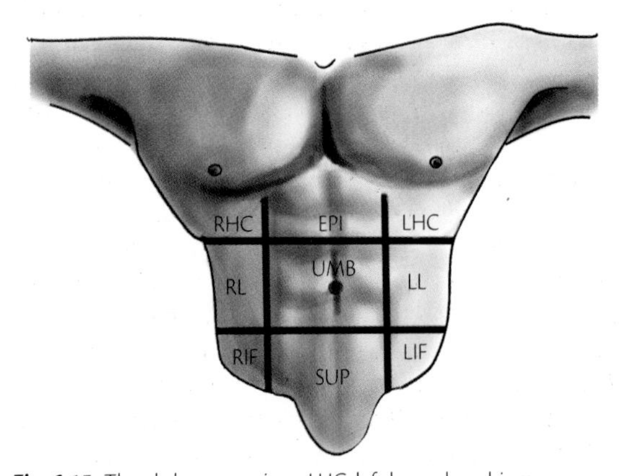

Fig. 6.15 The abdomen regions. LHC, left hypochondrium; LL, left lumbar region (or loin); LIF, left iliac fossa; EPI, epigastrium; UMB, umbilical region; SUP, suprapubic (or hypogastric) region; RHC, right hypochondrium; RL, right lumbar region (or loin); RIF, right iliac fossa.

Herniae

(DF 8/10.)

What are they?

A hernia is defined as the protrusion of an abdominal organ through an abnormal opening. They can be internal, for example, hiatus hernia (the stomach protrudes upwards through the diaphragmatic opening) or external, where they can be viewed with the naked eye. Herniae (*her-nee-ee*) are more localized bulges, which occur in areas of weakness in the abdominal wall. They tend to be labelled according to their site, for example, epigastric hernia. One characteristic of herniae is that their bulging increases with a rise in intra-abdominal pressure. This feature is exploited when you get the patient to cough. Herniae may disappear when the patient lies flat (the contents return to the abdominal cavity under the influence of gravity). If this happens the hernia is described as reducible. You may have to push the contents back yourself. If the contents cannot be returned, the hernia is irreducible. This occurs if there are adhesions between the hernial contents and the inner wall of the sac. A hernia becomes life threatening if it becomes strangulated. The likelihood of this happening increases the narrower the neck of the hernia. A narrow neck can constrict the blood supply of the abdominal contents leading to necrosis.

Causes

See Table 6.16.

TABLE 6.16 Factors in the causation of a hernia

Weakness of abdominal wall
Congenital
Obesity
Cachexia
Multiparity
Surgical incision
Repeated rise in intra-abdominal pressure
Chronic cough
Respiratory disease
Constipation (straining)

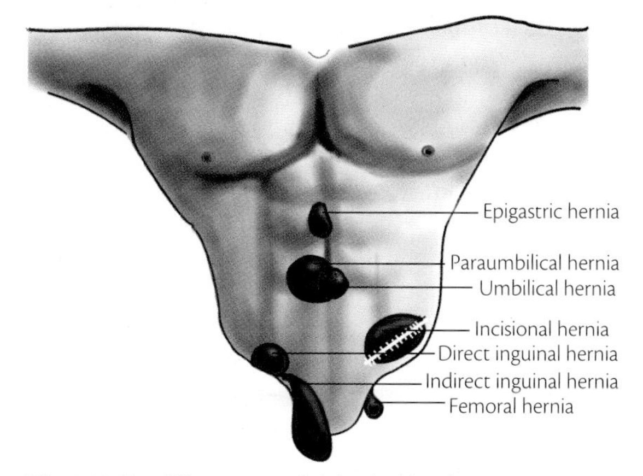

Fig. 6.16 The different types of abdominal herniae.

Types

See Fig. 6.16.

- **Epigastric.** This is a small protrusion through the linea alba (*lin-ee-a-al-ba*) (the central part of the rectus (*wrecked-us*) abdominus muscle. It can occur anywhere along the linea alba above the umbilicus and usually contains extraperitoneal fat. For a small hernia it can be quite painful.
- **Umbilical (*um-billy-cull or um-be-like-al*).** The swelling here is localized to the navel and is common in babies.
- **Paraumbilical.** This occurs just above or below the umbilicus. It occurs in obese people and in women who have had multiple childbirths. It has a narrow neck and is therefore prone to strangulation.
- **Divarication of recti (*die-varry-cay-shun-of-wreck-tie*).** This is again common in obese people and in women who have had multiple childbirths. In each case the abdominal musculature is weak and the linea alba bulges in a vertical line between the rectus abdominus muscle (see Fig. 6.17).

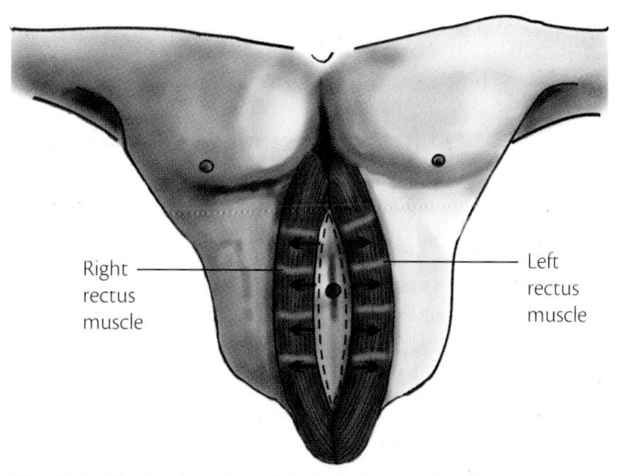

Fig. 6.17 Divarication of recti. A rise in intra-abdominal pressure causes a characteristic bulge in the midline of the abdomen forcing the inner border of the recti muscles apart.

- **Incisional.** Any surgical incision is a potential site of abdominal weakness. Sometimes a hernia can develop in a portion of a scar or along its whole length.
- **Direct inguinal.**
- **Indirect inguinal.** See p. 72.
- **Femoral.**

How to examine

You may notice a localized swelling on the abdomen as the patient undresses. As you do a general look, keep an eye on the swelling as the patient lies down. If the swelling enlarges (the act of lying down raises the intra-abdominal pressure) this can give you an early clue that you are dealing with a hernia. Do not worry if you miss this, as you will have the chance to check the swelling's response to intra-abdominal pressure in a little while. With any swelling you must assess it carefully, with regards to size, consistency, and so on (see p. 162). If you suspect that you are dealing with a hernia, then either get the patient to sit up or get them to cough. The rise in abdominal pressure will cause the swelling to bulge. Having diagnosed a hernia you must check to see if it is reducible. Do this by pushing the hernia gently with your fingers back into the abdomen. With any luck it should slide back. If it does not then the swelling is irreducible. You should then auscultate to see if you can hear bowel sounds over the swelling. If the hernia has become strangulated, the patient will be ill and in pain. The hernia itself will be tender and will lose its cough impulse.

Scars

(DF 3/10.) As in the cardiovascular examination, finding scars on the abdomen can be useful. Sometimes the information is just 'fodder' for interest but at other times it can be very relevant, for example, the patient with an appendectomy scar (gridiron incision) who has right iliac fossa pain. Their pain cannot be due to appendicitis and you need to think again.

Types of incisions

- **Median.** This type of incision gives access to most intra-abdominal organs. It is used in an emergency especially if the cause of the surgical emergency is not clear (the operation is called a laparotomy (*lap-a-rot-tummy*)). Some surgeons dub this the 'incision of indecision'.
- **Paramedian.** This used to be the incision of choice for older surgeons for a laparotomy. However it can lead to poor access to organs on the opposite side of the incision.
- **Kocher's (*cockers*).** (*Emil Theodor Kocher (1841– 1917), Swiss surgeon.*) This incision is found below and parallel to the right costal margin. It allows access to the liver and biliary tract (on the left a similar incision allows access to the spleen).
- **Transverse.** This is used to gain good exposure of the upper abdominal organs. This is another incision that is not often used these days.
- **Gridiron.** This incision is used for access to the appendix.
- **Rutherford-Morrison.** This incision is used primarily for access to the kidneys
- **Pfannenstiel (*fan-en-steal*).** (*Hans Hermann Johannes Pfannenstiel (1862–1909), German gynaecologist.*) This is a transverse incision just below the pubic hairline. It is used mainly for access to the uterus.
- **Umbilical.** Laparoscopy (note that small laparoscopic scars can be found almost anywhere on the abdomen because of the improvements in and desire to use laparoscopic techniques for certain operations). These laparoscopic operations require a good deal of skill and training to be effective.

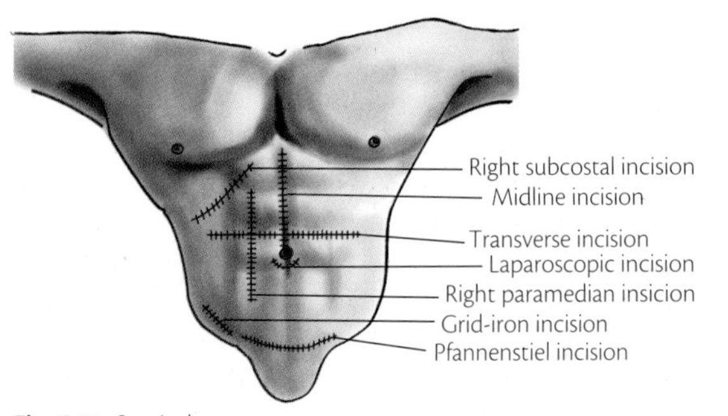

Fig. 6.18 Surgical scars

CASE 6.11

Problem. You see a 36-year-old woman who complains of central colicky abdominal pain for many years. She is bitter that nobody has been able to sort her out. She has seen many specialists including surgeons and she shows you her abdomen, which has a number of surgical scars on it. What is the diagnosis?

Discussion. Sometimes in medicine we cannot always make a diagnosis (unlike the slick TV doctors of films and soaps). If we cannot come to a diagnosis we owe it to the patient to make sure their condition is not life threatening and to ease discomfort and reassure where possible. With this patient you need to get her old notes if possible to see what tests have already been performed. If common things have been excluded, now is the time to plumb the depths of your mind (or textbook) to dredge up the rarer causes of abdominal pain such as acute intermittent porphyria, lead poisoning, and so on. If this fails, do not be afraid to seek a second opinion from a colleague. A fresh mind can sometimes unearth a clue that you may have overlooked (with the pressures of work there is no shame in this).

Sadly, there are times when a patient's history cannot be trusted. They may be malingerers, drug addicts, or alcoholics who do not want to face the truth. This patient may have Munchausen's (*munch-house-en*) syndrome (*Baron Karl Friedrich Hieronymus Frieherr von Munchausen (1720–1797), German soldier and traveller* famed for his outrageously fabricated tales). This is an ill-understood condition where the person enjoys the attention of being in hospital and will manufacture symptoms (sometimes to textbook standards) to achieve this end. They tend to be reliable at first but you find great difficulty in corroborating their story as they flit from hospital to hospital (especially if they feel that they are about to be exposed). They will even endure repeated surgery to remain in the hospital domain. Never ever diagnose this condition without investigating the patient thoroughly (although be suspicious in the right circumstances) or if you get good evidence about the person circulated from other hospitals. There is currently no cure for this condition.

How to examine

See Fig. 6.18. Scars may be difficult to see, especially old ones or those concealed in skin creases, for example, Pfannenstiel incision for caesarian sections or hysterectomy. You must look carefully and do not be afraid to get down close to look at scars. Also remember to lean over the patient and look at the left flank for a nephrectomy scar (Rutherford–Morrison). You can gain a rough idea of the age of the scar from its colour. A purply-red scar (in a Caucasian) indicates a recent scar (usually within a year of operation). A silvery-white scar indicates an older incision.

Striae

(DF 3/10). See Fig. 6.19. Striae are stretch marks. They indicate a recent decrease in the girth of the abdomen (especially a distended one). This can occur after pregnancy (striae gravidarum), following drainage of ascitic fluid, or an obese person who has lost weight. They tend to be salmon pink in colour (older ones tend to be silvery white). Striae can also occur in Cushing's syndrome (*Harvey Cushing (1869–1939), American neurosurgeon*) except in this condition they are reddy purple in colour and are more substantial. Striae are not just seen in the abdomen but can be seen on the shoulders, upper arms, back, thighs, buttocks, and so on.

Pulstations

(DF 4/10.) Pulsations in the abdomen are usually due to the abdominal aorta. They are a normal finding in the epigastrium of thin patients. However any pulsation especially in an obese patient raises the spectre of an aneurysm (*an-your-ism*) of the abdominal aorta. Make a mental note of any pulsation you see as you will need to palpate the area more fully during your examination.

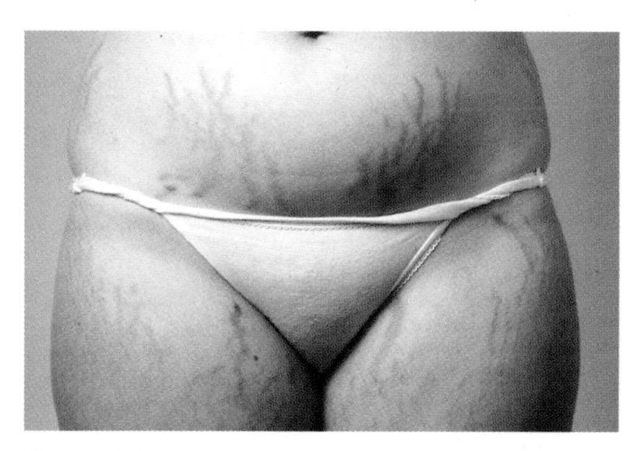

Fig. 6.19 Striae.

Peristalsis

(DF 9/10.) Peristalsis (*perry-stal-sis*) is the term used to describe the waves of contraction that propel food and gut contents along the bowel. Normally these waves are not visible (except in some thin patients). However if a patient develops an obstruction in the stomach or intestine, the waves of contraction become more pronounced as the gut tries to overcome the blockage. In small bowel obstruction, waves of peristalsis can be seen in the centre of the abdomen. With pyloric (*pie-lor-rick*) stenosis, where the outflow to the stomach is blocked, a peristaltic wave can be seen rippling from the left hypochondrium to the right (if the stomach is distended the wave can travel down past the umbilicus before ascending to the right hypochondrium). To clinically confirm pyloric stenosis, it was said that you should perform a 'succussion (*suck-cush-ion*) splash', that is, if you grasped the patient by the lower chest bilaterally and shook them vigorously from side to side, a sloshing sound can be heard (due to the copious contents of the stomach). However this sound can be heard in normal people up to 2 h after a meal and as it is not a very dignified test it is not recommended. If you have good clinical reasons to suspect pyloric stenosis, proceed with gastroscopy.

Distended veins

(DF 7/10.)

Significance

Normally there are very few distended veins on the abdominal wall. There are two important situations when distended veins are a prominent feature, portal hypertension in chronic liver disease and inferior vena caval obstruction (IVCO). In both cases the normal flow of blood back to the heart is impeded. To try and overcome this, blood is diverted through veins called collaterals to provide an alternative route back to the right side of the heart. As the volume of blood is large, the collaterals distend to accommodate the increased load. The abdominal veins represent a visible and important group of collaterals.

How to examine

First look at the distribution of the enlarged veins. Veins radiating from the umbilicus in a star-like fashion (termed the caput medusae) suggest portal hypertension (Fig. 6.20). Veins coursing vertically up the abdomen suggest IVCO. The next step is to work out the direction of blood flow, which is different in the two conditions. In portal hypertension the blood flow is away from the umbilicus and in IVCO the flow is upwards. To determine the blood flow, you need to press on a vein with the index finger of one hand. Place

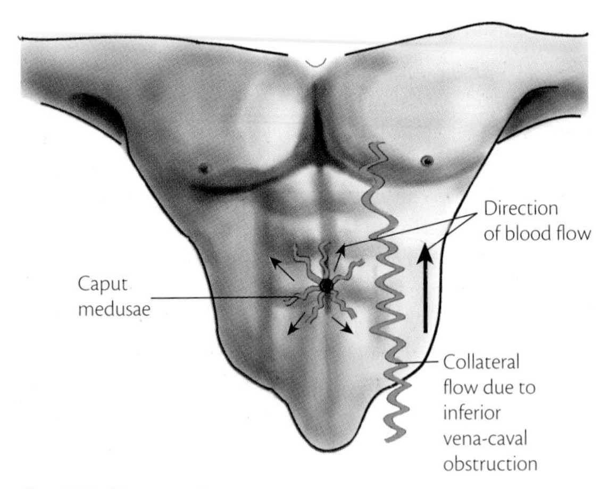

Fig. 6.20 Caput medusae.

the index finger of the other hand next to it and milk the blood out of the vein by sliding your finger about 3–5 cm in any direction. Lift up the finger of the milking hand and if the vein refills, then the blood flow is opposite to the direction of milking. If you lift up the milking finger and the vein does not distend then the blood flow is in the direction of milking and is being dammed back by your non-milking finger. See Fig. 6.21.

Palpation of the abdomen

14. Ask the patient if they have any tender areas before commencing light palpation. Palpate the abdomen lightly, mapping any areas of tenderness and note any masses (DF 4/10). Watch the patient's face for signs of pain!

(a)

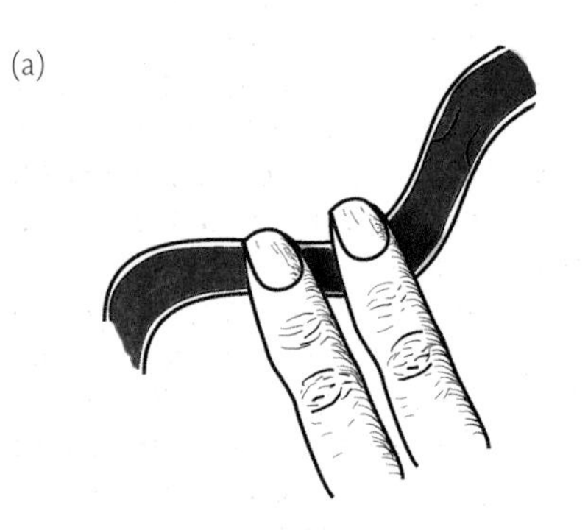

Place index fingers on the vein.

(b)

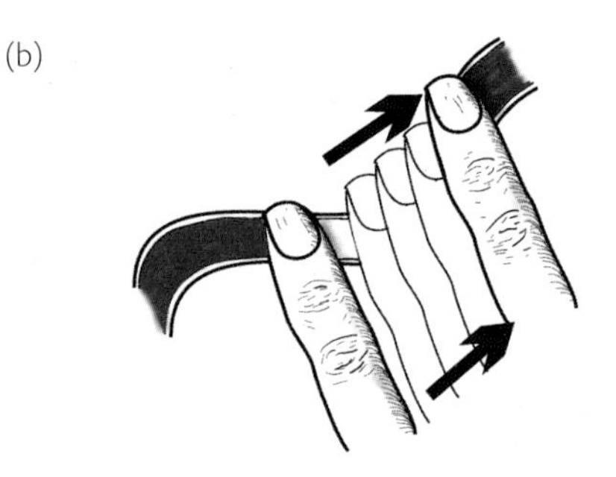

Milk in one direction.

(c)

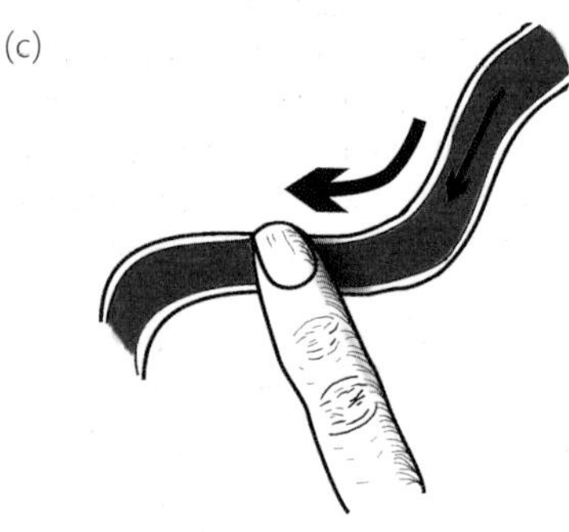

If vein refills the direction of flow is indicated by the arrow.

(d)

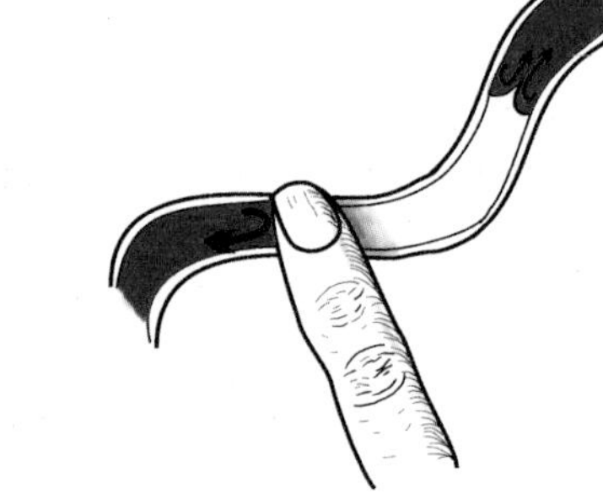

If vein does **not** refill see (e).

(e)

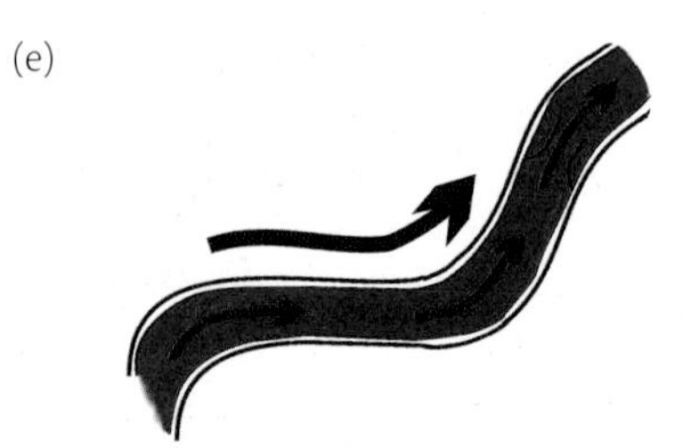

Direction of flow is indicated by the arrow.

Fig. 6.21 Sequence of drawings demonstrating direction of flow.

Keypoints

- Abdominal distention may be due to the 'five Fs': fat, flatus, faeces, foetus, and fluid.
- Herniae increase in size with an increase in intra-abdominal pressure (except if strangulated).
- Always get the patient to cough when examining for a hernia.
- No examination for a hernia is complete without getting the patient to stand and cough.
- The narrower the neck of a hernia the more prone it is to strangulate.
- Distended veins on the abdomen may signify impeded blood flow along the major veins back to the heart. The distribution of veins and the direction of blood flow give clues to the underlying problem, for example, caput medusae—portal hypertension, upward flow of blood—IVCO.

You are aiming to get a superficial overview of the abdomen and are looking specifically for tender areas and masses. There are varying degrees of tenderness, ranging from mild discomfort to the extreme pain associated with peritonitis. In addition, there are a number of phenomena that you need to be able to spot as they herald life-threatening complications. These are guarding, rebound tenderness, and rigidity.

Peritonitis

(DF 6/10.) This is inflammation of the peritoneum. The cause is usually a bacterial infection or irritation from bowel contents following leakage into the abdominal cavity. This can follow perforation of an organ, for example, perforated gastric ulcer. Other causes include penetrating injuries, for example, stabbing or after surgery, which will be obvious from the history and rarely blood-borne sources, which may be difficult to spot. Peritonitis is life threatening and must be recognized. The patient is usually ill and clammy with a rapid thready pulse and may exhibit guarding, rebound tenderness, or rigidity.

Guarding

(DF 7/10.) This is the instantaneous contraction of muscle overlying an inflamed organ or peritoneum. This reflex contraction attempts to guard the inflamed area from being prodded further. Guarding is usually associated with marked tenderness.

Rebound tenderness

(DF 7/10.) This is another sign of an inflamed peritoneum. This time the pain is experienced after quickly lifting your hand off the affected area. Sometimes the inflammation is so severe that rebound pain can be elicited in the affected area by lifting your hand of an area remote from it.

Rigidity

(DF 6/10.) Severe inflammation of the peritoneum can lead to generalized rigidity of the abdomen. The pain associated can be so intense that the patient can only lie still. Even breathing can exacerbate the pain, so that the abdomen is held totally rigid as the patient takes rapid shallow breaths using chest movements only.

How to examine

Always ask the patient if they have any tender areas before starting. You should also follow up by saying 'Let me know if anywhere is tender when I press' (it is amazing how many patients will wince in silence, so as not to cause a fuss). Make sure your hands are warm before touching the patient. If you touch a patient with cold hands (this is an unprofessional act!) they will tense up or shout out and you may have to conduct the rest of your examination on the ceiling! Begin by kneeling down by the bedside (you can stoop but this can be tiring) (see Fig. 6.22). Place your hand flat on the abdomen away from any tender areas. Keeping your hand flat, press gently with the pulps of your fingers. Do this by flexing with straight fingers from your metacarpophalangeal joints (the knuckles). Watch your patient's face for signs of pain. Work your way around the abdomen palpating in this manner. Try to be systematic, so that you cover the whole abdomen efficiently. As a guide you can palpate each of the nine regions in turn. Any tender areas should be assessed for guard-

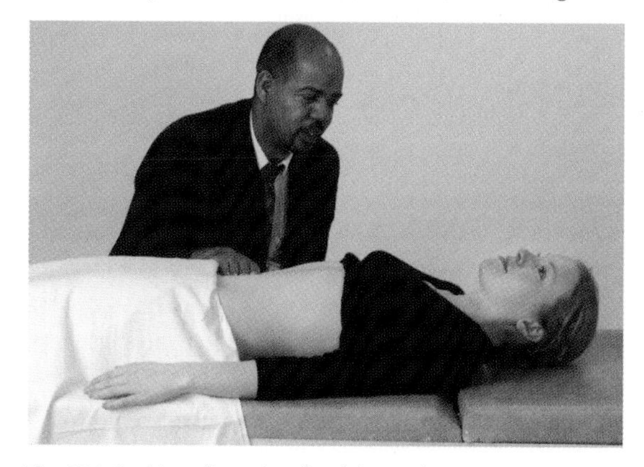

Fig. 6.22 Position of examiner for abdominal examination. Crouch or kneel beside the patient and do not forget to observe the face for signs of pain.

ing or rebound tenderness. As well as checking for tenderness you should be on the look-out for any unusual masses. At this stage do not try to work out what the mass is. Simply note the region it is in.

15. Palpate more deeply and assess any masses felt in more detail (DF 7/10).

Now you need to palpate more deeply. If there is marked tenderness, guarding, rebound tenderness, or rigidity this is unnecessary (and unkind). Palpation is done using the same technique as light palpation but by pressing down more firmly (some people achieve this by placing their free hand on top of the palpating hand).

If there were no abnormalities found on light palpation then retrace the areas you felt pressing more deeply this time. There are potential pitfalls when palpating the abdomen. There is the possibility of missing any abnormal structures and there is also the possibility of misinterpreting normal organs as abnormal (see Fig. 6.23). Normal structures you may encounter include the descending colon (this feels like a tube you can roll under your hand in the left lower quadrant) and the caecum in the right iliac fossa (this feels soft and ill defined and often squelches when pressed). The abdominal aorta is sometimes prominent in thin people (a pulsating tube found in the epigastrium). It is sometimes possible when palpating the epigastrium to be fooled into thinking that a contracting rectus muscle is a swelling. Be aware of this and if you are suspicious, try to get your patient to relax. The swelling should disappear with relaxation. In all cases you need to be aware of these pitfalls before you classify any mass as abnormal. If you do encounter an abnormal mass, you need to assess it in more detail. All the features listed below need to be examined.

Assessment of an abdominal mass

- **Site.**
- **Size.** Measured with a tape measure.
- **Border.** Hard, irregular? This suggests cancer.
- **Consistency.** Hard, irregular? This suggests cancer. Nodular? This suggests cancer or in the liver possibly cirrhosis.
- **Tenderness.** Suggests inflammatory process or distended capsule of an organ.

CASE 6.12

Problem. You examine a patient on the ward who seems well but when you examine their abdomen there is generalized rigidity. Has the patient developed peritonitis?

Discussion. No! But your cold, clammy hands may be sufficient to cause a generalized contraction of the rectus muscle of the abdomen. If you are unsure, quickly test your palpating fingers on the back of your other hand. Make sure your hands are warm. Another possible explanation is a very anxious patient. Sometimes they may contract their muscles before you lay a hand on them. Try to defuse their anxiety by getting them to relax. Sometimes taking deep breaths help. Occasionally you meet athletic people with impressive abdominal musculature (they are often proud of their 'six-pack'). Sometimes they have an increased resting tone that can make it difficult to appreciate any structures beneath (even with relaxation and deep breathing). It should also be pointed out that you do not need a rigid abdomen for peritonitis to be present. Some elderly patients have been known to be pyrexial with some tenderness in their abdomen but with no rebound, guarding, or rigidity and have been shown at post-mortem to have undiagnosed peritonitis.

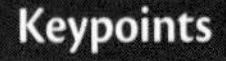

Keypoints

- Ask the patient if they have any tender areas before beginning palpation.
- Make sure the patient is comfortable.
- Watch the patient for signs of pain
- Severe tenderness, rebound tenderness, guarding, and rigidity are markers of serious pathology and will need surgical evaluation.

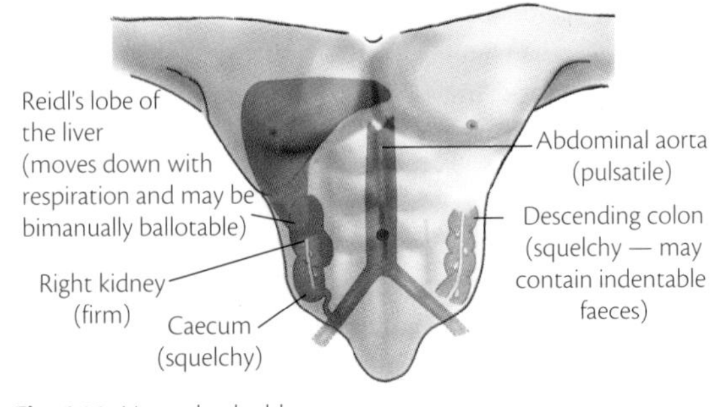

Fig. 6.23 Normal palpable structures.

- **Mobility.** Parts of the bowel are attached to mesentery and are mobile. Bowel tumours may become fixed if they spread and invade adjacent organs or skin. Some organs are permanently fixed, for example, the pancreas.
- **Movement with respiration.** See p. 166.
- **Percussion note.** See p. 167.
- **Pulsatility.** This suggests a vascular cause (beware transmitted pulsations).
- **Overlying temperature.** Warm? May suggest underlying imflammation, for example, abscess or infected cyst.
- **Bruit.** Suggests a vascular cause.

This information will help you to build an identikit picture of the mass and enable you to make a reasoned guess as to what it is. A knowledge of the anatomy of the abdomen will also help you in working out the potential origins of the mass. See Fig. 6.24.

Epigastric mass

See Table 6.17.

Right iliac fossa mass

See Table 6.18 and Fig. 6.25.

Left iliac fossa mass

See Table 6.19 and Fig. 6.26.

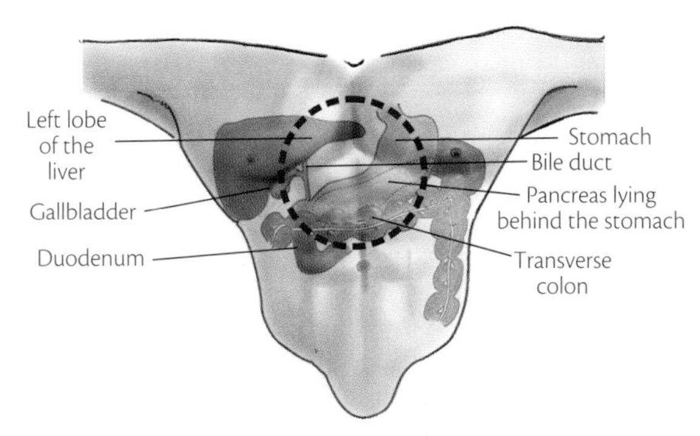

Fig. 6.24 Epigastric structures.

TABLE 6.17 Causes of an epigastric mass

Stomach	Cancer, pyloric stenosis
Liver	Enlarged left lobe
Pancreas	Pancreatic cysts, pancreatic pseudocyst (fluid in the lesser sac), cancer head of pancreas
Gallbladder (distended)	Mucocoele/empyaema

CASE 6.13

Problem. You see a 56-year-old man who complains of anorexia, vomiting, and weight loss. When you examine him he appears cachexic (emaciated). You notice he has a hard irregular lymph node in his left supraclavicular fossa and an irregular mass in his epigastrium. What is the diagnosis?

Discussion. This case reeks of cancer. The lymphadenopathy fits the description of Virchow's node (see p. 154) and the site of the mass in the epigastrium together with vomiting and weight loss is highly suggestive of stomach cancer.

TABLE 6.18 Causes of a right iliac fossa mass

Caecum	Carcinoma, Crohn's disease, tuberculosis
Appendix	Appendix abscess
Ovary	Cyst, carcinoma
Psoas muscle	Psoas abscess
External iliac artery	Aneurysm
Pelvic kidney	

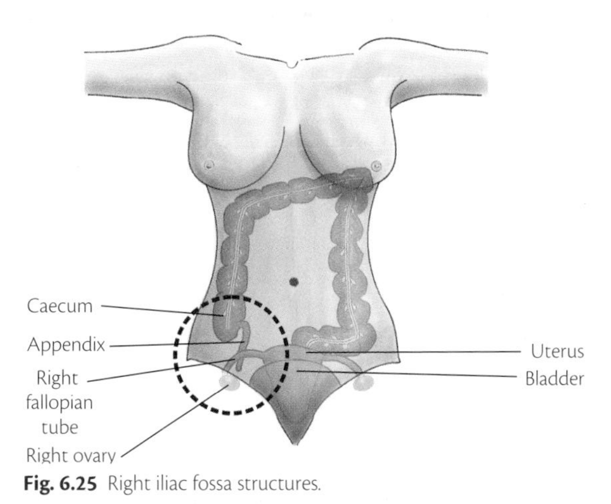

Fig. 6.25 Right iliac fossa structures.

Hypogastric mass

See Table 6.20 and Fig. 6.27. The most common cause of a hypogastric mass is an enlarged bladder and it usually occurs in elderly men with enlarged prostates that obstruct the flow of urine (see Fig. 6.28). The bladder can extend upwards as far as the umbilicus. If it occurs acutely it is an intensely painful condition. It can occur chronically over many weeks in the absence of pain. As

CASE 6.14

Problem. A 28-year-old man is admitted with abdominal pain. Initially the pain was peri-umbilical and colicky in nature. Later it localized to the right iliac fossa. He had tried to grin and bear the pain for 24 h but it did not subside. Furthermore he began to notice a tender swelling in the right iliac fossa. What is the diagnosis?

Discussion. The initial history is typical of appendicitis, with colicky pain starting around the umbilicus and later localizing to the right iliac fossa. The swelling developing in this area suggests that he has developed a complication of appendicitis, a local appendix abscess. This will be tender and fluctuant on examination.

CASE 6.15

History. You see an obese 86-year-old woman on the ward who was admitted with a fall. She normally walks with a zimmer frame because of osteoarthritis of the hips and knees and tends to sit in a chair most of the day. She does not seem to have sustained any serious injuries but when you examine her abdomen you find a left iliac fossa mass. It is firm, mobile, and non-tender. What are the possibilities?

Discussion. Any of the causes listed in the Table 6.19 are possible except an external iliac artery aneurysm, which would be pulsatile. Check the temperature chart to make sure she does not have a swinging pyrexia which would suggest an underlying abscess. However in this case the patient is relatively well apart from poor mobility and there is no suggestion of weight loss or any other obvious signs or symptoms. A little bit of lateral thinking might help here. She has osteoarthritis that limits her mobility and probably causes her a lot of pain. She may be on painkillers containing opioids, which can lead to constipation. Feel the mass again and this time apply firm pressure into the mass with your fingers. If it indents then it is likely that this mass is faecal loading of the sigmoid colon due to constipation. Once the bowel is cleared with laxatives or enemas the mass should disappear.

TABLE 6.19 Causes of a left iliac fossa mass

Sigmoid colon	Cancer, diverticular abscess
Ovary	Cyst, carcinoma
Psoas muscle	Psoas abscess
External iliac artery	Aneurysm
Pelvic kidney	

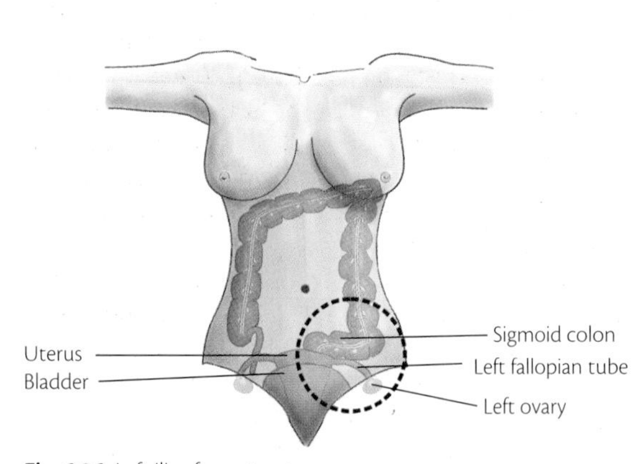

Fig. 6.26 Left iliac fossa structures.

TABLE 6.20 Causes of a hypogastric mass

Enlarged bladder
Ovarian cyst
Uterine fibroids/pregnancy
Tumour of sigmoid colon

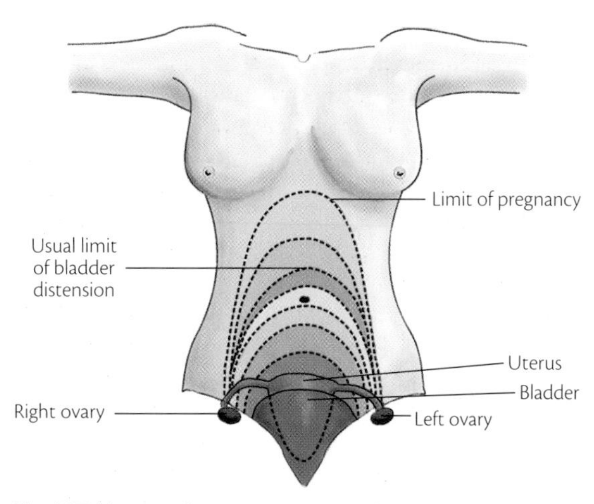

Fig. 6.27 Hypogastric structures.

it arises out of the pelvis you cannot get below it to feel its lower margin. It is also dull to percussion. These features are also shared by ovarian cysts and uterine

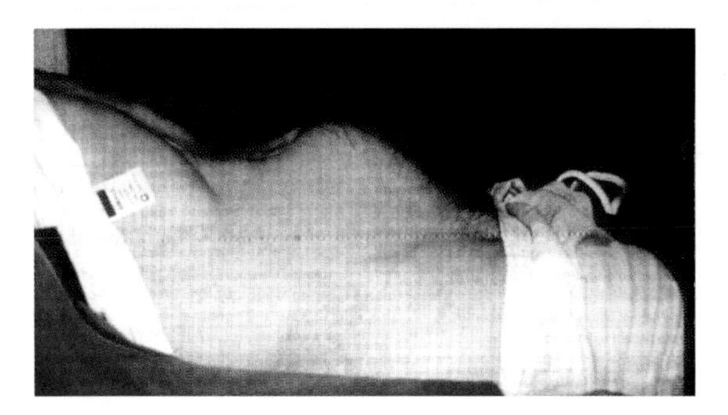

Fig. 6.28 Distended bladder. This is acute retention and requires immediate catherization.

fibroids. If you encounter an enlarged bladder you need to pass a catheter to drain the excess urine (in the acute situation this is accompanied by great relief for the patient). Sometimes if you are unsure about a hypogastric mass, passing a catheter may help. If urine drains and the mass decreases in size you can be sure you are dealing with an enlarged bladder. If little urine drains and the size of the mass is unaffected then the mass is not a bladder.

Tip

With the advent of portable bladder scanners the status of this organ can be assessed non-invasively.

Other masses

Aortic aneurysm

(DF 7/10.) This is the dilatation of the aorta, which usually occurs because of atherosclerosis. It is found in the mid-line in the centre of the abdomen. As an aneurysm enlarges the risk of it rupturing increases with possible catastrophic consequences. Therefore it is important that you are able to detect one. To do this you use a key feature of any artery, that is, its expansibility. If you find a pulsatile mass, place both your hands on either side of it and let your fingers rest gently against both borders. With each pulsation your fingers should be pushed up and outwards if it is an aortic aneurysm. This is important because a mass overlying the aorta can transmit its pulsation and give the illusion that it is a vascular structure. In this case, if you straddle the mass with your hands as before, your fingers will be lifted upwards but not outwards. See Fig. 6.29.

Gallbladder

(DF 9/10.) The gallbladder is only palpable occasionally. Gallstones are the commonest pathology to affect the gallbladder and this usually leads to a thickened fibrotic organ, which is impalpable. This observation is the basis of Courvoisier's Law (*Ludwig Georg Courvoisier (1843–1918), French surgeon*). This states that in the presence of jaundice a palpable gallbladder is unlikely to be due to a gallstone (exceptions do occur). If a gallbladder is palpable, other causes are more likely, for example, carcinoma of the head of pancreas, where the common bile duct is obstructed leading to distention of a normal gallbladder. A palpable gallbladder in the absence of jaundice can be due to a gallstone obstructing the cystic duct. The flow of bile is obstructed and in time the bile pigments trapped in the gallbladder are absorbed. Mucus is continually secreted by the gallbladder epithelium leading to distention. This is called a mucocoele (*mew-co-seal*) of the gallbladder. If this material becomes infected this creates an empyaema (*em-pie-ee-ma*) of the gallbladder.

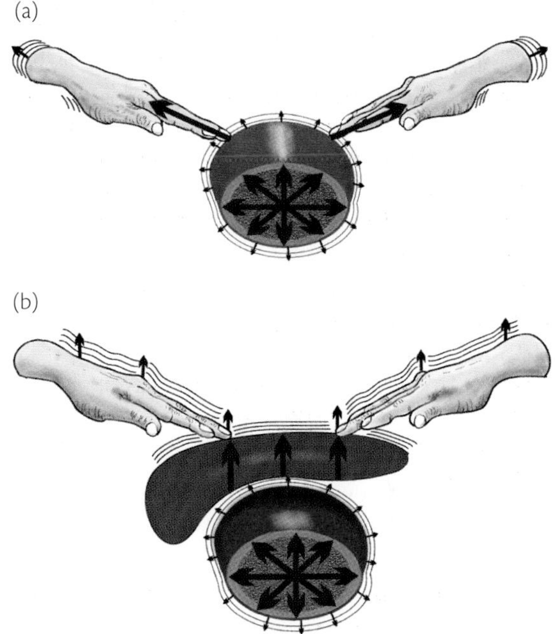

Fig. 6.29 Differentiating between expansile pulsation and transmitted pulsation of an aortic aneurysm. (a) The expansile nature of an aortic aneurysm: the fingers are pushed out laterally, (b) transmitted pulsation from an aortic aneurysm: in this case an enlarged liver transmits the pulsations upwards, elevating the hand.

16. Palpate specifically for enlarged organs: liver—commence in the right iliac fossa and move upwards towards the right costal margin while getting the patient to take deep breaths; spleen—commence in the right iliac fossa and move upwards towards the

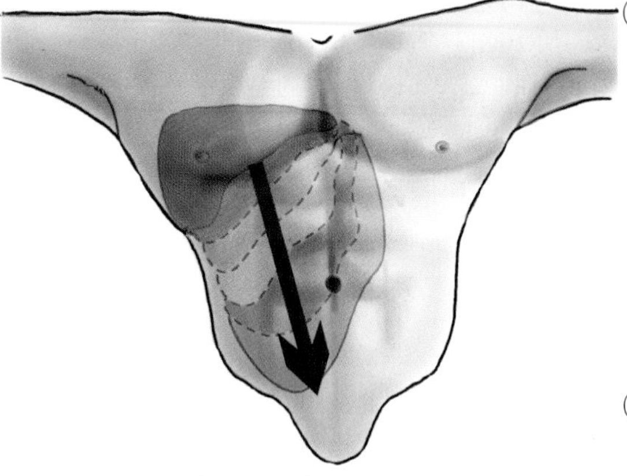

Fig. 6.30 Sequence of hepatic enlargement.

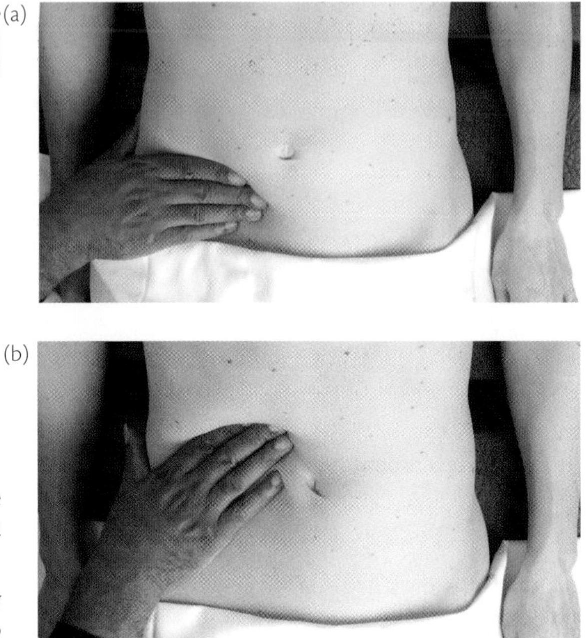

Fig. 6.31 Examining for a liver (see text for a full explanation).

left costal margin while getting the patient to take deep breaths; kidneys—commence in the flanks and 'bimanually ballot' them.

The liver, spleen, and kidneys are always routinely examined for. They are the most common organs to become palpable following disease and they have unique features that identify them. You must know them and be able to recognize them in your patient. In medical speak an enlarged organ has the suffix 'megaly' added to it, for example, hepatomegaly (enlarged liver) and splenomegaly (enlarged spleen).

Liver

(DF 7/10.) The liver is normally found under the right costal margin and is not normally palpable (a liver edge can sometimes be felt at the right costal margin). As it enlarges the liver edge can be felt in the right hypochondrium. With some diseases the liver can become massively enlarged and descend right down into the right iliac fossa. See Fig. 6.30.

How to examine

See Fig. 6.31. Remain kneeling down. You should always start off in the right iliac fossa so as not to miss massive hepatomegaly. Place your hand flat on the abdomen with your fingers angled up towards the patient's head. You will need to exert firm but gentle pressure into the abdomen while keeping your hand flat. It is the tips of the second and third fingers that are seeking the liver edge. Some people prefer to use the distal half of their index finger and the liver edge is felt against the radial border (the edge facing the thumb) of the digit.

The key to palpating for a liver is that it descends in the abdomen with inspiration. Ask your patient to take a deep breath and hold your hand still. You need to apply some pressure so that your hand is not displaced with the respiratory effort. You are feeling for an 'edge' that should descend to meet your fingers. This 'edge' is not always sharp but may be a feeling of a 'fullness' or 'something' bumping into or running under your fingers. If you do not feel anything, as the patient exhales move your hand a few fingerbreadths up towards the right costal margin and then hold your hand steady. Ask your patient to take another deep breath. Repeat this until you feel a liver edge or you reach the costal margin. A common mistake to make is to move your hand up towards the costal margin 'seeking' a liver during inspiration. If a mass is encountered, this movement of the hand may give the illusion that it is the mass itself that has moved to meet the fingers, so keep your hand still.

If you palpate a liver, feel its substance all the way to the costal margin. You should not be able to feel an upper border of the liver as it is under the lower ribs. It is said that you cannot get above the mass. This is a second very important characteristic of the liver. If you do feel an upper margin to a swelling then you are not dealing with a liver. Assess the liver and note if it feels smooth or irregular and whether it is tender or not. Also get some idea of the size of the liver. You can do this accurately by using a measuring tape from the costal margin to the liver edge or crudely by using fingerbreadths below the costal margin. Finally you need to percuss for both the upper and lower border of the liver, as occasionally in emphysema a normal liver can be pushed down by a hyperinflated lung. The liver is usually dull to percussion and therefore first percuss below the liver in an area that should be resonant. Percuss upwards and when the liver is encountered the note should become dull. Now percuss for the upper margin of the liver (this is normally in the sixth interspace). Start percussing just above the nipple on the right hand side of the chest (in a man) and percuss downward. The resonant note should become dull in the sixth interspace. If it remains resonant then suspect emphysema (look for other features) and downward displacement of the liver.

Causes of hepatomegaly

See Table 6.21.

Spleen

(DF 8/10). The spleen lies under the left costal margin along the ninth, tenth, and eleventh ribs and does not extend beyond the mid-axillary line in the adult. As it enlarges it can be felt in the left hypochondrium. In some diseases it can become massively enlarged and cross the mid-line into the right iliac fossa. See Fig. 6.32.

How to examine

You will need to stand to examine the spleen. You should always start off in the right iliac fossa so as not to miss massive splenomegaly (the identical position to Fig. 6.31(a)). Place your hand on the abdomen with your fingers aimed towards the patient's left shoulder. This time only the tips of your second and third fingers can be used to feel a splenic border. Now reach over with your non-palpating hand and pull up on the left lower ribs. This manoeuvre is meant to accentuate a spleen that is only just palpable. The key to palpating the spleen (like the liver) is that it descends in the abdomen with inspiration. Use exactly the same technique you used for the liver, but this time work your hand towards the left costal margin. If you palpate a spleen feel its substance all the way to the costal margin. You should not be able to 'get above it', to feel its upper border. This is the second distinguishing feature of the spleen. If you can get above it, you are not dealing with a spleen. Now feel the consistency of the spleen, note if it is tender and pay close attention to the splenic border. If you find a notch in it, this is the third unique feature of the spleen. Measure the size of the spleen with a tape measure or by gauging the number of finger-breadths below the costal margin. Finally percuss the lower border of the spleen starting well below the edge from an area of resonance. The percussion note should be dull when the spleen is encountered.

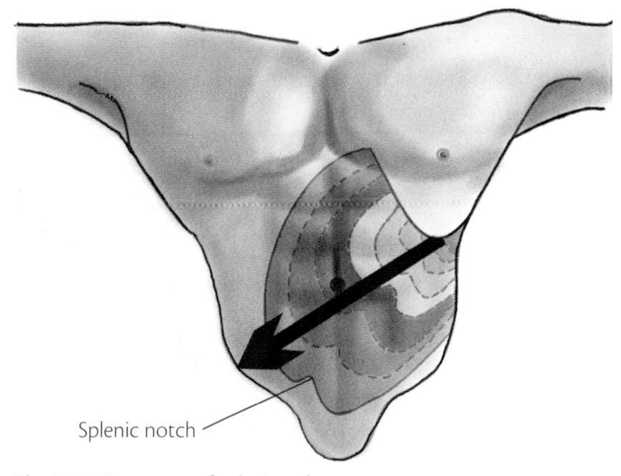

Fig. 6.32 Sequence of splenic enlargement.

TABLE 6.21 Causes of hepatomegaly

Cardiac	Congestive cardiac failure, tricuspid incompetence, hepatic vein thrombosis (Budd–Chiari syndrome*)
Infective	Viral (e.g. hepatitis A, B, or C, glandular fever), bacterial (e.g. brucellosis), parasite (e.g. hydatid disease), protozoal (e.g. amoebic abscess)
Haematological	Lymphoma, leukaemia (especially chronic granulocytic leukaemia), myelofibrosis, haemolytic anaemia
Infiltrative	Gaucher's disease†, amyloidosis

* George Budd (1808–1882), UK Physician, Hans Chiari (1851–1916), Austrian pathologist.

† Phillipe Charles Ernest Gaucher (1854–1918), French dermatologist.

There may be times when the spleen may only just be palpable. A technique called 'tipping the spleen' may help in this circumstance. Get your patient to roll onto their right hand side, with their left knee bent upwards. Ask the patient to reach over with their left arm and to rest it on your left shoulder. Put your hand right up to the left costal margin and get the patient to take a deep breath. If the spleen is just palpable you may be able to 'tip' it in this position (see Fig. 6.33). Sometimes you cannot palpate the spleen and the only clue to its enlargement is a dull percussion note in Traube's space (*Ludwig Traube (1818–1876), German physician*). This is the region in the ninth intercostal space that lies anterior to the anterior axillary line. Normally this area is resonant but as the spleen enlarges it occupies this space and the percussion note becomes dull.

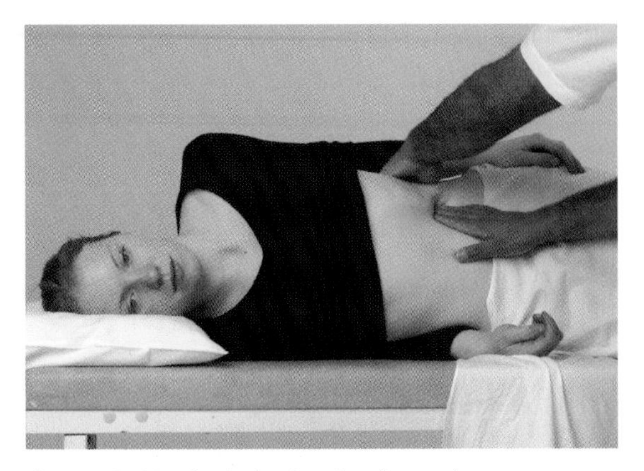

Fig. 6.33 Position for tipping the spleen (see text).

Causes of splenomegaly

See Table 6.22.

Kidneys

(DF 9/10.) The kidneys can prove very difficult to palpate especially if your technique is not spot on. In normal people they are impalpable (very occasionally the right kidney can be felt in thin people).

How to examine

See Figs 6.34 and 6.35. You need to stand up to examine the kidneys and you will need both hands to palpate (bimanual palpation). To examine the right kidney you must place your left hand under the patient in the renal angle. This is below the twelfth rib, above the posterior iliac crest and not as far in as the spine and paravertebral muscles. If you are too near any of these positions the area will feel hard and firm. You may have to move your hand around until you feel the right area, which should feel soft and yielding under your fingers. Now place your right hand flat on the abdomen on the right flank, lateral to the rectus muscle. This hand should be lying over the lower hand, with the patient's flank sandwiched between the two. Now press down with your right hand while flexing upwards with the fingers of your left. If the kidney is large enough you can feel it bumping against the right hand. This is called ballotting. As this movement is very brisk there may not be enough time to gauge the consistency and size of the kidney, unless the kidney is very large. In polycystic disease of the kidneys, they can be large and irregular and these features are readily appreciated and unforgettable. Now percuss over the kidney. It should be resonant over the kidney because of overlying gas-filled bowel.

TABLE 6.22 Causes of splenomegaly

Infective	Viral (e.g. hepatitis A, B, or C, glandular fever), bacterial (e.g. sub-acute bacterial endocarditis (SBE)), protozoal (e.g. malaria), parasite (e.g. hydatid disease)
Haematological	Leukaemias (especially chronic granulocytic leukaemia), myelofibrosis, lymphoma, haemolytic anaemias
Cirrhosis of the liver	
Infiltrative	Gaucher's disease, amyloidosis

CASE 6.16

Problem. You examine your patient and find a mass in the left hypochondrium. You feel an edge about four fingerbreadths below the costal margin but there is no notch in its border. The mass moves downwards with inspiration and you cannot get above it. The percussion note over the mass is resonant. What is it?

Discussion. Your intuition probably tells you this is a spleen but there is no notch and it is resonant to percussion. If something is not immediately straightforward you have to weigh up the evidence for and against your conclusions. It is in the right place to be a spleen, it moves downwards with inspiration, and you cannot get above it. Against it being a spleen is the absence of a notch and the resonant percussion note. However when you consider that you could easily miss a notch and that a spleen enlarged up to 6 cm can sometimes sound resonant, then the case against it being one is much weaker. A mass in the left hypochondrium that moves downwards with inspiration and you cannot get above is very likely to be a spleen.

Keypoints

- The spleen is normally found in the left hypochondrium.
- As the spleen enlarges it extends down and across the abdomen until a massive spleen can reach the right iliac fossa.
- You cannot palpate its upper margin.
- The spleen has a notch in its anterior border.
- The spleen moves downwards with inspiration.

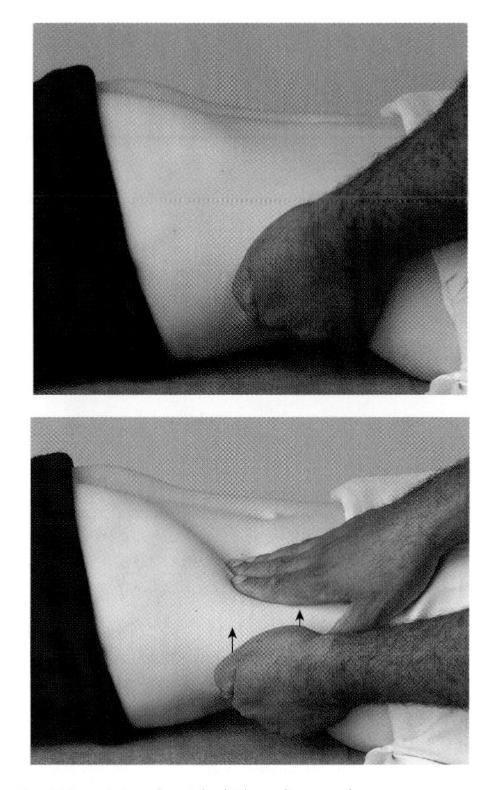

Fig. 6.34 Examining the right kidney (see text).

Palpating the left kidney can be very tricky. Remain standing and lean over your patient so you can slide the palm of your left hand around and then under the patient into the left renal angle. This may feel awkward at first so keep persevering. Check that the area above your fingers is soft and yielding to indicate that you are in the renal angle. Now place your right hand on the left flank aiming to overlap the fingers of both hands and produce the sandwich of the left flank. Now ballot the left kidney. This will need a lot of practice before you will feel comfortable doing it. It is interesting to note that the kidney does move downwards with respiration (just at the end of inspiration) but this property is not used in palpating for the kidneys.

Causes

See Table 6.23.

TABLE 6.23 Causes of an enlarged kidney

Polycystic kidneys
Tumours
Hydronephrosis
Amyloidosis

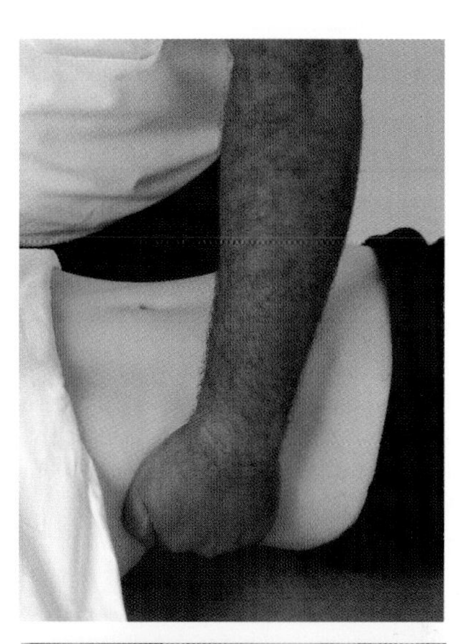

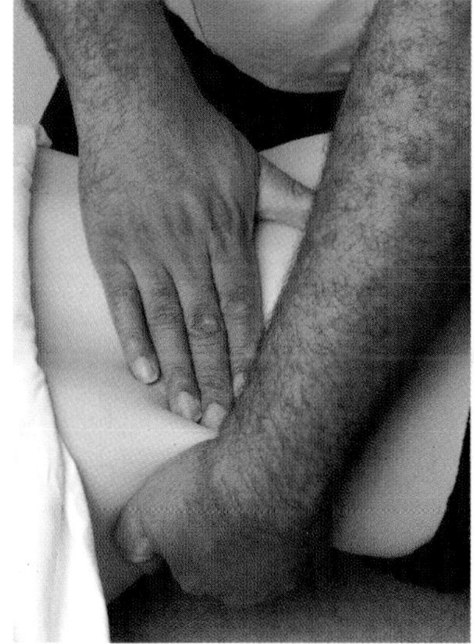

Fig. 6.35 Examining the left kidney (see text).

Percussion

17. Percuss over any masses or organs felt. Check for ascites. If the percussion note is dull in the flanks, go on to demonstrate shifting dullness (DF 7/10) or a fluid thrill (DF 6/10).

The general principle here is that any solid organ will sound dull and any gas-filled structure (usually bowel) will sound resonant. If any enlarged organ lies beneath bowel the percussion note above it will be resonant, for example, kidney. Usually your percussion will follow automatically if you find an enlarged organ or mass (as above). Even if you do not find anything you should still percuss carefully below the costal margins as a dull note

CASE 6.17

Problem. During your examination of a patient who looks well, you notice a mass in the right flank. It is bimanually ballotable but dull to percussion. When you did your routine to palpate the liver you thought you felt an edge meeting your fingers in the flank also. What is going on?

Discussion. You need to weigh up the evidence to hand. A mass in the right flank that is bimanually ballotable suggests an enlarged kidney but the percussion note is dull. You also thought that you felt a liver edge descend on inspiration. It might be worth rechecking this. This is perfectly acceptable to do if you are unsure (except in an exam setting). Your re-examination confirms a liver edge. It is possible that the patient has both an enlarged liver and kidney (if the patient is young and has polycystic enlargement of both organs). However in a well-looking adult it is more likely that they have a Riedel's lobe of the liver (*B. M. C. L. Riedel (1846–1916), German surgeon*). This is a congenital extension of the right lobe of the liver into the flank. This variant of liver anatomy is completely harmless and the liver functions normally (see Fig. 6.23).

Keypoints

- The kidneys are normally found in the flanks.
- When the kidneys enlarge they are bimanually ballotable
- Both an upper and a lower border can be palpated
- The kidneys move downward with late inspiration (this feature is not normally exploited when palpating)
- The percussion note over the kidneys is resonant

can inform you of a liver edge or splenic border that you may have missed on palpation. Percussion has an additional role in differentiating between some causes of abdominal distention. It is used particularly for eliciting ascites.

Ascites

What is it?

It is the abnormal collection of free fluid in the abdominal cavity. Traditionally it is divided into a transudate or an exudate depending on the protein content. If it is less than 30 g/l it is a transudate and if it is greater than 30 g/l it is an

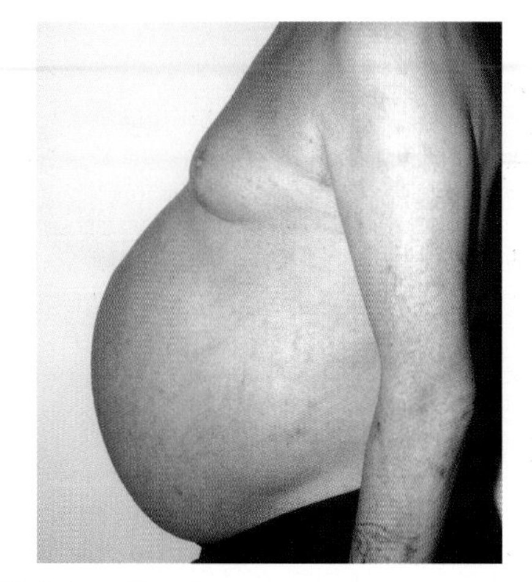

Fig. 6.36 Patient with ascites.

exudate (you may read different figures in other textbooks, for example, 20 g/dl or 25 g/dl, but the principle of high protein—exudate and low protein—transudate remains the same). Recently it has been recognized that the concentration of protein can vary with respect to the plasma protein and hence a modified definition states that ascitic fluid is a transudate if it is less than 10 mg/l **less** than the plasma albumen. Therefore if a patient has a plasma albumen of 25 mg/l and has ascitic fluid with a concentration of 19 g/l, this is still an exudate (despite being in the transudate range in the original definition). Ascitic fluid (like any liquid) will flow to the most dependent levels in a patient (see Fig. 6.36). In the supine patient this will be the flanks. Also loops of bowel will float uppermost in the centre of the abdomen. This distribution of fluid and bowel is exploited by examining the percussion note from the centre of the abdomen to the flanks.

Causes

See Table 6.24.

TABLE 6.24 Causes of ascites

Transudate
Congestive cardiac failure
Chronic liver disease
Nephrotic syndrome
Constrictive pericarditis
Hypoproteinaemia

Exudate
Intra-abdominal malignancy
Bacterial peritonitis
Tuberculous peritonitis

How to examine

See Fig. 6.37. Percuss the centre of the abdomen. The note should sound resonant. Now percuss in steps out towards the left flank. If abdominal distention is due to flatus the flanks will remain resonant. Sometimes the distention is so great that the percussion note is termed tympanitic (like a kettle drum). If the percussion note is dull in the flanks (and there is no splenomegaly) then it is likely that ascites is present. This requires confirmation by looking for shifting dullness. Having elicited a dull note in the flank, keep the percussed finger firmly on the flank and ask your patient to roll towards you (making sure your finger does not move). Allow the patient about 20 s to settle on their right side (this allows time for the fluid to redistribute and to shift down to the right). Now percuss your finger again. This time the note should be resonant. Some people prefer to make a mark on the flank with a pen to denote the area of dullness (get the patient's permission first) and to percuss over the mark once the patient has turned on their side.

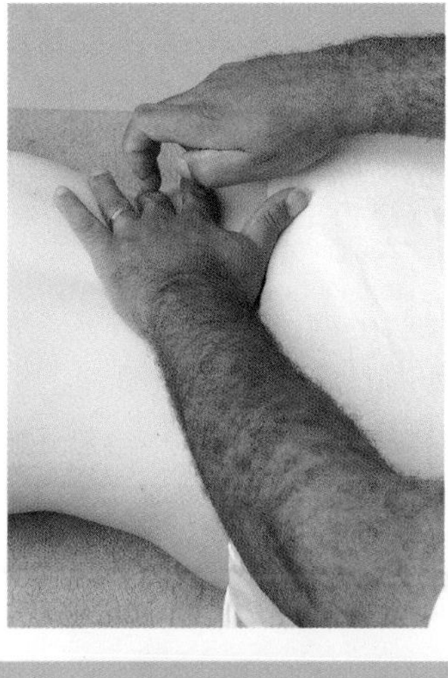

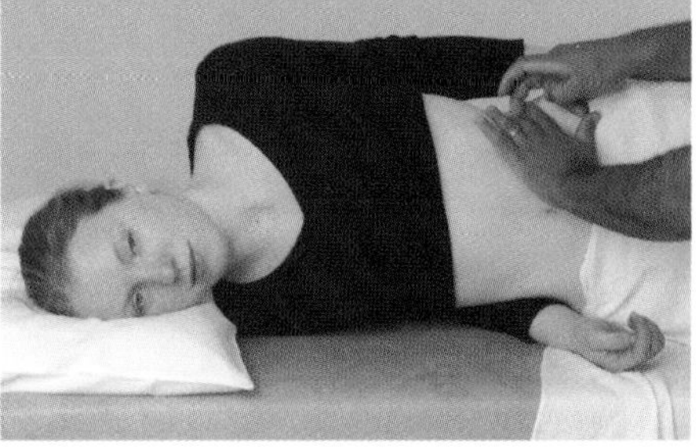

Fig. 6.37 Percussing for ascites (see text).

> **Tip**
>
> When eliciting shifting dullness always get your patient to roll onto their right side **towards you.** This allows you to ensure their safety. You can demonstrate shifting dullness with the patient rolling away from you but it is harder to control their position and it has been known for patients to roll out of bed and injure themselves.

Another method of demonstrating ascites is to elicit a fluid thrill. This technique is particularly good in the presence of large amounts of ascitic fluid. The aim here is to tap a flank with your fingertips (flicking with your finger can be painful) and the resulting impulse is conducted through the fluid to the opposite flank where you can observe or palpate it. As this wave can also be transmitted along the subcutaneous fat of obese patients you should get the patient (or any helpful person handy) to place a hand vertically in the mid-line so that the ulna border is pressed firmly into the abdomen.

One final method that you might be taught is the puddle sign. This is performed with the patient kneeling on all fours. In this position the fluid gravitates to the centre of the abdomen. This area should sound dull to percussion. It was said that this particular technique was sensitive and could detect small amounts of fluid. However this has been shown not to be the case. As this is an undignified test for both patient and examiner it is not recommended.

An important point to note is that a large amount of ascites can obscure masses or enlarged organs within the abdomen. In these circumstances a technique called dipping may be useful. Rather than palpating with the flat of your hand you dip your fingers into the abdomen with a sharp, rapid movement. If a mass is present you may feel something impact on your fingers for a brief moment. This technique can only alert you to the presence of something unusual within the abdomen because there is little opportunity to assess the features of any structure in such a brief instant.

Many people are baffled as to how this technique works. It works on the principle of inertia. If the same force is applied to objects of different masses in the same direction, the one with the lighter mass will move first, followed shortly by the heavier one (because of its greater inertia). When you dip your hand into an abdomen with ascites, the object with the lighter mass will move first, that is, the fluid. The fluid flows away from your fingers (and around any underlying mass). A heavier object such as a bowel cancer may remain motionless long enough (due to inertia) for your hand to feel it before it moves away also.

Keypoints

- If the percussion note is dull in the flanks look for shifting dullness (especially if there is abdominal distention).
- Always roll the patient towards you when checking for shifting dullness.
- Dipping is a crude method of determining the presence of organomegaly in the presence of ascites.

Auscultation

18. Auscultate for bowel sounds (DF 8/10) (and for bruits and rubs if necessary) (DF 9/10).

The first time you hear bowel sounds you will instantly recognize them. They are gurgling sounds that can be heard approximately every 10–20 s. If bowel sounds are absent (you sometimes have to auscultate for up to 1 min), this can represent a paralytic ileus or if the abdomen is rigid, peritonitis. These sounds usually become more plentiful after a meal. Bowel sounds are even more exaggerated with diarrhoea and can become loud enough to be audible to the unaided ear. Audible bowel sounds are called borborygmi (*bor-be-rig-me*). In mechanical obstruction of the bowel, the distended bowel can add a tinkling quality to the bowel sounds, which is pathognomonic (they are called tinkling bowel sounds funnily enough). Other sounds to listen for include renal artery bruits, which can be heard just above and lateral to the umbilicus in either flank. Bruits can sometimes be heard over an enlarged liver in alcoholic hepatitis or a hepatoma. Very rarely rubs (like a pleural rub) can be heard over the liver and spleen due to infarcts (these are so rare the author has yet to find someone who has heard one).

19. Examine the groins for lymphadenopathy and herniae (ask the patient to cough) (DF 8/10).

Now is the time to expose the groins. Take some time to inspect before you launch into palpation. Note any swellings in the groin and observe the testicles in men. In chronic liver disease there is loss of pubic hair (or change to female distribution in men and testicular atrophy. Now feel along the inguinal ligament. A small amount of irregularity is normal, as are small shotty lymph nodes that are less than 1 cm in diameter. Large lymph nodes should make you suspicious. Unilaterally enlarged nodes may herald skin malignancy of a leg. Unilateral or bilateral lymph nodes may be due to a lymphoma (look for nodes elsewhere and hepatosplenomegaly).

Keypoints

- Absent bowel sounds (not heard after 1 min) suggest a paralytic ileus.
- Tinkling bowel sounds suggest a mechanical obstruction of the bowel.
- Rubs and bruits are part of your auscultation routine for the abdomen but these sounds are very rare in practice.

Herniae

The principles of herniae have been described earlier. There are three main types of herniae to be found in the groin; the indirect inguinal hernia, the direct inguinal hernia, and the femoral hernia. The knowledge of the anatomy of this region is crucial to understanding the difference between them. See Fig. 6.38. The inguinal canal is an oblique canal that runs from the internal ring (a hole in the transversalis fascia) to the external ring (a defect in the external oblique aponeurosis). It allows the passage of the spermatic

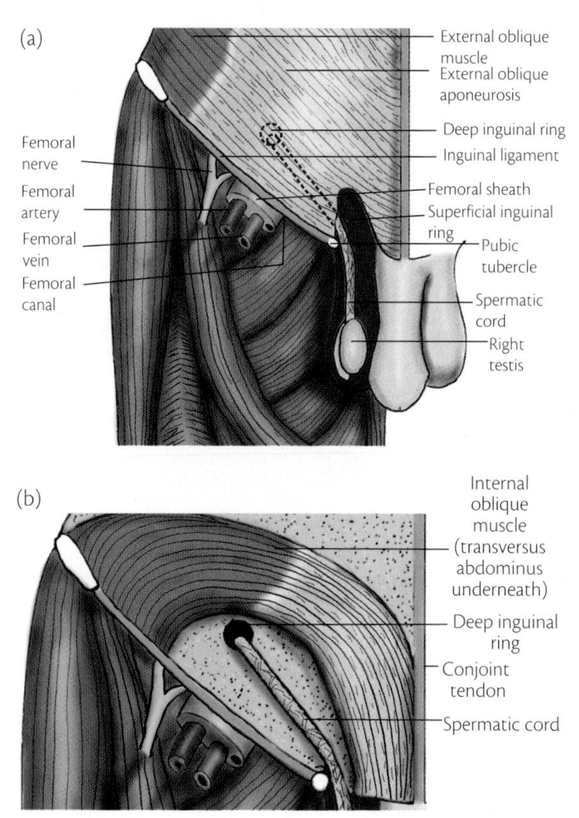

Fig. 6.38 The anatomy of the inguinal region; (b) with external oblique removed.

cord in men and the round ligament of the uterus in women, together with the ileo-inguinal nerve. The femoral canal runs beneath the inguinal ligament, under its medial aspect. On its lateral aspects lies first the femoral vein, then the femoral artery, and then the femoral nerve. The femoral canal only contains a lymph node and some fat.

Indirect inguinal hernia

This is the most common hernia in the groin. The hernial sac and contents pass through the internal ring into the inguinal canal. If the hernia is large enough it can pass through the external ring and descend into the scrotum or labium majora. As the internal ring is narrow there is potential for the hernia to strangulate.

Direct inguinal hernia

This hernia bulges forward directly through the posterior wall of the inguinal canal. As the hernial neck is wide this hernia rarely strangulates.

Femoral hernia

A femoral hernia passes down the femoral canal into the upper thigh. If large enough the hernial sac can emerge through the canal and turn upwards sometimes extending beyond the inguinal ligament. Because of the very narrow canal this hernia is very prone to strangulation.

See Fig. 6.39 for a diagram showing the relationship of indirect, direct, and femoral herniae.

How to examine

You may have already noticed a swelling in the groin. Even if you do not see one get your patient to cough. A bulging may betray the presence of an occult hernia. Get your patient to repeat the cough and this time place your hand over the swelling and feel the impulse. If you still have not found a hernia ask your patient to stand up before coughing again. Look and palpate as before. To distinguish between the different herniae you need to identify the pubic tubercle. Place your index finger in the crease of the groin at the beginning of the pubic hair. If you press firmly you should feel the inguinal ligament. Run your finger medially towards the scrotum or labium until you feel the bony knub of the pubic tubercle (do this quickly and professionally or you could get some worried looks from your patient). If the neck of the hernial sac is above and medial to the pubic tubercle it is an indirect inguinal hernia. If it is

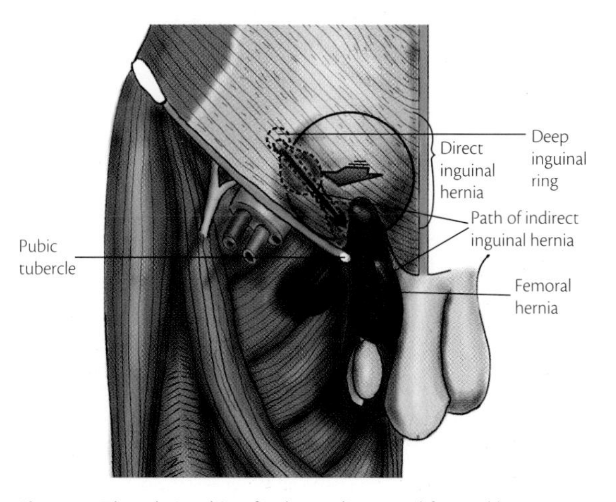

Fig. 6.39 The relationship of indirect, direct, and femoral herniae.

CASE 6.18

Problem. A normally fit 60-year-old man on your ward who was admitted with a pneumonia becomes ill. He complains of colicky lower abdominal pain and vomiting three times. He has not had his bowels opened all day and is unable to pass any wind. He has never had any previous surgery. The patient is seen by the house officer who finds that his pulse is 120/min and thready and the BP is 100/60. The abdomen is tender especially in its lower half and there are tinkling bowel sounds. The house officer thinks they are dealing with peritonitis but is unsure. Can you help them out?

Discussion. The history is typical of intestinal obstruction. If you visualize the bowel as a hollow tube then you can picture some of the symptoms you might get if it becomes blocked. Intestinal contents cannot get past and so the patient will vomit back faeculant matter. There will be colicky pain as the bowel tries to squeeze its contents passed the blockade. There will be absolute constipation even to flatus. The tinkling bowel sounds add weight to the diagnosis of intestinal obstruction. The next step is to work out why this man has developed the obstruction. He has had no previous surgery to suggest adhesions and there is nothing in his history to suggest he may have a cancer. When the cause is not obvious it is always worth looking in the patient's groins. A strangulated femoral hernia can easily be hidden here. This patient had a small, painful swelling in the groin, which was below and lateral to the pubic tubercle. It had no cough impulse. Find this swelling and you will have earned the thanks of the house officer and the consultant (not to mention the patient).

Keypoints

- When inspecting the groin of men, check for female distribution of pubic hair and testicular atrophy.
- Lymph nodes greater than 1 cm are pathological and you need to search for a cause.
- The neck of an indirect inguinal hernia is found above and medial to the pubic tubercle, while that of a femoral hernia is found below and lateral to the pubic tubercle.
- A femoral hernia is the most prone to strangulation, followed by an indirect inguinal hernia. A direct inguinal hernia rarely strangulates.

below and lateral to the pubic tubercle, it is a femoral hernia. You should now try to reduce the hernia with firm pressure. This manoeuvre will help you distinguish between an indirect inguinal and direct inguinal hernia. Once reduced an indirect hernia can be controlled by a finger over the internal ring (this can be found approximately half an inch above the pulse of the femoral artery). As the direct inguinal hernia is a forward bulge through the abdominal wall a finger will be unable to control it.

Wash your hands

20. Wash your hands.

Be obsessive or develop the insanity of the insanitary.

Presentation of findings

21. Now say, 'I would like to examine the external genitalia and perform a rectal examination.' Present findings.

Having felt for lymphadenopathy in the groin stand up straight and say, 'I would like to examine the external genitalia and perform a rectal examination.' The examiner will usually indicate that this is not necessary.

Then start the presentation. The exact style of presentation depends on your findings. If you findings point to an exact diagnosis, then be confident and mention this up front. For example, 'This man has chronic liver disease. He has hepatomegaly, which is three fingerbreadths below the costal margin and I could just tip a spleen. He has, in addition, jaundice, leuconychia, palmar erythema, and Dupuytren's contracture. There was no abdominal distention and I could not demonstrate any ascites.'

If your findings are inconclusive, detail them, give a differential diagnosis, and if you are unsure of an abdominal mass or organ or its aetiology suggest an abdominal ultrasound. For example, 'This man is jaundiced and has a mass in the right upper quadrant. It moves downward with inspiration and is dull to percussion. This man therefore has hepatomegaly, which could be due to liver metastases, lymphoma, cirrhosis of the liver, or congestive cardiac failure. Ultrasound will be helpful to confirm hepatomegaly and in defining its cause.' Here the student has missed the subtle signs, which would have clinched the diagnosis. They were also less certain as to the identity of the right upper quadrant mass but by listing its properties (and remembering the jaundice), quickly deduced that this had to be a liver. They then put together a reasonable differential diagnosis.

Tip

Do not forget to mention the rectal examination.

Other abdominal signs

Grey-Turner's sign

(DF 9/10.)

What is it?

Grey-Turner's sign (*George Grey-Turner (1877–1951), English surgeon*) is a subtle discoloration in the flanks that looks like a faint bruise. See Fig. 6.40.

Significance

Caused by bleeding into the abdominal cavity, with blood tracking into the subcutaneous layer of skin. Causes include haemorrhagic pancreatitis, a ruptured aortic aneurysm, or a ruptured ectopic pregnancy.

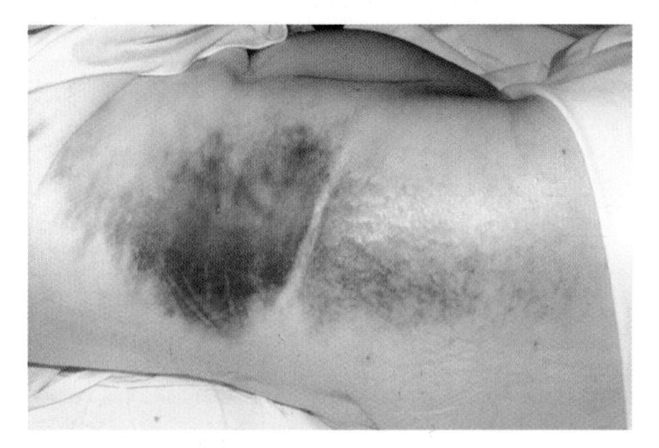

Fig. 6.40 Grey-Turner's sign.

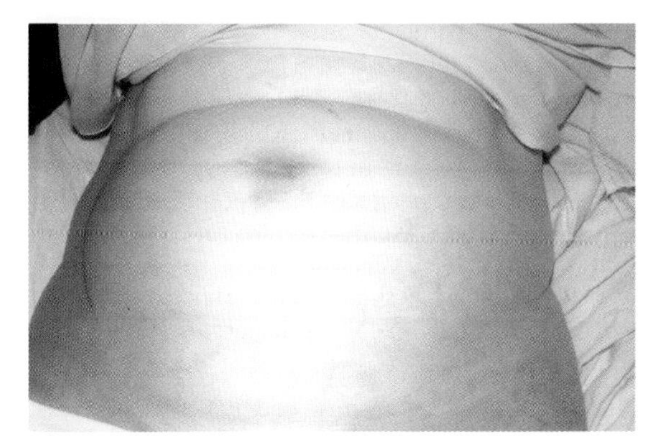

Fig. 6.41 Cullen's sign.

Cullen's sign

(DF 9/10.)

What is it?

Cullen's sign (*Thomas Stephen Cullen (1868–1953), American gynaecologist*) is a similar discoloration to Grey-Turner's sign, which occurs around the umblicus. See Fig. 6.41.

Significance

Same as for Grey-Turner's sign.

Murphy's sign

(DF 5/10.)

What is it?

Murphy's sign (*John Benjamin Murphy (1857–1916), American surgeon*) is the sudden pain elicited when palpating in the region of the gallbladder.

Significance

It denotes an inflammatory process of the gallbladder such as cholecystitis.

How to examine

You need to locate the area where the gallbladder normally lies (on the underside of the liver). Its position is located where the lateral border of the rectus muscle intersects with the right costal margin. As you get the patient to take a deep breath you slip your finger under the costal margin at this point. If the sign is positive the patient will cry out in pain or freeze in mid-breath in obvious discomfort. You can look for this sign deliberately if you suspect gallbladder disease but sometimes you may elicit this sign incidently when you are palpating for a liver.

CASE 6.19

Problem. You are on the ward when a 72-year-old man who is visiting a relative collapses. He had been overheard complaining of bad back pain for several hours before suddenly clutching his abdomen in obvious pain. He rapidly becomes pale, cyanosed, and sweaty. While the nurse runs to get a doctor you take his pulse and blood pressure. The pulse is 130/min, weak, and thready and the blood pressure is unrecordable. While you are waiting for help you use your initiative and palpate the man's abdomen. You notice a pulsatile mass in the centre of the abdomen. The crash team arrive and insert venflons and attach him to a cardiac monitor. You shrink into the background but as you do so, you notice faint bruising discoloration in the flanks. The leader of the crash team shouts out if anyone knows anything about this man. What do you say?

Discussion. Pluck up the courage and say what you know. You cannot be faulted for trying and every scrap helps. In fact in this case you may hold the key to this mans survival because as he loses his blood pressure the pulsatile nature of the aneurysm can be lost. You would be deemed very impressive if you said something like, 'I believe this man has a ruptured aortic aneurysm. He has a large pulsatile mass and is developing Grey-Turner's sign. He collapsed suddenly, went pale, cyanosed, and clammy, his pulse rate was 130/min, weak, and thready, and his blood pressure was unrecordable prior to you arriving.' This sounds very hard to do in a stressful situation. However as doctors we need to keep our wits about us and remain as cool and analytical as we can in an emergency. When the emergency has passed it is useful to evaluate your performance (and the other members of the team) to see if your responses can be improved. Never forget to document everything that you have done. Only then can you collapse in a heap. This patient was resuscitated with fluids and underwent emergency surgery. There is a high mortality associated with a ruptured aortic aneurysm and sadly despite all efforts this patient did not survive.

Abdominal diseases and investigations

In the earlier parts of this chapter, various medical conditions have been mentioned. In this section I now describe these. In general these descriptions are brief though certain aspects not well described in other textbooks are discussed in some detail.

Pharyngeal pouch

In old textbooks, this is sometimes referred to as Zenker's diverticulum (*Friedrich Albert Von Zenker (1825–1898), German pathologist*). This is an outpouching of the oesophagus that develops most commonly in elderly men. It causes dysphagia, sometimes accompanied by noisy gurgling sounds. At night there is often the regurgitation of undigested food, which may lead to aspiration pneumonia. Treatment is by excision, either by surgery or by endoscopic means.

Mallory–Weiss tear

This is a tear in the mucosa of the oesophagus, which occurs after repeated retching or vomiting. Bright red blood is seen in subsequent vomits.

Achalasia of the oesophagus

This condition is a cause of dysphagia. It can be primary (cause unknown) or secondary to conditions such as malignancy of the oesophagus. The primary condition is thought to be due to the degeneration of nerve cells in the myenteric plexus of the oesophagus. Dysphagia is caused through a combination of factors: decreased or absent peristalsis and increased resting pressure of the lower oesophageal sphincter, which fails to relax when food is swallowed.

Oesophageal varices

Varices (dilated veins) are found in chronic liver disease (of any cause) when portal hypertension develops. Normally blood flows from the gut along the hepatic portal vein to the liver (portal circulation) and from there to the inferior vena cava and hence to the heart (systemic circulation). When portal hypertension develops, blood flow is reversed away from the liver and has to find another way back to the systemic circulation. This occurs via collaterals (these are minor blood vessels that carry only a small proportion of blood in the same direction as the main blood supply). If blood flow is blocked in the main vessel, the body compensates by diverting the flow along these minor channels, which dilate with the increased blood volume. In portal hypertension there are four main clinical collaterals, called porta-systemic anastamoses (see Table 6.25). The most important of these are the ones that form oesophageal varices. Clinically if they rupture they can be the site of torrential bleeding.

Pancreatitis

This is a painful inflammatory condition of the pancreas, which can be acute or chronic. The most common predisposing causes are gallstones and heavy alcohol ingestion. The inflammation is caused by the pancreas's own enzymes. This can set off a sequence of metabolic events, which can have systemic effects and possibly lead to multi-organ failure. An acute attack is suggested by a rise of serum amylase to three times the upper limit of normal (a lower level does not exclude it). A chronic pancreatitis may result from repeated acute attacks (the serum amylase rise may be slight or non-existent). Malabsorption may result with chronic pancreatitis.

Gallstones

These can be made from cholesterol, bile pigments, or both. Most are asymptomatic and are found by chance on X-ray or ultrasound examination. If a stone impacts in the common bile duct it can cause biliary colic, jaundice, or ascending cholangitis. Stones in the gallbladder can provoke cholecystitis. The definitive treatment for symptomatic gallstones is surgery. It is also possible to dissolve certain gallstones with bile acid or to shatter them with lithotripsy (focused sound wave therapy).

Cholecystitis

This is inflammation of the gallbladder and is a complication of gallstones in the gallbladder. If a stone impacts in the gallbladder outlet, the gallbladder wall becomes inflamed by the increasing concentration of

TABLE 6.25 Porta-systemic anastomoses

Portal circulation	Systemic circulation	Clinical result
Oesophageal branch of left gastric vein	Oesophageal veins draining middle third of oesaphagus to azygous vein	Oesophageal varices
Paraumbilical veins	Superficial veins of anterior abdominal wall	Caput medusae
Superior rectal veins	Middle and inferior rectal veins	Haemorrhoids
Veins of ascending colon, descending colon, pancreas, duodenum, and liver	Renal, lumbar, phrenic veins	

bile. A secondary bacterial infection may occur. Repeated attacks of inflammation can cause fibrosis of the gallbladder (chronic cholecystitis). Occasionally cholecystitis can occur in the absence of gallstones. This is termed acalculous cholecystitis.

Jaundice

Knowledge of bilirubin metabolism will help you understand jaundice (see Fig. 6.42). The liver is the key because it is at the centre of bilirubin metabolism and all the causes of jaundice can be related to it, for example, pre-hepatic, hepatic, and post-hepatic jaundice. Bilirubin is formed by the breakdown of old or damaged red blood cells in the reticuloendothelial system. it is not soluble in water and is therefore bound to plasma protein and transported to the liver (at this stage bilirubin is described as unconjugated). The bilirubin is taken up by the liver and made water soluble by conjugating it with glucuronide. This process is facilitated by the enzyme glucuronyl transferase (you may see its full name, UDP-glucuronyl transferase, in other textbooks). The conjugated bilirubin is secreted in the bile and eventually passes into the duodenum. In the gut bacteria convert bilirubin to urobilinogen, which is later converted to stercobilins, which give faeces its characteristic brown colour. Some urobilinogen

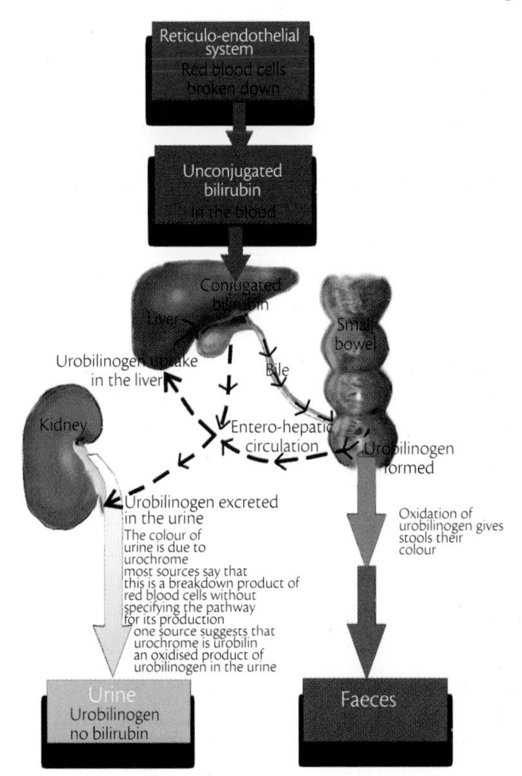

Fig. 6.42 The normal production and metabolism of bilirubin.

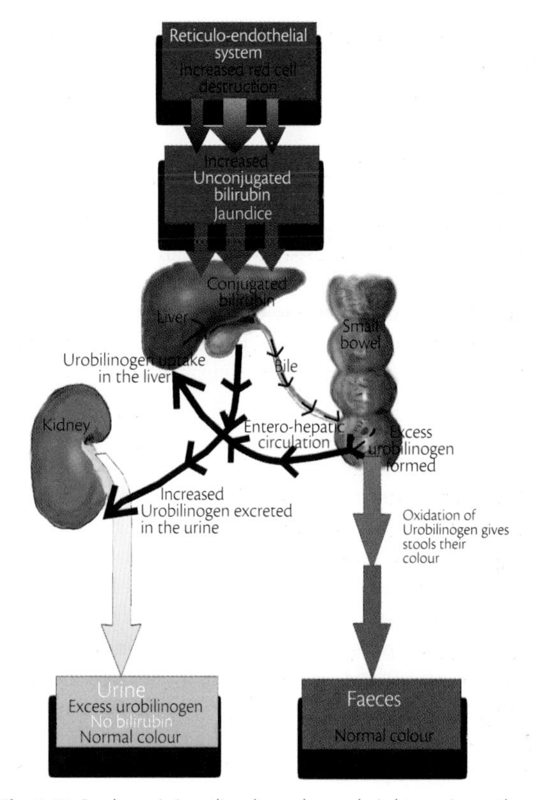

Fig. 6.43 Pre-hepatic jaundice due to haemolysis (unconjugated bilirubin).

is absorbed by the ileum into the portal blood, which transports it to the liver. Here the majority of urobilinogen is secreted into the bile and back into the gut. This recycling of urobilinogen is termed the enterohepatic circulation. Small amounts of urobilinogen escape into the general circulation and are eventually filtered by the kidney and excreted in the urine.

Pre-hepatic jaundice

Overall pre-hepatic causes are not common. The two circumstances you should know about are haemolytic anaemia and Gilbert's syndrome (see Fig. 6.43).

Haemolytic anaemia

There are various forms of haemolytic anaemia but in all cases there is the premature destruction of red blood cells. This leads to a greater amount of bilirubin being formed and causes jaundice when the concentration exceeds 30 μmol/l. The bilirubin is conjugated in the liver as normal but the liver is overwhelmed by the excess amount produced by haemolysis and hence the build-up of unconjugated bilirubin in the blood. The jaundice is usually mild and rarely exceeds 100 μmol/l. All the other aspects of bilirubin metabolism continue as normal, for example, the secretion of conjugated bilirubin in the bile, the formation of urobilinogen in the gut, the recycling of urobilinogen through the enterohepatic circulation, and the passage of urobilinogen in the urine. The only difference is that larger quantities of bilirubin are processed leading to greater quantities of urobilinogen in the gut and urine. As a result the colour of the stools and urine are unchanged.

Gilbert's syndrome

Gilbert's syndrome (*Nicolas Augustin Gilbert (1858– 1927), French physician*) is one of the familial hyperbilirubinaemias. It is the most common and can affect 2–7% of the population. A number of minor defects in bilirubin metabolism cause mild unconjugated jaundice. These are a decrease in uptake of bilirubin by the liver, decreased activity of glucuronyl transferase, and mild haemolysis. The key fact is that the liver is normal, which is reflected in normal liver function tests and the prognosis is excellent. The jaundice becomes more noticeable following alcohol ingestion, starvation, or intercurrent illness. Otherwise Gilbert's syndrome is usually found by chance when liver function tests show a mildly elevated bilirubin with normal levels of liver enzymes (should be confirmed by ruling out haemolysis as a cause of jaundice). A rare form of familial hyperbilirubinaemia is Criggler–Najjar syndrome (*John Fielding Crigler (born 1919), American paediatrician, Victor Assad Najjar (born 1914), Lebanese-born American paediatrician*). This is due to an absence of glucuronyl transferase (fatal in childhood); a milder form with reduced activity of glucuronyl transferase is compatible with survival into adulthood. The only treatment for this condition is liver transplantation.

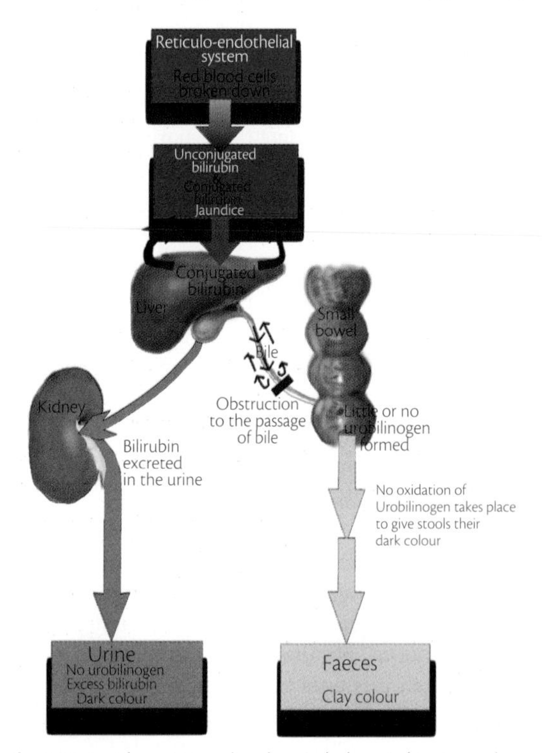

Fig. 6.44 Post-hepatic jaundice due to cholestasis (conjugated bilirubin).

Hepatic jaundice

There are many hepatic causes of jaundice. In this context, it can also be called hepatitic or hepatocellular jaundice. The causes can be acute, for example, drugs and viruses or chronic, for example, alcohol and other drugs and viruses. Any damage to the liver cells can interfere with their ability to take up bilirubin, to conjugate it, or to secrete it into bile. In addition, there is sometimes a cholestatic phase to the jaundice, that is, conjugated bilirubin is not secreted into bile but refluxes back into the blood stream. This is called intrahepatic cholestasis and the mechanism for this is not known. This cholestatic phase can be recognized clinically by pale, clay-coloured stools and dark orange/ brown urine (see later).

Post-hepatic jaundice

The causes of post-hepatic jaundice are easy to understand. There is obstruction to the flow of bile beyond the liver. This is often termed extrahepatic cholestasis and can occur anywhere in the biliary system from the liver to the duodenum. The bilirubin is unable to reach the small intestine and as a result, little or no bilirubin is converted to urobilinogen and hence the stools become pale (clay coloured). In addition, excess conjugated bilirubin refluxes back into the blood stream (levels can reach >100 μmol/l) and is deposited in the skin (yellow colour and itching) and sclera (yellow colour) and is also excreted in the urine, which becomes a dark orange colour (see Fig. 6.44)

Chronic liver disease

This is simply any liver disease that is present for more than 6 months. Some patients have acute attacks, which then go on to become chronic, for example, hepatitis B. Others are asymptomatic and are only discovered on blood tests. When followed up they may remain well for years before exhibiting symptoms, for example, primary biliary cirrhosis. Other patients may be asymptomatic until they present with a complication such as ascites or bleeding oesophageal varices when portal hypertension supervenes.

Cirrhosis of the liver

Cirrhosis is strictly a pathological diagnosis. Although it can be suspected clinically, it can only be confirmed following histological examination of a biopsy specimen.

It is the irreversible endpoint of a variety of insults; alcohol is the most common cause in the UK. Sometimes students make the mistake of using cirrhosis and chronic liver disease interchangeably. Cirrhosis is one form of chronic liver disease (other examples include hepatitis B and malignancy) although it may be the final endpoint for many causes of chronic liver disease.

Primary biliary cirrhosis

This form of cirrhosis is more common in females. The cause is unknown although an immunological mechanism is strongly suspected. Greater than 95% of sufferers have anti-mitochondrial antibodies.

Cholangiocarcinoma

This is an adenocarcinoma that arises from the biliary ducts. It is a rare cancer that usually presents with cholestatic jaundice. It may also cause abdominal pain, anorexia, and weight loss. It has a poor prognosis and treatment is usually palliative, that is, placing a stent by endoscopic retrograde cholangio-pancreatogram (ERCP) (a stent is a hollow structure placed within the lumen of an obstructed vessel to allow the free flow of fluid through it).

Sclerosing cholangitis

This is an inflammatory process of the biliary tree resulting in fibrosis and narrowing of the tract. It can be primary or secondary to other causes such as previous bile duct surgery, gallstones, or acquired immunodeficiency syndrome. Although there is no known cause for primary sclerosing cholangitis, there is a strong association with inflammatory bowel disease.

Inflammatory bowel disease

This term is used to describe a family of diseases that have in common an inflammatory infiltrate of the bowel of unknown cause. It is often used to describe ulcerative colitis or Crohn's disease although microscopic colitis is also embraced by the term. There are other causes of an inflammatory infiltrate in the bowel, for example, infection, radiation, and ischaemia, but these are not classified as inflammatory bowel disease.

Ulcerative colitis

This condition primarily affects the large bowel. The inflammatory infiltrate usually affects the mucosa. It usually presents with bloody diarrhoea. Other symptoms include anorexia, weight loss, fever, and abdominal pain relieved by defaecation. A rare complication is toxic megacolon, where the gut dilates and eventually perforates in a severe attack. It also has complications outside the gut, including (1) in the joints—arthritis, ankylosing spondylitis; (2) in the eyes—episcleritis; (3) in the skin—erythema nodosum and pyoderma gangrenosum; and (4) in the biliary tree—sclerosing cholangitis. There is a risk of cancer developing in some patients (usually those with extensive disease involving the whole of the large bowel—pancolitis) and in those who have had the disease a long time. The risk is quoted as 5–10% at 15–25 years in those with a pancolitis. These people are kept under surveillance by colonoscopy.

Crohn's disease

This condition can affect any part of the bowel from mouth to anus. The inflammatory infiltrate usually affects the submucosa. It also commonly presents with bloody diarrhoea and has similar symptoms to ulcerative colitis. The unusual feature with Crohn's disease is that it can affect some areas of the bowel and have normal bowel in between (the affected areas are called skip lesions). It can also lead to fistulae formation (a fistula is an abnormal connection between two epithelial surfaces, for example, between small bowel and large bowel or between bowel and skin). Ileal involvement may lead to malabsorption. It can also lead to similar extra-intestinal manifestation as ulcerative colitis although the frequency of complications differs.

Microscopic colitis

This is a form of inflammatory bowel disease where the bowel looks normal on colonoscopic or barium enema examination. However if biopsy samples are examined with microscopy they have characteristic histological appearances. Patients usually present with watery diarrhoea (bleeding PR is unusual).

Mesenteric ischaemia

This can be acute or chronic. It is difficult to diagnose, as there are few clinical signs and no diagnostic tests (plus doctors do not often think about the possibility). The acute form is usually caused by an embolus or thrombosis occluding the gut supply (although it can occur due to decreased perfusion in cardiogenic or hypovolaemic shock). With infarction of the bowel peritonitis may develop leading to increased abdominal pain with the signs of peritonism. Chronic ischaemia leads to abdominal pain up to an hour after a meal (this has been called intestinal claudication or angina, the analogy being drawn from coronary heart disease or peripheral vascular disease). Always think of this diagnosis in elderly patients, smokers, and those who have atrial fibrillation or other cardiovascular pathology, for example, stroke, ischaemic heart disease, and peripheral vascular disease.

Ischaemic colitis

This is a form of inflammatory disease of the bowel due to ischaemia that usually afflicts the elderly. It usually presents with left-sided abdominal pain and diarrhoea. Bleeding PR is unusual. It can be diagnosed on colonoscopy (biopsies may be needed to clinch the diagnosis) and changes tend to centre around the splenic flexure (the splenic flexure is the watershed between the superior mesenteric artery supply and the inferior mesenteric artery supply).

Acute intestinal obstruction

There are four main symptoms with intestinal obstruction: colicky abdominal pain, abdominal distention, faeculant vomiting, and absolute constipation (even to flatus). It can occur because of an obstruction in the lumen of the bowel, for example, tumour; because of an obstruction in the wall of the bowel, for example, stricture; or because of compression from outside the bowel, for example, adhesions following previous surgery.

Diverticular disease

A diverticulum is an outpouching of the bowel wall. It occurs because of the high pressures created within the lumen of the bowel during muscular contraction. This forces pockets of bowel through areas of weakness (usually where blood vessels enter the bowel via the mesentery). The presence of diverticulae scattered throughout the bowel is called diverticulosis. If inflammation occurs within a diverticulum, this is called diverticulitis. The whole spectrum of presentations associated with diverticulae is called diverticular disease. Other complications include diarrhoea and constipation, bleeding PR, abscess formation, and fistulae formation. If diverticulae occur in the jejunum, bacteria may multiply in the pockets in sufficient numbers to cause malabsorption of fat (the bacteria deconjugate bile salts preventing the absorption of fat).

Polyps

Polyps are small outgrowths from a mucous membrane surface. In the gut they can be sessile (flat and slightly elevated from the gut surface) or pedunculated (attached to the gut by a stalk). The majority of polyps are found by chance following bowel investigations. Others cause bleeding or iron deficiency anaemia. The importance of polyps lie in the malignant potential that some possess. These include some adenomas and inherited conditions such as Peutz–Jehger's syndrome, Gardner's syndrome, and familial polyposis coli.

Haemorrhoids

Internal haemorrhoids are also known as 'piles'. They are varices of the superior haemorrhoidal veins (also called the superior rectal veins). With your patient in the lithotomy position (think of the (undignified) position that women get into for a cervical smear), if you were to view the anus from the front (this gets worse) and you were to regard it as a clock, then haemorrhoids appear at 3, 7, and 11 o'clock. There are three categories of haemorrhoids:

(1) first-degree haemorrhoids (confined to the anal canal);

(2) second-degree haemorrhoids (prolapse from the anus following defaecation but return spontaneously or can be replaced with a finger);

(3) third-degree haemorrhoids (prolapse from the anus and cannot be replaced).

All three categories are painless unless thrombosis occurs. They usually cause bright red bleeding PR following defaecation or on the toilet paper. Predisposing causes include constipation, compression by a pregnant uterus, compression by other pelvic tumours, and rarely, portal hypertension.

Angiodysplasia

Angiodysplasia ('angio'—blood, 'dysplasia'—loss of differentiation of cells) are malformations of blood vessels in the gut that are susceptible to bleeding. They are more common in the elderly. The best investigation to identify them is colonoscopy where the lesions can be cauterized. Rarely, if bleeding is excessive or the lesions extensive, the patient may need resection of the affected bowel.

Endoscopy

This is a test using a flexible fibre-optic instrument, which can be passed within the body cavities to visualize the internal organs. Modern equipment has evolved to enable a variety of procedures to be undertaken via the endoscope. These include

(1) biopsy (taking a sample of tissue for histological analysis);

(2) diathermy (passing an electric current to control bleeding);

(3) suction for removing secretions or washings for analysis;

(4) inserting stents;

(5) using a variety of baskets for removing foreign bodies or unwanted material.

Endoscopy is a generic term that covers all the medical fibre-optic procedures (the prefix 'endos' means inside). Often the prefix is changed to denote the organ being investigated, for example:

- gastroscopy—stomach
- colonoscopy—colon
- sigmoidoscopy—sigmoid colon
- cystoscopy—bladder
- hysteroscopy—uterus.

Try to work out the organs that are visualized from the following:

- bronchoscopy
- laparoscopy
- mediastinoscopy
- arthroscopy
- proctoscopy.

Endoscopic retrograde cholangio-pancreatogram

The ERCP is a special form of endoscopy where the instrument is passed into the second part of the duodenum. The ampulla of Vater is cannulated (the common exit point of the common bile duct and the pancreatic duct). Radio-opaque dye is introduced into the duct system and the patient screened under X-ray control. This allows the diagnosis of biliary and pancreatic disease. The instrument can also be used therapeutically, for example, to remove stones or introduce stents.

Carcinoid syndrome

Carcinoid syndrome is a collection of symptoms due to high levels of circulating 5- hydroxytryptamine (5-HT) secreted from tumours of neuro-endocrine origin. The symptoms include flushing, wheezing due to bronchospasm, hypotension, tachycardia, and diarrhoea. Tumours can be found in the gastrointestinal tract, bronchus, thyroid, and testis. Gut tumours only manifest their symptoms if there are liver metastases because the 5-HT is normally metabolized in the liver. The rare bronchial carcinoid does not need this prerequesite as the 5-HT is secreted into the general circulation. Diagnosis is aided by finding the breakdown product, 5-hydroxyindoleacetic acid (5-HIAA) in the urine.

Zollinger–Ellison syndrome

This condition is due to a gastrinoma (a tumour secreting the hormone gastrin), which is usually found in the pancreas. The gastrin causes a hypersecretion of acid in the stomach, which causes severe peptic ulceration, in the stomach, duodenum, and even jejunum. Diarrhoea is also a common feature and the increased acidity in the small intestine can be sufficient to inactivate the pancreatic enzymes and precipitate malapsorption. Occasionally this tumour can be associated with multiple endocrine neoplasia type 1, which also includes pituitary tumours and hyperparathyroidism.

Acute intermittent porphyria

This is a rare disorder of haem synthesis (the haem part of the haemoglobin molecule). An enzyme porphobilinogen deaminase involved in the formation of haem has reduced or no activity, leading to a build-up of by-products in the blood. This causes severe abdominal pain (sufferers have been known to have undergone surgery in the mistaken belief that they have had an acute abdomen). Other features include hypertension, tachycardia, peripheral neuropathy, encephalopathy, and coma.

Hypercalcaemia

(The prefix 'hyper' means increased or excessive.) Hypercalcaemia may be caused by a number of conditions. The most common are hyperparathyroidism (the parathyroids glands are tiny glands within the substance of the thyroid, which are responsible for calcium metabolism) and malignancy. Hypercalcaemia can cause abdominal pain, constipation, thirst, polyuria, and urinary stones. This has led to the expression 'moans, groans, and abdominal stones' with respect to the symptoms of hypercalcaemia.

Diabetic ketoacidosis

This is a serious complication of diabetes mellitus. It can occur due to sepsis, starvation, or a diabetic failing to take insulin. Occasionally a person may present with this complication for the first time. Ketoacidosis occurs because the patient is unable to use glucose for energy (as occurs normally). Instead they use fat as an alternative energy source, which leads to the production of ketones (acetoacetate and hydroxybutyric acid) in the blood and urine, where they can be detected. The patient suffers thirst (polydipsia), polyuria, and weight loss due to excessive dehydration. The acidosis stimulates an increase in the breathing rate called 'air hunger' or 'Kussmaul's respiration' and the sweet acetone smell of ketones can be detected on the breath. The condition is insidious and if undetected can lead to confusion, coma, and death. Abdominal pain is an unusual method of presentation. Initial treatment involves fluid replacement and intravenous insulin.

Urinary tract infection

This is a non-specific term describing an infection anywhere in the urinary tract (it includes cystitis—infection of the bladder and pyelonephritis—infection of the kidneys). A patient may experience a fever, dysuria, and urinary frequency (the elderly may be non-specifically unwell or become confused).

Finals section

In this section, as with the previous chapters, issues dealing with Finals will be discussed. For revision read the examination summary (p. 143) and the keypoints throughout the chapter and do the questions on pp. 183–4.

If the CVS is at the heart of general medicine then the abdominal system is the guts of the specialty (sorry!). Many of the more common gastro-intestinal pathologies, for example, gastro-oesophageal reflux disease, peptic ulcer, and irritable bowel syndrome produce minimal signs and do not present a serious challenge for the short cases. Most Finals short cases will involve a palpable mass or organ, jaundice, or ascites. Each one will present a challenge to your clinical skills. Many of these can also be used as long cases. Some masses can be difficult to identify even with the 'perfect' clinical technique, so do not panic if you do not know the answer. As long as your technique is sound and you can come up with a reasonable differential diagnosis, then you will be given credit. Common cases are shown in Tables 6.26 and 6.27.

Key diagnostic clues

In real life many of the common conditions do not produce diagnostic signs. However with all abdominal conditions and in particular those associated with pain, **palpation** is the key. Signs of acute surgical complication, for example, guarding, rigidity, and rebound tenderness, constitute an emergency. With regards to short cases, where masses and organomegaly predominate, **palpation** again provides the most important clues.

TABLE 6.26 Finals cases

Jaundice
Hepatomegaly
Splenomegaly
Chronic liver disease
Hepatosplenomegaly
Ascites
Abdominal mass/palpable kidney

TABLE 6.27 Day-to-day cases

Abdominal pain
Dyspepsia
Diarrhoea/constipation
Inflammatory bowel disease
Any of the finals cases

Key signs of common palpable abnormalities

1. **Hepatomegaly.** Enlarges into the RHC, massive hepatomegaly can reach the RIF, moves downward with inspiration, a hard irregular edge suggests malignancy (rarely a polycystic liver), dull to percussion. **Always percuss down the right chest side of the chest to rule out displacement of the liver by emphysema.**
2. **Splenomegaly.** Enlarges into the LHC, massive splenomegaly can reach the RIF, it has a notch in its border, moves downward with inspiration, dull to percussion.
3. **Chronic liver disease.** Leuconychia, palmar erythema, Dupuytren's contracture (alcohol), spider naevi, purpura, jaundice, loss of axillary hair, testicular atrophy, caput medusae, hepatomegaly, splenomegaly, ascites.
4. **Ascites.** Abdominal distension, everted umbilicus (sometimes), fluid thrill, dull percussion in flanks, demonstrate shifting dullness.
5. **Enlarged kidneys.** Palpable in flanks using bimanual technique, moves down minimally with inspiration, resonant to percussion.

Some advice relating to examination problems

General

Use the abdominal system examination routine given on p. 143.

The instruction

The examiner will usually ask you to 'examine the abdominal system' or to 'examine the abdomen'. With the second command students feel obliged to dive straight onto the tummy. Resist this! Both commands mean the same thing so be thorough and start with the hands (following your inspection). Sometimes the examiner is more specific and may say 'palpate the abdomen.' Do exactly this. However be vigilant and keep your eyes peeled for other clues such as jaundice or spider naevi. These may help you to a final diagnosis.

Problem. You are still unsure whether to do a full examination or to concentrate on the abdomen.

Solution. If there is any doubt, do the full examination. This at least shows that you are thorough and if the examiners want you to concentrate on the abdomen, they will stop you and direct you to it (do not get upset by any irritation they might display, just concentrate on your performance).

General look

Fit this in while you introduce yourself to the patient and get them into position. It is recommended that the first thing checked for in an abdominal case is jaundice. If you spot this, you know immediately there is a problem in the hepatobiliary system (this is usually the case in a Finals examination but do not forget haemolytic jaundice, drugs, and so on). Check for lesions that may be spider naevi, for bruising, and for abdominal distention (you could make a diagnosis of chronic liver disease before you even start examining the patient, but make sure you are methodical and find **all** the features).

Positioning

Whatever position the patient is in make sure you lie them flat. Ask the patient's permission before doing so. If the patient is already flat quickly check they are comfortable (the elderly or those with musculoskeletal problems of the neck may need two pillows).

Hands

Problem. You always miss leuconychia and palmar erythema.

Solution. You must be **aware** of their possibility particularly in an abdominal case. If you keep thinking about them, you are less likely to miss them.

Face

Problem. You have seen red spidery marks on the hands and face and told your examiners they are spider naevi, yet they seem dissatisfied.

Solution. You must always demonstrate blanching before your examiners will accept the diagnosis of spider naevi. Your clinicals are like a driving test, you must be **seen** to do the right things no matter how obvious they seem.

Problem. You have missed the lesions of Peutz–Jehger or HHT syndromes.

Solution. Do not fret if you miss these. These conditions are rare and if you get a case you are more likely to be up for an honours mark. Your examiners are more concerned that you do not miss common and easy signs that could put a life in jeopardy. The answer here is the same as for leuconychia. You must be aware of the syndromes. Pay particular attention to the lips. If you are suspicious, get your patient to open their mouth and inspect the buccal mucosa (with HHT inspect their tongue, including the underside, for lesions).

The abdomen

Now you have got to the abdomen do not rush to get your clammy hands on it. Step back and inspect it from a distance. Does it move quietly with respiration? Is it distended? Does it have distended veins on its surface? Never rush into palpation and when you do start, be methodical.

Palpating the abdomen

Problem. After getting permission to palpate, the patient winces when you touch them. Should you continue?

Solution. It depends. It could have been a surprise or your cold clammy hand that could have provoked them. So apologize to the patient for causing discomfort and ask them if the area is normally tender. If it is, ask if you can feel the area albeit gently (the same applies even if it is not normally tender). If the patient still flinches with pain despite the gentlest of touches again apologize and abandon the examination. State to your examiners that you cannot proceed because of the obvious pain the patient is experiencing. For extra credit, also add that you would normally check for guarding or rebound tenderness to make sure the patient is not developing a surgical complication.

Presentation

Always offer to check the external genitalia and perform a rectal examination. Try to be confident and avoid the words seem or might.

Problem. You always find you forget one or two small but relevant features during your presentation (especially the numerous signs of chronic liver disease).

Solution. There are two possible solutions. The first is to know all the signs like the back of your hand so that you are less likely to forget them when you recite your findings to the examiner. The second is to give a running commentary as you go along. 'On examining the hands I have noticed leuconychia and palmar erythema. I have just noticed red spidery lesions on the arms, face, and upper trunk that are reminiscent of spider naevi. I shall now attempt to blanch them ... and yes they do blanch; they are spider naevi.' It is up to you to find the technique you prefer.

Good luck!

Questions

The more stars, the more important it is to know the answer.

1. How many signs of chronic liver disease can you name? ****
2. What are spider naevi? **

3. What is Virchow's node? ***
4. What are the causes of a right iliac fossa mass? ****
5. Where is the normal upper margin of the liver on the body surface? *
6. What are the causes of hepatomegaly? ****
7. What are the causes of splenomegaly? ****
8. How do you differentiate between an enlarged kidney and a spleen? ****
9. What are the causes of a liver bruit? **
10. What is globus hystericus? *
11. What are the causes of a left iliac fossa mass? ****
12. What is dyspepsia? **
13. What are the causes of a hypogastric mass? ****
14. What is haematemesis? ***
15. What are the causes of ascites? ****
16. What is a Mallory–Weiss tear? **
17. What methods do you know to demonstrate ascites? ****
18. What is melaena and what are the causes? ****
19. How do you distinguish clinically between pre-hepatic jaundice and post-hepatic (cholestatic) jaundice? ***
20. What is Charcot's triad? *
21. What is dysuria? **
22. What is spurious diarrhoea? **
23. What is Duputryen's contracture and what are the causes? ***
24. What are the 'five Fs' that cause abdominal distention? ****
25. How do you elicit a flapping tremor? ***
26. What is oliguria? **
27. What is Osler–Weber–Rendu syndrome? *
28. What are the causes of gynaecomastia? ****
29. How do you differentiate between an indirect inguinal hernia and a direct inguinal hernia? ***
30. How do you differentiate between an indirect inguinal hernia and a femoral hernia? ***
31. What are striae? *
32. What is a Pfannenstiel incision? *
33. How do you distinguish between a reducible hernia and an obstructed hernia? ****
34. How do you confirm an abdominal mass is an aortic aneurysm? ***
35. What is cirrhosis of the liver? **
36. What clinical manouvre distinguishes a hernia from other abdominal swellings? **
37. What is inflammatory bowel disease? ***
38. How do you detect peritonitis clinically? ****
39. What five properties does an enlarged liver possess? ****
40. What six properties does an enlarged spleen possess? ****
41. What do tinkling bowel sounds represent? ***
42. What is Grey-Turner's sign? *
43. How do you assess an abdominal swelling found on palpation? *****
44. What is diverticular disease? **
45. What is the relevance of absent bowel sounds? **
46. How does irritable bowel syndrome present? ***
47. What are the causes of a peptic ulcer? ****
48. What is Murphy's sign? **
49. What are the symptoms of intestinal obstruction? ****
50. What are the clinical manifestations of iron deficiency anaemia? ***

Score. Give 4 marks for 4 stars, 1 for 1 star, and so on. At the end of the third year, you should be scoring 70-plus and by Finals, 90-plus; 110-plus is very good.

Further reading

Dawson C, Whitfield H. *ABC of urology*. London: BMJ Publishing Group; 1997.

Rhodes JM, Tsai HH. *Clinical problems in gastroenterology*. London: Mosby-Wolfe; 1995.

Sewell DP, Chapman RGW, Mortenson N. *Ulcerative colitis and Crohn's Disease, a clinician's guide*. Edinburgh: Churchill Livingstone.

Silen W. *Cope's early diagnosis of the acute abdomen*. 2nd edn. Oxford: Oxford University Press; 2000.

Smith ME, Morton DG. *The digestive system, basic science and clinical conditions*. Edinburgh: Churchill Livingstone; 2001.

CHAPTER 7

Rectal examination

Chapter contents

Introduction

The rectal examination (per rectum (PR) examination) is a test that is guaranteed to send shudders through any student (and their patient). Unfortunately it is not the kind of thing, like brain operations, which only qualified doctors are allowed to do. Students are not only allowed but are expected to do PR examinations. Many of our hang-ups about this examination revolve around our fear of contact with faeces or subjecting our patient to such an invasive test. Even today, some qualified doctors often think of excuses to get out of doing them. Yet a PR examination is quick and easy to do and is usually painless. In fact, the hardest part of the examination can be putting your gloves on. Because of the intimate nature of this examination you will not be expected to perform this in a student or Finals examination.

The importance of the rectal examination

A great deal of information can be gained from a PR examination. The more common reasons for doing one are as follows.

1. Assessment of gastrointestinal disturbance, for example, constipation, diarrhoea, tenesmus, or bleeding per rectum (PR).
2. Assessment of the prostate in men.
3. Assessment of the acute abdomen.

Occasionally a PR examination can be used for unusual reasons such as searching for a cause in a pyrexia of unknown origin or the assessment of anal tone in a neurological examination. As with any test a doctor has to weigh up the advantages of doing the test against the potential harm it may cause. If there is any doubt about the need for a PR examination it might be useful to remember the old surgical saying, 'Put your finger in it before you put your foot in it.' There is no point sparing the patient's feelings if in the long run you have missed a potentially treatable lesion such as an early rectal carcinoma.

Rectal examination summary

1. Introduce yourself to your patient and explain why you want to perform a PR examination.
2. Ask for permission to perform the PR examination.
3. Get a chaperone/helper.
4. Ensure equipment is at hand and ready.
5. Position the patient.
6. Put on gloves.
7. Put lubricant on your index finger.
8. Warn the patient that you are about to perform the test.
9. Inspect the perianal region.
10. Introduce your finger into the anal canal.
11. Examine the rectum in a logical sequence.
12. Take your finger out and inspect the glove for faeces, blood, and so on.
13. Clean the perianal region.
14. Tell your patient you have finished and allow them to get dressed.
15. Wash your hands.
16. Report your findings.

Rectal examination in detail

1. Introduce yourself to your patient and explain why you want to perform a PR examination.

Say, 'Hello I'm Marjory Warren, a fifth-year student.' Extend your hand for shaking. Explain why you are doing the test. Communication is essential in preventing a mildly uncomfortable procedure from becoming a traumatic one. There are still instances where patients are bewildered because they went to their doctors with what seemed a trivial complaint and end up with a finger rampaging up their rear end. **You** might see the logical need for a PR but a patient has not shared your training. For example, a patient goes to his general practitioner (GP) and complains, 'I feel tired doctor'. The GP quickly notices the patient looks clinically pale and knowing that gastrointestinal blood loss is the most common cause of anaemia, rushes to do a PR examination. Under pressure to see a large number of patients he does not fully explain his motives. Later, in the pub, the man recounts his tale of horror to his mates. 'I was only feeling a bit tired and the next thing the doctor is sticking his finger up my ****.' One of his mates replies, 'He sounds like a pervert, I would complain if I were you.' There are two messages here. Always give a full and frank explanation of why you are doing things and no matter how busy you are, make sure that you have access to a chaperone who can back you up in case of complaints.

2. Ask for permission to perform the PR examination.

This will follow on from your explanation. Say something like, 'Do you mind if I examine your back passage?' Hopefully your patient will understand what you mean. If however they wonder why you have taken an interest in their house, you may have to elaborate further by using another word such as anus, rectum, or tail end. At this stage you need to alleviate any anxiety. Ask 'Have you had this done before?' If the answer is 'no', resist the temptation to say 'Me neither.' Be reassuring and say something like, 'Don't worry! I am just going to examine with a finger. It will be over in seconds and it is not normally painful.' If the patient has had it before and it was uncomfortable, try saying, 'I **will** be quick!'

3. Get a chaperone/helper.

For a male doctor examining a female patient, you **need** a female chaperone. For a female examining a male patient, either a male or female chaperone will do. Technically you don't need a chaperone if you are examining a patient of the same sex, although having a helper present can be useful, particularly if your patient is elderly and can be reassuring for some patients. There are some patients who might object to a chaperone. In these cases gently try to persuade them the reasons why a chaperone is necessary (for both parties). If they are still insistent it may be better to postpone the examination for another time (or another person) rather than run the risk of litigation.

4. Ensure equipment is at hand and ready.

The equipment is usually kept on a tray. You should have lubricating gel, disposable gloves, and some tissues or swabs to clean your patient afterwards. There is nothing more embarrassing than being stranded with

Tip

It is also sensible to have a disposable sheet, which you can place under the patient's bottom, just in case there is any faecal leakage.

your finger up a patient's bottom and realizing that you have nothing to clean them with and no means of getting to it (especially if you have no chaperone handy).

5. Position the patient.

Ask your patient to lie on the bed on their left side with their back facing you (see Fig. 7.1). It is helpful if they are near the edge, close to you. Pump the bed up to a height that will not put a strain on your back. Now ask your patient to bend their knees up towards their chest. It is helpful if you have an assistant, particularly for an elderly patient.

6. Put on gloves.

This is not as easy as it sounds. The big disposable gloves are the easiest to put on. The surgical-type rubber gloves can be difficult. Often there is only one size available (a nightmare for those of you with large hands) and they can be hell to put on if your hands are sweaty (a usual occurrence with your first few attempts).

7. Put lubricant on your index finger.

Just a small blob on the tip of your finger will do. Avoid the temptation to swamp your finger with the lubricant and get it everywhere.

8. Warn the patient that you are about to perform the test.

Prepare your patient by saying, 'you are going to feel some cold jelly and then my finger.'

9. Inspect the perianal region.

Prior to your digital examination, get your head down close to the perianal area, 'cheek to cheek' as it were, and inspect. If the bed cannot be raised high enough, then bend at the knees and keep a straight back. Use the fingers of your left hand to separate the buttocks. Your inspection should be brief so that there is little delay between your warning and the PR examination itself. You need to look for skin tags, prolapsed haemorrhoids (piles), or rarely evidence of fistulae (*fist-you-lee*) (see p. 179). A raw excoriated area may be found in someone with diarrhoea leading to frequent wiping with toilet paper and in the elderly you may notice pressure sores in someone who is bed bound.

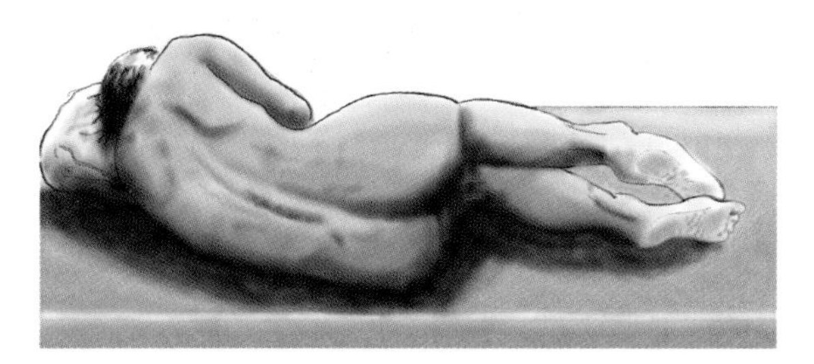

Fig. 7.1 Position for the rectal examination.

10. Introduce your finger into the anal canal.

See Fig. 7.2. If the anal sphincter is tight (your patient may be anxious) this manoeuvre can be aided if you ask your patient to take a deep breath or ask them to bear down or strain as if they are going to the toilet. The passage of your finger might feel a little uncomfortable but if your patient shouts out in pain, **stop the examination**. Such a painful rectum may indicate the presence of an anal fissure (*fisher*).

11. Examine the rectum in a logical sequence.

Once your finger is in the rectum you need a strategy for your examination. It does not matter what order you do things in so long as you are thorough and do not miss pathology. Knowing the anatomy of the region is essential (see Fig. 7.3). Developing a set routine will also stop you ferreting with your finger in a random and hopeful manner and decrease the likelihood of raised eyebrows from your anxious patient. The routine adopted by the author is to feel the posterior wall first (see Figs 7.4 and 7.5). This is because the posterior wall of the rectum naturally faces your finger following insertion. Simply flex your wrist and curl your index

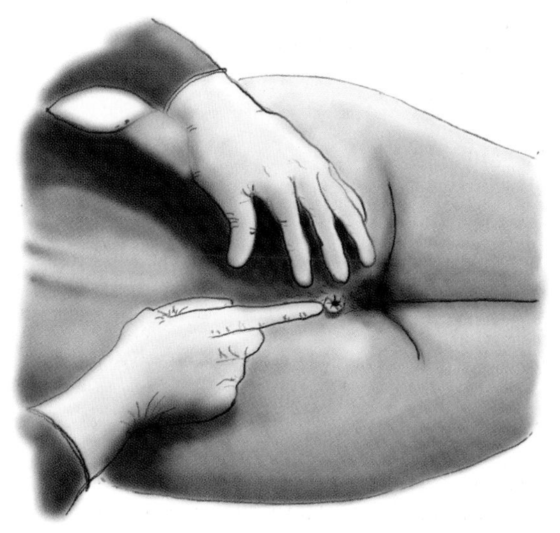

Fig. 7.2 Preparing to introduce finger into anus.

CASE 7.1

Problem. You attempt to insert your finger in the rectum of your patient but are having great difficulty.

Discussion. The likeliest explanation is that your patient is anxious and has a 'tight' sphincter. Try the manoeuvres outlined above, for example, get the patient to take a deep breath or push down as if going to the toilet. The resistance to your finger should lessen and your finger should slide into the anal canal (the sphincter should have an elastic feel around your finger). Occasionally difficulties can arise due to an anal stricture, a tumour near the anal verge or with an anal fissure. With an anal fissure, the associated pain may be so great that the sphincter can go into spasm.

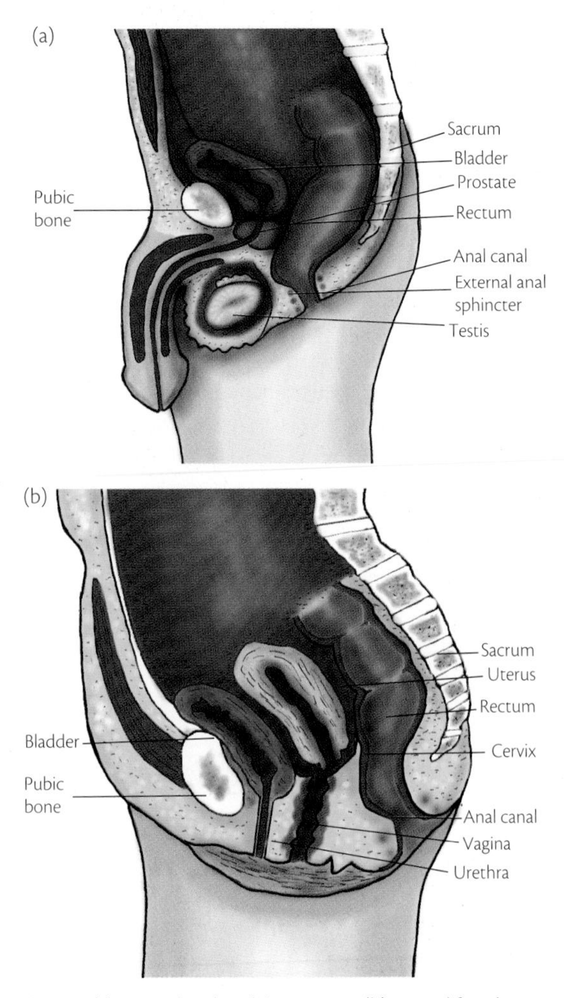

Fig. 7.3 (a) Normal male pelvic anatomy, (b) normal female pelvic anatomy.

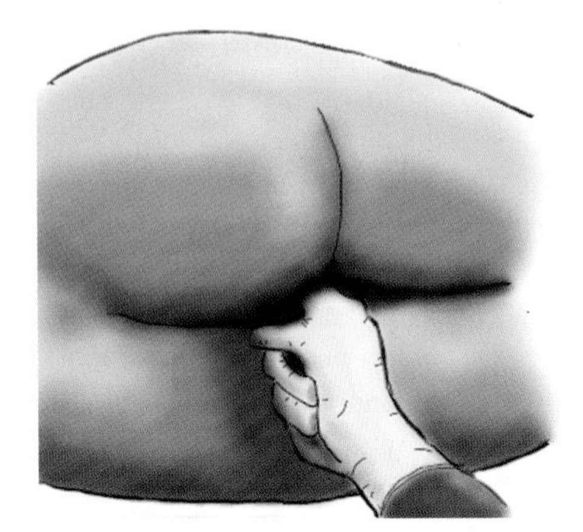

Fig. 7.4 Palpating the posterior wall of the anal canal.

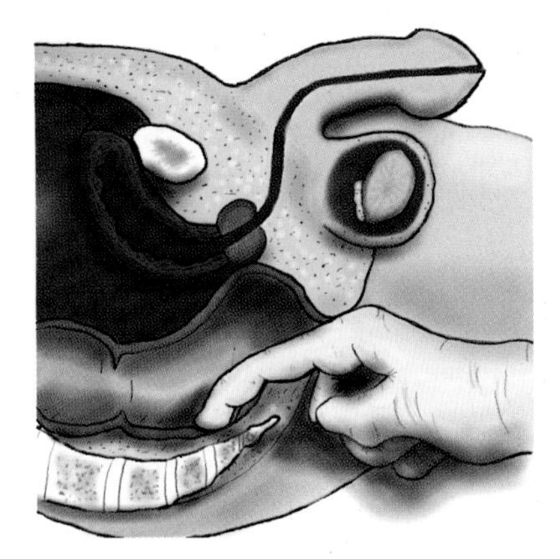

Fig. 7.5 Palpating the posterior wall of the anal canal of a man in cross-section.

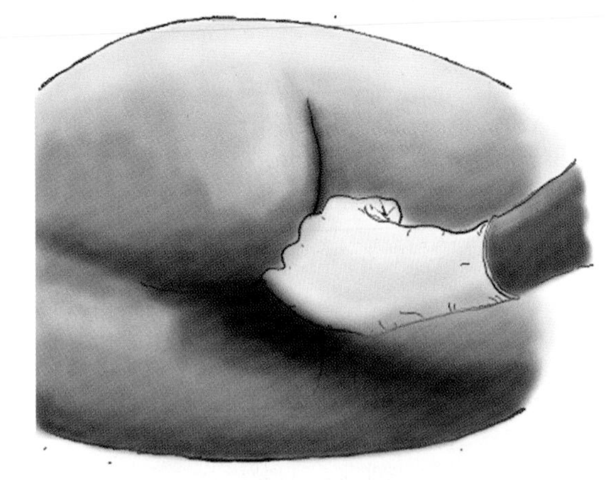

Fig. 7.6 Palpating the anterior wall of the anal canal.

finger and you will soon feel the back wall. It usually feels hard because of the sacrum (*say-crumb*) and coccyx (*cock-sicks*) directly behind it. Nevertheless if you sweep your finger along the surface of the wall it should feel smooth. Next, rotate your finger by pronating your wrist. Now your finger will be lying against the left lateral wall of the rectum (the pulp of your finger will be facing down to the couch). Again run your finger over the mucosal surface. Now supinate your wrist fully. Your finger should travel back in the direction it came and rotate a full 180°. You will now be examining the right lateral wall (the pulp of your finger should now be facing up to the ceiling). Finally rotate your finger back in the direction you have just come as if you were going to re-examine the left lateral wall but this time you need to continue to rotate your finger through a further 90°. To achieve this, you will naturally have to bend your trunk down to the left while rotating your right elbow up so that it lies above your examining wrist. This is an awkward position but the only way to examine the anterior wall (Fig. 7.6). Through the anterior wall you can assess the prostate in a man and appreciate the cervix in a woman (this is not a standard means of assessing the cervix) (see Figs 7.7 and 7.8).

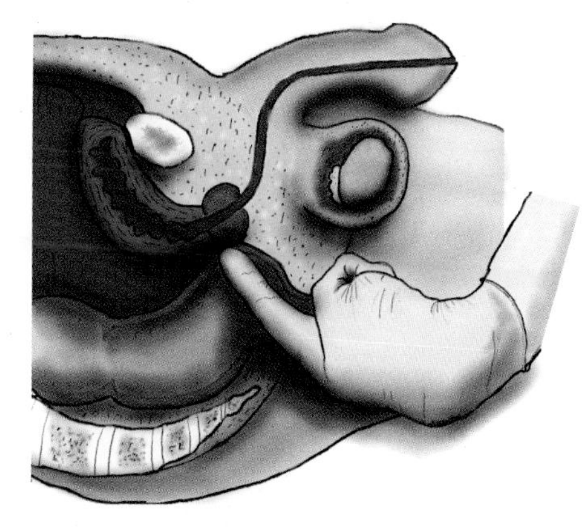

Fig. 7.7 Palpating the anterior anal canal of a man in cross-section.

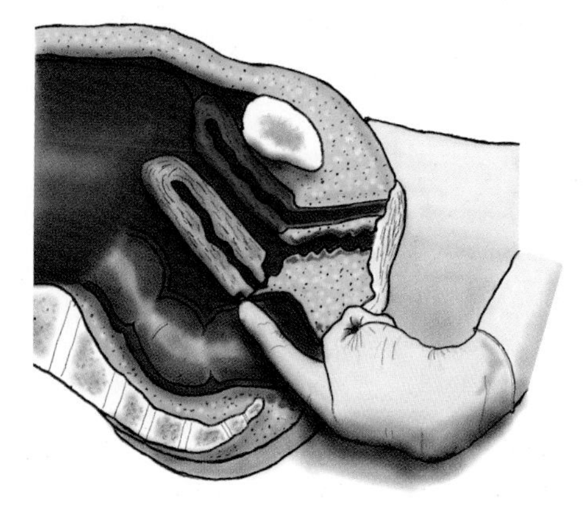

Fig. 7.8 Palpating the anterior anal canal of a woman in cross-section.

The most likely diagnoses are

- a normal examination
- faecal loading (see Fig. 7.9)
- benign prostatic hypertrophy (BPH)
- prostatic carcinoma (see Fig. 7.10)
- rectal carcinoma (see Fig. 7.11).

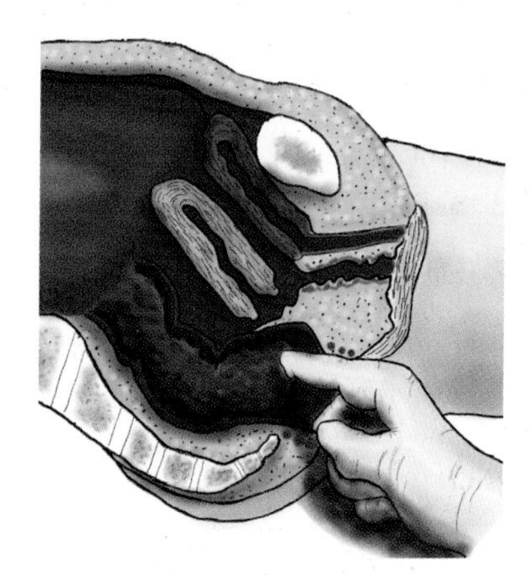

Fig. 7.9 Faecal loading.

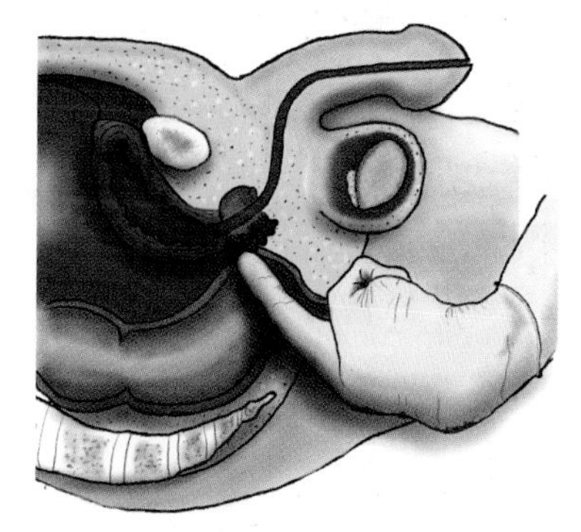

Fig. 7.10 Prostatic carcinoma.

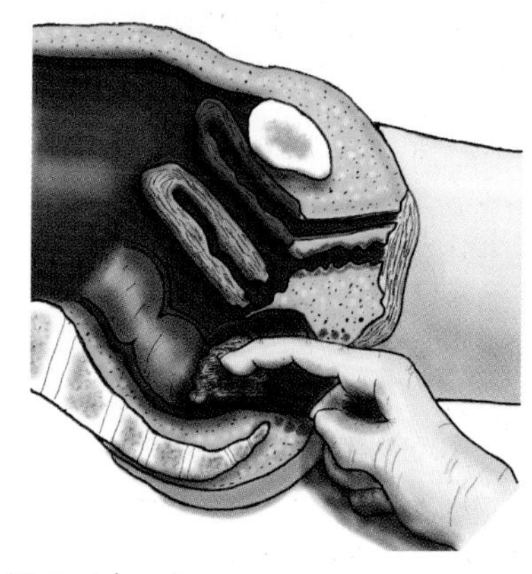

Fig. 7.11 Rectal carcinoma.

1. **A normal examination.** This is the most common finding. Only by doing plenty of PR examinations will you be able to appreciate this (as well as knowing when something is abnormal).
2. **Faecal loading.** This may be found particularly in the elderly. Your finger may pass easily through soft faeces or may impact upon hard faeces. A patient in this situation may complain of constipation or paradoxically complain of diarrhoea (called spurious diarrhoea) with bouts of faecal incontinence of which they have no sensation. The exact mechanism why liquid faeces are produced around a hard faecal mass is not known. The treatment required includes adequate hydration, increased fibre in the diet, exercise, and laxatives. In the case of impacted faeces a stool softener is recommended. Faeces may mimic a rectal tumour. However you will be able to indent a faecal mass and separate it from the rectal wall. You will not be able to do this with a rectal tumour.
3. **Benign prostatic hypertrophy.** BPH is not easy to appreciate at first. You have to do plenty of PR examinations to be familiar with the dimensions of the normal prostate. In a normal young man you will feel a rubbery swelling with a groove in the centre. On either side of this groove are the lateral lobes of the prostate, which should feel smooth and firm. In BPH these lobes can be very large and pronounced but the median groove usually remains palpable. It is important to note that a normal sized prostate can still cause obstruction to the flow of urine and conversely a large prostate may cause little in the way of obstruction to the flow of urine.
4. **Prostatic carcinoma.** Any hard lumps felt in the substance of the prostate is highly suggestive of a prostatic carcinoma. Another clue to the possibility of cancer is the obliteration of the median groove due to tumour growth.
5. **Rectal carcinoma.** This is usually readily apparent to the finger and often protrudes into the lumen (Some can ulcerate through the mucosa). Always check that the mass is part of the rectal wall and not adherent faeces.

12. Take your finger out and inspect the glove for faeces, blood, and so on.

Do not simply take your finger out thinking your ordeal is over. Your examination is not complete until you observe your index finger. You are looking for traces of faeces so that you can check the colour. A black residue might suggest a stool due to iron consumption or if it looks tarry, melaena. Is there bright red blood on the glove or mucus?

13. Clean the perianal region.

It is only courtesy for you to clean your patient of any smears, stains, or excess lubricant.

14. Tell your patient you have finished and allow them to get dressed.

This will be their cue to pull up their underwear and to get dressed while you reflect on your findings.

15. Wash your hands.

This is the most under-rated clinical skill.

16. Report your findings.

After subjecting your patient to this examination they will be keen to know what you have found. In most cases you can reassure them that everything is normal. You should also document your findings in the case notes. As a student you should never be put in the position where you find something abnormal without a

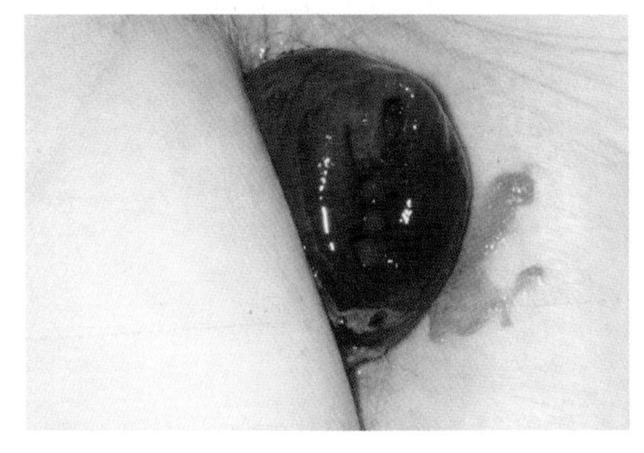

Fig. 7.12 Rectal prolapse.

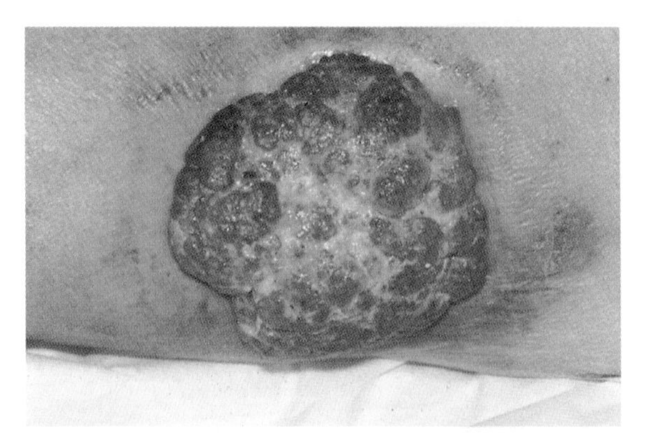

Fig. 7.13 Squamous cell carcinoma of the anus.

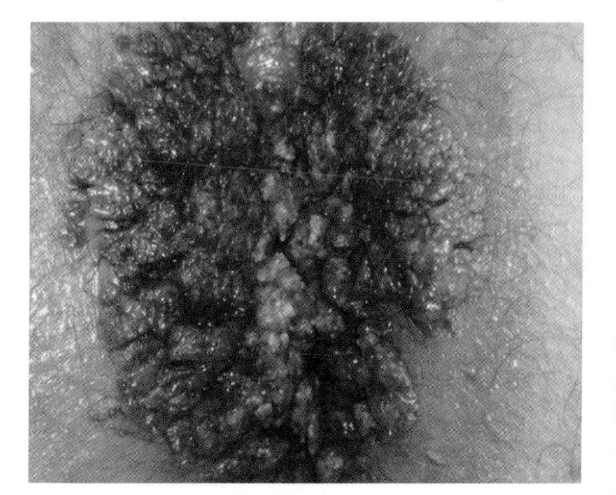

Fig. 7.14 Perianal warts.

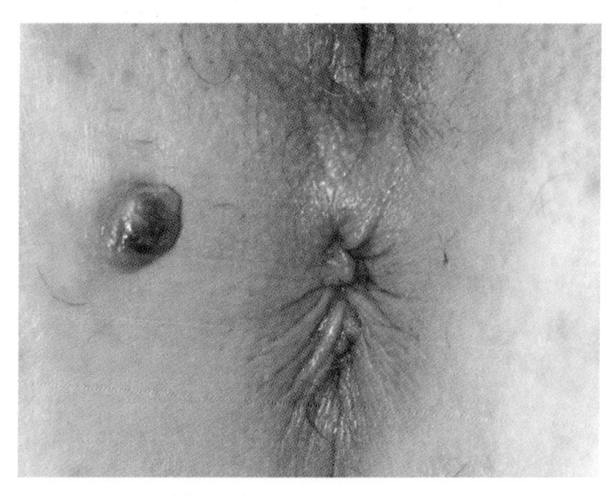

Fig. 7.15 Perianal fistula.

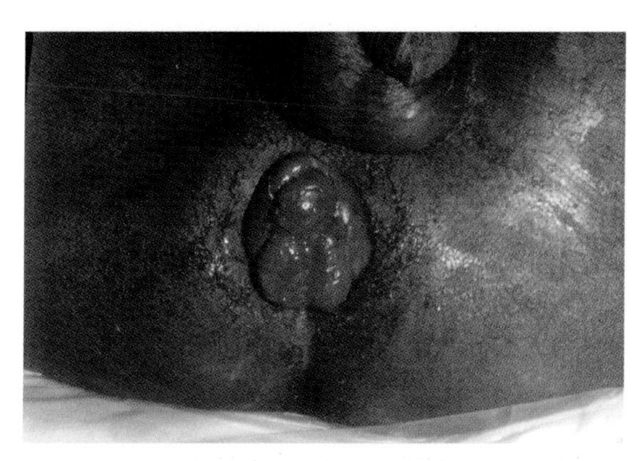

Fig. 7.16 Thrombosed haemorrhoid.

CASE 7.2

Problem. You perform a PR examination, which is uneventful until you withdraw your finger and notice some bright red blood. What is the cause?

Discussion. The likeliest cause is haemorrhoids (piles). Typically they cause bright red bleeding to be noticed in the toilet or on toilet paper. However, before accepting that they are the cause of bleeding you must take a full gastrointestinal history, particularly asking about features such as diarrhoea, constipation, tenesmus, and so on because there are many causes of bright red bleeding PR (usually from the left side of the large bowel such as the descending and sigmoid colon). Some causes of bleeding PR include

- anal fissure
- carcinoma of the colon
- inflammatory bowel disease
- diverticular disease
- angiodysplasia (*an-jio-dis-play-zia*) of the colon
- upper gastrointestinal bleeding, for example, from a peptic ulcer (can cause fresh bleeding PR if it is a large bleed with rapid transit through the gut).

Haemorrhoids can be confirmed as the source of bleeding by performing proctoscopy. This instrument allows a visual inspection of the rectum. If haemorrhoids are not seen or there are potential doubts about the source of bleeding (for example, other symptoms in the history) then you must go on to investigate the rest of the large bowel.

qualified doctor present. Usually you will be told to do a PR examination on someone who is already aware of their diagnosis.

You will need to report your findings to a doctor for feedback. They will want to know about the following:

- external abnormalities (see Figs 7.12–7.16)
- rectal masses
- prostate in men
- faeces.

Here is an example: 'On rectal examination there is a small anal tag externally. There are soft faeces in the rectum but no evidence of masses. The prostate is enlarged and firm.'

A further point to make once you begin your practice after passing your Finals is that you should always record in the notes if you do **not** perform a PR examination following an examination of the abdomen. In some cases this will not be relevant, for example, in a patient with a simple chest infection. However if a PR examination is relevant and not performed you must give a good reason why it was not performed, for example, patient refused consent.

Keypoints

- Always explain why you are doing a PR examination and ask permission.
- Always have a chaperone present (particularly male doctors).
- Examine a logical sequence, check for masses and faeces, and assess the prostate in men.
- Stop the examination if it is painful for the patient.
- Always inspect the glove after withdrawing your finger.
- Always record your findings in the patient's notes.

CHAPTER 8

Arms

Chapter contents

Introduction

When asked to examine the upper limbs, in the majority of cases the underlying diagnosis will be a neurological one. It is important to have some basic knowledge of neuroanatomy and this will be covered in this chapter. The neurological examination is one that often fills medical students (and some doctors) with a sense of dread. In fact it is one of the easiest examinations to perform and has the added benefit that all the signs elicited are very obvious; for example, the presence of a tremor or a brisk reflex. This is in contrast to those elusive diastolic murmurs in the cardiovascular system or that palpable splenic tip in the abdominal system.

Basic neuroanatomy

The two important subdivisions of the peripheral nervous supply to the limbs are the motor and sensory systems. In the motor system, impulses originate in the cerebral cortex and terminate at a muscle in the periphery to initiate movement, whereas the sensory system operates in the opposite direction, carrying information from receptors in the skin for example, up to the brain.

Motor pathways

Impulses from the motor cortex in the cerebral hemispheres travel along upper motor neurones (UMNs) in the corticospinal tracts to the internal capsule. This is an area

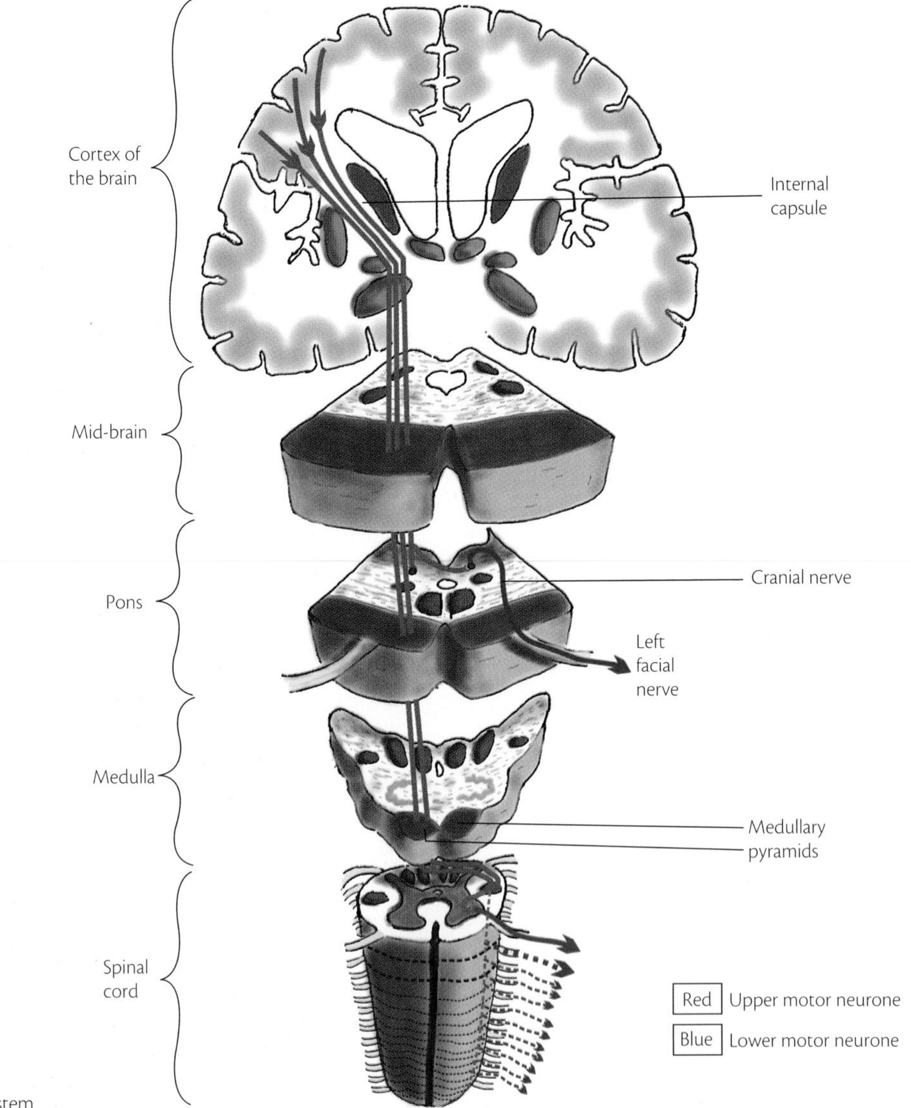

Fig. 8.1 The pyramidal system

of the brain where nerve fibres become tightly packed. From here, they travel through the mid-brain, pons (*ponz*), and medulla (*med-duller*) (collectively known as the brainstem). The majority of fibres cross the mid-line of the medulla in a process called 'decussation' (*de-cuss-ay-shun*). More precisely this occurs in an area called the pyramids of the medulla and hence the corticospinal tracts are also known as the pyramidal (*pi-ram-id-al*) tracts.

Having crossed over, the corticospinal tracts descend to different levels within the spinal cord. Some end in the cervical cord to supply the arms whilst others continue to the lumbar levels to supply the legs. They terminate in the 'anterior horns', which are projections of the grey matter within the spinal cord as seen on transverse section. Here they synapse with anterior horn cells, the axons of which are known as lower motor neurones (LMNs). These transmit impulses along the limbs to the target muscle. This pathway is important for control of movement by the cerebral cortex. Other descending tracts are also involved but the corticospinal pathway is the only one you need to know in detail. See Fig. 8.1.

Differentiating upper and lower motor neurone lesions

As illustrated above, the two main components of the motor pathway are the UMN, originating in the cerebral cortex and the LMN, originating in the anterior horns of the spinal cord; UMN and LMN lesions produce very different clinical pictures, although weakness is common to both. See Table 8.1 for a comparison of UMN And LMN lesions.

Upper motor neurone lesions

The UMN, under cortical control, acts to modify the activity of the LMN. It can stimulate the LMN to achieve voluntary movement, but has predominantly inhibitory effects at rest. If the UMN is damaged then loss of this descending inhibition from the cortex leads to increased reflexes and tone, mediated by the spinal reflex (see next section). Wasting is mild and occurs late in UMN lesions since the muscle is still innervated by the LMN. Upper motor neurone or 'pyramidal' weakness has a characteristic distribution, being more pronounced in weaker muscle groups. Hence in the arms, the relatively weak action of triceps is overcome by the biceps, leading to a flexor posture of the limb. By contrast, pyramidal weakness in the legs results in an extensor posture of the limb due to the extensor power of the quadriceps being greater than the flexor action of the hamstrings. Two further neurological signs, which are found in UMN but not LMN disease, are the plantar response (one of the superficial reflexes) and clonus (*clone-us*). These will be described in the chapter on the legs (Chapter 10).

Lower motor neurone lesions

The LMN forms the final common pathway to the muscle. If it is damaged, no impulses reach the target muscle, which becomes wasted and flaccid. Reflexes are diminished or absent because the muscle cannot contract. Visible contractions of muscle fibres known as fasciculations (*fa-sick-you-lay-shuns*) may be present. These are a characteristic feature of motor neurone disease. In contrast to UMN lesions, LMN pathology causes weakness that tends to predominantly affect the distal musculature.

TABLE 8.1 Comparison of upper and lower motor neurone lesions

	Upper motor neurone lesion	Lower motor neurone lesion
Inspection	Wasting, often mild. No fasciculations	Wasting more marked. Fasciculations may be present
Tone	Increased	Reduced/normal
Distribution of weakness	Extensors >flexors (arms), flexors >extensors (legs)	Distal>proximal
Reflexes	Increased	Reduced
Plantar response	Extensor	Flexor/absent

Spinal reflex

See Fig. 8.2. Although the pathway from the motor cortex to the target muscle seems long, it takes less than a second from initiation of a thought to contraction of a muscle. Occasionally even more rapid responses are required, so there are shorter pathways that do not travel up to the cortex. These form a local reflex arc between the muscle and the spinal cord, enabling the body to perform swift protective movements without requiring conscious thought.

Mechanism

Voluntary muscle contains 'spindle fibres'—adapted muscle fibres that act as sensory organs. When the tendon is tapped, stretching of the spindle fibres occurs, stimulating sensory impulses. These impulses pass along sensory afferent tracts to the spinal cord ('afferent' indicates that the tracts are entering the spinal cord). These directly synapse with the efferent fibres (that is, fibres leaving the spinal cord), which are LMNs,

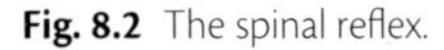

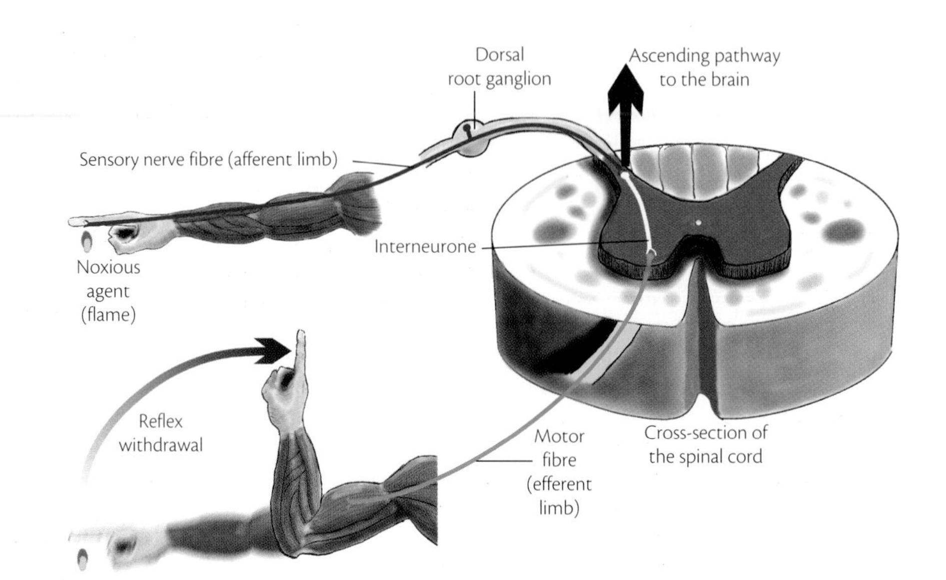

Fig. 8.2 The spinal reflex.

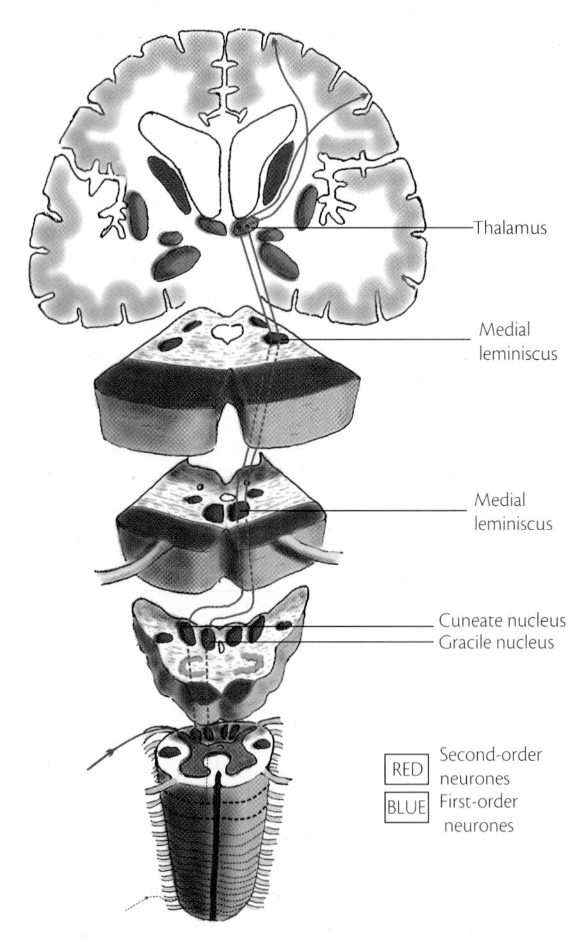

Fig. 8.3 The dorsal columns.

resulting in muscle contraction. This type of reflex is known as a 'stretch reflex', because reflex contraction of the muscle is triggered by stretching of the spindle fibres. This is in contrast to 'superficial reflexes', which are triggered by sensory receptors in the skin (for example, the plantar reflexes).

Control of movement

When voluntary movements are initiated by the cerebral cortex, other areas of the central nervous system are activated to ensure that muscle contraction is smooth and co-ordinated. The two most important of these are described here.

The cerebellum

The cerebellum (*serry-bell-um*) is located posterior and inferior to the cerebral hemispheres. It also consists of two hemispheres, each involved with control of movement of the **same** side of the body. They are linked by a mid-line structure called the vermis (*ver-miss*). The latter is concerned with the function of the trunk muscles and is involved in the maintenance of posture.

The basal ganglia

The basal ganglia are a group of structures situated within the cerebral hemispheres, deep to the cortex. They consist of the corpus striatum (*core-puss-try-ate-um*), the substantia nigra (*sub-stan-sha-nigh-gra*), and the subthalamic nucleus. The function of the basal ganglia is less well understood than the cerebellum, but they are also involved in normal muscle function. Diseases affecting these structures will be described later.

Sensory pathways

There are two main sensory pathways. One is the dorsal column system, which, as its name suggests, transmits impulses in the dorsal part of the cord relating to vibration, joint position sense, and pressure (see Fig. 8.3). The other is the spinothalamic (*spy-no-tha-lam-ick*) pathway, which carries pain and temperature information (see Fig. 8.4). Light touch is carried by both pathways, but principally in the dorsal columns. In the dorsal columns, impulses from receptors pass along the peripheral nerve to the spinal cord and ascend on the 'ipsilateral' side (meaning the same side) of the cord before crossing at the medulla. In contrast, the spinothalamic tracts decussate much earlier, either at the same level as their entry into the cord or a few segments above. They then ascend in the 'contralateral' (opposite) half of the cord. Impulses from both tracts pass to the sensory cortex of the cerebral hemispheres, via the thalamus (*tha-la-muss*). Damage at any point in these pathways may lead to abnormalities in the appreciation of sensation.

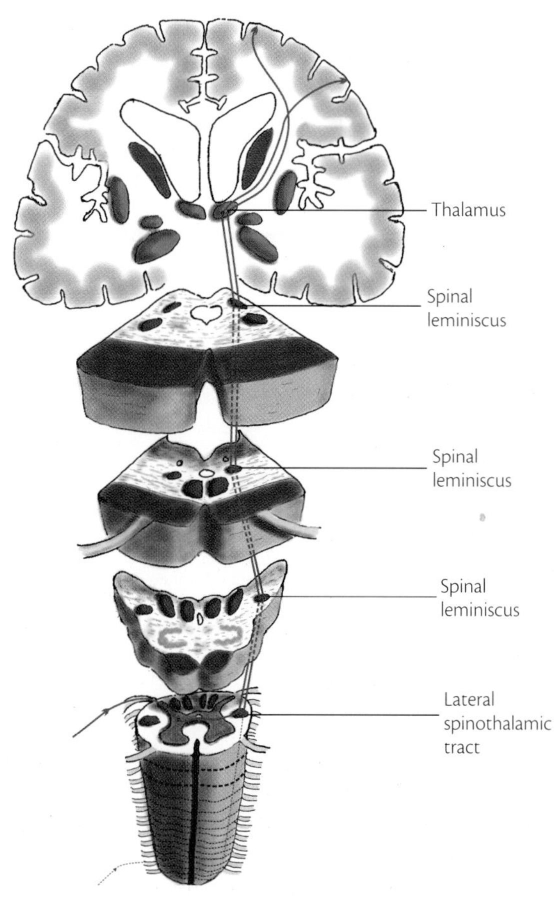

Fig. 8.4 The spinothalamic tracts.

> **Tip**
>
> Students often forget which tract travels on which side of the cord. The mnemonic **disc** will help: **d**orsal tracts are **i**psilateral; **s**pinothalamic tracts are **c**ontralateral.

Dermatomes

The skin can be divided up into areas known as dermatomes (*der-mat-omes*), each supplied by a specific spinal cord segment. For example, the skin over the tip of the shoulder lies within the C5 dermatome, because impulses from here will enter the cord at the fifth cervical segment (see Fig. 8.5). Unfortunately for students, it is important to have some idea about the distribution of dermatomes. This is because if there is a sensory disturbance that conforms to a dermatomal distribution it gives a clue as to where the lesion is.

Symptoms

As history taking is similar for the arms and legs, this section is the combination of symptoms for the chapters on both the arms and the legs (Chapter 10).

There is only a limited range of neurological symptoms. Unfortunately this does not mean that taking a history is any easier. You still need to be systematic and thorough in checking all aspects of the history to build up a 'disease profile' of your patient. Any information you glean will guide your examination and subsequent investigations and hopefully point you towards the diagnosis. When you take your history there are a few of points to bear in mind.

1. The neurological system has been divided up arbitrarily into smaller chunks (cranial nerves, arms, hands, and legs) and therefore any information you glean has to be interpreted together with information from these areas also.
2. Although you are concentrating on the limbs, you need to be aware of nearby structures (especially the legs) such as bowels, bladder, or spine, either for a potential cause (for example, a herniated lumbar disc causing sensory and motor loss of a particular nerve root) or for complications (for example, constipation and urinary retention due to spinal cord compression).

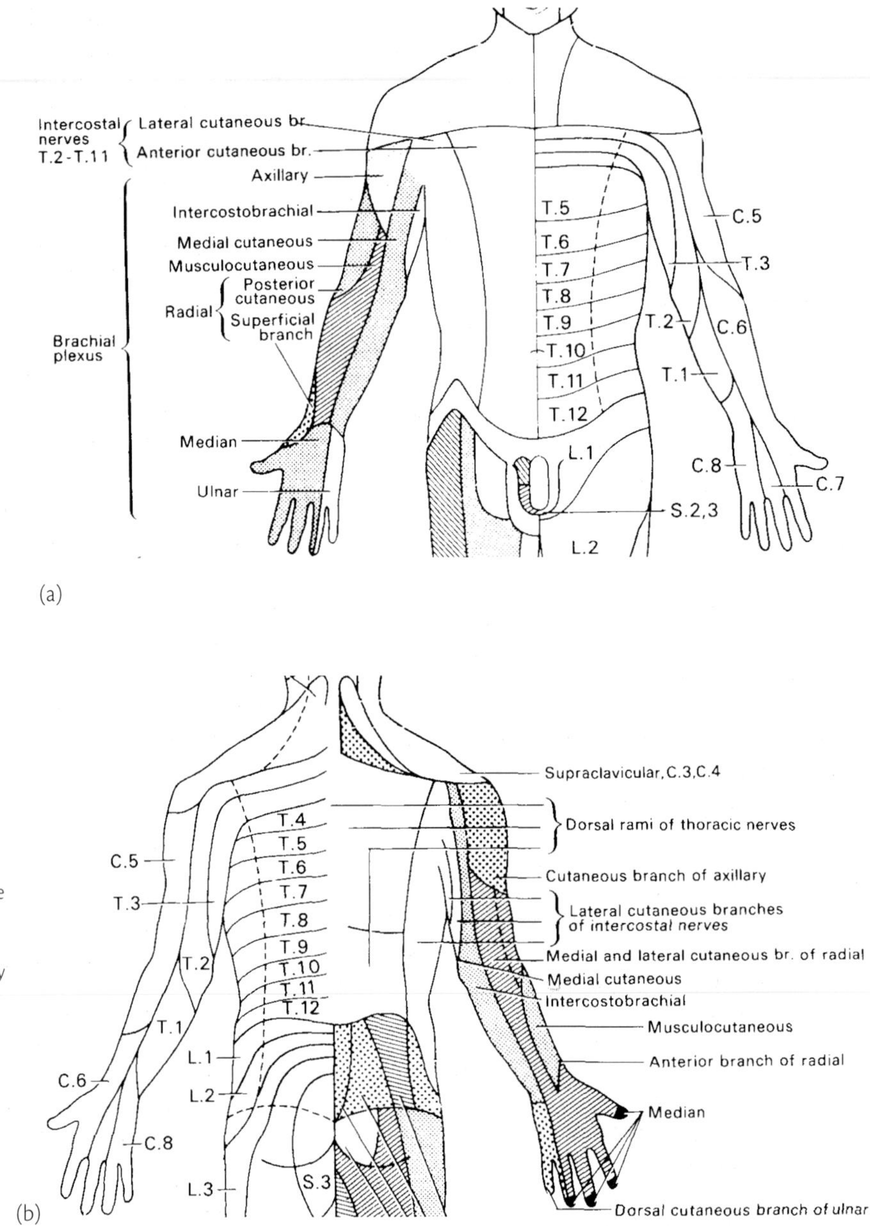

Fig. 8.5 The dermatomes of the upper limbs (a) Anterior view, (b) posterior view. Adapted by permission of Oxford University Press from **Fig. 1(a)** and **(b)** (pp. 21.110 and 21.112), *Oxford textbook of medicine* (2nd edn, Vol. 2), edited by Weatherall, D. J. *et al.* (1987), reproduced by permission of Oxford University Press from *Brain's clinical neurology* by R. Bannister.

3. Be alive to symptoms in other systems (that is, perform your review of systems) because some neurological diseases may produce symptoms elsewhere (for example, Friedreich's ataxia (*freed-ricks-attacks-ya*) (*Nikolaus Friedreich (1825–1882), German neurologist*) is associated with diabetes and hence polyuria, polydipsia, and so on) and diseases in other systems can cause neurological complications, for example, diabetes mellitus and peripheral neuropathy.

The main neurological symptoms are pain, paraesthaesia, numbness, and muscle weakness.

Pain

The subject of pain, especially of neurological origin (neurogenic (*new-roe-jen-ick*) pain) is a complicated one and there are whole textbooks devoted to the problem. The following represents a simplified means of dealing with pain in the spine and limbs.

Local pain

Local pain arises from the pain-sensitive structures involved in the spine, pelvis, and legs. These include soft tissue such as ligaments, muscles, and joints as well as the bones themselves. There is usually a clear relationship with trauma, which is often volunteered by the patient. The pain can be superficial, where it has a sharp 'light' quality and is easily localized by the patient. It does not interfere with muscle function. Deep pain tends to be dull and not so readily localized. In addition there may be decreased muscle activity around any inflammation or even frank spasm to protect the area. Further neurological problems can occur if nearby nerves are involved in an injury, for example, a fracture at the head of the fibula may damage the common peroneal (*peh-roe-knee-al*) nerve. This can lead to a foot-drop and loss of sensation of the anterior and lateral aspect of the leg and the dorsum of the foot.

Referred pain

This is even more difficult to localize as the area where the pain is experienced is remote from its site of origin. Pain can be referred from the spine, the pelvis, and even the abdominal or pelvic viscera. The pain can assume almost any character depending on the structure involved. The importance of referred pain is the potential for misdiagnosis.

Neuropathic pain

This is pain caused as a result of nerve damage in the central nervous system. Sometimes the term 'neurogenic pain' is used and means practically the same thing. Neuralgia (*new-ral-ja*) also means nerve pain although in latter years it has been tagged on to the end of specific nerves to represent a particular condition, for example, trigeminal (*try-jemmy-nal*) neuralgia. Neuropathic pain tends to be burning in nature, diffuse, and poorly localized. It can also be symmetrical in the case of a peripheral neuropathy. It can be difficult to treat but some patients do respond to the anti-depressant amitriptyline (*am-ee-trip-ta-lean*) or the anti- convulsant carbamazipine (*car-ba-maz-ee-peen* or *car-ba-maze-ee-peen*).

Radicular pain

This is a form of neuropathic pain with characteristic qualities. It is an episodic, shooting pain, which is conducted along a narrow path. When this form of pain is particularly severe it is described as lancinating. The best example of this form of pain is sciatica. Protrusion of an intervertebral disc (prolapse) can irritate adjacent nerve roots. As well as some localized pain at the site of the prolapse there is also transient shooting pain usually felt down the back of the leg. Manoeuvres like coughing, straining, stretching, or sneezing can irritate the nerve roots and provoke the pain.

There are other aspects of neuropathic pain that you may encounter occasionally in your reading.

1. **Allodynia (*allo-din-nia*).** This is an abnormal and unpleasant sensation produced by normal stimuli. This is sometimes called dysaesthesia (*dis-as-theez-ya*).
2. **Hyperalgesia.** This is where the pain threshold is lowered, so that the slightest stimulation can cause pain, for example, blowing on the skin can evoke pain.
3. **Hyperpathia.** This is where the pain threshold is elevated, so that a painful stimulus is not felt until it becomes very forceful. When it is experienced the full magnitude of the noxious stimulus is felt.

What to ask

With regards to neurogenic pain it is best to concentrate on questions regarding the pain itself. Begin with an open question, for example, 'tell me about your pain!' But be prepared to ask some supplementary questions.

1. 'Where is the pain?'
2. 'How long did it last?'
3. 'Did it come on suddenly or gradually?'
4. 'Is the pain constant or intermittent?'
5. 'Can you describe the pain?' Give some examples to help, for example, sharp, burning, shooting, or aching.
6. 'Does the pain radiate anywhere?' For example, down the back of the leg or the front of the leg.
7. 'Did anything bring the pain on?' For example, trauma or movement of a limb.
8. 'Does anything aggravate the pain?' For example, coughing, sneezing, or bending.
9. 'Does anything relieve the pain?'

The responses to these questions may suggest neurogenic pain. If so, ask about associated neurological symptoms (see later) As with many symptoms you also have to decide whether your patient is exaggerating the degree of pain or underplaying it. This is a skill you will learn to develop through your training.

Keypoints

- Neuropathic pain tends to be diffuse and burning in nature.
- Trauma may cause neurological dysfunction through damage to nearby nerves.
- Always bear in mind the possibility of referred pain so as to avoid the dangers of misdiagnosis.
- Radicular pain is a transient shooting pain that is conducted in a narrow band.

Paraesthesia

This is the feeling of pins and needles or a continual prickly feeling. It is usually caused by damage to larger myelinated fibres. Most people have experienced this at some point, for example, if they have slept on their arm overnight. This example also demonstrates that a non-neurological cause of paraesthesia exists, that is, disruption of arterial blood supply. Be aware that some patients have difficulty describing the sensation of paraesthesia and may call it pain instead. This phenomenon is not necessarily accompanied by objective sensory impairment and it is therefore difficult to localize the source of the lesion (an exception to this is the radicular distribution of paraesthesia in shingles).

Keypoints

- Paraesthesia can sometimes be described as pain by some patients.
- It has poor value in localizing a neurological lesion.
- Non-neurological causes exist, for example, disruption of the arterial supply.

Numbness

This is a decrease or absence of sensation and is usually accompanied by a loss of proprioception (*pro-pree-owe-sep-shun*). Always ask the patient what they mean when they say numb. Several expressions are often used by patients to explain numbness, for example, heaviness, dead feeling, cold, no sensation, 'it does not feel the same as the other leg', and so on. It is useful to ask further questions to define the problem further. Ascertain the following.

1. Can they feel their pyjamas, gloves, socks, or tights when they wear them?
2. Can they tell the difference between hot and cold materials?
3. Can they tell the difference between different surfaces on the floor, that is, carpets, tiles, or wooden floor?

Sometimes patients will volunteer that it feels as if they are walking on cotton wool or eggshells. Any loss of pain sensation in the long term can lead to burns, scars, or trophic ulcers. If pain sensation is profound this can lead to deranged joints (Charcot's (*shark-owes*) joints) (*Jean Martin Charcot (1825–1893), French neurologist*). The patient will be unaware of any of these injuries at the time they occur but may notice the changes later on or if relatives or friends draw their attention to it.

A sudden loss of sensation indicates an acute lesion and the possible causes include vascular events affecting the sensory cortex, sub-cortical structures, or even the spinal cord. Demyelination (*de-mile-lin-ay-shun*), such as with a transverse myelitis (*mile-eye-tiss*) or multiple sclerosis may also be possible (this is true of any neurological abnormality). A more gradual onset of numbness that ascends up the arms or legs over a period of time may suggest a peripheral neuropathy especially if it occurs in a 'glove and stocking' distribution. It is well known for patients with spinal cord compression to have a band of numbness, paraesthesia, or hyperaesthesia at the proximal limit of sensory loss.

Keypoints

- Always ask what a patient means by numbness.
- The patient may complain that they are walking on cotton wool, eggshells, and so on.
- Chronic loss of sensation can predispose to burns, scars, trophic ulcers, and even deranged joints (Charcot's joints).

Muscle weakness

Muscle weakness is an important and distressing symptom. The first thing to decide is whether there is true muscular weakness. Some people use the term to describe fatigue. Other patients will claim they have weakness in their arms or legs but in fact it is pain that limits their movement. If there is true muscle weakness, find out if it is the proximal or distal muscle groups that are affected. If it is an asymmetrical weakness is there a specific muscle group or muscle that is affected? One characteristic form of weakness occurs with myasthenia gravis (*my-ass-theen-ia-grah-vis*). The patient may start the day with full strength but become easily fatigued as their levels of neurotransmitter become depleted. Ascertain the following.

1. How long has the weakness has been noticed?
2. Does it affect all limbs or just the arms or legs?
3. Does it affect one or both arms (or one or both legs)? (nerve or root lesion?)
4. Does the weakness affect the proximal muscles or the distal muscles? Do they have difficulty combing their hair or have difficulty rising from a chair (proximal myopathy)? Do they have difficulty gripping objects or unscrewing jam jars? (peripheral neuropathy?)
5. Can the patient stand?
6. Can the patient stand on one leg?
7. Is the patient able to walk without difficulty?
8. Does the patient drag their leg when walking?
9. Does the patient feel as if they are drunk when they walk? (This suggests a balance problem although some patients may feel that this is weakness.)
10. Does the weakness vary substantially throughout the day? If yes follow this up and determine whether it is a dramatic weakness following activity (myasthenia gravis) or merely just a normal response to exhausting everyday tasks.
11. What other activities do they have difficulty with?

Keypoints

- Determine if there is true muscular weakness.
- Ask how the weakness affects their activities and abilities.
- Is there a pattern of weakness, for example, proximal >distal, asymmetry.
- If a patient experiences dramatic fatiguability in muscular function consider myasthenia gravis.

To complete your neurological history you need to know the patient's past medical history

1. Have they had any recent viral illnesses? This may suggest causes such as transverse myelitis or Guillain–Barré (*ghee-on-ba-ray*) (*George Charles Guillain (1876–1961), French neurologist, Jean Alexandre Barré (1880–1967), French neurologist*) syndrome.
2. Do they have important current illnesses, for example, diabetes mellitus or rheumatoid arthritis, which may predispose to nerve injury such as peripheral neuropathy or mononeuritis (*mono-new-right-iss*) multiplex?
3. Is there a history of trauma?
4. Have they had previous operations that may have damaged nearby nerves or a laminectomy involving the spine, which may suggest previous back problems such as a prolapsed intervertebral disc?
5. A drug history is always important.
6. Some drugs are notorious for causing injury:
   (1) **isoniazid** (***ice-so-nigh-a-zid***)—treatment for tuberculosis—peripheral neuropathy;
   (2) **rifampicin** (***riff-amp-i-sin***)—treatment for tuberculosis—peripheral neuropathy;
   (3) **penicillamine** (***penny-sill-am-mean***)—treatment for rheumatoid arthritis—peripheral neuropathy;
   (4) **gold**—treatment for rheumatoid arthritis—peripheral neuropathy;
   (5) **vincristine** (***vin-christine***)—chemotherapy.
7. A family history may be important for some conditions, for example, Huntington's chorea (*cu-rear*) (*George Sumner Huntington (1851–1916), American physician*)—autosomal dominant and Duchenne muscular dystrophy (*do-shen-muscular-dis-truffy*) (*Guillaume Benjamin Amand Duchenne (1807–1875), French neurologist*) (see p. 265)—X-linked recessive.
8. Always perform a review of systems looking for possible clues, for example, multi-system disorders or malignancy that may have effects in other systems as well the neurological system.
9. Also pay attention to the bowels and bladder, particularly if you suspect spinal cord compression where there may be constipation and urine retention. There are other conditions that may predispose to constipation and urine retention, for example, Parkinsons's disease (*James Parkinson (1755–1824), English physician*), stroke, and so on, either primarily through the disease process or through its treatments. However these do not present the emergency that spinal cord compression does.

Examination of the arms summary

1. Preparation.
2. Introduce yourself to the patient and ask for permission to examine.

Keypoints

- Always take a drug history.
- Ask about medical conditions that the patient has (or has suffered in the past).
- Do not forget to enquire about bowel and bladder function.

3. Position the patient and expose the arms. You may need to help!
4. Whilst doing 1–3, have a 'general look' Pain/ discomfort? Mood? Are they unsteady? Is there generalized wasting? Is there a walking aid nearby?
5. Inspection: look for wasting (DF 4/10), fasciculations (DF 6/10), and involuntary movements (DF 7/10).
6. Assess muscle tone at the wrist, elbow, and shoulder (DF 6/10).
7. Test power, proximally to distally (DF 5/10).
8. Test reflexes: biceps (DF 5/10), supinator (*soup-in-ate-or*) (DF 7/10), and triceps (DF 6/10).
9. Test co-ordination: finger–nose test (DF 6/10) and alternating hand movements (DF 4/10).
10. Assess sensation: light touch (DF 7/10), pain (DF 6/10), proprioception (DF 6/10), and vibration sense (DF 5/10).
11. Assess function: undoing buttons, writing, and so on.
12. Other signs.
13. Make sure your patient is comfortable and thank them for their time.
14. Wash your hands.
15. Analysing your findings.
16. Presenting your findings.

Examination of the arms in detail

1. Preparation.

Get your equipment ready. You will need

- tendon hammer
- 'neuropins'
- cotton wool
- tuning fork (128 Hz).

It is worth carrying the last three items in a receiving bowl for convenience.

2. Introduce yourself to the patient and ask for permission to examine.

Introduce yourself whilst shaking their hand. For example, 'Hello, I'm James Parkinson, a second-year medical student. Do you mind if I examine your arms?' This is one occasion where the handshake itself can give a rare diagnostic clue. If your patient has difficulty releasing their grip following the handshake they may have a condition called myotonica dystrophica (*my-owe-tonic-a-dis-trophy-ca*) (see p. 221), where there is a difficulty in relaxation of muscles.

3. Position the patient and expose the arms. You may need to help!

See Fig. 8.6. Ask the patient to get on to the bed, if not already on it and ask them if they would mind removing their top. It is not sufficient for your patient to roll up their sleeves. Adequate exposure is vital and if you fail to do this you will miss important clues. A woman patient can keep their bra on. Traditionally the arms are examined with the patient sitting up.

4. Whilst doing 1–3, have a 'general look' Pain/ discomfort? Mood? Are they unsteady? Is there generalized wasting? Is there a walking aid nearby?

Your general look as always has to be brief but packed with as many clues as you can digest. Does your patient look in pain or discomfort? Pay particular attention to their mood. This is important for any system but particularly for a neurological examination. Depression may be the end result of a chronic problem or may conversely be the cause of multiple non-specific symptoms.

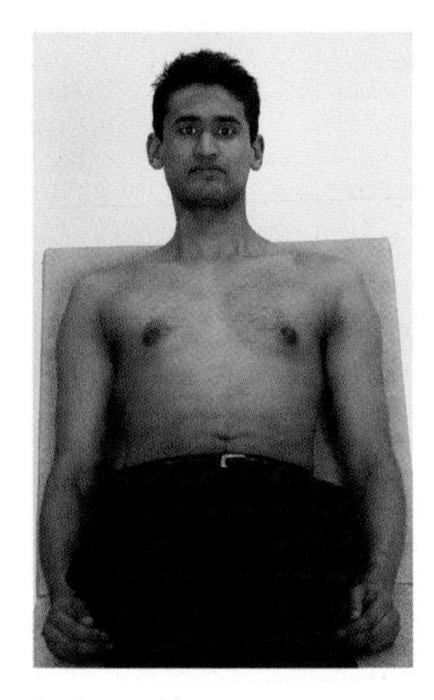

Fig. 8.6 Examination position.

A euphoric patient may have a frank psychiatric disorder but may occasionally have conditions in which emotional lability is a recognized feature, such as multiple sclerosis or stroke. Look for kyphoscoliosis (see p. 381), as there is an association with certain neurodegenerative conditions, for example, Friedreich's ataxia (see p. 221). Also watch the patient as they get on to the bed. Are they unsteady? This could suggest weakness in the legs or a cerebellar lesion (see p. 219). Also look for clues around the bed, for example, a diabetic sticker (peripheral neuropathy, mononeuritis multiplex (see p. 264), or diabetic amyotrophy (*ay-my-ot-roe-fee*) (see p. 265), a walking aid such as a walking stick, or even a wheelchair.

5. Inspection: look for wasting (DF 4/10), fasciculations (DF 6/10), and involuntary movements (DF 7/10).

Your general look should now become more focused as you concentrate on the arms and a more neurological theme (this does not mean you should not be alive to conditions outside this system which may cause neurological disease). This is initially performed standing at the foot of the bed. From here you can get a good look at the whole patient and will be able to identify any asymmetry. Now move in closer and inspect the arms in greater detail.

Wasting

Look specifically for wasting. Generalized wasting could be simply the result of any debilitating illness including cancer. In a neurological context wasting may suggest motor neurone disease or any other pathology affecting the LMNs. Some malignancies can cause neurological effects, usually via direct compression, for example, vertebral metastases causing spinal cord or nerve root compression. Local infiltration of nervous tissue can also occur, the classical example being an apical lung tumour invading the brachial plexus causing wasting of the small muscles of the hands and sensory disturbance at T1. A brain metastasis is a third example; a common presentation would be as a stroke. Tumours may also exert remote effects through so-called paraneoplastic syndromes. These can involve any organ system in the body. In the neurological system the most common presentations include proximal myopathy, peripheral neuropathy, mononeuropathy, and cerebellar dysfunction. The underlying mechanism is poorly understood, but may be related to cytokine release.

Fasciculations

These occur in LMN lesions and represent spontaneous discharges from motor units. They are visible as small contractions that look like the transient writhing of a worm under the skin. You may have to observe the arms for several minutes before you see one.

> **Tip**
>
> If you have not spotted any fasciculation within 30 s I would suggest you continue with the rest of your examination but keep a wary eye out for them as your patient relaxes momentarily between your assessments and even at the end of your examination.

Involuntary movements

These are important conditions that can cause a patient distress because of their lack of control over these movements and the subsequent embarrassment this can cause in public. As they are dynamic, a one-dimensional description cannot do them justice but they will make sense once you see examples during your training. The main categories of involuntary movements are

- tremor
- chorea
- athetosis (*ather-toe-sis*)
- hemiballismus (*hemi-ba-liss-muss*)
- dystonia (*dis-tone-ia*)
- myoclonus (*my-owe-clone-us*)
- tics.

Tremor

What is it?

This is a rhythmical trembling of a part of the body. Usually the hands are affected, but the feet, head, lips, tongue, and eyelids can be involved. They can be divided into resting tremors, postural tremors (physiological,) and intention (action) tremors, according to the situation that demonstrates them the best.

Resting tremors

As the name suggests these occur when the person is sitting or lying comfortably. The most important cause is Parkinson's disease (see p. 219). A parkinsonian tremor is sometimes described as a 'pill-rolling' tremor because the thumb oscillates back and forth across the palm as if a pill is being rolled between the thumb and index finger (see Fig. 8.7). This tremor is not always obvious and you may have to watch for some time before you see it. Be sure to look at both hands and focus particularly on the thumb movement. You must also be aware that a parkinsonian tremor can affect the wrist

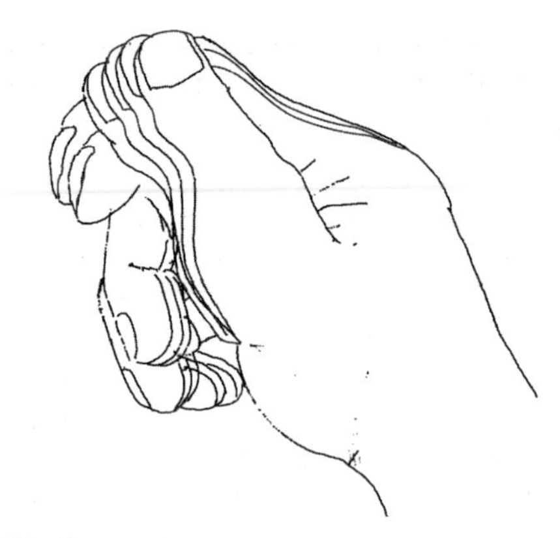

Fig. 8.7 Pill-rolling tremor

causing repeated pronation and supination, or flexion and extension. It may affect a foot causing it to tap up and down repeatedly and occasionally the head may also be affected causing it to nod repeatedly (called titubation). Resting tremors tend to diminish or disappear with movement of the limb; however sometimes they may be marked enough to be present during movement when they can be mistaken for intention tremors (see later).

Postural tremors

These are sometimes called physiological tremors because they are exaggerations of the normal physiological tremor that everybody possesses (which is usually too fine to be seen). They are very common; you may have had experience of tremors related to anxiety or fear (observe the hands of your fellow students at exam times). These tremors can be seen at rest but they become more apparent if you ask your patients to hold out their hands in front of them. They can be caused by

- fear or anxiety
- fatigue
- caffeine-containing drinks, for example, coffee
- drugs, for example, ventolin
- lithium
- theophylline (*thee-off-ee-lin*)
- withdrawal of alcohol
- thyrotoxicosis (see p. 350).

Intention tremors

The hallmark of an intention tremor is that it is absent when the limb is at rest but becomes evident on movement. It behaves differently to other tremors in that its amplitude does not remain constant. As a movement begins the limb may demonstrate small horizontal oscillations, which can quickly progress to much larger oscillations (in some conditions the limb can swing back and forth very wildly indeed). In the less dramatic cases the tremor may diminish or vanish altogether as the movement progresses and may re-emerge as the arm nears its target. A true intention tremor signifies a cerebellar disorder (see p. 219). The patient will have other cerebellar signs including inco-ordination and, past-pointing, all of which will be detailed later in the chapter.

Chorea

What is it?

These are irregular, jerky movements that can affect most muscle groups in a random sequence. In old textbooks the movements are often described as 'quasi-purposeful' which means the movements **almost** seem intentional. Many sufferers will go to great lengths to disguise these movements by making them seem **totally** intentional. Therefore if they are seated and their leg jumps, they will 'hijack' this movement and cross their leg and make it look like a planned manoeuvre. Similarly, if their arm jerks upwards, they may use the movement to scratch their nose. This behaviour may be so successful that people do not suspect the patient has chorea. The first thing you might notice is that your patient may seem a little fidgety or restless. You might even feel that their behaviour is a little eccentric. This should alert your mind to the possibility of chorea. Look at the face: is there a lot of grimacing and frequent changes of expression? Ask the patient to put out their tongue. They will be unable to maintain it in a constant position. Instead, it moves in and out repeatedly and for this reason it is called a trombone tremor of the tongue. Now look at the limbs. Are they constantly moving? Is your patient constantly changing posture? When you shook hands with your patient did you notice if their grip fluctuated? This waxing and waning of the grip has been likened to a milkmaid's grip (those of us who are not cows can only guess what a milkmaid's grip must be like). Finally do not forget your ears in your evaluation of someone with chorea. Sometimes you may hear the patient grunt and this is due to the involuntary contraction of the diaphragm, which forces air out through the larynx. Chorea can be caused by

- Huntington's chorea
- Sydenham's chorea (associated with rheumatic fever) (*Thomas Sydenham (1624–1689), English physician*)
- thyrotoxicosis
- polycythaemia (*polly-sigh-theme-ia*) rubra vera
- pregnancy
- systemic lupus erythmatosus (SLE).

Athetosis

What is it?

This is a slow 'snake-like' writhing movement that tends to affect the peripheries, including the hands, feet, and face. Sometimes chorea and athetosis co-exist and the resulting condition is known as 'choreoathetosis'.

Hemiballismus

What is it?

This abnormal movement is so violent that it causes the flailing of one or both limbs on one side of the body. The cause is a lesion of the contralateral sub-thalamic nucleus (a component of the basal ganglia). Thankfully this condition does not occur very often in clinical practice.

Dystonia

What is it?

Part of the body assumes an abnormal posture due to a sustained contraction of a particular muscle group. It may be focal, affecting one or a few muscle groups only, or generalized.

Focal dystonias

These may be familiar through their colloquial names, for example, writer's cramp and wry neck (spasmodic torticollis (*taut-i-coll-iss*)). With writer's cramp the muscles of the hand and forearm contract as the person attempts to write. They may manage to write a few lines (or even less) before the task has to be abandoned. This used to be thought of as a psychiatric disorder until recently. Spasmodic torticollis is the (sometimes) painful contraction of the sternomastoid muscle, which twists the neck to one side (torticollis) (see Fig. 8.8).

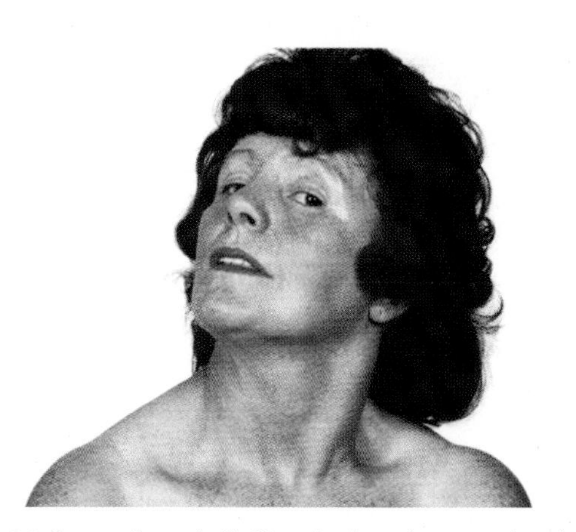

Fig. 8.8 Spasmodic torticollis. Note the dystonic contraction of the left sternomastoid leading to the abnormal posture of the head. Reprinted from **Fig. 6.52** (p. 6.18), *Atlas of Clinical Neurology* (2nd edn), by G. David Perkin, Fred Hochberg, and Douglas C. Miller (1993), Mosby Publications, with permission from Elsevier.

Sometimes other neck muscles can be involved leading to forward flexion (antecollis) or backward extension (retrocollis).

Generalized dystonias

These tend to be seen more commonly in children as a result of birth trauma, metabolic, or neurodegenerative disorders. An idiopathic form exists, idiopathic torsion dystonia (old name, dystonia musculorum deformans (*dis-tone-ia-mus-cue-lore-um-de-four-mans*)), which may have a genetic basis. Again, this is seen more commonly in childhood. Sufferers may exhibit a torticollis, the back may twist or arch backwards and the arms typically rotate inwards and extend, with the wrists flexed. They may walk with their feet plantarflexed and inverted, forcing them to walk stiffly on tiptoes. These extreme postures can be held for hours and in advanced cases only disappear during sleep.

Myoclonus

What are they?

These are brief, shock-like jerks that may be restricted to a muscle group (focal) or be more generalized, the latter usually as a component of juvenile epilepsy. They are distinct from chorea in that they are usually rhythmical and do not flit from one muscle group to another. Myoclonus can occur in normal people, for example, on falling asleep. The small number of beats that affect the legs can be sufficient to cause the affected person to wake.

Tics

What are they?

These are irregular jerky movements that are repeated continually. They differ from other forms of involuntary movements in that they can be voluntarily suppressed. These movements tend to affect the face and upper body and common movements include exaggerated blinking, grimacing, sniffing, shoulder shrugging, and so on. One disorder that exhibits complex tics is gilles de la Tourette (*jeel-de-la-tour-ett*) syndrome (*George Albert Édouard Brutus de la Tourette (1857–1904), French neurologist*). It has captured the medical imagination because of the outrageous behaviour that can be seen with this syndrome. Some tics can be repetition of obscene gestures. Sufferers also exhibit vocal tics, which include grunting, barking, and in some cases swearing.

Tone

6. Assess muscle tone at the wrist, elbow, and shoulder (DF 6/10).

Keypoints

- Wasting (in the absence of malnutrition, cachexia, or disuse) is a manifestation of an LMN lesion.
- Fasciculations are also LMN phenomena.
- Always check for involuntary movements, which may give useful clues.

What is it?

Tone is the resistance felt when moving a joint through its range of movement.

Significance

In a normal individual there is very little resistance as any joint is moved through its range of movement. In pathological circumstances there can be an increase in the resistance (hypertonia) as the joint is moved or a decrease (hypotonia).

Hypertonia

Hypertonia may have characteristics that point to the underlying nature of a lesion. Upper motor neurone lesions cause what is known as 'clasp-knife' rigidity (also called spasticity). The increased tone is felt throughout the majority of the range before the tone 'gives way' in much the same way that a clasp knife does when it is opened. In Parkinson's disease, two types of increased tone are seen, the typical one being 'cogwheel' rigidity, which is similar to the intermittent resistance felt when turning a cog wheel. The other is 'lead-pipe' rigidity, named because the resistance felt is said to be similar to that when bending a lead pipe (!), that is, sustained resistance throughout the range of movement (at last medical terms that are self-evident!).

Hypotonia

Hypotonia is subtle and is due to an LMN lesion. There is practically no resistance to movement (sometimes described as flaccidity).

How to examine

See Fig. 8.9. Before you start testing you need to make your patient as relaxed as possible. Say something like, 'I am going to move your arm about and I need you to be as relaxed as you can. Don't try to help me, just stay as loose as you can.' Muscle tone is tested at the wrist by holding the fingers of the arm being tested and gently flexing and extending the wrist. Now assess tone at the elbow. Maintain your grip on the fingers and pronate (palm downwards) and supinate (palm upwards) the forearm, followed by flexing and extending at the elbow. Finish off by abducting and adducting the (flexed) arm at the shoulder. Although each joint is described individually the aim is to create a continuous movement of the arm that will allow each joint to be

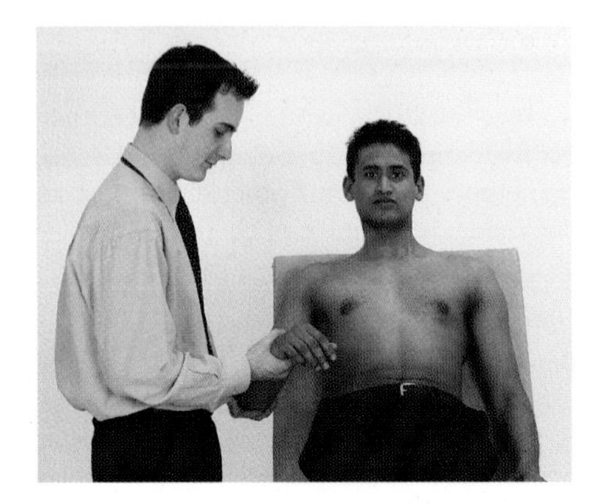

Fig. 8.9 The assessment of tone. The starting position before moving the joints through their range of movement.

Tip

Try to be unpredictable with your movements across all the joints. Make some movements small, some much greater, some a little slower, and some rapid. This will lessen the chances of your patient 'second guessing' you and trying to help you.

CASE 8.1

Problem. You are assessing the tone of your patient's upper limbs and you are unsure if it is increased.

Discussion. The most common cause of a slight increase in tone is an unrelaxed patient, which can fool the unwary. Some patients will contract their muscles in a bid to help you move the arm. The resistance you feel is the opposing force of the muscle when you reverse the movement of the arm. Stress to the patient that they need to relax. You also need to monitor the arm carefully. Feel the weight of the arm: does it flop into your arm when you take it? Watch the arm carefully and make sure no muscles contract during your assessment. If they do, your assessment of tone is invalid. If the patient still cannot relax, try distracting them. Ask them to move the opposite arm or leg up and down, while you quickly assess tone in the arm. Usually if the tone is pathologically increased, there will be other signs to support this, for example, mild weakness and hyper-reflexia.

CASE 8.2

Problem. You have assessed the tone of a patient and are unsure if there is hypotonia.

Discussion. This one is difficult. The difference between a normal patient and one with hypotonia is very subtle. Here it is speculated that if you asked a sample of physicians to diagnose pathological hypotonia with blindfolds on, the number of correct responses would be close to what you would expect by chance. The author would only diagnose it in the context of other LMN signs, for example, weakness, wasting, fasciculation, and decreased or absent reflexes.

Keypoints

- Make sure your patient is relaxed (and remains relaxed) when testing tone.
- Hypertonia indicates a UMN lesion.
- Hypotonia indicates an LMN lesion.
- Hypertonia is easier to detect than hypotonia.

assessed sequentially (experienced neurologists are so adept at this that it sometimes looks like they have created a Mexican wave on one side of the body). As you gain in confidence you will find that you can switch your attention rapidly from one joint to the next.

7. Test power, proximally to distally (DF 5/10).

It is important to remember that your assessment of power has to take into account what you would normally expect for that individual. So a healthy little old lady would score just as well as Arnold Schwarznegger. The most common standardized scale used to grade power is the MRC scale.There are five grades of power: 0 = nil; 1 = flicker of movement; 2 = movement if gravity is eliminated; 3 = movement against gravity but not against resistance; 4 = movement against resistance but abnormally weak; and 5 = normal.

There are several ways to test power, but the best technique is to demonstrate exactly what you want the patient to do and get them to copy you. First, ask them to hold their arms outstretched (palm upwards) in front of them. This is a good screening test for any mild weakness. A UMN lesion of one arm will cause it to drift downwards and pronate. Now test each muscle group in turn, starting at the shoulders. Always compare the two sides.

Shoulder abduction and adduction

Demonstrate by holding your arms out to the side in a horizontal position, with the elbows flexed: 'Put your arms up like this; now, don't let me push them down' (abduction, using nerve roots C5 and C6; see Fig. 8.10). During this movement, you need to provide resistance by pressing on the mid-shaft of the upper arms. If your patient has full strength it will be difficult to budge the arm (grade 5/5). If you can move the patient's arm with a little difficulty the patient has grade 4/5 power. If the patient can just about abduct their arm but are unable to resist your opposing force their power is grade 3/5. If the patient cannot abduct their arm against gravity you need to alter the position of your patient. Ask them to lie flat and then to abduct their arm. This eliminates the effect of gravity because the movement required is now parallel to the floor. If they are now able to perform this movement they have a power grading of 2/5. If they cannot and only a flicker of movement occurs, the grade is 1/5. If no flicker of movement occurs the grade is 0/5. Repeat your assessment for adduction

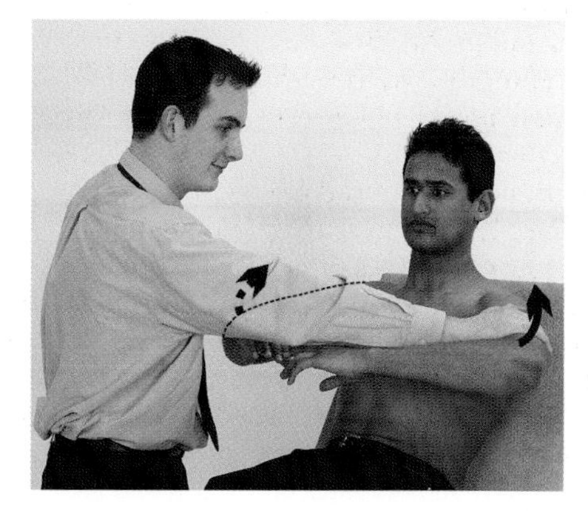

Fig. 8.10 Testing the power of shoulder abduction. Note the arrows represent the direction of force generated by the patient.

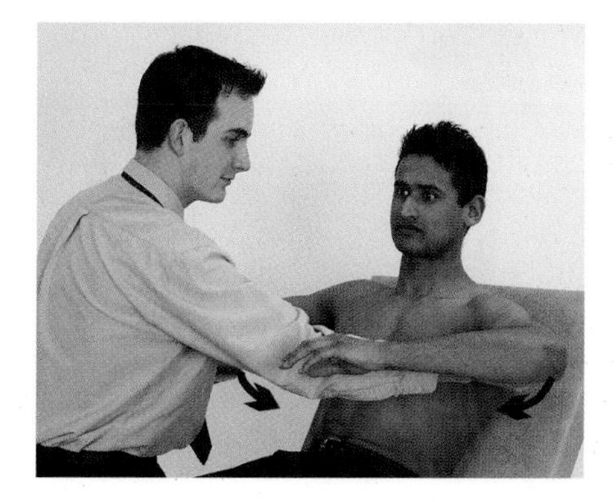

Fig. 8.11 Testing the power of shoulder adduction.

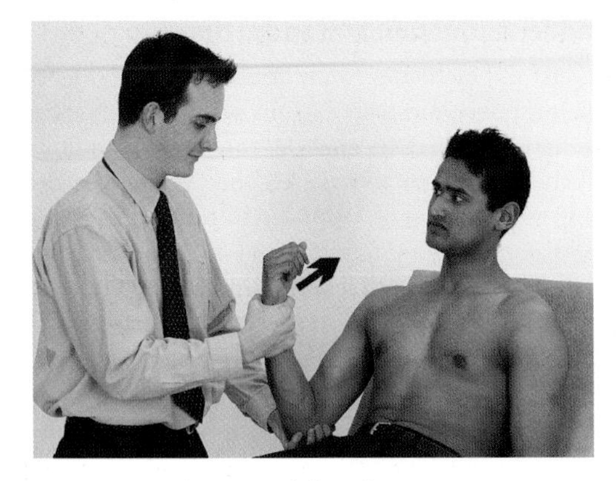

Fig. 8.12 Testing the power of elbow flexion.

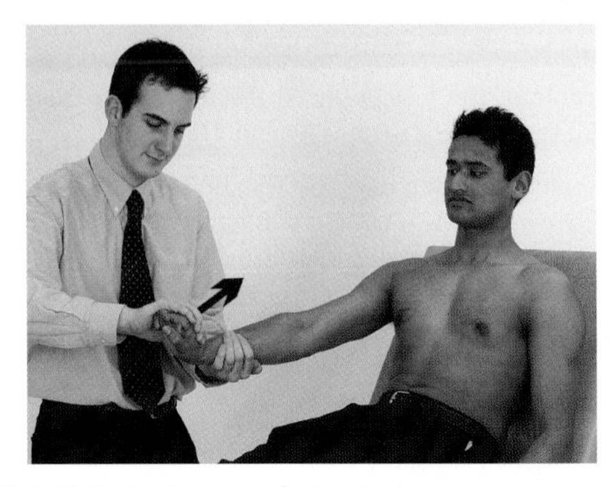

Fig. 8.14 Testing the power of wrist extension.

(adduction, C6, C7, C8; see Fig. 8.11). Ask your patient to adopt the same position as for abduction but this time, put your arms under your patient's and say, 'Now try to press your elbows in to your waist.' Grade the power as before but note that adduction will occur with the help of gravity in this position. Therefore for grades 2/5–3/5, you have to make an educated guess as to the grade of power (rather than suspend your patient upside down to test adduction against gravity). As you assess more and more patients this guess will become more precise within the subjective limits of the scale.

Elbow flexion and extension

Ask your patient to put their fists up like a boxer: 'Bend your elbows in front of you like this; now pull me towards you' (elbow flexion, C5, C6; see Fig. 8.12). 'Now push me away' (elbow extension, C7, C8; see Fig. 8.13). Grade the power as before. If your patient has grade 2/5 power, that is, they cannot flex the arm against gravity, you will have to hold their upper arm and abduct it to 90°. With the arm horizontal, flexion will take place without gravity and you can grade the power according to the response. As with shoulder adduction, extension of the elbow will occur with the **aid** of gravity. Therefore you will have to make a reasonable guess for grades 2/5–3/5. It is also important that when you assess extension you make sure the patient's palms are facing their face, otherwise you will not just be testing triceps (C7) but getting extra help from brachioradialis (*bray-kio-ray-di-ay-liss*) (C5, C6) as well.

Wrist extension (dorsiflexion) and wrist flexion (palmar flexion)

Check each wrist in turn, holding the forearm steady with your left hand and providing resistance with your right hand. Say to your patient 'Make a fist. Now cock your wrists up like this; don't let me bend them down' (wrist extension, C5, C6, C7; see Fig. 8.14). As the patient extends their wrist, apply downward pressure with your right hand. If your patient is unable to do this, turn the wrist into a semi-pronated position to eliminate gravity, then repeat. When you have assessed

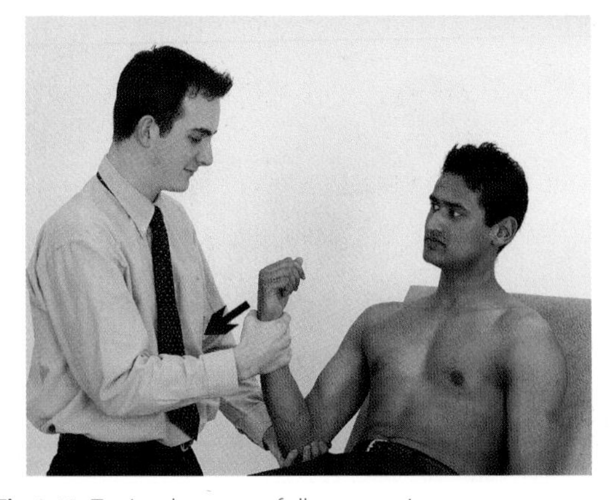

Fig. 8.13 Testing the power of elbow extension.

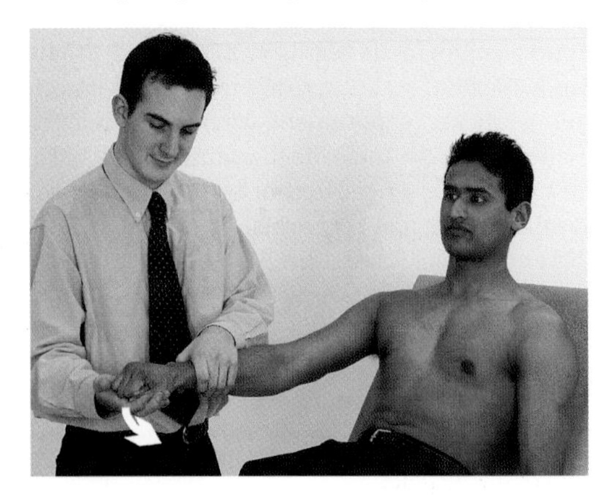

Fig. 8.15 Testing the power of wrist flexion.

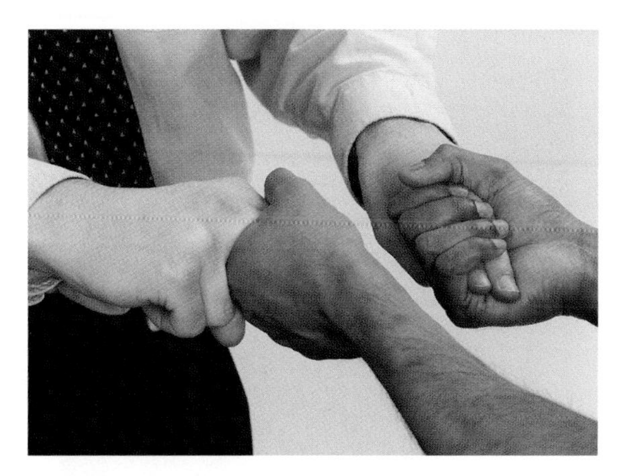

Fig. 8.16 Testing grip strength.

extension keep their wrist cocked and place your right hand underneath it. Say 'Push down against my hand' (wrist flexion, C6, C7, C8; see Fig. 8.15). Use your left hand to hold their forearm so that they are only using the wrist flexors to push against you rather than their entire arm. As with shoulder adduction and elbow extension, wrist flexion is also aided by gravity.

Grip

Ask the patient to grip your index and middle fingers, testing both hands together (C8, T1; see Fig. 8.16). This is a rather non-specific test, but it does enable you to make a general assessment of the strength of distal muscles compared to the proximal ones, which is useful if a proximal myopathy is suspected. Finally, grip strength is vital in performing activities of daily living, so you are also making an assessment of function. For further assessment of hand function see Chapter 9.

Keypoints

- Assessing power is subjective and you need to judge what is normal for an individual (for example, pensioner compared with Arnold Schwarzneggar).
- Try to remember the root values of the muscles tested as this may help in localizing a lesion.
- Compare the power in both arms and proximally versus distally to detect patterns of weakness.
- Make sure the patient's performance is not modified by pain.

8. Test reflexes: biceps (DF 5/10), supinator (DF 7/10), and triceps (DF 6/10).

When assessing the reflexes, you need to look for a contraction in the muscle concerned as well as movement of the arm itself, because the latter may not be obvious if the contraction is weak. The left-sided reflexes are more difficult to elicit and require more practice. In all cases the patient should have their arms in a relaxed posture. The best position is with both arms folded across the upper abdomen.

Biceps

See Figs 8.17 and 8.18. Hold the tendon hammer loosely at the end with your right hand (if you are right handed) and place your left thumb just below and parallel to the skin crease in the antecubital (*anti-cube-it-al*) fossa. The right biceps tendon will be palpable here as a thick cord. Extend your right wrist, then flick it gently into flexion and let the heavy end of the hammer swing down with gravity to hit your left thumb. You do not need to apply any force. If the reflex is elicited then there is no need to

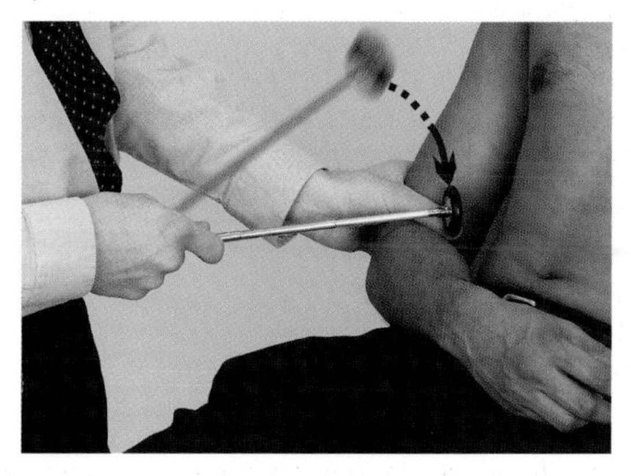

Fig. 8.17 Eliciting the right biceps reflex. Make sure your patient is adequately relaxed.

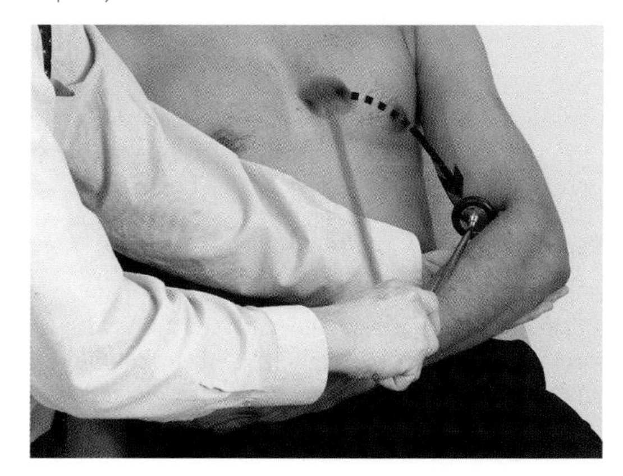

Fig. 8.18 Eliciting the left biceps reflex.

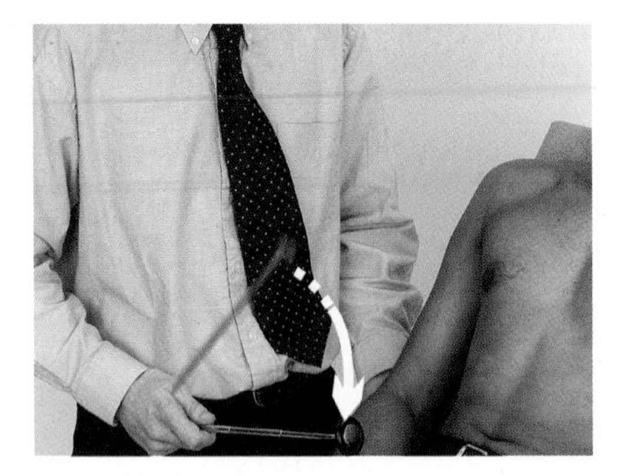

Fig. 8.19 Eliciting the right supinator reflex.

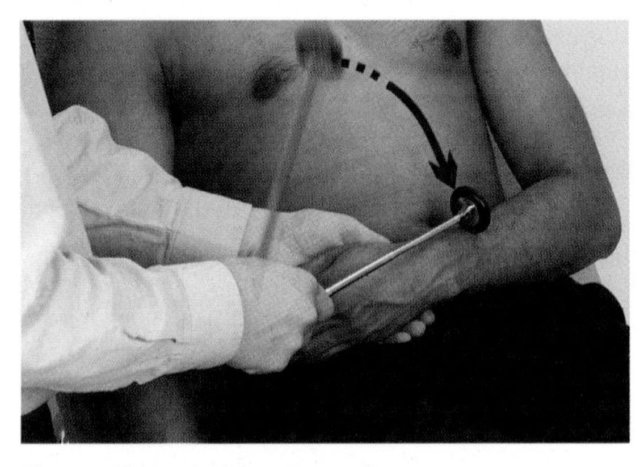

Fig. 8.20 Eliciting the left supinator reflex.

give the patient repeated wallops to make sure. Repeat on the left biceps tendon to compare directly.

Supinator

See Figs 8.19 and 8.20. Place your left index and middle fingers at the site of the tendon, which is three-quarters of the distance along the forearm from the antecubital fossa, on the radial aspect. The tendon itself can be difficult to feel but do not panic, the reflex is likely to be elicited despite this. The hammer is used in exactly the same way as for the eliciting the biceps reflex. Now check the opposite side.

Triceps

See Figs 8.21 and 8.22. This is a flat tendon that can be palpated running vertically upwards from the posterior aspect of the elbow tip just above the bony prominence (the olecranon *(oh-leck-ran-on)*). This time, the tendon is tapped directly rather than with your fingers interposed. The left side is particularly tricky and the arm needs to be pulled across the chest towards you to enable you to elicit the reflex. As you cannot directly see the tendon you will have to aim in the general direction just above the elbow. If you can carry off the procedure without slapping the patient in the face, you are doing well.

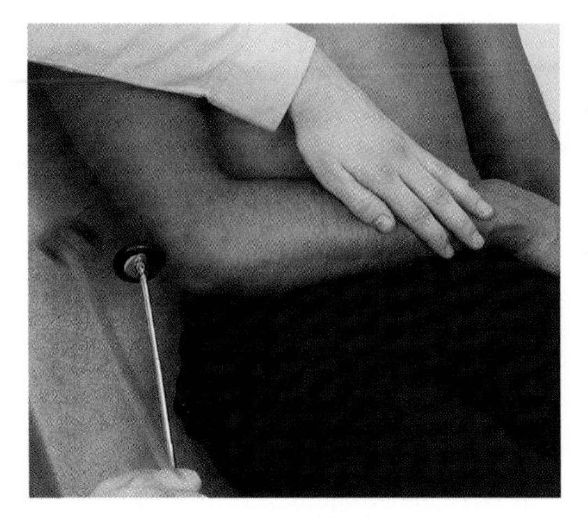

Fig. 8.21 Eliciting the right triceps reflex.

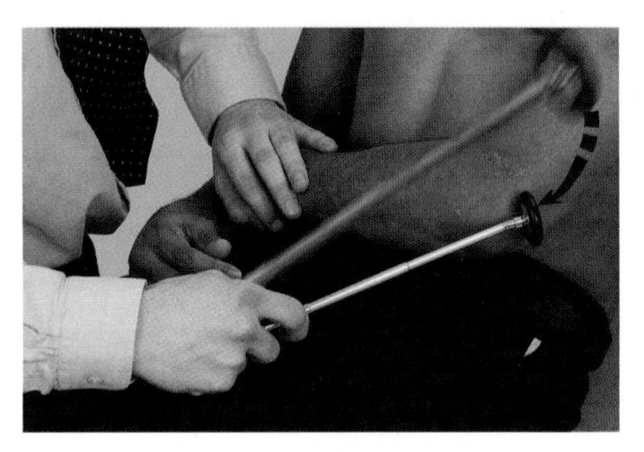

Fig. 8.22 Eliciting the left triceps reflex.

Reinforcement of reflexes

See Fig. 8.23 and Table 8.2. If you are unable to elicit a reflex then it is acceptable to try once more. If you still cannot demonstrate it, you need to attempt reinforcement. Explain to the patient that they need to relax and when you say 'Now!' they need to clench their teeth (providing they have got their teeth in, of course). Timing is essential here. You need to time the swing of the hammer so that you strike the tendon as the patient clenches their teeth (or gums). This manoeuvre is important because you cannot say a reflex is absent until you have been unable to elicit it with reinforcement. This part of the examination is often forgotten. If hyper-reflexia is elicited there are various other reflexes

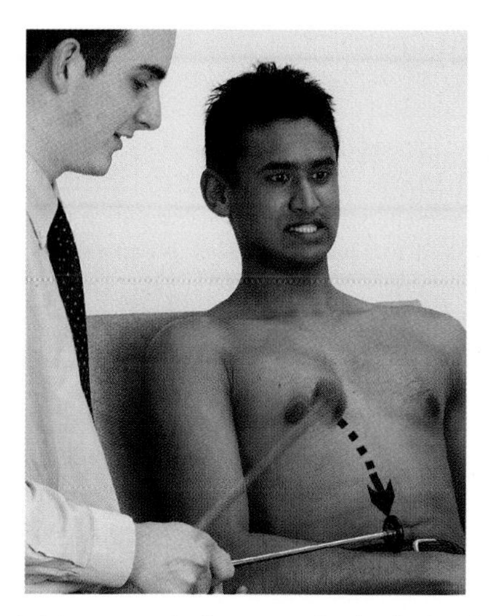

Fig. 8.23 Reinforcement of reflexes. Note the clenched teeth just at the point of contact of the hammer with the tendon.

TABLE 8.2 Grading of reflexes

–	Absent
–/+	Present with reinforcement
+	Normal
++	Brisk but normal
+++	Abnormally brisk (hyper-reflexia)

CASE 8.3

Problem. When you elicit the biceps reflex the right one seems brisker than the left. Is this significant?

Discussion. It may be, but before you can say it is, you need to satisfy certain criteria. Was the patient relaxed when you tested each reflex? If they were relaxed for the right biceps but tense for the left this could lead to the discrepancy you observed. Therefore make sure your patient is relaxed throughout your assessment. The other factor to consider is your technique. You need to make sure the tendon hammer strikes each tendon with equal force. If you actively tap the tendon (rather than let it swing down with gravity) it is possible that you may have hit the right biceps tendon harder than the left. Practise letting gravity take over the down-swing and in time you will be assured that you are eliciting each reflex with an equivalent stimulus. With experience you will control these factors and make a valid comparison of the reflexes.

CASE 8.4

Problem. You are trying to elicit the reflexes in the arms but cannot get them, why?

Discussion. This could be due to a number of factors. Your technique may be faulty, for example, you might not be striking the tendons precisely (the supinator can be easy to miss at first), so double-check that you are controlling the tendon hammer and aiming correctly. A common cause of absent reflexes is a tense patient. So make sure the patient is relaxed and keep monitoring for signs of muscle activity (as for assessing tone). You may have to persevere for several minutes before complete relaxation is achieved. Only when you are satisfied that the reflexes are unobtainable with your patient fully relaxed should you attempt to elicit them with reinforcement. If they are absent with reinforcement, then this suggests LMN pathology such as a peripheral neuropathy.

CASE 8.5

Problem. You have been told to go and examine a patient who has just been admitted acutely with a left hemiplegia (*hemi-plea-jah*). You find that he has no movement of the left arm (grade 0/5), the tone is not increased, and you are unable to elicit any reflexes in that arm. You are confused because you know a stroke is the cause of a UMN lesion but your findings are completely the opposite of what you would expect.

Discussion. If you see a patient in the very early stages of a stroke, they often have a flaccid paralysis, that is, decreased tone, absent reflexes, and lack of plantar response. Over the next few hours or days you will see the classic signs of a UMN lesion emerge, that is, increased tone, hyper-reflexia, and an upgoing plantar. The same phenomenon can be seen shortly after an acute injury to the spinal cord.

which you can go on to test, including Hoffman's, the pectoral, the deltoid, and the finger reflexes (see p. 215).

9. Test co-ordination: finger–nose test (DF 6/10) and alternating hand movements (DF 4/10).

There are two main tests involved. It is worth noting that these are difficult to interpret if the patient has marked limb weakness, so do not waste time attempting them if the power is grade 3 or less.

Keypoints

- Make sure your patient is relaxed throughout the examination.
- Try to remember the root values of the reflexes tested as they can help to localize a lesion.
- Hyper-reflexia is due to a UMN lesion.
- Arreflexia is due to an LMN lesion.
- Always perform reinforcement before declaring that a reflex is absent.

Finger–nose testing

See Fig. 8.24. Hold your index finger at arm's length from the patient. Ask them to touch it with their right index finger then to touch their nose. It is worth doing a dry run by grasping the patient's finger and guiding them to each target so they get the idea. Tell them to repeat the sequence several times, as quickly and accurately as possible. Note that if your index finger is held too close to the patient, you may miss subtle inco-ordination. Your instructions must be clear, otherwise you run the risk of the patient lurching towards you to touch your nose! If the patient has a cerebellar lesion the finger–nose test may bring out an intention tremor. In other words the tremor occurs when the patient attempts to carry out skilled actions such as aiming for a target at arm's length. This is in contrast to a parkinsonian tremor, which occurs at rest. The patient may also exhibit 'past-pointing' (dysmetria (*dis-met-ria*)) in which they miss the target altogether.

Alternating hand movements

Demonstrate what you want your patient to do, that is, tap your right hand on to your left, first with the palm then with the dorsal aspect. Continue to alternate quickly. In cerebellar lesions, this test will be carried out slowly and clumsily and is called dysdiadochokinesia (*dis-die-owe-dough-co-kin-easier*) (see Fig. 8.25). A simpler form of this is to ask the patient to tap the back of one hand repeatedly as fast as they can using the fingers of the other hand. Similar results will be obtained.

In another technique you might see occasionally, the examiner will ask the patient to hold their arms out in

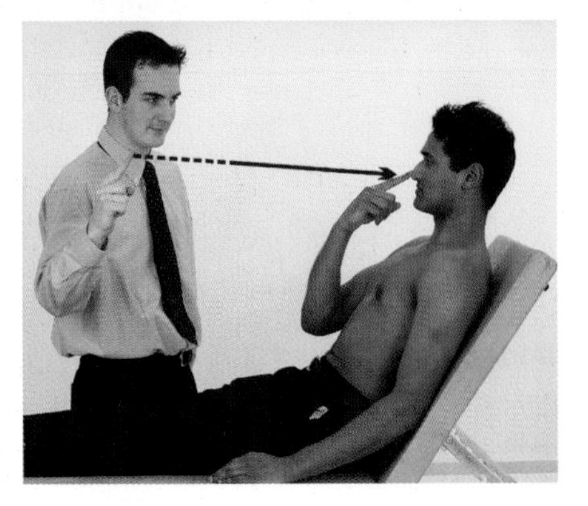

Fig. 8.24 The finger–nose test.

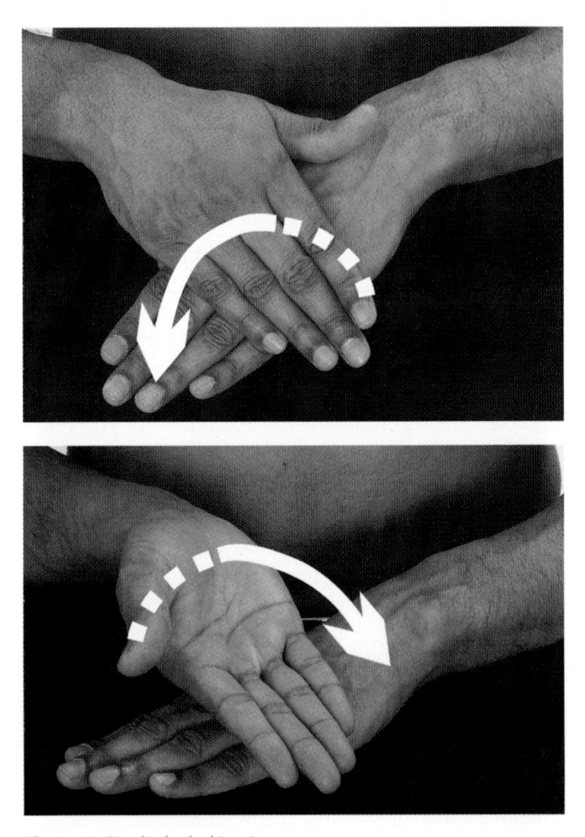

Fig. 8.25 Dysdiadochokinesia.

Tip

Ask if the patient is right or left handed, because the non-dominant hand is often slightly more clumsy than the dominant one.

front of them with their eyes closed and maintain that position even when the arms are pushed down. The examiner then gently pushes down on one of the forearms. A normal person will resist this movement and quickly restore the arm to roughly its former position. A patient with cerebellar dysfunction may bounce their arm up and down and oscillate it about its original position in a bid to restore its posture.

Keypoints

- Do not test co-ordination in the presence of limb weakness (grade 3/5 or less) or in the presence of involuntary movements.
- An intention tremor, past-pointing, and dysdiadochokinesis indicate a cerebellar lesion.
- The non-dominant hand is usually clumsier than the dominant hand.

10. Assess sensation: light touch (DF 7/10), pain (DF 6/10), proprioception (DF 6/10), and vibration sense (DF 5/10).

By convention, each part of the sensory examination begins distally, moving proximally up the arms. In practice it does not matter where you start assessing sensation so long as you are systematic and thorough. Remember that any sensory loss should fit into one of four main patterns.

- **Global sensory loss.** The entire limb is affected, for example, in stroke.
- **Peripheral neuropathy.** 'Glove and stocking' distribution.
- **Dermatomal sensory loss.** Often two or more adjacent dermatomes are involved, in which case the cause is a peripheral nerve lesion, for example, a median nerve. Occasionally just one dermatome is affected, usually due to compression of a single nerve root as it exits the spinal cord.
- **Dissociated sensory loss.** There is loss of certain modalities of sensation but preservation of others, for example, loss of pain and temperature sensation but intact appreciation of light touch and proprioception, as in syringomyelia (*si-ring-owe-mile-ia*) (see p. 220).

Light touch

Impulses for light touch travel principally up the dorsal columns in the spinal cord as described earlier. Damage to any component of the sensory pathway from the sense organs in the skin, along the course of the nerves in the limbs and the pathways in the spinal cord, up to the cerebral cortex can lead to disorder of light touch appreciation.

How to examine

Examination is performed using a piece of cotton wool. First, make one end into a wisp and then gently dab the skin (once only) over the top of the sternum. Ask the patient to confirm that they can feel it and that it feels soft, as they would expect cotton wool to feel (some patients may have altered perception while still being able to feel the stimulus). Next dab the skin of one of the fingers of the right hand. Instruct the patient: 'Say "yes" if you can feel this and if it feels the same as on the chest.' If an affirmative response is given continue in the same manner moving up the arm and alternating from the lateral to the medial aspects of the arm so that you can compare the stimulus across different dermatomes. Repeat the process in the left arm. An alternative method is to dab the same dermatome on each arm to directly compare, then move up the arms as before. There is no fixed number of times you need to dab, but an average number would be about eight for each arm. If an area of sensory loss is identified, dab once more to confirm your findings then attempt to map out its boundaries. This will help you to identify which of the four patterns of sensory loss the deficit corresponds to.

Pain

Pain, along with temperature sensation, travels principally along the spinothalamic tracts in the spinal cord to the brain (see p. 197).

How to examine

A pin-prick is used as a surrogate for pain. The assessment is performed using special 'neurotips', which are available on the wards. Never use venepuncture needles as these are more painful and may draw blood. Again, begin at the sternum. Warn the patient that you are now using something sharp and gently tap the skin with the tip. Ask them to confirm that it feels sharp. Then move on to the arms as before, but ask them to say 'sharp' each time they feel the pricking sensation; or 'dull' if this is the case. If a sharp sensation is perceived as dull then this either indicates that the appreciation of pain is abnormal or that you have been too timid with your stimulus, so be bold and try to achieve a similar 'tap' with each test. If the patient is unable to detect the stimulus at all, the area is said to be anaesthetic. Feel free to directly compare any area with the sternum again to verify your findings, particularly if they are subtle.

Proprioception

Proprioception is the ability of a person to sense the position of any of their joints in space without the aid of their eyes. Hence this is also called 'joint position sense'. Stretch receptors (see pp. 195–6) in joints send information about joint position via the dorsal columns to the brain.

How to examine

Ask your patient to watch what you are doing. Hold both sides of the proximal phalanx of your patient's thumb between your left index finger and thumb. Using your right hand hold the distal phalanx in the same way and flex the interphalangeal (*inter-falan-jeel*) joint. Tell them that this is 'down'. Next extend the joint and tell them that this is 'up'. Ask the patient to close their eyes. Wiggle the distal phalanx up and down a few times then stop in either position and ask the patient to say which position they think it is in. Repeat this a few more times using different positions. If they get them all correct, proprioception is normal and there is no need to test the arm further. If they answer incorrectly repeat the test to confirm your findings then go on to examine the next proximal joint, that is, the wrist, to assess how widespread the problem is. A crude method exists for screening for a proprioceptive loss in the hands. Ask your patient to put their hands out in front of them and close their eyes. Then instruct them to place each index finger in turn on their nose. A normal person will be able to locate their nose without any difficulty even with their eyes shut.

Vibration sense

Vibration sense is the ability to appreciate a vibrating stimulus. The physiological advantage of this is unclear but it is an observation that the medical profession has made use of. It is likely that the stimulus predominantly travels along the dorsal columns. It is one of the first modalities to be affected in certain conditions, for example, peripheral neuropathy. It is often absent distally in healthy, elderly people.

How to examine

Remember to use a 128 Hz tuning fork (the smaller 512 Hz fork is used for testing hearing). You should find the frequency value inscribed on the tuning fork. Try to avoid making the fork vibrate by hitting a hard surface such as the bedside locker. Sufficient stimulus can be achieved simply by springing the two prongs together with your thumb and index finger. Make the fork vibrate, then place the end on the sternum and ask the patient to confirm that they can feel it vibrating (or 'buzzing'). Make it vibrate again then touch the distal interphalangeal joint of their right thumb and ask, 'Can you feel the buzzing/vibration now?' If they can, then vibration sense is normal and you can proceed on to the left arm. If it is abnormal (they may feel the pressure of the fork but not the vibration) you need to move to the wrist (and then the elbow if necessary) and repeat the test. Note that testing is performed over bony areas because these are better for transmitting a vibrating impulse.

CASE 8.6

Problem. You are assessing proprioception in the right thumb. Sometimes your patient gets the position right and sometimes they get it wrong. Are they messing around?

Discussion. Very rarely will this be the case (although you do have to be aware of the potential malingerer). Patients with an intact dorsal column system are able to give the correct answer even with small increments in movement, so an inconsistent response suggests that your patient is guessing the answer. This is because patients often feel obliged to give a response even when they are unsure. Often in this situation you will be able to detect uncertainty in their expression and voice. If you suspect they are guessing do not be afraid to ask them if this is the case. The danger with a patient guessing is they may get it right by chance, throwing you off the scent. Also check if there is any difficulty with vibration sense and light touch if you have not done so already, as these modalities are mainly transmitted along the same tracts.

Tip

Always make sure you ask, 'Can you feel it buzzing?' because if you simply ask if they can feel the tuning fork, some patients will say 'yes' when they feel the pressure on the skin rather than the actual vibration. which is the focus of your assessment.

Other modalities of sensation

Temperature and two-point discrimination are not routinely tested.

Temperature sensation

Temperature sensation (DF 3/10) can be tested with test tubes of cold (approximately 7°C) and warm (approximately 40°C) water. Be quick while doing this test, as the temperature should be maintained relatively constant throughout the test. If the temperature is too hot or cold then you run the risk of stimulating pain fibres in addition, which will be unpleasant for your patient and confuse your results. In clinical practice the crude test of using the cold tines of a tuning fork is more commonly used.

Tip

Check briefly before placing the tuning fork on the patient's skin to make sure it feels cold because after a few exposures to the skin the fork will warm up, giving misleading results.

Two-point discrimination

Two-point discrimination (DF 7/10) can be tested using a paper clip opened out so that the two ends are 5 mm apart and can be used to touch the skin simultaneously. A normal result is where the patient can feel the two stimuli as two separate points on sensitive areas of the body such as the fingers. If the two ends are any closer they are usually perceived as a single stimulus. In disease states such as a peripheral neuropathy the distance at which two points can be perceived separately increases, in some cases to several centimetres.

Keypoints

- For any sensory modality (except proprioception) always compare the sensation elicited to that on the sternum.
- Also compare sensation in equivalent dermatomes of each arm and proximal to distal to discern patterns of sensory loss.
- Remember the root values of the dermatomes as this will help in localizing a lesion.
- Never use a venepuncture needle to assess pain.
- Always use a 128 Hz tuning fork for vibration sense.
- Make sure the patient appreciates the buzzing sensation in vibration testing rather than cold or pressure sensation.

11. Assess function: undoing buttons, writing, and so on.

If you have identified an abnormality in the examination so far, it is good practice to assess how disabled the patient is by it. For example, if you have found weakness or deforming arthritis in the hands, see if they are able to undo buttons or write. If you have found a proximal weakness ask the patient if they have difficulty combing their hair and see if they are able to stand from a sitting position.

Other signs of the arms

12. Other signs.

Hoffman's reflex

(DF 8/10.) See Fig. 8.26. Hoffman's reflex (*Johann Hoffman (1857–1919), German neurologist*) is elicited by holding the middle phalanx of the patient's middle finger between your left index finger and thumb, with their palm facing downwards. Their hand must be relaxed. Flick the distal phalanx downwards with your right thumb. If hyper-reflexia is present the patient's thumb will be seen to flex with the stimulus.

Finger jerks

(DF 9/10.) See Fig. 8.27. Place two fingers across the palmar aspect of the patient's proximal phalanges and take their weight with them. The patient's hand should be facing palm downwards. Swing the tendon hammer up to tap your own fingers. The impact should cause slight flexion of the patient's fingers. This reflex is not easily seen normally but becomes more prominent in hyper-reflexia.

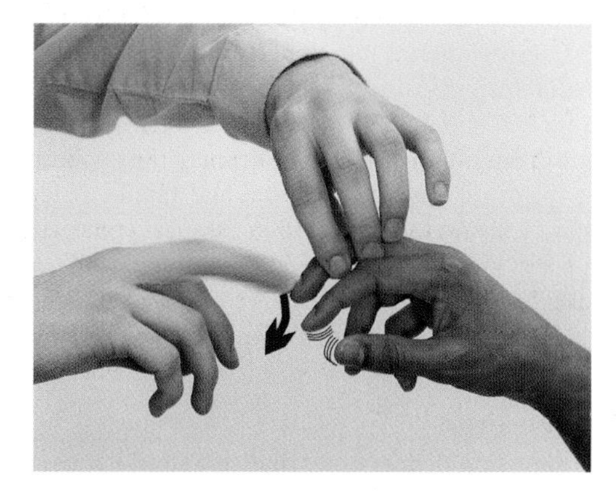

Fig. 8.26 Hoffmans reflex. Flicking the distal phalanx of the middle finger leads to the flexion of the index finger and thumb.

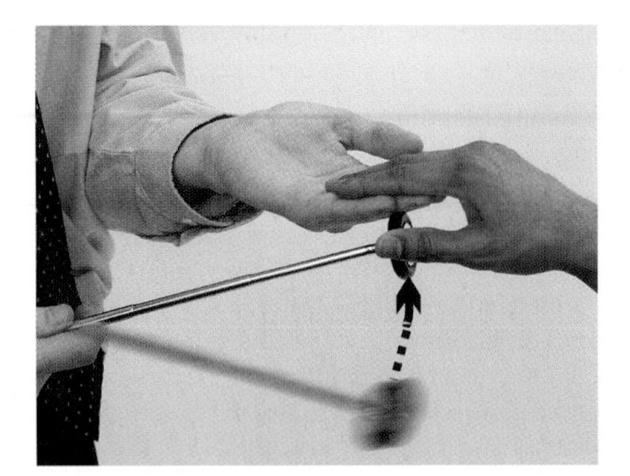

Fig. 8.27 Finger jerks.

Other tendon reflexes

Just about any muscle with a tendon that is accessible can be shown to have a reflex. The pectoral and deltoid reflexes are two examples. With the pectoral reflex, tapping on the lateral insertion of pectoralis major (by placing your fingers on the lateral chest wall and pressing them up to the shoulder just above the armpit) causes a slight muscle contraction, which jerks the shoulder forward and which becomes exaggerated in hyper-reflexia. The deltoid reflex is elicited by tapping the insertion of the deltoid muscle (by placing your fingers on the lateral aspect of the shoulder where the bulk of the muscle starts to converge on the upper humerus). Again the reflex becomes more exaggerated in hyper-reflexia.

Agnosia

What is it?

Agnosia (*ag-nose-ia*) is an inability of the cerebral cortex to recognize or interpret stimuli delivered from intact sense organs and pathways. The area responsible for this interpretation is mainly the parietal cortex of the non-dominant hemisphere. In over 90% of right-handed people and about 70% of left-handed people the right hemisphere is non-dominant. Clinically the two important forms of agnosia are visual and tactile. It is appropriate to test for agnosia if you suspect your patient has a disorder causing cortical dysfunction, such as a stroke. Tactile agnosia (sometimes called astereognosia (*ay-stereo-ag-nose-ia*)) is the inability to recognize familiar objects by touch.

How to examine

You must first demonstrate that sensation is intact in the hand being assessed. When you are satisfied in this regard you can begin testing by asking the patient to close their eyes and then putting a pen or key, for example, into the affected (usually left) hand. They will be unable to recognize it is until you put it into the right hand or let them open their eyes to see it.

Neglect

What is it?

In this condition the patient disregards, and in extreme cases denies, the existence of the affected side. It can also be caused by a lesion in the non-dominant parietal cortex (occipital lobe lesions may be associated with visual neglect).

How to examine

Again ensure that sensation is intact and ask the patient to close their eyes. Now touch the normal arm (again, usually the right arm) and ask them to tell you with which arm they felt the touch. They should be able to give the correct response. Repeat on the left arm and they may say that they feel the touch but are unable to localize it in the body. An extension of this test is to touch both arms simultaneously. Ask the patient to say on which side the touch was felt. A normal response would of course be 'both'. However a patient with neglect will only detect stimulus on the unaffected arm and will indicate that arm only. This inability to detect a stimulus in the presence of a competing stimulus presented at the same time is called 'sensory extinction' or 'sensory inattention'. A further way of demonstrating neglect is to ask your patient to draw a clock face and fill in the numbers representing the hours. With neglect they will only fill in one half of the clock (being totally unaware of the other half).

Apraxia

What is it?

Apraxia (*ay-pracks-ia*) is the inability to perform previously learned activities despite having intact (or only mildly impaired) motor function. It is again a feature of damage to the non-dominant parietal cortex.

How to examine

Having demonstrated that your patient has reasonable power (at least 4/5), ask them to perform an everyday task such as dressing or reading a book. They will be unable to do so and will appear lost, stopping frequently to ponder their next move; they may do bizarre things, for example, trying to put their trousers over their heads.

13. Make sure your patient is comfortable and thank them for their time.

> **Tip**
>
> It is important to be aware of the presence of parietal syndromes, such as agnosia, apraxia, and neglect when you qualify because they all have one other thing in common. The rehabilitation team recognizes that the patient has good motor or sensory function but are dismayed by the patient's lack of progress. They may wrongly stigmatize a patient and brand them as lazy and poorly motivated. This in turn can decrease the patient's morale, leading to further impairment of their rehabilitation, which rapidly becomes a vicious cycle. In fact these are the patients who often require more support and rehabilitation.

This is self-evident but easy to forget, especially if your mind is engaged in working out the solution to the clinical problem.

Wash your hands

14. Wash your hands

Be as scrupulous as a microbiologist. They wash their hands before going to the toilet.

Analysis of findings

15. Analysing your findings.

The aim is to try to fit your examination findings into a clinical pattern and you should try to analyse each sign as you find it. A detailed account of how to do this will be found in Chapter 10 (p. 260).

Presentation of findings

16. Presenting your findings.

This is difficult to do well and requires practice. In general it is best to talk about your findings in the order that you examined so that you do not miss out anything of importance. Relevant normal findings can be mentioned at the end. If the diagnosis is straightforward then state it and support it with your findings. For example, 'The patient has a left-sided hemiplegia. There is spasticity of the left arm with reduced power, grade 3/5. There is hyper-reflexia of the left arm but Hoffman's sign was negative. I also noticed that there is the suggestion of a VII nerve lesion of the left side of the face. Although I have not formally tested the nerve, in this context I would expect it to be an upper motor neuroneVII nerve palsy. The likely cause of these findings is a stroke.' The recognition of the VII palsy demonstrated to the examiners that the student was vigilant in noticing further clues outside their remit. They were also very canny in that they realized they could not say conclusively that the patient's VII nerve palsy was of upper motor neurone type because they had not assessed this properly.

If the diagnosis is not obvious do not panic. Students mistakenly believe that reaching a correct diagnosis is the single most important part of the examination. Your examiners are far more concerned with how competent your method of examination is and whether or not you have a courteous attitude to the patient. If you are unsure of the diagnosis then present your findings together with a reasonable differential diagnosis and possibly suggest further investigations, which may help resolve the situation. For example, 'There is increased tone in the arms bilaterally, with decreased power grade 4/5 in both arms. There is generalized hyper-reflexia in both arms with positive Hoffman's sign and finger jerks. This patient has evidence of upper motor neurone lesions in both arms and the possibilities include multiple sclerosis, motor neurone disease (although I did not see any wasting or fasiculations), a lesion in the cervical cord, or bilateral strokes. To try and determine the cause, I would normally take a full history and examine other aspects of the neurological system including legs and cranial nerves so as to guide my investigations. These might include a magnetic resonance imaging or computed tomography scan of the brain and cervical cord.' This final point is so important because it would be a waste of time and resources organizing a computed tomography (CT) scan of the brain if you elicit signs that point to lower motor neurone pathology.

Neurological diseases and investigations

In earlier parts of this chapter, various medical conditions have been mentioned. In this section these will now be described. In general these descriptions are brief though certain aspects not well described in other textbooks are discussed in some detail.

Stroke

This is one of the most common neurological cases. A stroke is defined as a sudden onset of focal neurological deficit due to a vascular event. Eighty per cent are due to thrombosis or thromboembolism (from a carotid artery plaque or the heart). Other causes you should be aware of include intracranial haemorrhage (for example, rupture of an intracerebral artery, subarachnoid (*sub-arack-noid*), subdural (*sub-due-ral*), or extradural haemorrhage or spontaneous haemorrhage in a patient taking aspirin or warfarin) and vasculitic disorders (including SLE, infective endocarditis, and temporal arteritis).

Risk factors

The risk factors are hypertension, hypercholesterolaemia (*high-per-coal-est-er-ol-eem-ia*), diabetes mellitus, smoking, increasing age, positive family history, and hyperviscosity states (for example, polycythaemia, oral contraceptive). In thromboembolic stroke important additional factors include atrial fibrillation and recent myocardial infarction. The primary risk factors for haemorrhagic stroke include hypertension, anti-platelet and anti-coagulant drugs, and bleeding disorders.

Symptoms

The symptoms depend on the area of brain affected and are described below. As mentioned earlier in the chapter, strokes tend to cause an absence of symptoms, so beware of diagnosing a patient with stroke disease if they present with 'positive' symptoms such as paraesthesia. Another common misconception is that strokes cause blackouts; this is rarely the case.

Classification of stroke disease

One method used is based on the duration of symptoms: transient ischaemic attack if duration <24 h, stroke if duration >24 h. A more recent method has attempted to correlate the clinical features with the blood supply to the brain, which will be outlined next. This classification is more useful because it gives a rough guide to the prognosis of a stroke patient and is simple enough to be used in research protocols.

Blood supply to the brain

The blood supply is categorized into anterior and posterior subdivisions. The anterior circulation is derived from the carotid arteries. These give rise to the anterior and middle cerebral arteries, which take part in a circle of anastomosing vessels on the base of the brain known as the circle of Willis. From this circle further vessels arise, which supply the substance of the brain. The posterior circulation is derived from the two vertebral arteries that ascend in the neck and join to form the basilar artery. Branches from this, for example, the posterior cerebral artery, form the posterior part of the circle of Willis.

Classification of stroke

1. **Total anterior circulation syndrome (TACS).** This is the result of infarction of the entire area supplied by the carotid circulation on one side. Clinically there is a triad of
   (1) contralateral motor or sensory loss;
   (2) hemianopia (hemi-an-owe-pia);
   (3) disorder of language (if the left hemisphere is involved) or neglect/agnosia (if the right hemisphere is involved).

Prognosis is poor and risk of recurrence is low.

2. **Partial anterior circulation syndrome (PACS).** This is the term used when only two of the above three clinical features are present.

Prognosis is more favourable than for TACS. Risk of recurrence is high, hence the importance of identifying and treating risk factors for stroke.

3. **Lacunar syndrome (LACS).** Unlike TACS or PACS, which are usually caused by large vessel thrombosis, a lacunar (*la-koon-ar*) infarct is caused by disease of a small vessel within the substance of the brain. A typical presentation would be an isolated motor or sensory loss or ataxia of a limb. However a significant deficit may nevertheless result, for example, a lacunar infarct of the internal capsule may cause a dense hemiparesis, via involvement of the pyramidal tracts.

Prognosis is good and risk of recurrence is high.

4. **Posterior circulation syndrome (POCS).** This refers to strokes occurring in the territory supplied by the vertebrobasilar (*ver-ti-bro-baz-ee-lar*) system. Typical symptoms include vertigo, vomiting, and nystagmus (*ni-stag-muss*) (due to involvement of the vestibular system), diplopia (*dip-low-pia*) (due to opthalmoplegia (*op-thal-mow-plea-jah*) caused by ipsilateral third or sixth cranial nerve paralysis), dysphagia (due to palsy of the cranial nerves supplying the palate), and contralateral sensory or motor loss.

Prognosis is variable and risk of recurrence is high.

Investigations

1. Blood tests, including full blood count (polycythaemia?), glucose (diabetes?), erythrocyte sedimentation rate (ESR) (vasculitis?), and urea and electrolytes (degree of hydration?).
2. Electrocardiogram (ECG)—myocardial infarction? atrial fibrillation?
3. Chest X-ray—intracerebral metastasis rather than stroke?

4. Carotid duplex (*due-plex*) is useful if your patient has had a stroke in the anterior circulation territory and would be fit for a carotid endarterectomy (*end-art-er-wreck-tummy*) in the future.
5. A cardiac ultrasound may be useful (particularly if your patient has atrial fibrillation).
6. CT scanning is useful in two situations: to rule out haemorrhage (if you are contemplating starting aspirin) and if you suspect a diagnosis other than stroke, for example, tumour or abscess.

Treatment

1. Aspirin for thrombotic and thromboembolic infarcts if the patient is able to swallow.
2. If the patient also has atrial fibrillation then warfarin is given after an interval unless there are contraindications.
3. Risk factors are treated.
4. Rehabilitation of the patient is undertaken via a multidisciplinary approach.
5. Prevention of complications (bedsores and contractures, aspiration pneumonia, and depression).

Parkinson's disease

This is caused by degeneration of the dopamine-containing cells in the substantia nigra of the basal ganglia.

Findings in the arms

1. Resting tremor, which improves with action.
2. Assessing tone will identify rigidity.
3. Check for bradykinesia (*braddy-kine-easier*) (slowness of movement) by asking the patient to tap a hand on to their lap as fast as they can.

Features elsewhere

The face is expressionless ('mask-like') and the voice is often monotonous and of low volume. Ask the patient to walk to demonstrate the stooped posture, shuffling gait, and lack of arm swing. You could also ask the patient to write; the words are often small and spidery (micrographia) (*my-crow-graph-ia*). Patients also have a tendency towards drooling (sialorrhoea) (*sigh-al-owe-rear*) and greasy skin (seborrhoea) (*seb-owe-rear*).

Treatment

L-dopa and similar drugs help restore the dopamine within the brain and are particularly useful for treating bradykinesia and rigidity. Tremor responds less well, but if this is the predominant symptom, patients may benefit from anti-cholinergic drugs.

Parkinsonism

As well as the idiopathic form of the disease, other conditions may mimic Parkinson's due to their involvement of the basal ganglia. Examples include stroke disease, certain drugs (neuroleptics), Alzheimer's disease (*Alois Alzheimer (1864–1915), German psychiatrist/neurologist*), head injury, Wilson's disease (*Samuel Alexander Kinnier Wilson (1878–1937), British neurologist*), and heavy metal poisoning. You should be alerted to the possibility of parkinsonism rather than Parkinson's disease if your patient has evidence of UMN signs (suggesting stroke disease) or dementia (suggesting Alzheimer's), although dementia is a late feature of Parkinson's. In addition, three syndromes exist that are known as the Parkinson plus syndromes.

1. **Steele–Richardson–Olsewski (*ol-chef-ski*) syndrome.** (*John C. Steele (twentieth century), Canadian neurologist, J. Clifford Richardson (born 1909), Canadian neurologist, Jerzy Olszewski (1913–1966), Polish-born Canadian neurologist.*) Parkinsonism plus failure of vertical gaze and pseudobulbar palsy due to degeneration of the upper brainstem.
2. **Shy-Drager (*shy-dray-guh*) syndrome.** (*George Milton Shy (1919–1967), American neurologist, Glenn Albert Drager (1917–1967), American neurologist.*) Parkinsonism plus autonomic failure (postural hypotension and atonic bladder). Also known as multi-system atrophy.
3. **Olivo-ponto-cerebellar syndrome.** Parkinsonism plus cerebellar and pyramidal involvement.

In general, parkinsonism responds poorly or even adversely to conventional anti-parkinsonian drugs.

Cerebellar syndromes

There is a range of diseases that can affect the cerebellum. They can be acute or chronic and may lead to incoordination and loss of balance. See pp. 211–12 for the clinical signs. The causes are

(1) multiple sclerosis (use the word 'demyelination' in front of patients until the diagnosis is confirmed);

(2) alcohol;

(3) stroke (within the cerebellum or affecting its tracts);

(4) tumour (primary, metastatic, or paraneoplastic);

(5) Friedreich's ataxia and other inherited neurodegenerative syndromes.

Multiple sclerosis

This is a disease of unknown aetiology characterized by two or more episodes of neurological dysfunction, which are separated both in time and site. These are attributable to multiple plaques scattered throughout the central nervous system. Always bear this diagnosis in mind when asked to examine a young patient's arms.

Findings in the arms

Cerebellar signs may be present, with or without UMN signs such as hyper-reflexia.

Features elsewhere

Eye movement testing may display nystagmus (due to cerebellar involvement) or ataxic nystagmus (due to involvement of the median longitudinal fasciculus), optic atrophy (see chapter 11), or spastic paraparesis (*para-par-ee-sis*).

Treatment

Treatment of an acute episode is with steroids (a short course of high-dose intravenous methyl-prednisolone). Interferon (*interfere-on*) has more recently been shown to have a modest beneficial effect but is not widely available. Baclofen (*back-low-fen*) is useful for treating spasticity.

Motor neurone disease

This is a disease characterized by progressive degeneration of motor fibres. There are three clinical patterns based on the motor fibres involved:

1. **Progressive muscular atrophy.** Anterior horn cell degeneration leading to LMN signs.
2. **Amyotrophic (*ay-myo-trow-fic*) lateral sclerosis.** Lateral corticospinal tract involvement, hence the name.
3. **Progressive bulbar palsy.** This affects the motor cranial nerves IX–XII. In practice, patients tend to have features of more than one of these clinical patterns.

Findings in the arms

There is often a mixture of UMN and LMN signs with a striking absence of sensory signs, for example, generalized wasting, fasciculations, with brisk reflexes. However pure LMN signs may be present.

Features elsewhere

Dysarthria, dysphagia, wasted fasciculating tongue (bulbar palsy), and spastic paraparesis (*para-par-ee-sis*).

Cervical spondylosis

This is a common disease, characterized by degeneration of the intervertebral discs, thickening of the ligaments surrounding the lower cervical spine, and osteophyte formation (new outgrowths of bone). These changes may result in compression of nerve roots as they exit the spinal cord, leading to LMN signs in the arms. C5, C6, and C7 are the roots most commonly involved. Encroachment on the spinal cord itself may also occur, involving the descending UMN tracts. The latter is sometimes known as cervical myelopathy (*mile-op-athy*).

Symptoms in the arms

Typically pain, paraesthesia, or clumsiness of the arms.

Findings in the arms

There may be LMN and sensory signs and sometimes UMN features, for example, wasting of the small muscles of the hand, sensory loss in a dermatomal distribution, and reflexes that may be brisk or absent depending on the level of spinal cord affected. There may be evidence of reflex inversion (to understand this concept it will help to first refresh your memory of the spinal reflex, discussed earlier in the chapter). In the case of the inverted biceps reflex, when the biceps tendon is tapped, the muscle spindle is stimulated and sensory impulses travel to the spinal cord at level C5, C6. Under normal circumstances this would lead to stimulation of C5, C6 motor fibres and subsequently biceps contraction. However if these motor fibres are damaged due to cervical spondylosis impinging on the C5, C6 nerve roots then biceps contraction does not occur. Instead, the sensory impulses entering the cord at this level stimulate adjacent spinal cord fibres, for example, those supplying triceps and the finger flexors, resulting in contraction of these muscles.

Syringomyelia

In this condition a fluid-filled cavity gradually expands within the central cervical cord. The spinothalamic fibres from the arms enter and cross the mid-line of the cervical cord, so these are the first tracts to be affected, leading to a loss of pain and temperature sensation in the arms. There is relative sparing of the dorsal columns because these are situated in the posterior part of the cord. This leads to a so-called 'dissociated sensory loss' because proprioception and vibration sense remain relatively preserved. Later features include LMN signs in the arms (via compression of the anterior horn cells in the cervical cord that supply the arms) and UMN signs in the legs (via involvement of the descending pyramidal tracts to the lower limbs). Magnetic resonance imaging (MRI) is the imaging investigation of choice and treatment is via surgical decompression.

Proximal myopathy

There is wasting and weakness of the shoulder girdle with relative sparing of the distal musculature, that is, grip strength is preserved. There are usually no other abnormal neurological signs. In particular the reflexes are normal, in contrast to UMN and LMN pathology. The legs are similarly affected, with proximal weakness leading to difficulty standing from a sitting position and a waddling gait. The important causes include polymyositis (*polly-my-owe-site-iss*), myasthenia, osteomalacia (*os-tea-owe-mal-ay-sha*), alcohol, and steroids. Treatment is of the underlying cause.

Myotonia dystrophica

This is an autosomal dominant condition of gradual onset usually in the third decade. Patients present with progressive muscle weakness involving the face and sternomastoids, giving rise to the typical long, sad-looking face, bilateral ptosis (*toe-sis* see p. 295), and dysarthria (*dis-are-thria*). Limb muscles are also affected. Myotonia is a characteristic feature and refers to delayed muscle relaxation, for example, the slowly relaxing handshake. Other associated findings include frontal balding, cataracts, cardiomyopathy, and intellectual impairment. No treatment slows the progression of the disease but phenytoin (*fenny-toe-in*) and procainamide (*pro-cain-a-mide*) have both been used to ameliorate the myotonia, with variable results.

Friedreich's ataxia

This neurodegenerative disease is one the most common inherited ataxias. The usual mode of transmission is autosomal recessive, although other forms have been described. The median age of onset is 12 years. Clinical features relate to the neural tissue involved: cerebellum and spinocerebellar tracts (ataxia, nystagmus, dysarthria, and incoordination), corticospinal tracts (spastic paraparesis and extensor plantars), and peripheral neuropathy (sensory loss and pes cavus (*pes-cave-us*)). Other features include optic atrophy, kyphoscoliosis, and cardiomyopathy. The disease is progressive and irreversible; patients inevitably become wheelchair bound and usually die in the fifth decade from the associated cardiac disease.

Electromyography

Electromyography (EMG) is the recording of electrical activity of muscle fibres for diagnostic purposes. A small needle electrode is inserted into the muscle to be tested. The needle tip detects signals from the surrounding muscle fibres. These signals are amplified and recorded on an oscilloscope.

Examples

1. **Motor neurone disease.** Muscle denervation leads to spontaneous depolarization of muscle fibres, producing 'fibrillation potentials' (sensory nerve conduction studies will be normal).
2. **Myopathic pattern.** Low-amplitude polyphasic action potentials and spontaneous fibrillation; for example, seen in proximal myopathy.
3. **Polymyositis.** Shows features of myopathy with denervation. Definitive diagnosis is via muscle biopsy.
4. **Myotonia dystrophica.** High-frequency discharges, which diminish in a repeated manner giving a characteristic sound known as 'dive-bomber discharges'.
5. **Myasthenia.** Unstable neuromuscular junction transmission leads to variability of muscle action potentials known as 'jitter'. Also see next section.

In practice, the findings are not always clear cut and the EMG should be used in conjunction with the clinical picture.

Nerve conduction studies

These also involve the use of electrodes, which are attached to the skin. The nerve under test is excited percutaneously by a 'stimulatory electrode'; the impulse is carried along the nerve and detected at a 'recording electrode' further along the nerve (for example, in the case of sensory neurones) or at the target muscle (in the investigation of motor neurones). Information gained includes action potentials (motor and sensory), motor latency, and conduction velocities (motor and sensory). Velocities are calculated by dividing the distance separating the two electrodes by the time taken for the impulse to travel between them.

Nerve conduction studies are useful in differentiating between the different types of peripheral neuropathies.

Axonal type

Features

Reduced amplitude of action potentials.

Examples

Nerve laceration, peripheral neuropathies due to diabetes mellitus, alcohol, and other toxins.

Demyelinating type

Features

Reduced conduction velocity and in extreme cases 'conduction block'.

Examples

Guillain–Barré syndrome and nerve entrapment syndromes (for example, carpal tunnel syndrome).

Sensory neuropathies

Features

May be axonal or demyelinating; motor conduction normal.

Examples

Diabetes, uraemia, and vitamin B deficiencies.

Motor neuropathies

Features

May be axonal or demyelinating; sensory conduction normal.

Examples

Some hereditary neuropathies, lead poisoning, and porphyria.

Neuromuscular junction disorders

Features

Repetitive nerve stimulation shows a characteristic decrement in the muscle action potential.

Example

Myaesthenia gravis.

Computed tomography

This is a sensitive radiographic technique, which is a useful diagnostic aid. An X-ray beam is passed through the area to be imaged in consecutive horizontal 'slices', which are 2–10 mm apart. The information obtained is processed by a computer, which constructs two-dimensional images. Further information is obtained when intravenous contrast is administered at the time of scanning. Computed tomography has uses throughout the body. In the brain, unenhanced scans (no intravenous contrast) are useful in demonstrating intracranial bleeds (which show up as abnormal white areas) or infarcts (provided the scan is performed after 24 h; before this time the scan is usually normal). Cerebral atrophy is seen as shrinkage of brain tissue with corresponding enlargement of the sulci (*sul-sigh*) and ventricles. Enlargement of the ventricular system alone is termed 'hydrocephalus'. Intravenous contrast will highlight vascular abnormalities such as tumours, abscesses (showing 'ring enhancement'), and arteriovenous malformations. However CT may miss very small lesions and is less adept than MRI at demonstrating pathology in the brainstem. In the chest, CT can identify masses too small to be detected by conventional X-ray and gives further information relating to abnormalities shown on X-ray. Abdominal CT is used to stage tumours and in situations where ultrasound has been unable to assess deep structures, notably the pancreas, which is often obscured by overlying bowel gas.

Magnetic resonance imaging

This technique employs magnetism rather than radiation to produce images. An area of the body is exposed to a magnetic field leading to excitation of hydrogen nuclei (remember that the body is composed of 70% water). The signals produced by this process are computed, resulting in transverse images similar to CT; in addition a mid-line sagittal (*saj-it-al*) image can be obtained, which are useful in the diagnosis of brainstem and cervical cord pathology such as multiple sclerosis or syringomyelia. The use of magnetism, however, precludes its use in patients who have cardiac pacemakers and the screening process is performed in a small, enclosed chamber, which is most unpopular with claustrophobics!

Electroencephalography

Electroencephalolography (*elect-roe-en-kef-allo-graffy*) (EEG). Put simply, this is the brain's equivalent of an ECG. Multiple electrodes are put in strategic, internationally agreed positions. These record the electrical activity of the brain and deductions can be made, depending on the patient's characteristics, for example, age, medication, arousal, and so on. Four main brain rhythms may be identified: alpha rhythms (frequency of 8–12 Hz), usually seen when the eyes are closed; beta rhythms (faster rate, frequency 20–22 Hz), seen in anxious individuals and with sedative medication; delta rhythms (slower waves 1–4 Hz), which can be found in children but are normally pathological in adults; and theta rhythm (5–7 Hz), found in children. Interpretation of the EEG should only be done in conjunction with the patient's history and examination. It can be used to investigate seizures, blackouts, confusion, and sleep disorders. Various physiological challenges can be used to try and unmask a latent condition (usually epilepsy), for example, hyperventilation or the use of strobe light. There are limitations to the use of the EEG and neurophysiologists who perform them will take these into account when analysing any trace. For example, an epileptic may have a normal EEG between attacks. Also large intracerebral lesions may not register any electrical abnormality, whereas small lesions (invisible on the CT scan) can cause widespread electrical changes.

Finals section

For revision read the examination summary (p. 201) and the keypoints throughout the chapter and try the questions on pp. 204–5. See Tables 8.3 and 8.4 for day-to-day and Finals cases, respectively. The most common

TABLE 8.3 Day-to-day cases

Neurological	Non-neurological
Stroke	Rheumatoid arthritis
Parkinson's disease	Psoriasis
Cervical myelopathy	Purpura
Multiple sclerosis	

TABLE 8.4 Finals cases

Neurological	Non-neurological
Day-to-day cases	As for Table 8.3
Cerebellar syndromes, for example, multiple sclerosis	
Motor neurone disease	
Median/ulnar nerve palsy	

neurological problem you will see is stroke, although there are moves to concentrate these patients on designated stroke units rather than on general wards (as this improves survival and recovery). Other conditions include multiple sclerosis and Parkinson's disease. If you are lucky enough to have an attachment on a neurology ward you may see more exotic diseases. These may sometimes be used for Finals examinations because they are rich in neurological signs.

Key diagnostic clues

Perhaps this section should be called 'key localizing clues' because many of the signs you look for will point you to the site of the lesion rather than indicate the diagnosis. With motor loss, tone and reflexes give the most diagnostic information. With sensory loss, it is the pattern of loss that gives the most diagnostic information. It is helpful to categorize neurological signs into the following (see Chapter 10 (p. 260) for a fuller account of how to analyse your findings).

Motor

1. **UMN.** Little wasting, increased tone, decreased power, hyper-reflexia (clonus, upgoing plantar, spastic or hemiplegic gait in the legs).
2. **LMN.** Wasting, decreased tone, decreased power, decreased or absent reflexes (downgoing plantar in the leg).
3. **Extrapyramidal.** Involuntary movements, increased tone rigidity, (abnormal gait in the legs).
4. **Cerebellar.** Intention tremor, past-pointing, incoordination, dysdiadochokinesis, nystagmus in the eyes, ataxic gait in the legs.

Sensory

Patterns of sensory loss

1. The whole arm (cortical lesion?)
2. Dermatomal (root lesion? peripheral nerve lesion?)
3. Distal arm greater than proximal arm (peripheral neuropathy?)
4. Dissociated sensory loss (spinal cord lesion?)

Remember that the above classification of motor and sensory deficits is somewhat arbitrary and many of the categories can co-exist. A fuller explanation of how to localize a lesion can be found in Chapter 10.

Some advice relating to examination problems

General

Use the neurological examination routine for the arms given on p. 201.

The Instruction

The examiner will usually ask you to 'examine the arms neurologically' or just to 'examine the arms'. The latter command is apt to cause confusion because the case may not be neurological. Do not waste time dithering in this situation. The key to this problem is a quick visual survey. The intended focus of the case may be a skin rash or deformity of the wrist or elbow. If nothing leaps to the eye on inspection (or if you see wasting, fasciculations, and so on) then start a neurological examination.

Follow up non-neurological findings

This is quite difficult to do because it requires thinking on your feet. For example, if a scaly rash is present on the back of the elbow (suggesting psoriasis) you should go on to check the contralateral elbow for involvement, plus other sites such as the scalp. If you really want to impress your examiners, check for nail pitting and arthropathy, which are associations of psoriasis.

General look

This is important so do not forget it. It is probably easiest to fit this in during your focused inspection of the arms. A sly glance at the face and the rest of the body may give you a vital clue, for example, an expressionless face and a hunched posture may suggest Parkinson's disease and this may alert you to look for a pill-rolling tremor and cog-wheel rigidity.

Relax the patient

It is vitally important that your patient is relaxed throughout the examination (particularly when assessing tone and reflexes). It will help your cause if you can be as relaxed as possible too!

The neurological examination

The next dilemma you face is which aspect of the neurological system to test first, that is, sensory or motor system. In the absence of any leading clues I would advocate starting with the motor system as this is relatively quick to do (tone, power, reflexes, and coordination), whereas the sensory system can be more time consuming (light touch, pin-prick, vibration, and proprioception). Very often if you select the wrong system or the wrong aspect of the neurological system, your examiners will usually guide you to the relevant part so as not to waste valuable time.

Analyse as you go

As you examine do not simply elicit signs and then try to make sense of all of it at the end (in front of impatient and off-putting examiners). Try to analyse the significance of each sign as you go along. This will guide your subsequent examination, for example, looking for supplementary signs that may support a diagnosis as well as helping you to come to a conclusion more quickly.

Tone

Do not waste time agonising whether or not the tone is increased. If it is increased it is usually obvious (so long as you have practised sufficiently). If you are unsure, work through the rest of your examination looking for further clues. If you find hyper-reflexia, then it is likely that the tone is increased.

Power

This is straightforward. Look for assymetry of power (stroke? root lesion? nerve lesion?) and whether power is weaker proximally compared to distally (proximal myopathy?). There is always some debate as to whether testing of the muscles of the hands should be part of the arms examination. Generally speaking, if the abnormality you were supposed to pick up was in the hands, you would have been asked to examine these from the start.

Reflexes

Make sure you are competent at eliciting reflexes in the left arm.

Problem. You have found hyper-reflexia (and hypertonia) and are unsure whether to demonstrate Hoffmann's sign, finger jerks, deltoid reflexes and so on (see 'Other signs of the arms').

Solution. If hyper-reflexia is obvious it is probably not necessary but you are in an examination and so you want to demonstrate that you know more than the average. If you are confident, then perform Hoffman's sign and the finger jerks as these will add weight to the findings of hyper-reflexia (if you are not confident do not attempt them). I would draw the line at eliciting the deltoid and pectoral reflexes, as this could be seen as 'gilding the lily' and not adding too much more to your present state of knowledge. Remember, if you cannot elicit reflexes then you must try to elicit them with reinforcement! Often at this stage you will be stopped by the examiner and asked to present your findings. If this does not occur then you need to proceed to testing sensation. Contrary to popular belief this is not a disaster waiting to happen. Just remember that if there is a sensory deficit it will be blindingly obvious.

Sensation

Be systematic when assessing sensation. Aim to compare both arms. The proximal and distal portion of one arm and the radial and ulnar aspect of one arm. If you find a deficit try to elicit the pattern of loss. Is the whole arm affected (cortical lesion?)? Is the distal portion of both arms affected (peripheral neuropathy?)? A difference between the radial and ulnar borders may suggest a root lesion (radial border C6, ulnar border T1). Does it conform to a dermatomal distribution or to a peripheral nerve distribution? If you can answer these questions you are on the way to localizing where a lesion might be.

Presentation

Always mention that you would normally perform a full neurological examination and not just the arms in isolation, as there may be clues elsewhere that would help pinpoint the source of a lesion. Try to be confident—avoid the words 'seems' or 'might'!

Good luck!

Questions

The more stars, the more important it is to know the answer.

1. What are fasiculations? In which circumstances may they occur? ***
2. What are the causes of muscle wasting? **
3. In stroke classification how would you differentiate a total from a partial anterior circulation infarct? ****
4. What are the causes of parkinsonism? ****

5. What does apraxia mean? Where is the likely site of the lesion? ****
6. What is a dermatome? **
7. What information do the dorsal columns of the spinal cord transmit? ***
8. What are the causes of increased muscle tone? ****
9. What is syringomyelia? **
10. What are the causes of a cerebellar syndrome? ****
11. How would you demonstrate the Hoffman's reflex? What does it indicate? ***
12. What is sensory neglect? How does it affect a patient's recovery from stroke? ****
13. What would you expect to see on the magnetic resonance imaging scan of a patient with multiple sclerosis? **
14. What do you understand by the word proprioception? What is an alternative name for it? Name two diseases in which proprioception is altered. ***
15. What would be the diagnostic investigation of choice for motor neurone disease? ***
16. What is dysdiadochokinesia? **
17. What does the term dissociated sensory loss mean? **
18. What are the causes of a proximal myopathy? ***
19. Which structures within the brain are involved in the control of movement? ***
20. What are the key features of Parkinson's disease? ****
21. Which neurological diseases may be encountered in the arms of a diabetic? ****
22. Which clinical picture may result from an infarct in the right subthalamic nucleus? **
23. Describe the spinal reflex arc. ****
24. Which neurological disease is associated with a slow-relaxing grip? *
25. Name the two types of muscle rigidity that may be seen in Parkinson's disease. **
26. What do you understand by agnosia? ****
27. What are the common causes of a peripheral neuropathy? Which is the most common? ****
28. How would you differentiate between upper and lower motor neurone lesions? ****
29. Which drugs may cause a tremor? ***
30. What are the risk factors that predispose to a stroke? ****
31. What does a power grading of 3/5 indicate? **
32. What are the three clinical patterns seen in motor neurone disease? ****
33. Give some common examples of dystonias. **
34. Which nerve roots supply the biceps muscle? **
35. What do contralateral and ipsilateral mean? **
36. Which structures comprise the brainstem? **
37. What does paraneoplastic mean? **
38. What is chorea? Give some examples. ***
39. What does decussation mean? Where in the nervous system do the pyramidal tracts decussate? **
40. Explain the concept of reflex inversion. ****

Score. Give 4 marks for 4 stars, 1 for 1 star, and so on. At the end of the third year, you should be scoring 70-plus and by Finals, 90-plus; 110-plus is very good.

Further reading

Crossman AR, Neary D. *Neuroanatomy, an illustrated colour text*. Edinburgh: Churchill Livingstone; 2000.

Fuller G, Manford M. *Neurology, an illustrated colour text*. Edinburgh: Churchill Livingstone;1999.

Parsons M. *A colour atlas of clinical neurology*. 3rd edn. London: Wolfe; 1992.

Patten J. Neurological differential diagnosis. 2nd edn. London: Springer; 1995.

Perkin G. *Mosby's colour atlas and text of neurology*. 2nd edn. London: Mosby-Wolfe; 2002.

Ross RT. *How to examine the nervous system*. London: Lange 1998.

CHAPTER 9

Hands

Chapter contents

Introduction

The hands are of great functional importance. The complicated fine movements we make with our hands distinguish us from the rest of the animal kingdom and so a disproportionately large area of the brain is dedicated to supplying the motor and sensory function of the hand. Examination of the hands is very important as it can provide diagnostic clues to systemic, rheumatological, neurological, and dermatological diseases. A brief inspection of the hands is therefore a fundamental starting point in any general physical examination. In this chapter the focus will be on neurological signs and symptoms, which will complement the previous chapter on the arms (Chapter 8). The neuroanatomy of the arms is relevant to the hands as are many of the symptoms. This chapter will concentrate on areas specific to the hands.

Symptoms

Anaesthesia, paraesthesia and dysaesthesia, and muscle weakness

See Chapter 8 for definitions and what to ask.

Tremor

What is it?

A tremor is an involuntary movement that usually affects the limbs, most commonly the hands. It is a repetitive rhythmic movement. A tremor can be coarse or fine. There are four main types of tremor (see Table 9.1).

1. **Postural tremor.** We all have a fine, 5–8 Hz physiological tremor, which is normally invisible (Hz = hertz, that is, one cycle per second). This can become exaggerated for various reasons when it is known as a postural tremor. It occurs at rest and can be demonstrated clinically by getting your patient to stretch their arms out in front of them. It can also be inherited as an autosomal dominant trait and is called benign essential tremor. This tremor is often improved by alcohol and can be treated with β-blockers. It differs from other postural tremor in that it can be quite coarse in nature and has often been mistaken for Parkinson's Disease.
2. **'Pill-rolling' tremor.** This is a slow (4–6 Hz), fine, resting tremor. The name derives from the repetitive movement of finger and thumb, as if a pill were being rolled between them. A pill-rolling tremor is typical of parkinsonism. Parkinsonism is a syndrome comprised of the triad of a resting tremor, rigidity (increased tone or stiffness), and bradykinesia (slow movements). Parkinsonism can be idiopathic, when it is known as Parkinson's disease. It can also be caused by drugs (dopamine antagonists, for example, metoclopramide and haloperidol) and viral encephalitis.
3. **Intention tremor.** This occurs during movement and is absent at rest. It is a fine tremor (3 Hz) and is often associated with past pointing (dysmetria). An intention tremor is a feature of cerebellar disease. Other associated signs are ataxia, dysarthria (slurred speech), and nystagmus. (Common causes of cerebellar signs in an examination are cerebrovascular disease or multiple sclerosis.)
4. **Flapping tremor.** Also called asterixis (*ass-stir-ix-iss*), this is an important sign in hepatic encephalitis, renal failure, and type II respiratory failure. Type II respiratory failure is when the patient hypoventilates (breathes insufficiently) causing the carbon dioxide level in the blood to increase.

TABLE 9.1 Causes of tremor

Postural tremor	Old age, anxiety, drugs (β_2 agonists, caffeine, steroids), exercise, hyperthyroidism, hypoglycaemia, inherited
'Pill-rolling' tremor	Parkinson's disease, drug-induced parkinsonism, viral encephalitis, cerebrovascular disease
Intention tremor	Cerebellar pathology, eg. multiple sclerosis, cerebrovascular disease
Flapping tremor	Hepatic failure, type II respiratory failure, uraemia

What to ask about a tremor

1. When did the tremor start? Was it a gradual or sudden onset? A gradual onset may be due to a progressive disease like Parkinson's disease. An acute onset could be caused by a stroke or starting a new drug.
2. Is it worse at any particular time of day? An early morning tremor may be due to alcohol withdrawal. A benign essential tremor can be exaggerated by tiredness and therefore be more pronounced in the evening.
3. Is there anything that makes it better? Alcohol may improve benign essential tremor. Holding an object in the hand can improve a pill-rolling tremor.
4. Is there anything that makes it worse? Many tremors can get worse with anxiety especially if the patient is conscious of being closely observed.
5. How does it affect the patient? Does it prevent them from doing certain tasks?
6. Does the patient have any other symptoms? Dysarthria, poor balance, and intention tremor are associated with cerebellar disease. Stiffness, difficulty standing up, turning over in bed, and increased incidence of falls are associated with parkinsonism.

7. Is there any family history of tremors? Benign essential tremor can be inherited as an autosomal dominant trait, so one of the parents should have the disease. There are genetic conditions that can affect the cerebellum, for example, Freidrich's ataxia, which have a variable inheritance.

See also the section on involuntary movements in Chapter 8.

Keypoints

- The commonest tremor is a postural tremor.
- A flapping tremor is a sign of hepatic encephalopathy, renal failure, or type II respiratory failure.
- A pill rolling tremor is diagnostic of parkinsonism.

The importance of examining the hands

Learning to examine the hands is of supreme importance as it can provide clues to disease in any system. If the eyes are the windows of the soul, then the hands are the windows to a diagnosis. Even the fingernails can provide vital signs that can point towards disease. The majority of times an assessment of the hand will lead to a rheumatological, neurological, or dermatological condition. However any physical examination should begin with an examination of the hand.

Examination of the hands summary

1. Introduce yourself to the patient and ask for permission to examine.
2. Ask the patient if they have any pain in their hands or arms.
3. Position the patient and expose their hands and arms.
4. Whilst doing 1–3, be having a 'general look'.
5. Observe the posture of the hand.
6. Inspect the dorsum and then the palmar aspect of both hands and look for any obvious abnormalities.
7. Inspect the muscles for wasting or fasciculation.
8. Examine for a tremor.
9. Assess tone.
10. Assess muscle power.
11. Test sensation.
12. Assess function by asking the patient to write, to undo then do up a button, and to pick up a coin from a flat surface. Test the patient's speed doing repetitive fine movements.
13. Wash your hands.
14. Presentation.

Examination of the hands in detail

1. Introduce yourself to the patient and ask for permission to examine.

Say something like 'Hello, I'm Maurice Raynaud, a fourth-year medical student. Do you mind if I examine your hands?'

2. Ask the patient if they have any pain in their hands or arms.

This is a very important question to ask, so remember it! The patient may have very tender hands, for example, in acute rheumatoid arthritis. Inflicting pain on a patient can ruin the doctor–patient relationship (and would look bad in an examination).

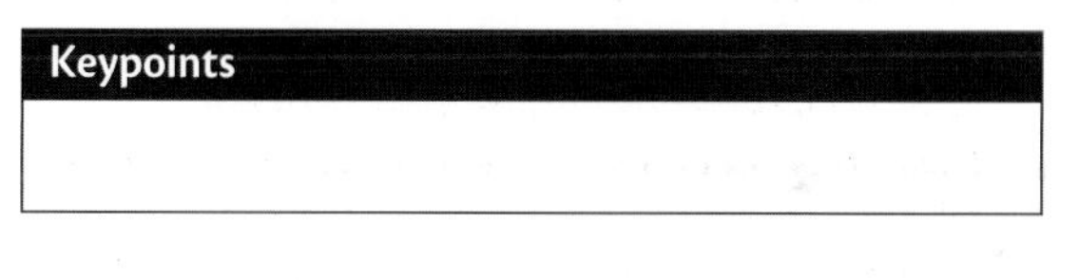

3. Position the patient and expose their hands and arms.

Ask the patient to get on to a bed or chair (if not already on) and make sure they are comfortable. Get the patient to expose their hands and arms. If you are doing a full neurological examination then the whole of the upper limbs and trunk will need to be exposed.

- **Has the patient got a typical facies?** A patient with myotonia dystrophica has a triangular-shaped face, with bilateral partial ptosis, wasting of the temporalis muscle, and frontal balding (see 'Diseases and investigations of the arms' (Chapter 8) and Fig. 11.2).
- **Is there an obvious rash?** A purpuric rash can occur with vasculitic conditions, for example, rheumatoid arthritis. Vasculitides (*vas-cue-lit-i-deez*) can also cause cutaneous ulcers. In polymyositis and dermatomyositis (*der-mat-owe-my-owe-site-iss*) the patient can get a lilac discolouration around the eyelids, which is known as a heliotrope (*he-leo-trope*) rash. It can be associated with increased photosensitivity of the skin.

3. **Also look at the local environment around the patient.** A walking stick or wheelchair suggests a degree of disability, possibly due to neurological or rheumatological disease. Other clues include specially adapted cups or cutlery.
4. **Whilst doing 1–3, be having a 'general look'.**
5. **Observe the posture of the hand.**

The posture of the hand may give a clue to an underlying condition. Here are some examples of characteristic appearances that herald an underlying diagnosis.

Claw hand

What is it?

See Fig. 9.1. The claw hand (main en griffe) (*man-on-griff*) is the clawed appearance of the hand as a result of hyperextension of the metacarpophalangeal (MCP) joints (especially the fourth and fifth joints) and flexion of the proximal interphalangeal (PIP) and distal interphalangeal (DIP) joints (especially the fourth and fifth joints).

(a)

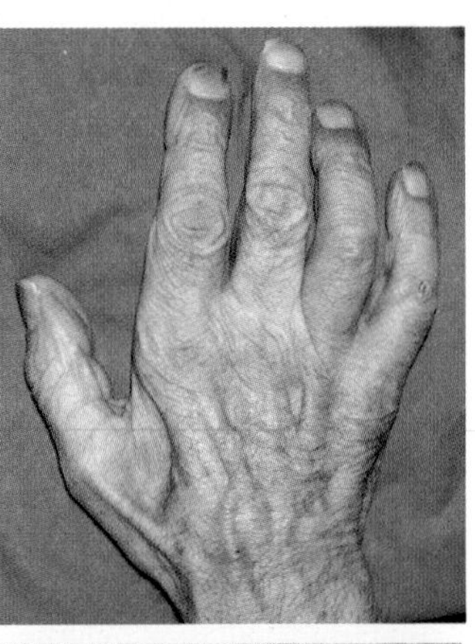

(b)

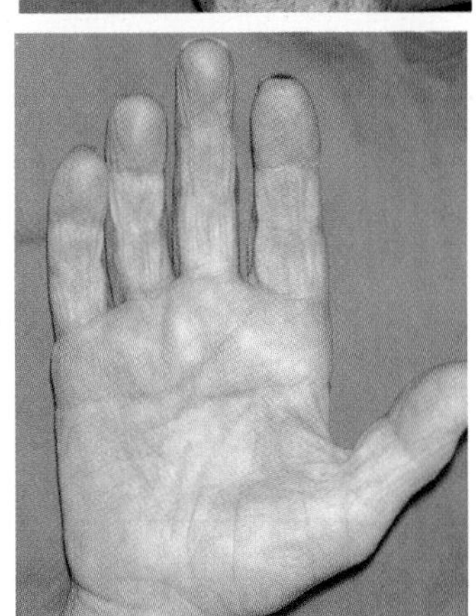

Fig. 9.1 Ulna claw hand (see text).

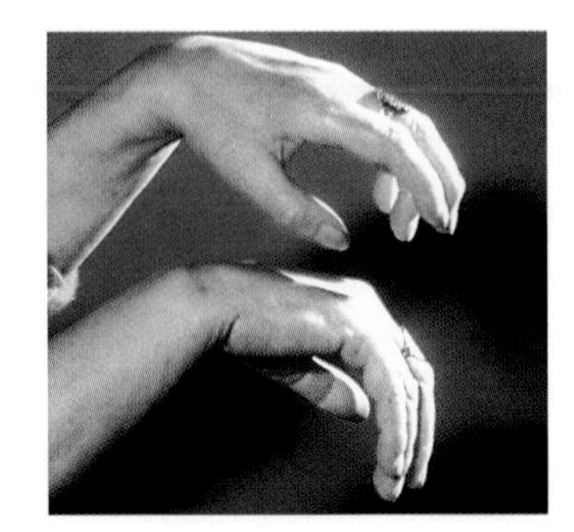

Fig. 9.2 Bilateral wrist drop.

Significance

The appearance is the result of an ulnar nerve lesion that has become chronic. There is also wasting of the hypothenar (*high-poe-thee-nar*) eminence and sensory loss over the medial half of the hand and medial one and a half digits (see later in this chapter).

Wrist drop

What is it?

See Fig. 9.2. The wrist of either hand (occasionally both) flops limply.

Significance

If this feature is persistent it suggests a radial nerve lesion, which leads to paralysis of the long extensor muscles of the forearm, and normally produces wrist and finger extension (see later in this chapter).

'Spastic hand'

What is it?

This is due to a chronic increase in tone of the affected limb. The fingers are tightly flexed into the palm and can only be prised open with difficulty. The wrist is also flexed.

Significance

This is caused by an upper motor neurone lesion affecting the limb. You will need to search for other signs of an upper motor lesion and for an underlying cause (see Chapters 8 and 10).

Dystonia

What is it?

The hand may adopt an abnormal posture due to sustained contraction of a particular muscle group or as part of a generalized dystonic phenomenon (see p. 205). This position can be maintained for minutes, hours, or even days (with respite only during sleep). Occasionally you may be faced with a patient who exhibits a bizarre hand posture for seconds only. This probably represents an elaborate handshake from a member of a secret society, for example, the Masons and is of no clinical importance.

There are non-neurological causes of an abnormal hand posture that can mimic a nerve injury and the conditions that can cause confusion include Dupuytren's (*dew-pit-rens*) contracture and Volkmann's (*voke-mans*) ischaemic contracture.

Dupuytren's contracture

The earliest indication of this condition may be the flexion of the ring finger towards the palm. As it progresses other fingers can flex towards the palm giving the hand a clawed appearance. It is associated with alcoholic liver disease and this should prompt a search for other stigmata of alcoholic liver disease (see Chapter 6 for other associations and a fuller description).

Volkmann's ischaemic contracture

What is it?

Volkmann's ischaemic contracture (*Richard von Volkmann (1830–1889), German surgeon*) is due to the contracture of the forearm muscles as a result of necrosis and replacement of muscle by fibrous tissue. There are three patterns of appearance depending on whether the long flexors or the long extensor muscles are predominantly affected.

- **Long flexors.** Wrist flexed, fingers extended. If the wrist is passively extended the fingers become flexed.
- **Long extensors.** Wrist and MCP joints extended, fingers flexed.
- **Both affected.** Wrist flexed, MCP joints extended, fingers flexed.

Significance

The ischaemia is a consequence of a fracture of the lower end of the humerus or of the radius and ulna. The brachial artery can go into spasm and interrupt the blood supply to the forearm muscles. This can also occur if a plaster cast is applied too tightly and this needs to be watched for following stabilization of the fracture.

6. Inspect the dorsum and then the palmar aspect of both hands and look for any obvious abnormalities.

Take a few seconds to make a general inspection of the hands. A swollen, deformed hand may suggest rheumatoid arthritis as the basis of a neurological problem.

Keypoints

- A clawed hand suggests an ulnar nerve lesion.
- Wrist drop is due to a radial nerve lesion.
- Dupuytren's contracture causes flexion of the ring finger initially.
- Abnormal postures of the hand may be due to dystonia.

Nail fold infarcts may suggest a vasculitic cause for any deficit. Rarely you may find purplish raised papules particularly over the knuckles, which may be Gottron's (*got-trenz*) papules of dermatomyositis. Neurofibromata (*new-roe-fie-bro-matta*) are subcutaneous nodules, which may be sessile (relatively flat and embedded in the skin) or pedunculated (attached to the skin by a narrow stalk). They occur in neurofibromatosis (*new-roe-fie-bro-mat-toe-sis*) and may be associated with café-au-lait patches and lipomata. Café-au-lait patches are pale brown or coffee-coloured patches found on the body. Up to five patches can be considered normal. Above this number may indicate neurofibromatosis. Lipoma are fatty deposits in the skin. Neurofibroma may arise from peripheral nerve roots or cranial nerves and cause neurological problems by compression of the nerve as they grow. They are usually benign tumours but occasionally they undergo sarcomatous (*sar-comb-a-tuss*) change and become malignant.

7. Inspect the muscles for wasting or fasciculation.
Look carefully at the hands. Is there loss of muscle bulk? Remember to examine both the dorsum and the palmar aspects of both hands. Sometimes it is difficult to assess the muscle on inspection and you need to palpate. The appreciation of subtle degrees of muscle loss by palpation will only come with practice. Is there any pattern to the muscle wasting? Are all the small muscles of the hand affected? Or is the loss of muscle bulk isolated to a group of muscles, like the thenar eminence? Are both hands affected or is it unilateral? Is there any associated deformity of the hand suggesting nerve damage? (See discussion on hand posture earlier.)

Tip

If you are unsure about the degree of wasting of the patient's hand muscles, compare them with the muscle bulk of your own hands.

Muscle wasting

- **Isolated wasting of the thenar eminence.** This is caused by a median nerve palsy. Although damage to the nerve can occur from the nerve root onwards, the most common cause is carpal tunnel syndrome (see Fig. 9.3).
- **Generalized wasting of the hand muscles with sparing of the thenar eminence.** This is caused by an ulnar nerve palsy (see Fig. 9.1). Classically there is wasting of the hypothenar eminence and the first dorsal interosseus (*in-ter-ross-ee-us*) muscle and guttering of the dorsum of the hand. There may also be associated muscle wasting of the forearm medially. An ulnar claw hand may develop, due to hyperextension of the fourth and fifth metacarpophalangeal (*met-er-car-po-fal-an-jeel*) joints and flexion of the interphalangeal (*in-ter-fal-an-jeel*) joints.

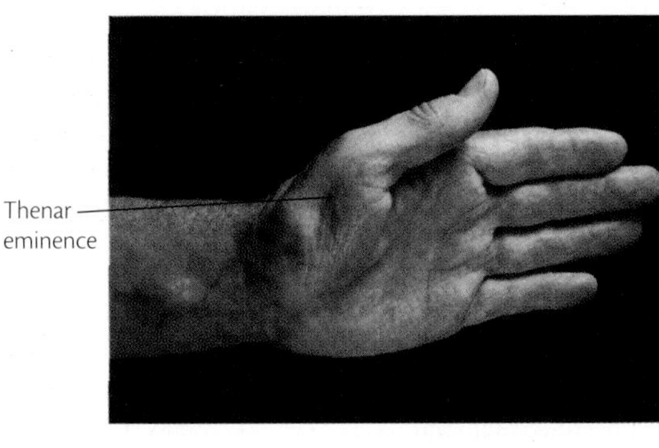

Fig. 9.3 Carpal tunnel syndrome. Reprinted from **Fig. 2.39** (p. 2.17), *Atlas of Clinical Neurology* (2nd edn), by G. David Perkin, Fred Hochberg, and Douglas C. Miller (1993), Mosby Publications, with permission from Elsevier.

TABLE 9.2 Causes of wasting of the small muscles of the hand

Anterior horn cell lesions	Motor neurone disease, syringomyelia, Charcot Marie Tooth, old polio (very rare, but still seen in examinations)
Cervical root lesions	Spondylosis
Brachial plexus lesions	Cervical rib, Pancoast's tumour*/other malignant infiltration, trauma
Ulnar and median nerve lesions	
Disuse of the muscles	Rheumatoid arthritis, old age
Generalized wasting	Dramatic weight loss of any cause

* Henry Khunrath Pancoast (1875–1939), US radiologist.

- **Generalized wasting of the small muscles of the hand.** There is wasting of both the thenar and hypothenar eminences and dorsal guttering. Chronically a claw hand may develop. See Table 9.2.

Tip

Be careful when presenting your differential diagnosis in front of a patient. If at all possible **do not**! If you must, avoid terms like cancer, motor neurone disease, and multiple sclerosis. Use mitotic lesion, anterior horn cell disease, and demyelinating disease respectively. Remember it looks bad to distress your patient in an examination or teaching session.

CASE 9.1

Problem. You examine the hands of a 62-year-old woman. There is dorsal guttering of the hand suggesting generalized wasting of the intrinsic muscles. There are no gross deformities of the hands although the metacarpal heads seem prominent and there is the suggestion of ulnar deviation. On palpation there is a boggy feeling at the MCP and PIP joints, which are warm and tender. Your patient can perform all the functional tasks you give her including undoing and redoing her buttons and twisting the lid off a jam jar although it is done with pain and difficulty. There is no sensory abnormality. What is the cause of the muscle wasting?

Discussion. Dorsal guttering is the description given to the channels in between the metacarpal bones, which are revealed when there is substantial wasting of the intrinsic muscles of the hand. The clue to the cause of the wasting is the soft boggy feeling around the MCP and PIP joints, which are warm and tender. There is an active sinovitis (*sign-owe-vie-tiss*) (see Chapter 13), which will cause pain and interfere with everyday functions as evidenced by the difficulty she has with manipulating her buttons or opening the jam jar. In addition there is the prominence of the metacarpal heads and the suspicion of ulnar deviation, which points towards an early presentation of rheumatoid arthritis. You should complete your examination by searching for rheumatoid nodules and also checking for plaques of psoriasis as one form of psoriatic arthropathy can mimic rheumatoid arthritis.

Fasciculations

Fasciculations are irregular, fine flickering movements of muscle fibres under the skin (see p. 203). They occur in lower motor neurone lesions. Muscle wasting and fasciculations are characteristic of motor neurone disease.

8. Examine for a tremor.

The different types of tremors and their possible aetiology have been discussed already in the 'Symptoms' section of this chapter. When examining a tremor you need to ask three questions: (1)When does it occur? (2) Is it coarse or fine? and (3)Does anything exacerbate it?

> **CASE 9.2**
>
> **Problem.** You are examining the hands of an 89-year-old woman. You notice there is generalized wasting of the intrinsic muscles of the hand with no fasciculation. The power is normal for all hand movements, there is no sensory abnormality, and there are no no joint deformities. What is the cause of the muscle wasting?
>
> **Discussion.** If it were not for the presence of the wasting of the intrinsic hand muscles, these would be normal hands. The only other clue here is the age of the patient. This pattern of loss can be seen in the frail elderly where there is often a global decrease in lean muscle mass. Day-to-day function is not affected by this form of muscle wasting (although there may be problems coping with extraordinary stresses including illness, trips, and so on.) Another cause to consider is cervical myelopathy. In this condition hand function can also be preserved. The key sign to elicit would be reflex inversion (see p. 220) and until her reflexes are assessed this remains a differential diagnosis.

> **Keypoints**
>
> - Isolated wasting of the thenar eminence is commonly caused by carpal tunnel syndrome.
> - Wasting of the small muscles of the hand associated with fasiculations is diagnostic of motor neurone disease.
> - Wasting of the small muscles of the hand may be due to old age, generalized wasting conditions, rheumatoid arthritis, or ulna nerve lesions.

> **Tip**
>
> A pill-rolling tremor may be accentuated by asking the patient to count backwards from 10 to zero.

- **Initially inspect for a tremor whilst the patient's hands are resting on a pillow or in their lap.** Is there a rest tremor? Is the tremor coarse or fine? A pill-rolling tremor is a fine tremor, which occurs at rest. It is characteristic of parkinsonism. The patient may also have an expressionless face described as a mask-like facies, have a small shuffling gait, and be bradykinetic.
- **Next ask the patient to hold their hands out in front of them, palms facing downwards.** The commonest tremor seen is a postural tremor. It can be demonstrated by placing a sheet of paper on the patient's outstretched hands.
- **If you suspect your patient has liver, renal, or respiratory failure, get them to dorsi-flex their wrists with their arms outstretched.** This will demonstrate a **flapping tremor** (see p, 219). If your patient has a flapping tremor you should look for other features of hepatic, renal, and respiratory failure.

> **Tip**
>
> When demonstrating a flapping tremor it is vital that the patient's arms are extended for long enough. It can take up to 1 min for the distinctive tremor to develop.

- **If you suspect an intention tremor then demonstrate this by performing the finger-nose test.** This is a fundamental part of the neurological examination and is therefore discussed fully on p. 212.

9. Assess tone.

Assess muscle tone by gently rotating, then flexing and extending the patient's wrist joint. Is there increased or decreased resistance to movement? Does the amount of increased resistance remain constant? This is known as lead-pipe rigidity (seen in parkinsonism). Or does the resistance suddenly give way? This is known as clasp knife spasticity (seen in upper motor neurone lesions). This is best appreciated at larger joints such as the elbow. Is there a cog-wheeling effect? This occurs in parkinsonism, due to the combined effect of a tremor and rigidity. It is usually most pronounced during flexion and extension at the wrist.

Tip

It is possible to make cog wheeling more pronounced. While passively flexing and extending their wrist, ask the patient to actively extend and flex the opposite arm at the shoulder.

After examining the wrist assess the other joints of the hand, by flexing and extending them. For a more detailed account of the assessment of tone review see p. 205.

Keypoints

- Lead-pipe and cog-wheel rigidity is characteristic of parkinsonism.
- Clasp knife spasticity is characteristic of upper motor neurone lesions.

10. Assess muscle power.

When examining muscle power your instructions to the patient should be clear and concise. You may need to demonstrate the action to the patient. Muscle groups should be tested bilaterally and sequentially. The strength in the two hands should be similar, although the dominant limb may be slightly stronger.

- **'Grasp my fingers as tight as possible.'** Offer the patient two of your fingers to hold. This assesses the strength of finger flexion. The muscles being tested are flexor digitorum profundus (*flex-or-digit-or-um–pro-fund-us*) and flexor digitorum superficialis (*soup-er-fishy-ale-iss*). They are supplied by branches from the median and ulnar nerves (their innervation is principally from spinal root C8) (opposition of the thumb is supplied by T1).

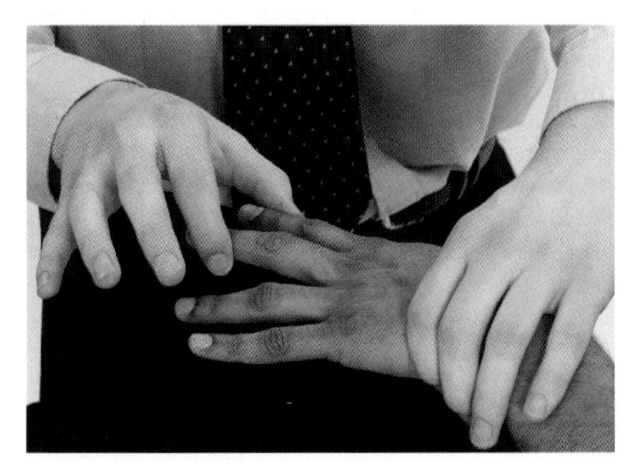

Fig. 9.4 Finger abduction.

- **'Hold your hand out straight, don't let me bend your fingers.'** This assesses finger extension. The muscle is extensor digitorum, supplied by the radial nerve fibres and is innervated chiefly from the root C7.
- **'Spread your fingers out wide, don't let me push your fingers together.'** This assesses finger abduction. This tests the dorsal interossei (*inter-ross-ee-eye*) muscles. Supplied by the ulnar nerve fibres, from spinal root T1 (see Fig. 9.4).
- **'Grasp this piece of paper between your fingers as tightly as possible. Stop me from pulling it out.'** Here you are assessing finger adduction. The muscles being used are the palmar interossei. Also supplied by the ulnar nerve, arising from spinal root T1 (see Fig. 9.5).
- **'Point your thumb towards the ceiling. Don't let me push it down.'** This is assessing abduction of the thumb. The muscle being tested is abductor pollicis brevis (*ab-duck-tor-polly-sis-brev-iss*), supplied by fibres from the median nerve arising from T1 (see Fig. 9.6).

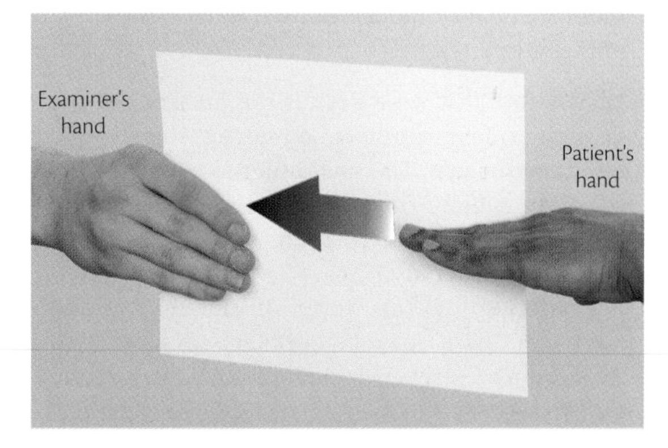

Fig. 9.5 Finger adduction.

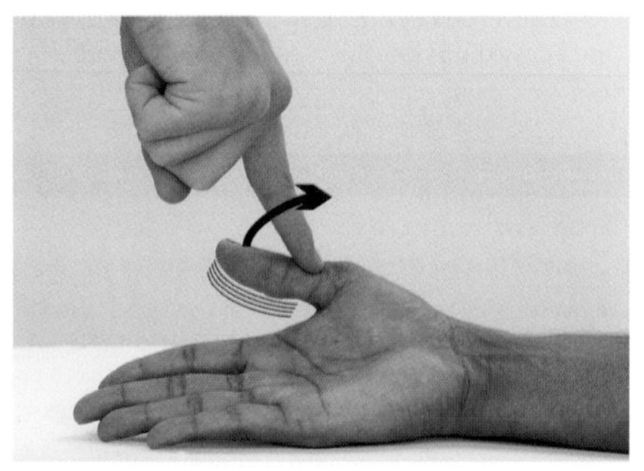

Fig. 9.6 Abduction of the thumb. The arrow represents the direction of force generated by the patient.

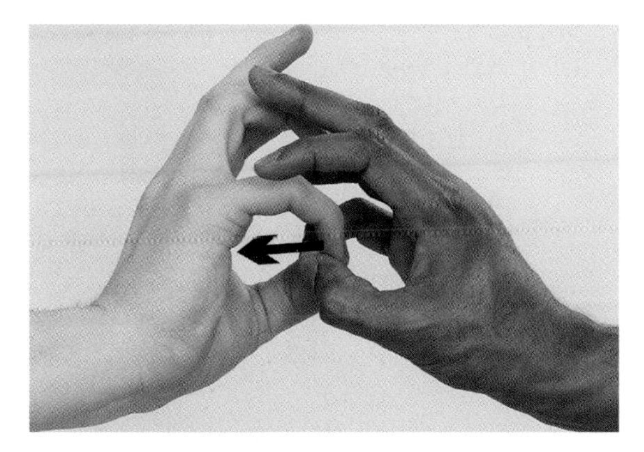

Fig. 9.7 Opposition of the thumb.

- **'Place your thumb and little finger together to form a ring. Don't let me pull them apart.'** This is assessing opposition between the thumb and little finger. The major muscle used is opponens pollicis (*op-poe-nens-polly-sis*), which is supplied by a branch of the median nerve (see Fig. 9.7) (root T1). Movement of the little finger is via a branch of the ulna nerve (C8).

11. Test sensation.

Test light touch, pin-prick, vibration, and proprioception as for the arms. Remember when testing sensation you need to continually think about the distribution of the sensory abnormality and whether it corresponds with

- an individual dermatome;
- the territory of a peripheral nerve;
- a sensory polyneuropathy—glove and stocking distribution;
- a cortical distribution.

(See Chapter 8.)

> **Tip**
>
> If a patient has **not** noticed any altered sensation you are unlikely to find any abnormality on examination.

12. Assess function by asking the patient to write, to undo then do up a button, and to pick up a coin from a flat surface. Test the patient's speed doing repetitive fine movements.

It is important to try and assess how the patient's function is affected by their condition. This can be illustrated by asking the patient to perform a few tasks. Here are some suggestions.

- Ask the patient to write their name and address on a piece of paper. In parkinsonism the patient develops micrographia: their writing becomes smaller as they progress across the page. This is a useful test to monitor the change in parkinsonism over time or the response of a patient to treatment.
- Then ask the patient to undo and do up a button on their shirt or pyjama top. Next get them to pick up a coin from a flat, firm surface like a table. These tests examine the patient's dexterity and ability to perform fine movements and many neurological (and rheumatological) diseases can impair them.
- Finally assess the patient's speed at repetitive fine movements, by getting them to place each of their fingers in turn in opposition with the thumb of the same hand. They should perform this as quickly as possible. This should then be repeated with the opposite hand. A lot of conditions affecting the hand can cause bradykinesia (slowing of movement). Parkinsonism causes bradykinesia, which characteristically becomes slower with repetitive movements. The bradykinesia of parkinsonism becomes more pronounced by asking the patient to count backwards from 10 to zero.

> **Tip**
>
> It is often easier for you to demonstrate the test for repetitive fine movements than to explain it to the patient.

> **Keypoints**
>
> - Always assess hand function.
> - Many neurological and rheumatological disorders can impair hand function.
> - Parkinsonism causes micrographia.
> - Parkinsonism causes a progressive bradykinesia.

Wash your hands

13. Wash your hands.

Keep it clean!

Presentation of findings

14. Presentation.

After completing your examination of the hands thank the patient and offer to assist in replacing clothes (in an examination you could be penalized for discourteous behaviour despite a flawless performance). If you know the diagnosis, begin your presentation with it and then support it with your findings. If you do not know the diagnosis, describe your findings and then offer a differential diagnosis. For example, 'The patient has an ulnar nerve palsy because she has a clawed hand with flexion more evident in the ring and little fingers. There is wasting of the hypothenar eminence and there is anaesthesia over the medial half of the hand and medial one and a half digits. There was no sign of injury at the wrist but there is a deformity of the elbow, which suggests there may have been an old fracture at this site leading to damage of the ulna nerve.'

Other signs of the hands

Tinel's sign

See Fig. 9.8. This is an additional test if you suspect a carpal tunnel syndrome. To elicit Tinel's (*tin-elz*) sign (*Jules Tinel (1879–1952), French neurologist*) you percuss over the median nerve as it runs through the carpal tunnel at the wrist. To locate the nerve get your patient to flex their wrist slightly. This accentuates the tendon of palmaris longus (*pal-ma-riss-long-us*). Roll your index finger laterally over the tendon and tap about an inch from the wrist crease (in those patients who lack this tendon, locate the radial artery and aim slightly medial to this position about an inch from the wrist crease). The test is positive if the patient feels tingling or pain over the first three and a half digits of the hand, that is, paraesthesia in the distribution of the median nerve.

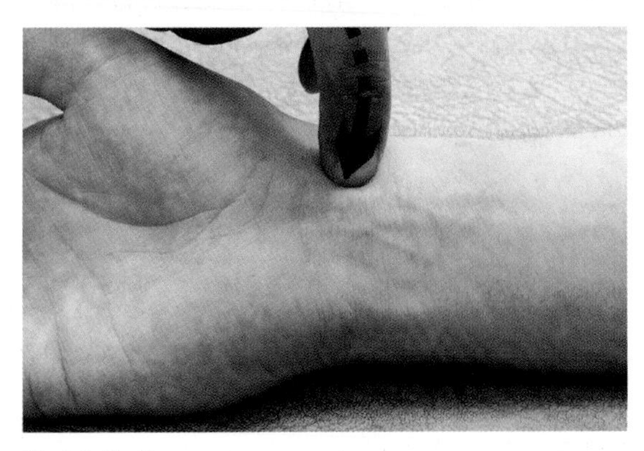

Fig. 9.8 Tinel's test.

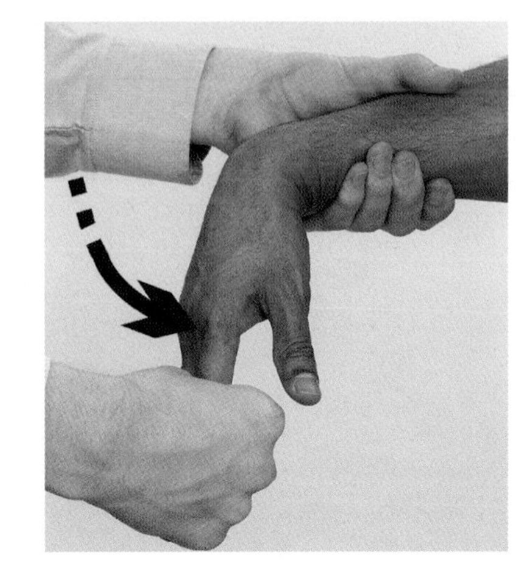

Fig. 9.9 Phalen's test.

Phalen's sign

See Fig. 9.9. Phalen's (*fail-enz*) sign (*George Phalen (1911–1998), American orthopaedic surgeon*) is a further test you can perform if you suspect carpal tunnel syndrome. Ask the patient to flex the wrist of the affected hand for a minute. Patients with carpal tunnel syndrome develop paraesthesia in the distribution of the median nerve. The symptoms resolve quickly when the wrist is relaxed.

Froment's sign

See Fig. 9.10. Froment's (*fro-ments*) sign (*Jules Froment (1878–1946), French physician*) is a test that demonstrates the inability of the thumb to adduct in an ulnar nerve lesion (see later). Ask your patient to grip a piece of paper between their thumb and index finger (this requires adduction of the thumb). In the presence of an ulna nerve palsy the grip is achieved by flexing the thumb.

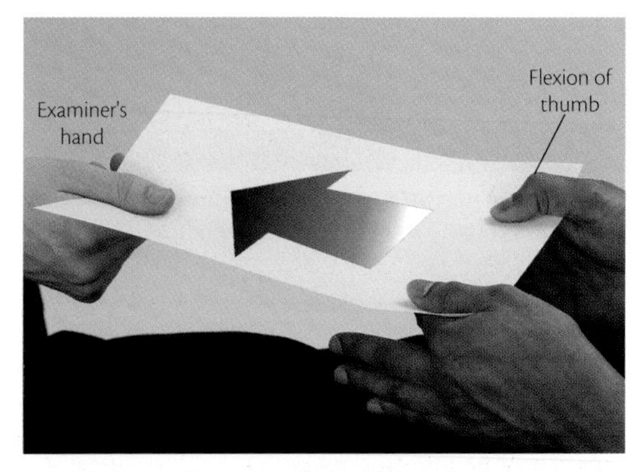

Fig. 9.10 Froment's sign. Note flexion of the patient's right thumb. This 'trick movement' is adopted because there is a paralysis of adductor pollicis brevis (supplied by the ulnar nerve).

CASE 9.3

Problem. You are in your Finals examination and are asked to examine the hands of a 43-year-old man with diabetes. They seem large and spade like (and felt 'doughy' when you shook hands earlier) and your first impressions were of a large hunched man with coarse facial features. As you concentrate on the hands you notice wasting of the thenar eminence but no other neurological abnormalities. Tinel's test was negative but Phalen's test was positive. What is the diagnosis and what questions would you like to ask?

Discussion. The wasting of the thenar eminence suggests carpal tunnel syndrome especially as there is no wasting of the intrinsic muscles of the hand to point to a T1 root lesion. You have obviously considered this as you have performed the supplementary tests of Tinel and Phalen. The positive Phalen's test adds further weight to the diagnosis. Ask, 'Do you ever get pins and needles?' If the answer to this is 'yes', ask, 'When does this symptom come on?' (it is usually worse at night) and 'Where do you get the pins and needles?' (this should be in the distribution of the median nerve including the lateral three and a half digits on the palmar aspect). If the answers are as above the clinical diagnosis is carpal tunnel syndrome. It is important to note that even if both Tinel's and Phalen's tests are negative you should not dismiss the diagnosis if you have a strong clinical suspicion of the syndrome. Go on to perform nerve conduction studies, which will give you the answer.

However you have not finished, as you need to establish a cause for the carpal tunnel syndrome. There are further hints in your first impressions of this patient (which are often easy to dismiss when you are concentrating on the task in hand). He has large spade-like hands, which feel doughy and you noticed his coarse facial features. These impressions conjure up the image of acromegaly (*a-crow-meg-alley*). So continue your questions. 'Have you needed a change in shoe, glove, or hat size?' An increase in size of any of these features points to acromegaly (in the absence of oedema). 'Have you had a persistent headache?' A pituitary tumour, secreting growth hormone, which produces the syndrome of acromegaly may cause a headache. 'Have you had any visual disturbance?' Patients develop a bitemporal hemianopia. 'When did you develop diabetes?' If this is recent then it could be caused by acromegaly (see later). This is an unusual cause of carpal tunnel syndrome but the unusual have a habit of cropping up in examinations!

CASE 9.4

Problem. A 52-year-old man who is a longstanding alcoholic is admitted to your ward following a fit. On recovery he is anxious and jittery and cannot give any coherent account of his activities for the last week. The only concrete information was that he had been unable to drink for 24 h before his fit. His other concern was the paralysis of his right hand, which had occurred since the fit. You conduct a full neurological examination and determine that he has a lower motor neurone lesion affecting his right wrist predominantly leading to a wrist drop and poor grip. The consultant conducts their round and decides in view of the fit and his continued paralysis he should have a computed tomography scan of his brain. Is this the correct course of action?

Discussion. This case highlights the difficulties of dealing with an alcoholic. Often the history can be scanty or unreliable and therefore you often have to make your best guess and back it up with investigations. Although the consultant's course of action is a safe one, it is an unnecessary and expensive one. Their worry is that he may have a space-occupying lesion (commonly a subdural haematoma in alcoholics) leading to his fit and a focal paralysis **but** the signs do not add up. You have discovered a lower motor lesion, which means the problem has to be at the spinal root, brachial plexus, or peripheral nerve level (see Chapters 8 and 10). A wrist drop suggests a radial nerve palsy and would interfere with his ability to grip (see later). Determining the cause however will be difficult without a decent history. A fracture of the shaft of the humerus can be ruled out as this would be evident clinically. It is possible that he could have dangled his arm over the back of a chair in a drunken stupor and the upward pressure from the back of the chair could compress the radial nerve in the axilla. Another mechanism is compression of the radial nerve in the spiral groove of the humerus (at the back of the arm), if he lay unconscious for any length of time on a hard surface, for example, a floor. Other possibilities include peripheral neuropathy (although alcohol tends to cause a sensory or a mixed motor and sensory neuropathy rather than a pure motor one) or a mononeuropathy secondary to a paraneoplastic syndrome. The most likely cause for a fit in this context would be alcohol withdrawal as he was unable to drink for 24 h and was showing some of the classic signs, for example, agitation and tremor.

Diseases and investigations of the hands

In the earlier parts of this chapter, various medical conditions have been mentioned. These are now described in this section. In general these descriptions are brief though certain aspects not well described in other textbooks are discussed in some detail

Polymyositis

This is a connective tissue disorder causing inflammation of the muscles. There is a progressive proximal weakness and sometimes tenderness of the muscles. It can result in swallowing and respiratory problems.

Dermatomyositis

This is the name given to polymyositis when there is a predominance of dermatological features. Characteristically the skin is photosensitive; there is a lilac heliotrope rash around the eyes and a purple rash across the knuckles known as Gottron's papules (*Heinrich Adolf Gottron (1890–1974), German dermatologist*). There is thought to be an association with certain malignancies.

Ulna nerve palsy

A palsy is an old-fashioned term for paralysis. The ulna nerve arises from the medial cord of the brachial plexus (a network of nerve fibres, in turn arising from the nerve roots C5, C6, C7, C8, and T1, which eventually supplies the upper limb). It provides the motor and sensory supply to the medial aspect of the forearm and hand. Its root value is C8, T1. It can be damaged (1) at the elbow, following a fracture or stab wound or (2) at the wrist, by a stab wound as the nerve runs superficial to the flexor retinaculum (*ret-in-ack-you-lum*) (a fibrous band of connective tissue that forms a roof over the carpal tunnel).

Injury at the elbow

It causes wasting of the small muscles of the hand (except the thenar eminence (the mound of muscle at the base of the thumb) supplied by the median nerve). **Motor**: paralysis of abduction and adduction of the fingers (they will be unable to keep a piece of paper between their fingers, see earlier) and paralysis of adduction of the thumb (adductor pollicis brevis is the only muscle of the thenar eminence supplied by the ulnar nerve). There will be a positive Froment's sign (see p. 236). The combination of weakness and wasting together with the unopposed action of non-paralysed muscle leads to the production of a clawed hand (see p. 230). **Sensory:** loss of sensation over the medial half of the hand and medial one and a half digits on both palmar and dorsal surfaces.

Injury at the wrist

As for the elbow except there is (1) no involvement of the medial forearm muscles and (2) sparing of the sensation over the medial half of the dorsum of the hand.

Function

Despite these deficits the hand is still useful because the thumb and index finger remain functional both in motor and sensory terms and the vital pincer grip can be maintained.

Radial nerve palsy

The radial nerve arises from the posterior cord of the brachial plexus. It mainly supplies the triceps muscle (producing extension at the elbow), the long extensors of the forearm (extending the wrist and fingers), and sensation over the posterior aspect of the arm, forearm, lateral half of the hand, and lateral three and a half digits. It can be damaged (1) in the axilla, due to upward pressure from a crutch or a drunk falling asleep with their arm dangling over the back of a chair or due to downward traction on the nerve following a fracture dislocation of the neck of the humerus or (2) in the spiral groove of the humerus. This is a groove in the posterior aspect of the shaft of the humerus. The radial nerve can be injured due to a fracture of the shaft of the humerus or due to pressure from callus formation following a fracture or to a tightly fitting plaster cast. It can also occur in an unconscious patient if the back of the arm rests against a hard surface for a long time.

Injury in the axilla

Motor: paralysis of the triceps muscle leading to loss of extension at the elbow and paralysis of the long extensors of the forearm leading to a wrist drop. **Sensory:** small area of anaesthesia over the posterior surface of the lower arm and forearm and a small variable area of loss over the lateral half of the dorsum of the hand and over the base of the thumb. Note that the area of loss is much less than expected due to overlapping innervation from neighbouring cutaneous nerves.

Injury in the spiral groove of the humerus

As above, except no paralysis of the triceps if the nerve is damaged in the distal part of the spiral groove and only a variable area of sensory loss around the root of the thumb.

Function

Motor function is affected adversely because of the wrist drop. In this position the long flexors of the forearm cannot flex the fingers and therefore grip is impaired. This can be overcome by passively extending the wrist, which allows the flexors to function and restore finger grip.

Median nerve palsy

The median nerve arises from the medial and lateral cords of the brachial plexus. It mainly supplies the long flexor muscles of the forearm (except the medial component, which is supplied by the ulnar nerve), the muscles of the thenar eminence (except adductor pollucis brevis, which is supplied by the ulnar nerve), and sensation over the lateral half of the palm and lateral three and a half digits (palmar surface only). It can be damaged (1) at the elbow following a supracondylar (*soup-ra-con-dill-are*) fracture of the humerus, (2) at the wrist following a stab wound proximal to the flexor retinaculum, or (3) at the wrist due to compression in the carpal tunnel.

Injury at the elbow

It causes wasting of the thenar eminence leading to a 'flattened' hand. **Motor:** wrist flexion is weak with deviation to the medial side due to the unopposed action of the flexor muscles under ulnar nerve control. There will be no finger flexion of the index and middle finger but there will be weak flexion of the ring and little finger because they have some innervation from the ulna nerve. The thumb is practically useless as flexion, abduction, and opposition is lost. **Sensation:** loss of sensation over the lateral half of the palm and the lateral three and a half digits (palmar surface).

Injury at the wrist at the wrist following a stab wound proximal to the flexor retinaculum

As above except the long flexors of the forearm are not affected.

Injury at the wrist due to compression in the carpal tunnel

See below.

Function

This is the most disabling nerve injury of the hand. The hand is rendered useless because of the loss of sensation over the thumb and index finger and the loss of the pincer grip.

Carpal tunnel syndrome

This is compression of the median nerve at the wrist as it travels under the flexor retinaculum (see pp. 232–7). It causes wasting of the thenar eminence and pain and tingling in the arm, hand, and lateral three and a half digits. This tends to be worse at nights and is relieved by shaking the hands on waking. See Table 9.3 for causes of carpal tunnel syndrome.

TABLE 9.3 Causes of carpal tunnel syndrome

Idiopathic
Pregnancy, menopause, oral contraceptive pill
Rheumatoid arthritis
Myxoedema
Acromegaly
Amyloidosis
Gout

Acromegaly

Acromegaly occurs due to excess production of growth hormone in adults. The most common cause is a pituitary adenoma (a benign tumour in the brain). It results in an overgrowth of the body's soft tissues. Individuals with acromegaly have a prominent supraorbital ridge, a large lower jaw resulting in a prognathism (*prog-nath-izm*), and large facial features. Their hands are large and spade shaped, their skin is thickened and greasy, there is a high incidence of diabetes mellitus, and they may have a bitemporal hemianopia due to the adenoma pressing on the optic chiasma (*kie-azma*).

Neurofibromatosis

This is also called Von Recklinghausen's (*wreck-ling-house-enz*) disease (*Friedrich Daniel Von Recklinghausen (1833–1910), German pathologist*). This is an autosomal dominant condition (therefore one of the parents will have some evidence of the disease). Neurofibromas are benign tumours that arise from peripheral nerves, spinal nerve roots, and cranial nerves. They can be few or numerous and may be sessile or pedunculated (*pee-done-cue-late-ed*) (which means they have a stalk). They cause neurological deficits as they grow (slowly) by compressing their nerve of origin. The most common cranial nerve affected is the VIIIth nerve. Those growing on spinal roots can cause spinal cord compression if they extend into the spinal cord. As they grow through the intervertebral foramina, this narrow opening gives the tumour a 'waist' and eventually a dumbbell appearance. There is also an association with café-au-lait spots. There are usually more than five of these brownish pigmented lesions. In a rare form of neurofibromatosis there can be an exuberant overgrowth of neurofibromas leading to gross deformities. It was initially thought that the 'elephant man' was a product of this rare variant. This is now disputed and another even

TABLE 9.4 Day-to-day and finals cases

Parkinsonism
Rheumatoid arthritis
Wasting of the small muscles of the hand
Carpal tunnel syndrome
Ulna nerve palsy
Median nerve palsy
Radial nerve palsy

rarer syndrome (proteus syndrome) has been suggested as the cause. About 1% of patients with neurofibromatosis will have phaechromocytoma (*fay-chrome-owe-site-owe-ma*) (a tumour of the adrenal medulla).

Finals section

The emphasis of this section is on the short cases as this format usually causes the most uncertainty. The Objective Structured Clinical Examinations (OSCEs) usually have more straightforward and standardized instructions. Despite the different formats the clinical approach remains the same. For revision read the examination summary (p. 229) and the keypoints throughout the chapter. See Table 9.4 for day-to-day and Finals cases.

Some advice relating to examination problems

General

Rheumatology cases tend to dominate in hand examinations! There are a wide variety of rheumatological conditions to choose from and patients are often well despite their illness. Despite this you should be on your guard for a neurological condition or the co-existance of the two possibilities in the same patient.

The instruction

The likeliest instruction will be 'examine this patient's hands'.

Problem. You are unsure when asked to examine the hands whether to check the joints or to perform a neurological examination.

Solution. Do not panic, your observation is the key. Quickly look at the hands and determine if there are any abnormalities. Thankfully most joint disease will be immediately obvious. Look for swelling or deformities. If these are spotted you are home free (but do not relax too much as there is still work to be done). If there are no obvious abnormalities visible **then** it is sensible to begin a neurological examination.

General look

Before you plunge into your examination of the hand, sneak a peak at the face and the rest of the body. A patient with a plethoric, round face with purpura on the arms may be cushingoid as a result of steroid treatment for rheumatoid arthritis. Do they have an apathetic face with frontal baldness and bilateral partial ptosis (suggesting myotonia dystrophica)? Is there a heliotrope rash of dermatomyositis? Are there café-au-lait spots or neurofibroamata?

Shake hands with the patient

You need to use some judgement here. If the patient's hand is deformed with joint swelling it may be better **not** to shake hands. If you feel it is safe to do so gently shake the patient's hand. Very occasionally in the examination setting you may be faced with a patient that has difficulty relaxing their grip. This patient may have myotonia dystrophica.

Position the hand

If there is obvious deformity, ask the patient if their hands are painful. If a pillow is handy get them to rest their palms on them. If no pillow is present hold the hands very carefully so as not to cause discomfort.

Observe the hand posture

Is there wrist drop? (radial nerve palsy). Is the hand clawed? (suggesting a possible ulna nerve palsy). Is there a flattened ape-like hand? (possible median nerve palsy).

Inspect

Look for evidence of vasculitis. Look at the muscles. Is there wasting of the thenar eminence? (possible carpal tunnel or other median nerve palsy). Is there wasting of the hypothenar eminence? (possible ulna nerve palsy). Is there generalized wasting of the intrinsic muscles of the hand? (possible ulna nerve palsy). Are there any fasciculations? (highly suggestive of motor neurone disease).

Palpate

Confirm that wasting has occurred in major muscle groups by palpation.

Tone

Check tone and be on the lookout for cog-wheel rigidity if you suspect parkinsonism.

Power

Check all muscle groups and do not forget specialist movements of the hand like opposition of the thumb.

Sensation

Does any sensory loss correspond with a dermatome, a peripheral nerve, peripheral neuropathy, or a cortical lesion?

Function

You need to perform a quick check of function. Get your patient to undo and do up their buttons, hold a pen and write, and so on.

Checklist of key signs for some Finals cases

1. **Parkinsonism.** Mask-like facies, pill-rolling tremor, bradykinesis, lead-pipe and cog-wheel rigidity. Complete your examination by asking the patient to walk. They may have difficulty getting out of a chair and be slow to initiate movement. Their gait will be slow, shuffling steps.

2. **Carpal tunnel syndrome.** Wasting over the thenar eminence, paraesthesia over the first three and a half digits, weakness of abduction and opposition of the thumb, positive Tinel's and Phalen's tests. Remember to look for any possible causes of carpal tunnel syndrome—rheumatoid arthritis, acromegaly.

3. **Radial nerve lesion.** Wrist drop (weak wrist extension), weak grip, altered sensation on the dorsum of the hand between the thumb and index finger.

4. **Ulnar nerve lesion.** Ulnar claw hand, wasting of the small muscles of the hand except over the thenar eminence, sensory loss over the little finger and half the ring finger.

5. **Rheumatoid arthritis.** Swelling and deformity of the wrist, MCP, and PIP joints, muscle wasting, peripheral nerve palsies, signs of vasculitis (p. 390), signs of long-term steroid usage. Complete your examination by looking for complications of rheumatoid arthritis: pulmonary fibrosis—auscultate the lung bases for fine crepitations; Sjogren's syndrome (see p. 391)—ask the patient if they have a dry mouth or eyes; Felty's syndrome—palpate for splenomegaly.

Presentation

Try to be confident—avoid the words 'seems' or 'might'!

Good luck!

Further reading

As for Chapter 8.

CHAPTER 10

Legs

Chapter contents

Introduction

When asked to examine the legs, the majority of cases will be neurological. The legs can also give valuable information in other systemic diseases, for example, congestive heart failure, musculoskeletal disorders, and endocrine diseases. to name a few. This chapter will concentrate on neurological aspects of the legs and includes history taking and eliciting neurological signs. As the spinal cord is important in transmitting neurological information to and from the legs, an analysis of the symptoms referred from the back are also included in this chapter.

Basic neuroanatomy

A basic understanding of the anatomy and physiology of the central and peripheral nervous system of the legs will help you analyse your findings and help you towards a diagnosis. The overview of the pathways described in the chapter on the arms (Chapter 8) is relevant here. I will concentrate on the lower spinal cord and nerve roots.

Motor pathways

The pathways described in Chapter 8 are relevant to the legs and many of the tracts in the legs represent a continuation of the descending tracts that have travelled the cervical and thoracic spinal cord. The lumbosacral segments of the spinal cord are responsible for the innervation of the lower limbs. The lumbar roots L2, L3, and L4 join outside the spinal canal to form the lumbar plexus and give branches that supply the anterior aspect of the thigh through the femoral and obturator (*ob-chew-rater*) nerves. The rest of the leg is supplied by the sacral plexus formed by L4, L5, and the sacral roots via the sciatic (*sigh-attic*) nerve and its branches and the tibial (*tib-i-al*) and common peroneal (*pe-roe-knee-al or per-owe-nial*) nerve.

A further point to note is that the spinal cord terminates at the level of the L1 vertebrae. Nerve roots below this point pass vertically downwards to supply the lower body and limbs. Collectively the nerve roots are referred to as the cauda equina (*cord-a-equine-a*). The dura mater (*dure-a-may-ter*), the protective sheath surrounding the spinal cord (and which is continuous with the dura mater covering the brain) continues downwards before terminating at the level of S2. This gap between spinal cord and dura mater is filled by cerebrospinal fluid (CSF), as well as the cauda equina and it is here that CSF can be removed by lumbar puncture for analysis in relative safety (there is a risk of damage to the spinal cord if this technique is performed at a level higher than L1). See Fig. 10.1.

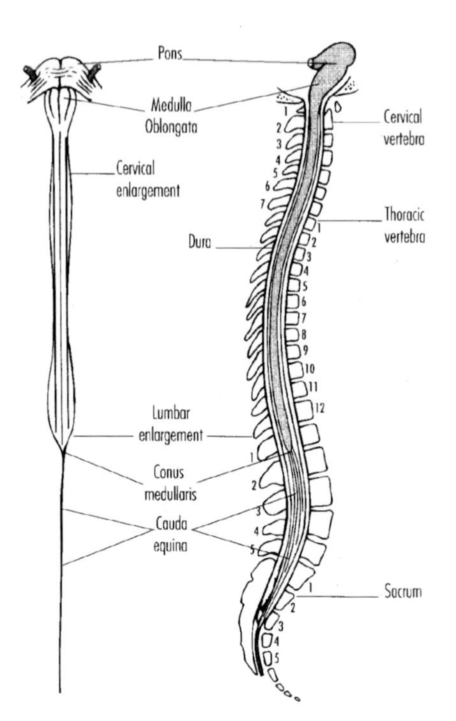

Fig. 10.1 The anatomy of the lumbar region demonstrating the termination of the spinal cord. Reproduced by permission of Oxford University Press from **Fig. 6.5** (p. 67), *Neurology*, by M Donaghy (1997).

Sensory pathways

See Fig. 10.2. All sensory information in the legs is conducted from specialized nerve endings in the legs via their cutaneous nerve supply. These in turn are the branches of the major nerves supplying the legs, that is, the femoral nerve, the obturator nerve, and the sciatic nerve. As with the arms, the nerve fibres conveying light touch and proprioception ascend in the dorsal columns of the spinal cord (see p. 196) and those carrying pain and temperature ascend in the lateral (and anterior) spinothalamic tracts. Vibration sense is probably transmitted along both dorsal columns and spinothalamic tracts.

Symptoms

See the 'Symptoms' section in Chapter 8.

The importance of examining the legs

No neurological examination is complete without examining the legs. Findings in the legs taken in conjunction with those from elsewhere help in the final localization of a neurological lesion. In fact important clues can be gained from simply watching a patient walk. Therefore as elsewhere, repeated practice is the key (in normal indi-

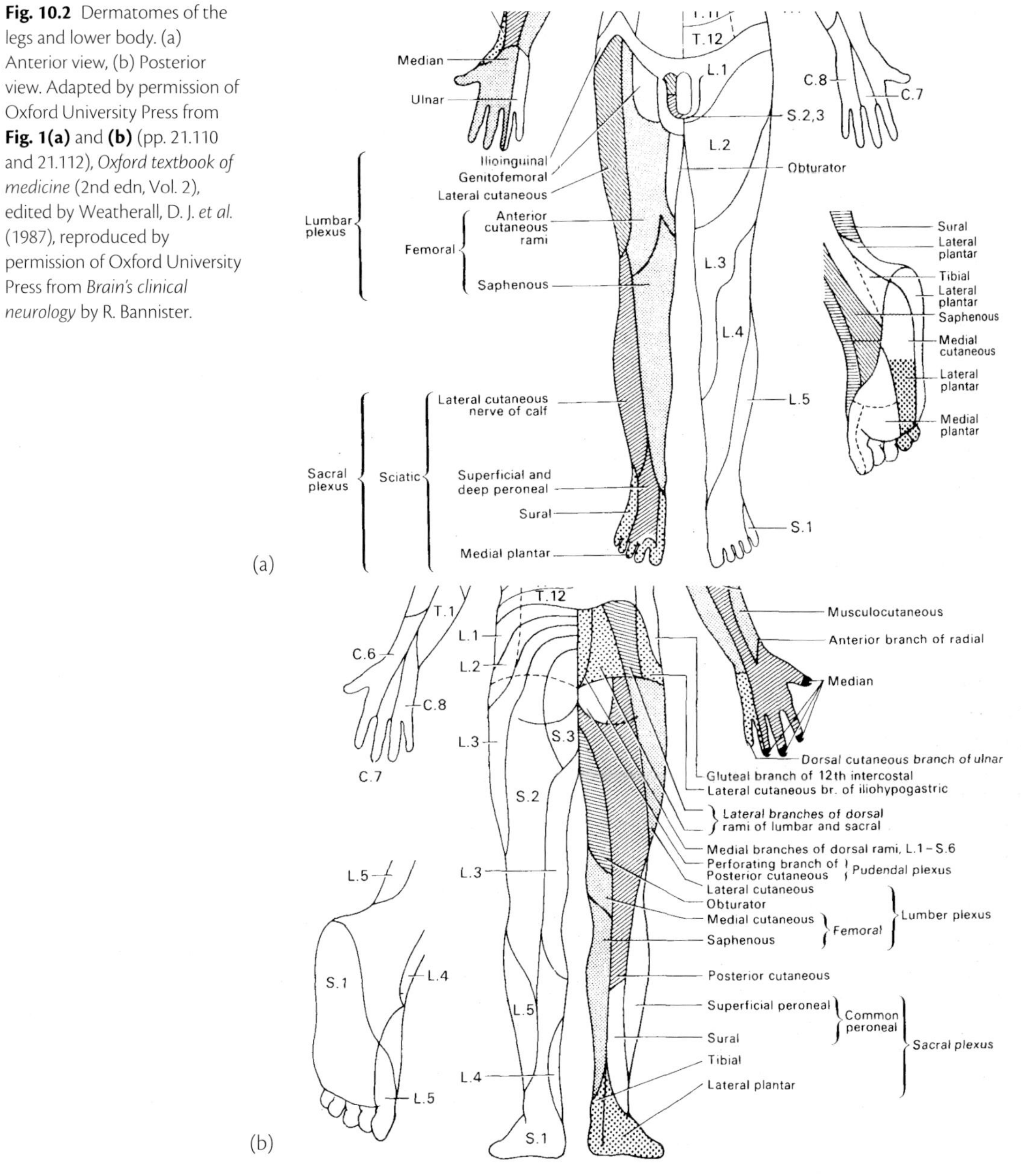

Fig. 10.2 Dermatomes of the legs and lower body. (a) Anterior view, (b) Posterior view. Adapted by permission of Oxford University Press from **Fig. 1(a)** and **(b)** (pp. 21.110 and 21.112), *Oxford textbook of medicine* (2nd edn, Vol. 2), edited by Weatherall, D. J. *et al.* (1987), reproduced by permission of Oxford University Press from *Brain's clinical neurology* by R. Bannister.

viduals as well as patients). Being proficient in neurological examination will not only help you with diagnosis but will guide further investigation and management.

Examination of the legs summary

1. Preparation.
2. Introduce yourself to the patient and ask for permission to examine.
3. Ask the patient to get on to the bed (if not already on the bed). You may need to help!
4. Ask the patient to strip to their underwear.
5. Whilst doing 1–3, have a 'general look' Pain/discomfort? Mood? Are they unsteady? Is there generalized wasting? Is there a walking aid nearby?
6. Inspection: look for wasting (DF 4/10), fasciculations (DF 6/10), contractures (DF 4/10), trophic ulcers (DF 5/10), and involuntary movements (DF 7/10).

7. Assess tone at the hip, knee, and ankle (DF 5/10).
8. Test for clonus (DF 6/10).
9. Test power, proximally to distally (DF 5/10).
10. Test reflexes: knee (DF 4/10) and ankle (DF 9/10).
11. Test plantar reflex (DF 8/10).
12. Test co-ordination: heel–shin test (DF 6/10) and foot tapping movements (DF 4/10).
13. Assess sensation: light touch (DF 7/10), pain (DF 6/10), vibration sense (DF 5/10), and proprioception (DF 6/10).
14. Get your patient to stand: perform Romberg's test (DF 5/10).
15. Assess gait (DF 7/10).
16. Make sure your patient is comfortable and thank them for their time.
17. Wash your hands.
18. Analysing your findings.
19. Presentation.

Examination of the legs in detail

1. Preparation.

Get your equipment ready. You will need

- tendon hammer
- 'neuropins'
- cotton wool
- tuning fork (128 Hz).

Carry the last three items in a receiving bowl for convenience.

2. Introduce yourself to the patient and ask for permission to examine.

Introduce yourself whilst shaking their hand; say something like, 'Hello, I'm Joseph Babinski, a second-year Polish exchange student. Do you mind if I examine your legs?'

3. Ask the patient to get on to the bed (if not already on the bed). You may need to help!

If the patient is unable to get on to the bed, offer your assistance or get help. However before you do this try and work out why the patient is having difficulty. Are they unsteady? Do they have weakness in their leg muscles or pain in their joints? If you are unsure do not be afraid to ask, as the reason may have direct relevance to the rest of your neurological examination.

4. Ask the patient to strip to their underwear.

Adequate exposure of the legs is important. The legs can be examined with the patient either sitting up or laid down in bed. Once in bed ask the patient to undress to their undergarments and ensure adequate exposure to chest level.

5. Whilst doing 1–4, have a 'general look'. Pain/discomfort? Mood? Are they unsteady? Is there generalized wasting? Is there a walking aid nearby?

You need to pick up as many clues as you can with your general look. Many of the features discussed in the 'general look' for the arms are relevant for the legs. This has to be brief but packed with as many clues as you can digest. Does your patient look in pain or discomfort? Pay particular attention to their mood. The spine is also important and a quick glance here as the patient is getting undressed and settling on the bed is very useful. Look for deformities such as kyphoscoliosis (see p. 381), as there is an association with some neurodegenerative conditions, for example, Friedrich's ataxia (see p. 221). Surgical scars may suggest previous operation (for example, laminectomy) and hint at a chronic back problem. Watch the patient as they get on to the bed. Are they unsteady? This could suggest weakness in the legs or a cerebellar lesion (see p. 219). A patient with proximal weakness will try and support their thighs with their hands and lift their legs onto the bed. Also look for clues around the bed, for example, a diabetic sticker (peripheral neuropathy, mononeuritis multiplex (see p. 264), or diabetic amyotrophy (see p. 265))? Aids such as a walking stick, zimmer frame, or wheelchair are major pointers to a difficulty with walking.

6. Inspection: look for wasting (DF 4/10), fasciculations (DF 6/10), contractures (DF 4/10), trophic ulcers (DF 5/10), and involuntary movements (DF 7/10).

Your general look should now become more focused. Stand at the end of the bed and begin inspecting the legs.

Wasting

As with the arms, if you detect any wasting, you need to know if it is generalized or confined to a specific muscle group. Is there asymmetry, which could suggest a root or a specific nerve lesion? Gross wasting and shortening of a limb of long standing may suggest previous poliomyelitis (the patient may wear a built-up shoe to compensate for the unequal leg lengths). Wasting of the thighs preferentially may suggest a proximal myopathy (any associated tenderness of the muscles should make you consider

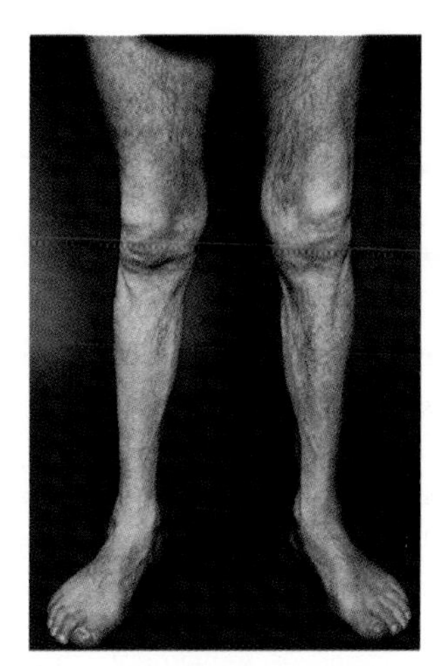

Fig. 10.3 Hereditary sensory motor neuropathy (Charcot Marie Tooth disorder). Reprinted from **Fig. 2.2** (p. 2.2), *Atlas of Clinical Neurology* (2nd edn), by G. David Perkin, Fred Hochberg, and Douglas C. Miller (1993), Mosby Publications, with permission from Elsevier.

poly/dermatomyositis). One characteristic pattern of wasting can be seen with Charcot Marie Tooth disease (*Jean Martin Charcot (1825– 1893), French neurologist, Pierre Marie (1853–1940), French neurologist, Howard Henry Tooth (1856–1925), English physician*) (also known as hereditary sensory motor neuropathy (HSMN)) (see Fig. 10.3). The wasting begins distally and spreads up the leg sometimes stopping mid-calf. The appearance produced is often likened to an inverted champagne bottle. It is also associated with pes cavus (an abnormally pronounced plantar arch), as is Friedrich's ataxia. Remember that most causes of wasting (if malnutrition is excluded) are due to lower motor neurone (LMN) lesions. Upper motor lesions seldom cause muscle wasting but if it is present it is often due to chronic disuse and is less marked. Do not be afraid to palpate the muscle bulk to confirm wasting. Wasted hypotonic muscle tends to be flabby, soft, and insubstantial (compare this with your own muscles).

Fasciculations

See the description on p. 203.

Contractures

These can result from any longstanding neurological disease. Contractures are a result of longstanding upper and lower motor lesions following chronic disuse and lead to a stiff deformed limb. This is due to shortening of structures such as tendons, muscles, joint capsules, skin, and connective tissue. The underlying pathophysiology is not known but the condition is preventable by regular 'passive' movement of a paralysed limb.

Trophic ulcers

These are usually found on the soles opposite the metatarsophalangeal joints, which are major pressure points during weight bearing. They indicate severe peripheral nerve injury and are seen most commonly in diabetes mellitus.

Involuntary movements

Refer to the section on involuntary movements in Chapter 8. The range of disorders described there can affect the legs also. I have also added a further two conditions here for completeness.

Extensor spasm

This is a non-specific feature of upper motor neurone (UMN) disease and is a sudden jerky movement (usually of the hip). It can be uncomfortable and even painful for the patient. It is thought to be due to the release of inhibitory impulses of the dorsal reticulo-spinal fibres on the LMNs.

Associated reactions

This can also occur in longstanding, UMN pathology (usually stroke). When a patient changes the posture of a limb or performs an involuntary act, for example, a yawn, there may be an accompanying movement of a normally paralysed limb, for example, a hemiplegic leg may flex in response to the yawn. Its importance lies in the false promise it conveys. A patient may feel that movement is returning in the limb and be filled with optimism, only to find their hopes dashed later on.

7. Assess tone at the hip, knee, and ankle (DF 5/10).

See Fig. 10.4. The principle of assessing tone in the legs is the same as in the arms. The key to getting reliable results is a comfortable and relaxed patient. Check that they do not have pain in their legs or joints prior to

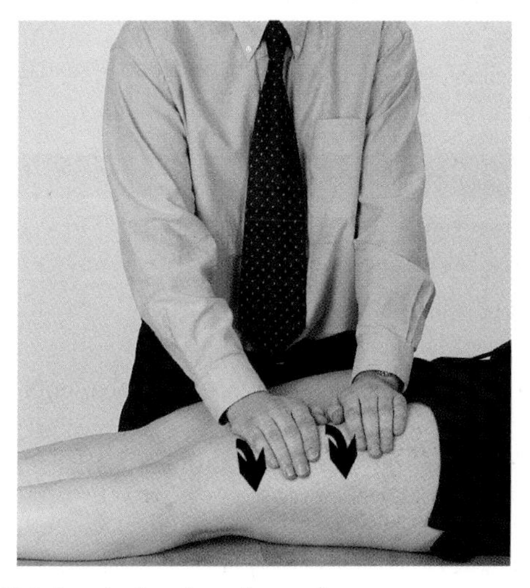

Fig. 10.4 Examination of tone (see text).

> **Tip**
>
> When assessing tone at the knee, pay particular attention to the leg just after you have flexed it upwards and have removed your displacing force. If the patient is relaxed the leg should flop back naturally on to the bed. However if they are not relaxed, the leg remains in the flexed position and does not flop back on to the bed. You should also see the telltale contraction of the quadriceps muscle and if this is the case your assessment of tone is void and needs to be repeated.

assessing. Say to your patient, ' let your leg go nice and floppy, just relax and let me do the moving.' Then place the flat of both your hands on your target leg and gently rotate it inwards and outwards (as if you were using a rolling pin to flatten dough). Now place both hands under the knee and quickly lift them about 6 inches and then let go (this movement should flex the knee partially). A normal leg should be rolled very easily; there should be little resistance when the knee is displaced upwards and it should flop back readily on to the bed (repeated practice on patients with normal tone should help you generate a 'feel' for this).

With a spastic leg there is much more resistance and the knee is difficult to flex. A hypotonic leg is floppy like a rag doll; it will be flexed quite easily and will readily flop back on to the bed. As with the assessment of tone in the arms try to make your movements of varying amplitudes and unpredictable.

8. Test for clonus (DF 6/10).

- **What is clonus?** This is a rhythmical jerking movement, which can be produced by applying a rapid stretch (and sustaining that stretch) to a muscle. The jerking represents an initial reflex contraction to protect the muscle, followed by relaxation. If you maintain a stretch on the muscle it will contract and relax again and may enter an iterative cycle of contraction and relaxation, which can be sustained for numerous beats (greater than five beats usually indicates pathology).
- **Significance.** The presence of sustained clonus implies the presence of an UMN lesion affecting the limb under test.
- **How to examine.** Clonus is traditionally demonstrated at the ankle or knee. To elicit ankle clonus, simply grasp the forefoot and dorsiflex it sharply (but not violently) and maintain some upward pressure at the end of the range of movement (this maintains a stretch on the tendon). If clonus is present you will feel the foot start to jerk up and down. Keep pressing up on the foot as this will provide the stretch that will maintain the phenomenon. See Fig. 10.5. To elicit knee clonus, grip the lateral borders of the patella (kneecap) between your thumb and other fingers. Now pull it down sharply as far as it will go and then maintain some downward pressure. If clonus is present the patella will jerk up and down rhythmically.

> **Keypoints**
>
> - Make sure your patient is relaxed (and remains relaxed) when testing tone.
> - Hypertonia indicates an UMN lesion.
> - Hypotonia is very subtle to detect.
> - Hypotonia indicates a LMN lesion.
> - If an abnormality of tone is found try to anticipate other possible findings, for example, hyperreflexia, clonus, extensor plantar, or hemiplegic or spastic gait (see below).

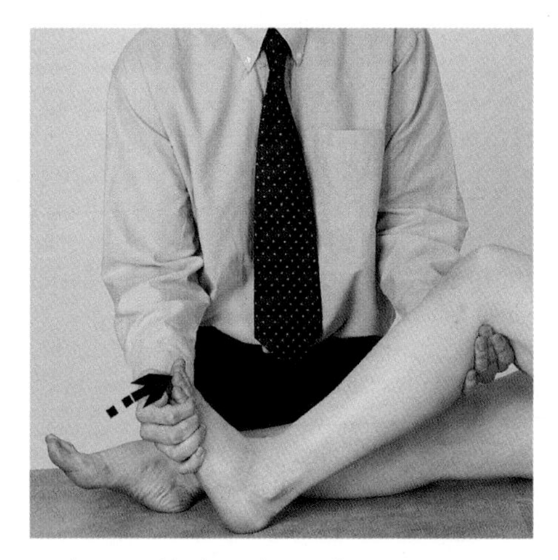

Fig. 10.5 Eliciting ankle clonus (see text).

> **Tip**
>
> A more elegant way of demonstrating knee clonus is to place your index finger at the top of the patella and to strike it gently downwards with a tendon hammer. Remember to maintain some downward pressure with your index finger at the end of the manoeuvre.

Keypoints

- Clonus can be demonstrated at the knee and ankle.
- The presence of sustained clonus indicates an UMN lesion.

9. Test power, proximally to distally (DF 5/10).

Test power as you did for the arms and use the Medical Research Council (MRC) scale to grade your findings. Also make sure that you double-check for the possibility of painful joints prior to your assessment.

Hip flexion and extension

See Figs 10.6 and 10.7. Say to your patient, 'lift up your leg, don't let me push it down' (hip flexion L1, L2, L3). As they raise their leg, place your hand on the top of the thigh and push down. If the patient is unable to raise their leg against gravity (by MRC definition, less than grade 3/5), get them to lie on their side to eliminate gravity from the movement (the side opposite to the leg being tested). Now get them to flex their hip again. If they can, this is grade 2/5. If they cannot and there is only a flicker of contraction, this is grade 1/5. No contraction is grade 0/5. Do the same for the other leg. Now put your hand under the thigh and say to your patient, 'push down with your leg' or 'pull your leg into the bed' (hip extension L5, S1). Remember that this movement is aided by gravity and therefore you also have to make an empirical judgement for grade 2/5–3/5. The purists may suggest that you lie your patient face down on the bed and raise their leg so that gravity is a factor again but this is not necessary and leads to your patient having to change position numerous times.

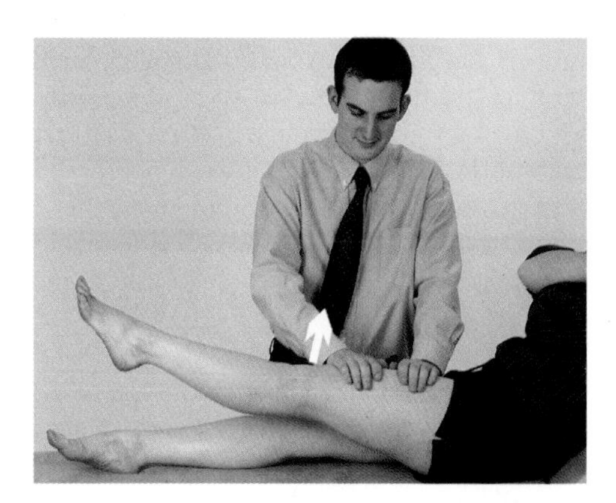

Fig. 10.6 Assessing the power of hip flexion. Arrows represent the direction of force generated by the patient.

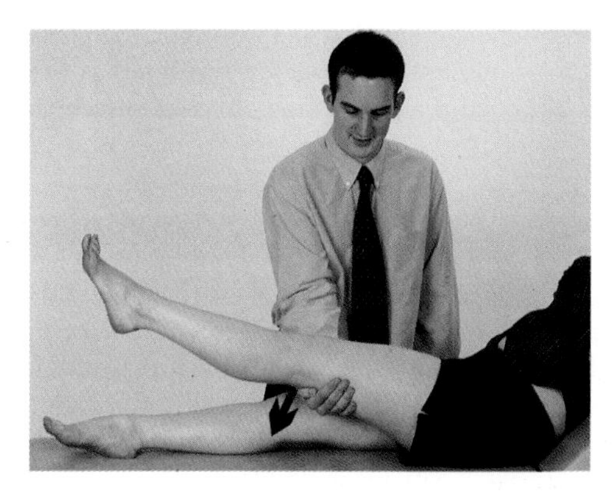

Fig. 10.7 Assessing the power of hip extension.

Hip abduction and adduction

Place your hands on the lateral aspect of each thigh and say, 'spread your legs apart and push against my hand' (abduction L4, L5, S1). Now place your hands on the inner aspect of each thigh and say, 'pull your legs together' (adduction L2, L3, L4). Compare both hip movements together and grade them. Gravity is not a major influence on these movements and therefore grades 2/5–3/5 will have to be estimated.

Knee flexion and extension

See Figs 10.8 and 10.9. Now get your patient to bend their knees up in the air. As they do this place your hand on the back of the calf and say, 'pull me towards you as hard as you can'or 'pull your heel in towards your bottom' (flexion L5, S1) and resist the subsequent movement. Now test the other leg. Then move your hand to the front of the shin and say, 'push me away now as hard as you can' (extension L3, L4) and resist it. Grade the power for both legs as before.

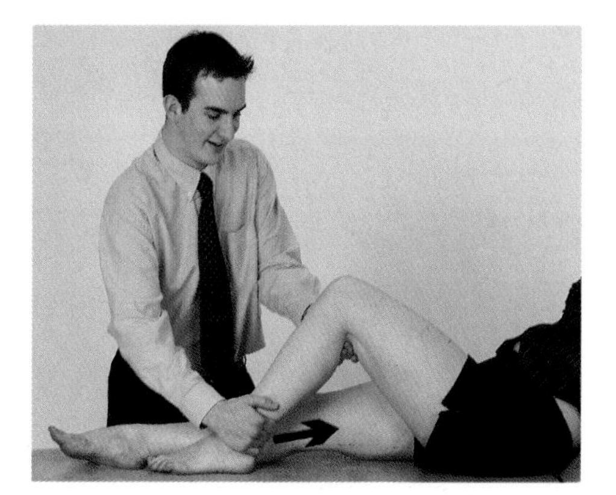

Fig. 10.8 Assessing the power of knee flexion.

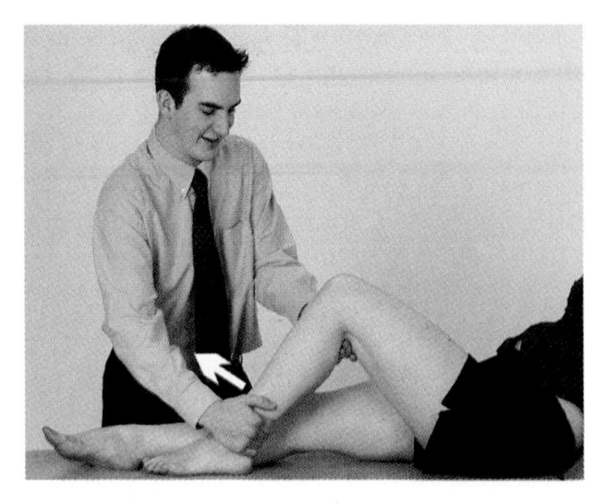

Fig. 10.9 Assessing the power of knee extension.

Dorsiflexion and plantarflexion of feet

See Figs 10.10 and 10.11. Say, ' cock your feet up.' When the patient has complied place your hands on the dorsum of the foot and say, 'don't let me push them down' (dorsiflexion L4, L5). Resist the movement. It is possible to assess both feet at the same time by placing the legs alongside each other and then providing resistance with the back of your hand and forearm on the dorsum of the feet. Now place your hands on the soles and say, ' push me away now' and resist the movement (plantarflexion S1). Grade all movements as before.

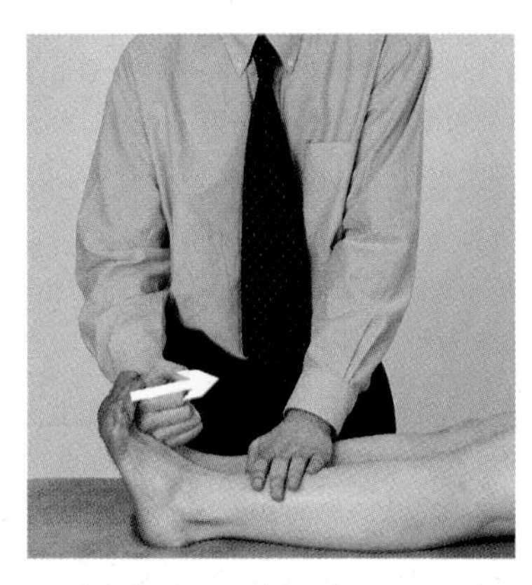

Fig. 10.10 Assessing the power of dorsiflexion.

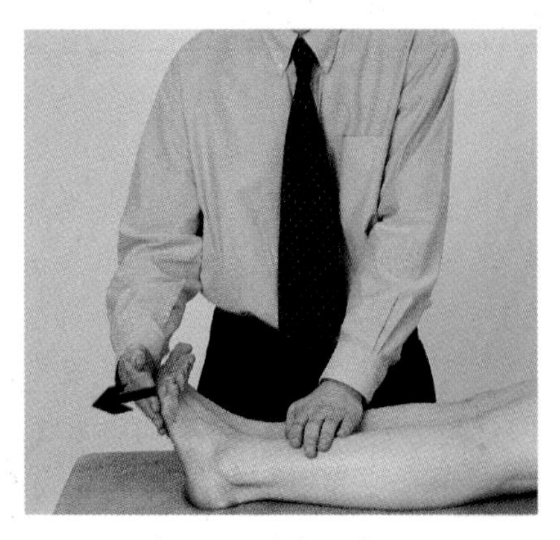

Fig. 10.11 Assessing the power of plantarflexion.

> **Tip**
>
> If a patient has a foot drop do not assume that they cannot plantarflex their foot. You will have to physically dorsiflex the foot before asking them to push their foot down. You may be surprised to find that this movement may be unaffected.

Inversion and eversion of the foot

These movements are not often tested but are useful if motor deficits have been found in your previous assessments. Ensure that the patient's leg is fully relaxed on the bed. Now place your fingers on the medial border of their sole and say, 'turn your foot in towards my fingers ... don't let me move it' (inversion L4). Remove your fingers and place them on the lateral border of the foot and say, ' turn your foot out towards my fingers ... don't let me move it' (eversion S1). Make sure that the only part of the leg that moves is the foot. Check both feet and grade accordingly and remember that both these movements are relatively weak compared to the larger muscle groups.

Toe extension and flexion

Place your thumb or index finger on the nail of the big toe and say, ' cock up your big toe' and resist the action (extension L5). Now place your digit on the sole of the big toe and say, ' push your toe away' and resist again (flexion S1).

10. Test reflexes: knee (DF 4/10) and ankle (DF 9/10).

The technique for eliciting and recording the results of the knee and ankle reflexes are the same as for the arms, although the positioning of the patient requires some attention.

> **Tip**
>
> While you are assessing power, every now and then glance at your patient's face and make sure that they are not grimacing with pain. If the power is limited it is worth asking whether it was pain or lack of power that restricted their performance because some patients will suffer in silence.

Keypoints

- Try to recall the root values of the muscles being tested as this will help in localizing the neurological lesion.
- Make sure your patient gives their maximum effort (but without resorting to a trial of strength).
- Make sure it is a lack of power and not pain which is reducing performance.

Knee jerk

(L3, L4.) See Fig. 10.12. Make sure your patient is lying relaxed and comfortable on the bed. Inform the patient about the test: 'I am just going to check your reflexes. Just relax your legs and let them rest in my hands.' Gently insert your hand underneath the knee and gently lift the knee off the bed. Check to make sure the full weight of the leg is resting on your arm. If it is not and you can see them contracting their quadriceps muscle, reinforce your request to relax. Strike the patellar tendon, which lies between the patella and its insertion at the tibial tuberosity (about 4–6 cm below). Watch for the leg jerking forward or if this is not obvious, the contraction of the quadriceps muscle above. Observe the response you get and grade it according to the scale on p. 211; then do the other knee and compare.

Ankle reflex

(L5, S1.) See Figs 10.13 and 10.14. The ankle jerks can be particularly awkward to demonstrate. First warn your patient, 'I am going to move your leg and I need you to stay completely relaxed.' Now flex the knee and laterally rotate the leg letting the leg flop naturally to the side (some people place the ankle on the opposite leg before rotating the leg under test). Dorsiflex the ankle with your non-dominant hand to put the achilles tendon on stretch and strike the tendon, just above its attachment to the heel. Observe for plantar flexion and also for contraction of the calf muscle. The left ankle jerk is even more fiddly as your non-dominant arm is forced up in an awkward arch as you dorsiflex the left foot and you have to swing your tendon hammer within this arch at an unusual angle to strike the tendon. The potential for tying yourself in an embarrassing knot has never been

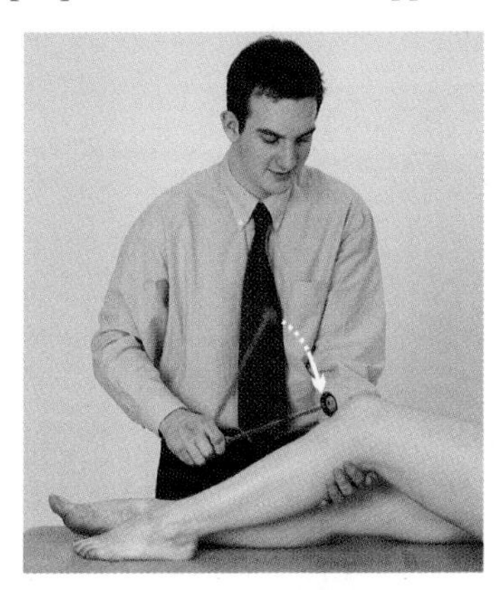

Fig. 10.12 Eliciting the knee reflex. The technique is the same for both knees.

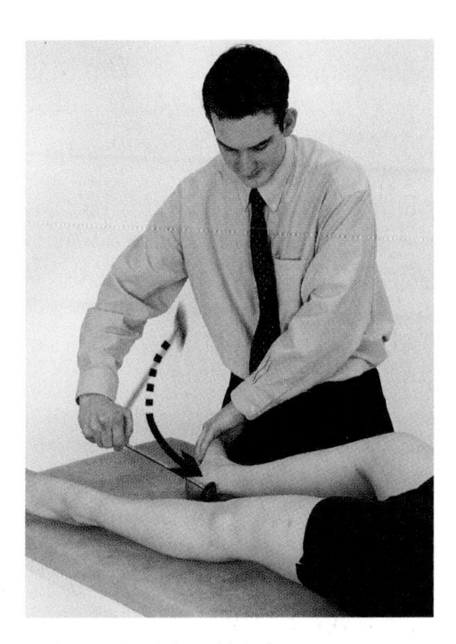

Fig. 10.13 Eliciting the right ankle jerk.

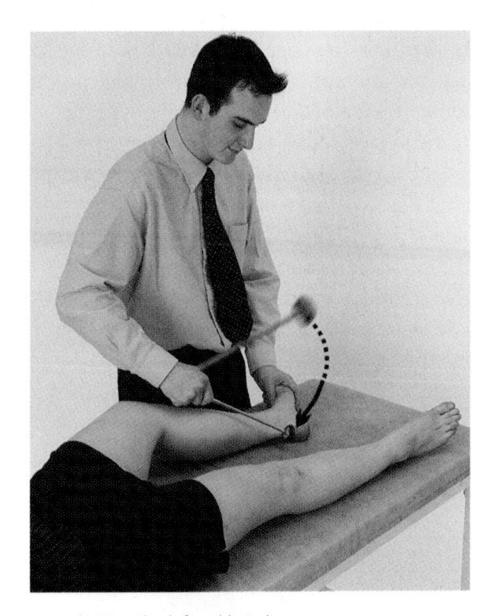

Fig. 10.14 Eliciting the left ankle jerk.

Tip

Another less elaborate way of eliciting the ankle jerks is to keep the legs relaxed and lying on the bed. You need to be standing on the right side of the bed facing towards the feet. In this position, you simply dorsiflex the foot with your non-dominant hand and then strike this hand with the tendon hammer. This procedure is not recommended for an examination situation (currently).

Tip

Learn to elicit the left ankle jerk well because it is used as 'quality assurance' for the standard of medical students' neurological examination by some examiners. If these examiners see that you cannot perform this proficiently they will automatically fail you so be warned!

so high, therefore, practice is the key. Grade the reflexes as before and attempt reinforcement if you cannot elicit a response (see below). The authors advocate walking around the bed or couch and performing the left ankle jerk as they do the right. It is simple to perform and at the end of the day it is the result that is crucial (providing the ankle jerk is elicited with an equivalent stimulus to the right to enable a valid comparison).

If any of the lower limb reflexes are absent despite adequate relaxation, then attempt them again with reinforcement. To do this, get the patient to interlock the fingers of both hands together (palms facing each other and the fingers of the topmost hand hooking into the curled up fingers of the hand below). Ask the patient to pull them apart when you give the word. Say, 'Now!' on the upswing of your tendon hammer. If your timing is right you should strike the tendon at the same time as your patient starts performing the manoeuvre. This is sometimes known as Jendrassik's *(jen-drass-icks)* manoeuvre *(Erno Jendrassik (1858–1921), Hungarian physician)* (see Fig. 10.15). Grade your response as on p. 211.

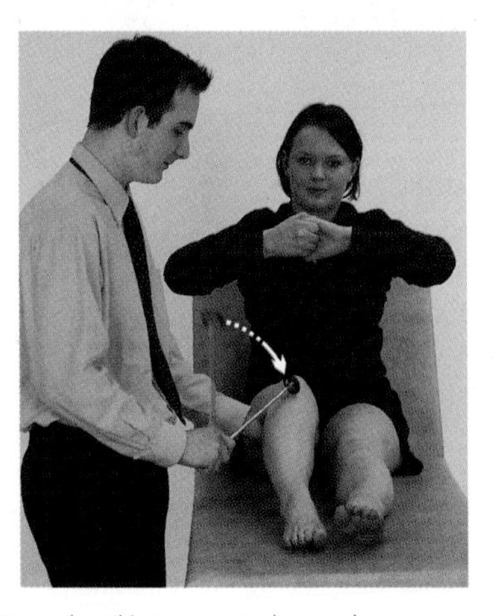

Fig. 10.15 Jendrassik's manoeuvre (see text).

Keypoints

- Make sure your patient is relaxed throughout the examination.
- Try to recall the root values of the reflexes as this will aid in the localization of the lesion, for example, knee jerk (L3, L4).
- Hyper-reflexia indicates an upper motor lesion above the level of the reflex arc.
- An absence of reflexes indicates a lower motor lesion at the level of the reflex arc.
- Make sure you are particularly proficient in eliciting the left ankle jerk.
- Always attempt reinforcement before saying a reflex is absent.

11. Test plantar reflex (DF 8/10).

See Fig. 10.16. This is the most important of the superficial reflexes. It is a reflex contraction that occurs as the result of a scratch-like stimulus to the skin. This reflex is tested using a firm stimulus on the sole of the foot. Warn the patient beforehand: 'I'm just going to scratch the bottom of your foot.' Using the blunt tip of a key or an orange stick, apply a firm stroke starting at the heel, moving upwards along the lateral border and across the metatarsophalageal joints of the toes taking care not to touch the ball of the big toe. This can cause

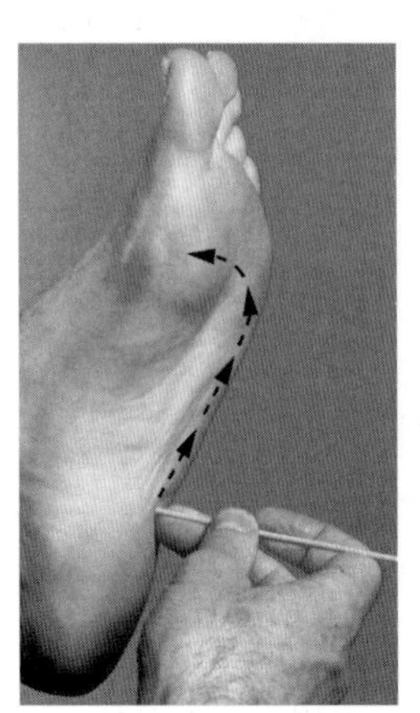

Fig. 10.16 Eliciting the plantar reflex. A normal flexor response is indicated by the arrow. Reproduced by permission of Oxford University Press from **Fig. 2.35(a)** (p. 31), *Neurology*, by M Donaghy (1997).

flexion of the big toe, sometimes called a withdrawal response. Observe the first movement of the big toe carefully. A normal response is a downgoing flexor response of the big toe. If the response is an upward extension of the big toe, this is abnormal and it is termed an extensor plantar or a positive Babinski response (*Joseph Jules François Felix Babinski (1807–1875), French neurologist of Polish descent*). A positive Babinski response is indicative of an UMN lesion (note that there is no equivalent 'negative Babinski response' for a normal flexor response). Some people advocate looking for a fanning movement of the other toes to help in deciding whether a plantar is upgoing but this can be misleading, so stick to observing the big toe only. An absent response is encountered in severe peripheral neuropathy due to severe sensory impairment, total paralysis, or even when the patient is tense.

12. Test co-ordination: heel–shin test (DF 6/10) and foot tapping movements (DF 4/10).

CASE 10.1

Problem. You are concluding your neurological examination and have found no abnormalities, but when you elicit the plantar reflex the toe goes upwards. Is this a positive Babinski response?

Discussion. The likely answer is no. You would only expect a positive Babinski response in the presence of an upper motor neuron (UMN) lesion, in which case you would elicit other related signs such as spasticity, clonus, or hyper-reflexia. You may also see a positive Babinski response in an unconscious patient or in someone with an encephalopathy, which is not the case here. The likeliest scenario is the withdrawal response. This is usually elicited in someone who is anxious or ticklish. A full-blown response includes an upgoing big toe accompanied by a rapid flexion at the knee as the leg is lifted away from the noxious stimulus. The key to the true plantar response is the very first movement of the big toe. This requires close observation of the big toe (pray that your patient has washed their feet). The very first movement is fleeting but is downgoing before the withdrawal response. Often this first movement is so difficult that many members of a medical team disagree. If you are faced with uncertainty, remember to weigh up the consequences of a positive sign in the context of other clinical features. In this case there were no other neurological features to make a positive Babinski response tenable.

Keypoints

- Make sure you use a blunt instrument such as a key or orange stick to elicit the plantar reflex.
- An upgoing plantar is consistent with an UMN lesion.
- The first direction of movement of the big toe is the crucial one.
- An upgoing plantar is termed an extensor plantar response or a positive Babinski sign.

Inco-ordination of leg movements as with the arms can indicate a lesion in the cerebellum or involvement of its tracts in the spinal cord or brainstem. Beware of making any judgement on co-ordination in the presence of spasticity or weakness of grade 3/5 or less.

Heel–shin

See Fig. 10.17. Make sure the patient is lying flat in the bed with both legs straight. Ask him to lift the leg and place the heel on to the opposite knee. Then get him to

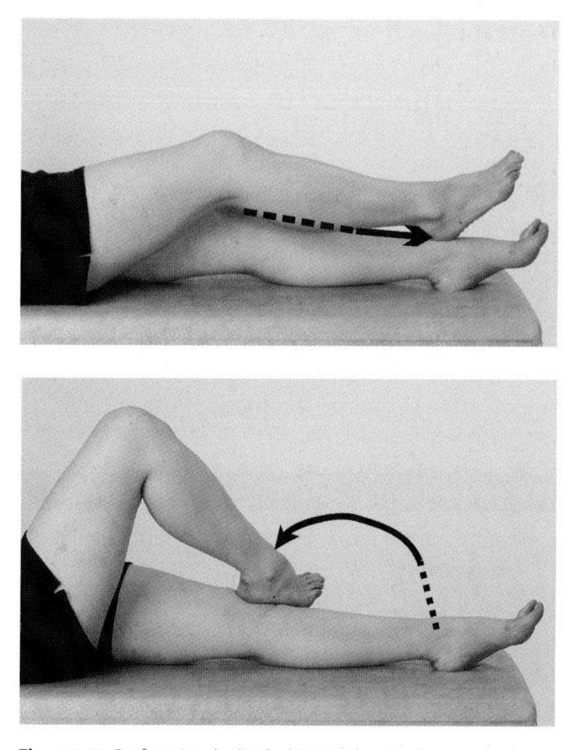

Fig. 10.17 Performing the heel–shin test (see text).

slide the heel along the shin until he reaches the ankle. Now ask him to lift the heel back up to the knee and repeat this cycle a few times (about three times is sufficient). It is useful to do a rehearsal by getting hold of the patient's leg and guiding it through the sequence of events. Once the patient has started it is also helpful to prompt them to remind them of their objectives, for example, 'slide down the shin ... to the ankle', 'now lift it up', ' go back to the knee', and 'slide down again'. A normal person can do this quickly and efficiently. A person with inco-ordination will find that their foot might shake on the shin and veer away from the ankle (you may see the heel drop off the shin before reaching the ankle). Sometimes people may make it to the ankle but the clue to some degree of inco-ordination is that the movement is slow, hesitant, and very deliberate. If you are suspicious of inco-ordination go on to check the patient's gait (see below) as well as looking for evidence of this in the upper limbs (and nystagmus). You can increase the sensitivity of this test by holding your finger about a metre above the patient's foot and asking them to touch it with their big toe after they have reached the ankle. If they are unable to locate your finger with their toe, this is further evidence that could support a cerebellar lesion. From this point they can begin the cycle again by putting their heel back on the knee. Go on to check the other leg.

Foot tapping

This is the lower limb's equivalent of tapping the back of your hand. Simply place the palm of your hand near the forefoot of the leg being tested. It should be close enough for the foot to make contact when it is plantarflexed. Say to your patient, 'tap your foot as fast as you can.' Although the foot is naturally clumsier than the hand a normal person can still tap fairly rapidly, that is, between three and five taps per second. Any slower than this suggests inco-ordination. The problem with this test is that it is not very specific for cerebellar disorder. The inco-ordination you demonstrate here could simply be natural clumsiness. However if other

Keypoints

- Do not make hasty judgements regarding inco-ordination of the legs in the presence of weakness (3/5 or less in the legs), spasticity, or involuntary movements.
- Mild inco-ordination in the legs may just reflect clumsiness. If you find inco-ordination, look for further evidence of cerebellar disease elsewhere.

CASE 10.2

Problem. A 45-year-old woman was admitted via casualty with difficulty walking. She had a 2-week history of progressive leg weakness and stiffness. In addition, she noticed some numbness in both legs. There were no bowel or bladder symptoms. When asked about previous symptoms she recalled a time in her twenties, where she experienced blurring of the vision in her right eye, which resolved after a few days. On examination, she was apyrexial and had evidence of inco-ordination, dysdiadochokinesia, and an intention tremor, with past-pointing in the left arm. She had increased tone in both legs, plus clonus in the right leg. Power was reduced to 3/5 in the right leg and 4/5 in the left leg. There was generalized hyper-reflexia. There was also sensory loss extending up the legs to the umbilicus (*um-be-like-us*). Her cranial nerve examination was normal except for nystagmus to the left. What is the diagnosis?

Discussion. At first sight this case seems a nightmare, overflowing with all sorts of neurological signs. You need to try and digest the information, breaking it up into smaller pieces and see if you can recognize any patterns. Start with the motor system. The collection of signs in the left arm (together with the nystagmus to the left in the cranial nerves) should make you think of a cerebellar lesion in its left hemisphere. The signs in the legs are different. They point to bilateral UMN lesions affecting the legs (this pattern is called a spastic paraparesis). However there are no UMN signs in the arms, which means that the lesion has to be below the nerve supply to the arms, which points to its location being at the thoracic level or lower in the spine. There are a number of causes of a spastic paraparesis but the presence of a sensory level is worrying. It suggests spinal cord compression and the level demonstrated on examination (up to the umbilicus) further localizes the lesion within a few spinal segments around the T10 level. This is a neurological emergency and urgent magnetic resonance imaging (MRI) (or a computed tomography (CT) myelogram) needs to be performed. However, spinal cord compression does not explain the left-sided cerebellar signs. To do this you would have to think of a second condition unrelated to the cord compression (for example, stroke) to explain every-

(*continue*)

CASE 10.2 (*continued*)

thing. Although this is possible the patient would be unlucky to have two different pathologies at the same time. A much better explanation for her condition is multiple sclerosis (MS). Plaques of demyelination can be found scattered throughout the central nervous system, which can lead to unusual patterns of neurological signs that are not easy to explain at first sight. Another characteristic of MS is its relapsing and remitting nature. This means that your patient may suffer a neurological deficit before it improves or disappears altogether. The episode in her twenties sounds suspiciously like optic neuritis (see p. 322) and is a common symptom of MS. Despite the high probability of MS in this case it is prudent to exclude spinal cord compression as mentioned earlier because mistakes have been made in similar circumstances, for example, patients assumed to have MS have later been found to have spinal cord tumours).

features of inco-ordination are present elsewhere this does provide some further evidence.

13. Assess sensation: light touch (DF 7/10), pain (DF 6/10), vibration sense (DF 5/10), and proprioception (DF 6/10).

All modalities should be tested with the eyes closed using the techniques described in Chapter 8 (see p. 213).

Light touch

Use a piece of cotton wool that is made into a wisp at one end. Dab first on the sternum and confirm that this is felt and feels soft as cotton wool would be expected to feel. Then go on to check the legs in the same fashion as the arms. Compare both legs at equivalent points and compare the dermatomes within each leg as well. Also check that the stimulus is roughly similar to the one on the sternum. Do not forget to examine the back of the legs. See Fig. 10.2 for the dermatomes (p. 245).

Tip

If you find sensory loss in the lower limbs you must always check the sensation around the anus (S4) and check the anal tone with a finger (a lax patulous anus may indicate an S5 lesion). You will also need to pay particular attention to the function of the bowels and bladder. Find out if they have become constipated or have had difficulty passing urine recently (and check for a palpable bladder). The latter two problems are associated with spinal cord compression.

Tip

A crude but rapid screen for the possibility of spinal cord compression involves searching for a sensory level with your finger. Quickly touch the sternum as your reference point and confirm that the patient can feel your finger. Then start at one toe and if the sensation is abnormal, run your finger slowly up the leg on to the abdomen. You should ask the patient to let you know when the sensation feels normal. This technique can alert you to other neurological deficits but you must always follow this up with a more conventional and thorough assessment as described above.

Pain

Always use the blunted 'neuro-pins' for testing pain. Follow the techniques used for assessing pain in the examination of the arms (Chapter 8). Again compare both legs at equivalent points, as well as the dermatomes within each leg and check with the reference pin-prick at the sternum. Always check the back of the legs. Checking temperature sensation is not usually required but a rapid screen or confirmation of a problem involving the spinothalamic tracts can be performed as on p. 215.

Vibration sense

See Fig. 10.18. Use a 128 Hz tuning fork to test vibration sense. Check the tuning fork works by testing it on your elbow before performing the test. Strike the tuning fork on the patella hammer or flip the tip using the

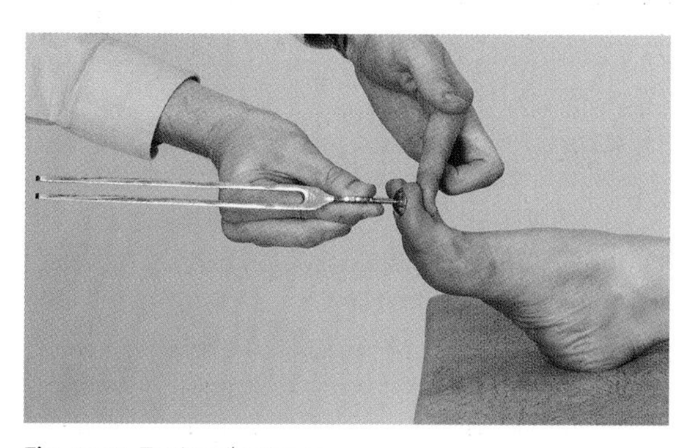

Fig. 10.18 Testing vibration sense.

thumb and index finger and place it on the sternum. Make sure your patient can appreciate the vibration. If they can, reactivate the tuning fork and place it on the plantar surface of the big toe. If they can appreciate the vibration there then this modality is normal. If they cannot then move the tuning fork up the leg. Try the medial or lateral malleoli of the ankle, followed by other bony prominences of the leg. This could be the shin, the tibial tuberosity near the top of the tibia, or the anterior superior iliac spine, which is the bony bit that you can feel at the front of the hip at waist level. Document the level where vibration is first perceived.

Proprioception

The interphalangeal joint of the big toe is usually used for testing joint position sense in the small joints. Again the technique is similar to the one used in assessing proprioception in the arms. Hold the proximal phalanx of the big toe with the thumb and index finger on either side of the digit and hold the distal phalanx with the thumb and index finger in a similar fashion. Move the distal phalanx up and down in the manner described on p. 214 and note the response. If joint position sense is impaired at the toe move to a larger joint, for example, the ankle and retest. Proprioceptive loss has to be severe for a person not to be able to appreciate the position of the foot at the ankle or the leg at the knee. Repeat the test on the opposite leg. A crude screen for proprioceptive loss is to ask the patient to close their eyes and to place their heel on the opposite big toe. If they cannot do this, this suggests there is impairment of joint position sense.

Keypoints

- For any sensory modality (except proprioception) always compare the sensation elicited to that on the sternum.
- Also compare sensation in equivalent dermatomes of each leg and proximal to distal, to discern patterns of sensory loss (do not forget the back of the legs).
- Remember the root values of the dermatomes as this will help in localizing a lesion.
- Never use a venepuncture needle to assess pain.
- Always use a 128 Hz tuning fork for vibration sense.
- Make sure the patient appreciates the buzzing sensation in vibration testing rather than cold or pressure sensation.
- If you suspect spinal cord compression, look for a sensory level.
- Anal sensation and anal tone are a valuable adjunct to sensory testing and should never be forgotten.

14. Get your patient to stand: perform Romberg's test (DF 5/10).

Watch carefully as your patient attempts to stand and notice the ease or difficulty with which they assume an upright posture.

What is Romberg's test? *(Moritz Heinrich Romberg (1795–1873), German neurologist.)* This is a test looking for sensory ataxia. This condition is the result of abnormal joint position sense in the feet and simply means that the patient has a tendency to be unsteady because of a lack of proprioception. This unsteadiness may not be initially apparent because vision is a very potent aid to balance and this test uses this fact to detect its presence.

How to examine. When the patient stands, ask them to put their feet fairly close together and to 'get their balance.' Stand close to the patient and extend your arms to the front and the back of the patient. Once they are steady ask them to close their eyes. A normal person will be able to maintain their balance without problem. Someone with sensory ataxia will begin to sway and may even fall over, hence the need to

CASE 10.3

Problem. You are preparing to perform Romberg's test on a patient. As they stand you notice that they seem unsteady and sway continually around their centre of gravity. When you ask them to close their eyes, they overbalance. You conclude that they have a positive Romberg's test but when you demonstrate this to the registrar on your firm, they say you are wrong. Why?

Discussion. The key to a true positive Romberg's test is that the patient should be steady before they close their eyes. If they are unsteady before they close their eyes this suggests a different pathology. Cerebellar ataxia can lead to unsteadiness and this will be exaggerated when the eyes are closed (look for other cerebellar features, for example, nystagmus, dysdiadochokinesia, incoordination, intention tremor, and past-pointing).

Keypoints

- Romberg's test checks for sensory ataxia.
- Make sure your patient is steady before getting them to close their eyes.
- If the patient becomes unsteady when the eyes are closed the test is positive and indicates sensory ataxia (due to loss of joint position sense).

have your arms ready to catch them should this look likely.

Gait

15. Assess gait (DF 7/10).

What is it?

This simply means the way in which a person walks (and not the mobile barrier in your garden fence).

Significance

No neurological examination of the legs is complete without watching a patient's gait. Walking is a complex activity dependent on many factors including muscles, joints, intact nerves, and higher brain centres. A problem in any one of these areas can lead to a change in the normal walking pattern. A doctor should be able to recognize the main patterns of abnormal gait as these can give useful insights into the possible underlying mechanisms. Once you are confident in spotting the major patterns you will find you will be able to predict the signs you should find in a neurological examination (a knack that will save time in the busy clinics that you will inherit in the future.)

How to examine

If you have not had the opportunity to see the patient walk (or if you are in an examination situation) it is useful to ask the patient, 'Do you have difficulty walking?' If they say 'no', observe them safely from a distance. If they say 'yes' then you have to supervise them closely. Get close enough so that you can catch them if they look as if they are going to fall over. This does have the disadvantage of restricting your observations. If after a number of steps the patient seems stable you can retreat further away so that you can get a better look at the overall walking pattern. Get your patient to turn round and to walk back. Turning is an even more complex manoeuvre and may unmask problems in people who may only be mildly affected by a disorder.

Most students can recognize a normal gait pattern as they have seen thousands (subconsciously) by the time they reach medical school. The key things to look for are as follows.

Tip

If the patient is prone to stumbling, it is worth getting someone else to be on hand to catch your patient (preferably out of your line of sight) so that you can be free to analyse the gait unhindered by safety concerns.

- **Stability.** Is your patient stable or unstable?
- **Stride length.** Are the steps taken regular or does the stride length vary? Are the steps taken short and shuffling?
- **Gait pattern.** This is the manner in which the patient walks, which will now be described.

Antalgic gait

Antalgic (*ant-al-jick*) gait is the pattern of walking readily recognizable as 'the limp'. Any cause of pain, in any part of the leg, which is severe enough, will force the sufferer to keep as much weight off the affected limb as possible.

Ataxic gait

This implies an unbalanced or unsteady gait. The usual cause is a cerebellar lesion (although vestibular (*vest-tib-you-lar*) or labyrinthine (*lab-i-rin-thine*) lesions are also possible). Look at the patient's stance before they start walking. They usually stand with their feet wide apart to maximize their stability (hence sometimes called a broad-based gait). Despite this, some patients remain unsteady and may sway or lurch to the affected side (that is, an ipsilateral cerebellar hemisphere lesion) and can be mistaken for drunks. In milder forms, when you get the patient to turn they may stagger (or even fall so beware). If you still suspect a cerebellar disorder but the patient has performed normally, put more stress on them by getting them to walk as if on a tightrope by putting the heel of one foot in front of the toe of the other foot. Normal people will be able to do this reasonably well but ataxic people will reel all over the place.

Hemiplegic gait

This is associated with a stroke and depends on its severity. The patient's posture will give some clues. Their stroke leg may be adducted and extended, with a plantarflexed foot. The arm on the same side may also be adducted, internally rotated, and with both the wrist and elbow flexed. As the hemiplegic leg is usually weak and stiff, the patient tends to swing it round in a circular movement (called circumduction) rather than lift it off the ground.

Spastic gait

This is basically a bilateral version of the hemiplegic gait (although the arms do not adopt the above posture in a spinal cord lesion). As both legs are adducted and plantarflexed, this gives the patient the appearance of a pair of scissors (the gait is sometimes called a scissors gait). Each leg has to sweep stiffly around the other adducted knee in turn. Sometimes the patient looks like they are wading through mud or quicksand. With milder disease the patient may just walk more stiffly than normal.

Steppage gait

This occurs with lesions causing foot drop, for example, lateral popliteal nerve palsy, L5, S1, root involvement, or peripheral neuropathy. The patient is unable to dorsiflex the foot to get it clear of the ground. Instead they have to raise their whole leg to achieve this before the foot is 'slapped' back onto the floor. This slapping gives a further audible clue to the trained observer. If the lesion is bilateral, the gait resembles a dressage horse performing an exaggerated canter.

Stamping gait

This resembles the high stepping gait but is due to sensory loss in the feet rather than a motor disturbance. The feet rather than slapping down passively are actively 'stamped' down by the patient. The patient has impaired joint position sense and is therefore unsure of where their feet are in space. Stamping provides a much greater stimulus, which increases the chance of proprioceptive feedback. In severe cases the patient has to look down at their feet to be sure of what their feet are actually doing.

Parkinsonian gait

The patient's posture is flexed and when they walk it is with short shuffling steps, with very little arm swing. Sometimes the patient has difficulty starting off and seems stuck in a pose. This is called freezing and can happen during the walk. Because of their flexed posture when they lean forward to start moving, their centre of gravity falls outside their base of support (that is, their legs), which makes them unstable. They then have to hurry to 'chase their centre of gravity' or they will topple over (this is called a festinant (*fest-in-ent*) gait). A useful analogy for this is the sprint start (try it yourself), where the athlete is in the set position. Their centre of gravity is well outside the support from their legs (but is inside that provided by the arms and legs). If you were to remove the arms the athlete will fall to the ground. They however overcome this instability at the start of the race by driving hard and fast with their legs until their centre of gravity is once again acting through the support provided by their legs.

Myopathic gait

This is due to proximal muscle weakness, which affects the hip girdle muscles. These muscles keep the pelvis horizontal as the other leg is swung through. However when they are weak the pelvis dips down on the side which is off the ground. Then when this leg is planted on the floor the pelvis is elevated on that side but dips down on the other side. This process repeats itself, leading to an oscillation of the pelvis that resembles the waddling of a duck (hence sometimes called a waddling gait).

Apraxic gait

This is a form of 'higher level' gait disorder which means that the centres in the brain responsible for automatic movements, for example, walking are dysfunctional. This is despite adequate power and co-ordination to fulfil the task. There is often difficulty in initiating the walk and the gait is wide based with the feet seemingly stuck to the ground. This gives the walk a shuffling quality that has been likened to skating on ice. The patient also tends to lead backwards and can fall in this direction also. With the initial freezing and shuffling, this gait can sometimes be mistaken for a parkinsonian gait. Other variations of this gait include taking small steps (given a French term 'marche àpetit-pas' (*marsh-a-pet-tea-pah*)) or having a variable step length, that is, taking some small and then some longer steps. The smooth pattern of walking is disrupted and the patient may even stop walking before setting off on the same leg they had just landed on. Also watch them turn. A normal person will execute this effortlessly but your patient will take several small steps to complete the turn. An analysis of the footprints made by such a person shows that they make up the points of a star and again this is given a French term (marche a l'etoile (*marsh-a-lay-twarl*)).

Hysterical gait

This can take many forms but the key feature is inconsistency (both in history and examination). The gait may change when repeated and often the underlying neurology is normal or does not fit the predicted gait pattern (an old-fashioned term for this is astasia abasia, which is a hysterical term for a hysterical gait).

Other signs of the legs

There are a number of alternative methods for eliciting an extensor plantar (see p. 252) although some of these are difficult to elicit and are often only present in severe disease. They are worth knowing for completeness.

Keypoints

- No neurological examination is complete without watching the patient walk.
- Familiarity with the different gait patterns can give major clues to the underlying problem.
- Always check if they have a problem walking beforehand (or if they need walking aids).
- When you watch a patient walk **make sure** you or someone else is on hand in case the patient stumbles.

1. **Gordon's sign.** (*Alfred Gordon (1874–1953), American neurologist.*) Squeezing the calf muscle leads to an extensor plantar in a UMN lesion.
2. **Chaddock's reflex.** (*Gilbert Chaddock (1861–1936), American neurologist.*) Stroking the lateral border of the dorsum of the foot leads to an extensor plantar in a UMN lesion.
3. **Oppenheim's** (*op-pen-high-ms*) **reflex.** (*Hermann Oppenheim (1858–1919), German neurologist.*) Pressure along the medial aspect of the shin with the thumb from above downwards, can cause an extensor plantar in an UMN lesion.

Abdominal reflex

(DF 5/10.) See Fig. 10.19. The abdominal reflex is another superficial reflex and is tested with a scratch provided by the tip of a patella hammer or key. First apply a scratch in the subcostal region parallel to the costal margin from the flanks towards the mid-line (D6–D8). Repeat again at the level of the umbilicus (D10), followed by a stroke parallel to the iliac crest in the iliac fossa (D11, D12). Also check the opposite side. A normal response is a brisk contraction of the muscles of the anterior abdominal wall directly below the stimulus. If this is absent it may suggest an UMN lesion above the root supply of the area stimulated. However this can be absent in an anxious patient and is therefore not a reliable sign. It has a minor role in supporting other UMN signs that you may have demonstrated.

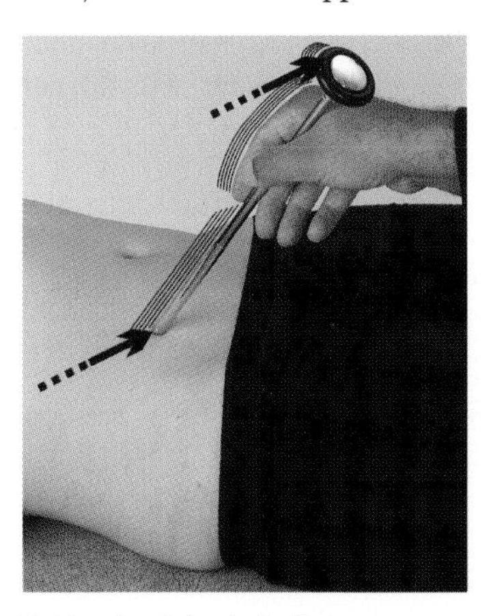

Fig. 10.19 Eliciting the abdominal reflex.

Cremastric reflex

(L1.) (DF 7/10.) In the male, stroking the inner thigh, gently, with the tip of a patella hammer tests for cremastric (*cream-ass-ter-rick*) reflex. Observe for the contraction of the scrotum on the same side. This is due to the contraction of the cremastric muscle.

Anal reflex

(S4, S5.) (DF 4/10.) If the skin around the anus is scratched lightly, the external sphincter contracts in response

Bulbocavernosus reflex

(S2, S3, S4.) (DF 8/10.) If the glans penis (the 'helmet' part of the penis) is gently squeezed, the bulbocavernosus (*bulb-owe-cavern-owe-suss*) muscle contracts in response. This is best appreciated by palpating the underside of the penis lightly with a finger to feel its contraction. This reflex is rarely tested and it goes without saying that if you are going to do it, you will need to explain it **very carefully**! (You do wonder about the motivations of those pioneering physicians who closely observed the first cremasteric, anal, and bulbocavernosus reflexes!)

Parietal lobe function

Some of the screening tests of parietal (*per-riot-al*) cortical function can be used on the lower limbs, for example, tactile neglect and extinction and graphaesthesia (*graph-ess-thee-zia*), although they do not add much more information than can be gained from the arms (see p. 216).

16. Make sure your patient is comfortable and thank them for their time.

This is only polite.

Wash your hands

17. Wash your hands.

Germs are no respecter, so please don't be a hospital vector!

18. Analysing your findings.

While you wash your hands you should continue to make sense of your findings (see below).

Presentation of findings

19. Presentation.

If you are sure of the diagnosis, mention it at the beginning, for example: 'this young gentleman has amyotrophic lateral sclerosis, motor neurone disease. He has a spastic paraparesis, as evidenced by the posture of both legs, increased tone bilaterally and ankle clonus. He has grade 3/5 power bilaterally, exaggerated knee and ankle jerks with bilateral extensor plantar response, gross bilateral wasting of distal and proximal muscles with fasciculations. He has preserved sensation and coordination and no bladder involvement. I would also like to examine the upper limbs and cranial nerves.'

If you are unsure of the diagnosis, present the findings, for example: 'this young lady has wasting of bilateral, gluteal (*glue-tea-al*) and thigh muscle wasting, normal muscle tone, grade 3/5 power of the proximal muscles bilaterally. She has a waddling gait. Her reflexes, sensation, and co-ordination are normal. She has proximal myopathy and I wish to offer a differential diagnosis and will complete my examination by examining the upper limb and look for evidence of other metabolic causes like hyperthyroidism and Cushing's syndrome. I would also like to know the family history to rule out hereditary limb-girdle syndromes.'

Analysis of findings

You should attempt to interpret your results as you go along. Try to work out the significance of the signs you have elicited and gradually build up a picture of possible diseases (much like a jigsaw or identikit picture). Refine your thoughts with the information gained from your history taking and do not be afraid to let your thoughts range beyond the neurological system. The neurology you unearth could be the result of disease in another system, for example, lung cancer with brain metastases or a paraneoplastic syndrome. As you learn more about neurological diseases you will automatically build on this framework and learn to spot emerging patterns that will guide you towards the location of a lesion if not the diagnosis itself. Although some diagnoses can be made from your neurological examination it is best to try and work out **where** the lesion is rather than what it is initially. Begin by asking the following.

1. Is the **motor** system affected or the **sensory** system affected? (If both are affected begin by analysing the motor system first—see below for the reason.)
2. If the motor system is affected, which of the following is it?
   1. A UMN lesion?
   2. An LMN lesion?
   3. A cerebellar lesion?
   4. An extrapyramidal lesion?

In the cases of 3 and 4 the location of the lesion is reasonably obvious but with 1 and 2 there is still some work to be done.

3. If it is a **UMN** lesion is it **unilateral** or **bilateral**? (UMN = hypertonia, clonus, hyper-reflexia, extensor plantar.)
4. If it is a lesion causing **unilateral UMN** signs, where in the central nervous system (CNS) is it? In both unilateral and bilateral UMN lesions you need to try and home in on the cause. The lesion can be anywhere from the spinal cord up through the brainstem to the cerebral cortex. The author finds the best way of 'pinning down' a unilateral UMN lesion is by analysing the pattern of weakness (in conjunction with other useful features) on either side of the mid-line.

(a) Cortical.

	R	L
Face	weak	normal
Arm	weak	normal
Leg	weak	normal

In this example the right side of the body is weak and as this is controlled by the contralateral cortex, the lesion is likely to be in the **left cerebral cortex**. Other features pointing to a cortical origin include disturbance of higher functions, including language, that is, dysphasias (dis-faze-ias), neglect (see p. 216), hemianopias (hemi-an-owe-pee-a) (see p. 286), decreased conscious level, and so on. The vascular territory affected will further influence the pattern of deficits (see p. 217).

(b) Internal capsule.

	R	L
Face	weak	normal
Arm	weak	normal
Leg	weak	normal

Another possible cause of this configuration is a lesion in the internal capsule (see p. 194). Here all the motor and sensory fibres converge into this narrow area and hence a small lesion can lead to a major deficit. As this area is 'subcortical' there is no hemianopia, dysphasia, and so on.

(c) **Brainstem.**

	R	L
Face	normal	weak
Arm	weak	normal
Leg	weak	normal

The key feature of a brainstem lesion is an ipsilateral deficit of a cranial nerve combined with a contralateral hemiplegia. In this example there is a lesion of the VIIth nerve on the **left-hand side**, which will be an LMN lesion as it is at the level of the VIIth cranial nerve nucleus. However at this level the corticospinal tracts have not reached their crossing point further down in the medulla and therefore the arm and leg on the right side will be affected. Other cranial nerves can be affected, for example, an ipsilateral IIIrd nerve palsy with a contralateral hemiplegia (Weber's syndrome).

(d) **Spinal cord.**

	R	L
Face	normal	normal
Arm	normal	normal
Leg	weak	normal

Any motor lesion below the brainstem (where the corticospinal tracts have crossed) will affect the limbs on the ipsilateral side. This example suggests a spinal cord lesion on the right side. As the arms are normal, this indicates that the lesion is below the level of its nerve supply. The likeliest position for the lesion is the thoracic cord (or possibly a high lumbar lesion). Additional sensory information will help in pin-pointing the lesion. If there is total involvement of one half of the spinal cord the resulting neurological pattern is called the Brown-Sequard (seck-card) syndrome (see Case 10.5).

5. If it is a lesion causing **bilateral UMN** signs, where in the CNS is it? The method recommended for homing in on a lesion causing bilateral UMN signs is to look at the pattern of reflexes.

(a) **Cortical.**

Jaw jerk	brisk	
	R	L
Arm	brisk	brisk
Leg	brisk	brisk
Plantars	↑	↑

For a cortical lesion to cause bilateral UMN lesions, it has to span the mid-line (called a parasagittal (para-saj-it-tal) lesion). The resulting bilateral UMN weakness is called a spastic paraparesis. The brisk jaw jerk is the key to the cortical origin here. It implies a bilateral UMN lesion that must be above the brainstem. However a normal jaw jerk does not exclude a cortical origin. Therefore a CT or MRI scan of the brain is recommended. Causes include bilateral CVAs, MS, and a parasagittal tumour.

(b) **High cervical cord**

Jaw jerk	normal	
	R	L
Arm	brisk	brisk
Leg	brisk	brisk
Plantars	↑	↑

This configuration suggests a lesion in the cervical cord. The brisk reflexes in the arms suggest the lesion is higher than its nerve supply. The normal jaw jerk suggests that the lesion is below the brainstem. However a normal jaw jerk does not exclude the possibility of a cortical lesion and so a CT or MRI scan of the head is important before focusing on imaging the cervical cord. A high cervical lesion eg transection of the cord following trauma can be fatal eg above C3 because this is the nerve supply to the diaphragms and would lead to respiratory failure. The paralysis of all four limbs is described as a quadroparesis or tetraparesis.

(c) **Cervical cord.**

Jaw jerk	normal	
	R	L
Arm	brisk/↓/absent	brisk/↓/absent
Leg	brisk	brisk
Plantars	↑	↑

This example suggests very strongly that the lesion is in the lower cervical cord. The mixture of brisk reflexes and diminished or absent reflexes (UMN and LMN signs) can lead to accurate localization. The diminished or absent reflexes (LMN) indicate the level of the lesion. The interrupted pyramidal tracts below this lesion will cause brisk reflexes in the area of supply, for example, an intervertebral disc pressing on the cord at the level of C5/C6 will cause LMN signs at C5/C6 (absent reflexes at C5/C6 = absent biceps/absent deltoid) and UMN signs at C7 and below (brisk reflexes at C7 = brisk triceps/brisk supinator).

(d) **Thoracic cord.**

Jaw jerk	normal	
	R	L
Arm	normal	normal
Leg	brisk	brisk
Plantars	↑	↑

This configuration suggests the lesion is below the level of the nerve supply to the arms, that is, below T1 of the thoracic cord. The brisk reflexes in both knees suggest that the lesion must be above L3/L4. This puts the lesion in the thoracic cord (more accurately between T1 and L3). Weakness that just affects the legs is called a paraparesis.

6. If it is a lesion causing LMN signs is it **unilateral** or **bilateral**? (LMN = wasting, fasciculations, hypotonia, diminished or absent reflexes, flexor plantars.)
7. If it is a lesion causing **unilateral LMN** signs, where in the peripheral nervous system is it? Again you need to try and home in on the cause. This is a little easier than for a UMN lesion. A lesion can be anywhere from the anterior horn cell in the spinal cord to the muscle end plates. It is easier to consider either a root lesion or a peripheral nerve lesion.
   (a) **Root lesion.** Spotting the difference between a root lesion and a peripheral nerve injury can be difficult as their presentations can be similar. The author tends to try and match the root values of the affected muscles with the root values of affected tendon reflexes and dermatomes. For example, **root lesion C5**—wasted and weak deltoid, supraspinatus (*soup-ra-spin-ate-us*), and infraspinatus:
   - **movement affected**—shoulder abduction through the full range of movement (180°);
   - **tendon reflexes affected**—deltoid (C5) absent and biceps (C5, C6) diminished or absent;
   - **dermatome affected**—C5 affected over the whole of the shoulder (see p. X) (there may also be pain experienced in this area).

Compare this with an **axillary nerve lesion**—wasted and weak deltoid (teres (*terry's*) minor is not accessible to testing):
   - **movement affected—**shoulder abduction **but** only after the first 90° of abduction;
   - **tendon reflexes affected**—none;
   - **sensory loss—**some sensory loss (or pain) over a small area of the shoulder tip.

Although many features are similar the distinguishing features are as follows.

	Root lesion	Axillary nerve palsy
Shoulder abduction	full 180° weak	second 90° weak
Tendon reflexes	absent deltoid	normal
	↓ biceps	normal

   (b) **Peripheral nerve lesion.** The previous example highlights the need to know the consequences of lesions to important nerve supplies to the limbs. This is the only way you can detect the patterns they produce (and sadly there are no shortcuts). The important nerves include the following.

Arms	Legs
Median	sciatic_common peroneal nerve
Radial	femoral
Musculocutaneous (*muss-cue-low-cute-ay-knee-us*)	
Axillary	

And this includes learning the lesions at different levels in the limbs and their common causes.

8. If it is a lesion causing **bilateral LMN** signs, what is it? The emphasis here is different. Instead of trying to localize the lesion, the emphasis is on recognizing the pattern and hence the type of lesion.
   (a) Bilateral proximal weakness affecting the arms and legs suggests a proximal myopathy (reflexes are unaffected and there are no sensory features).
   (b) Bilateral distal weakness affecting the arms and legs suggests a motor peripheral neuropathy (reflexes _ or absent).
   (c) It is a mixed motor/sensory peripheral neuropathy if there is an associated sensory loss in a glove and stocking distribution (do not forget that only the arms or the legs need be affected).
9. Is it a **sensory** lesion (or mixed)?
10. Analysing sensory impairment can be done for an isolated sensory lesion or a mixed motor/sensory lesion. In both cases the approach is the same. In mixed lesions it is recommended that the motor component is analysed first for the following reasons.
    (a) In the author's neurological routine the motor system precedes the sensory system.
    (b) The sensory examination is more subjective and can vary because of your technique (unequal stimuli) or the patient's personality (stoical versus obsessive).
    (c) In some areas the overlap of adjacent sensory nerves can reduce the sensory deficit you would expect (this is particularly true in the arms).
    (d) Sometimes an area of sensory impairment (or pain) can extend beyond the boundaries you would expect for a particular nerve supply.

The author simply separate sensory deficits into four main categories:

- affecting the whole limb (cortical/subcortical lesion?);
- affecting dermatomes (root lesion? peripheral nerve lesion?);
- distal limbs affected (peripheral neuropathy?);
- dissociated sensory loss (spinal cord lesion?).

See Fig. 10.20 for a flowchart summarizing the previous analyses.

Neurological diseases and investigations

In the earlier parts of this chapter, various medical conditions have been mentioned. In this section those conditions that have not been covered in the corresponding section in Chapter 8 will be described. In

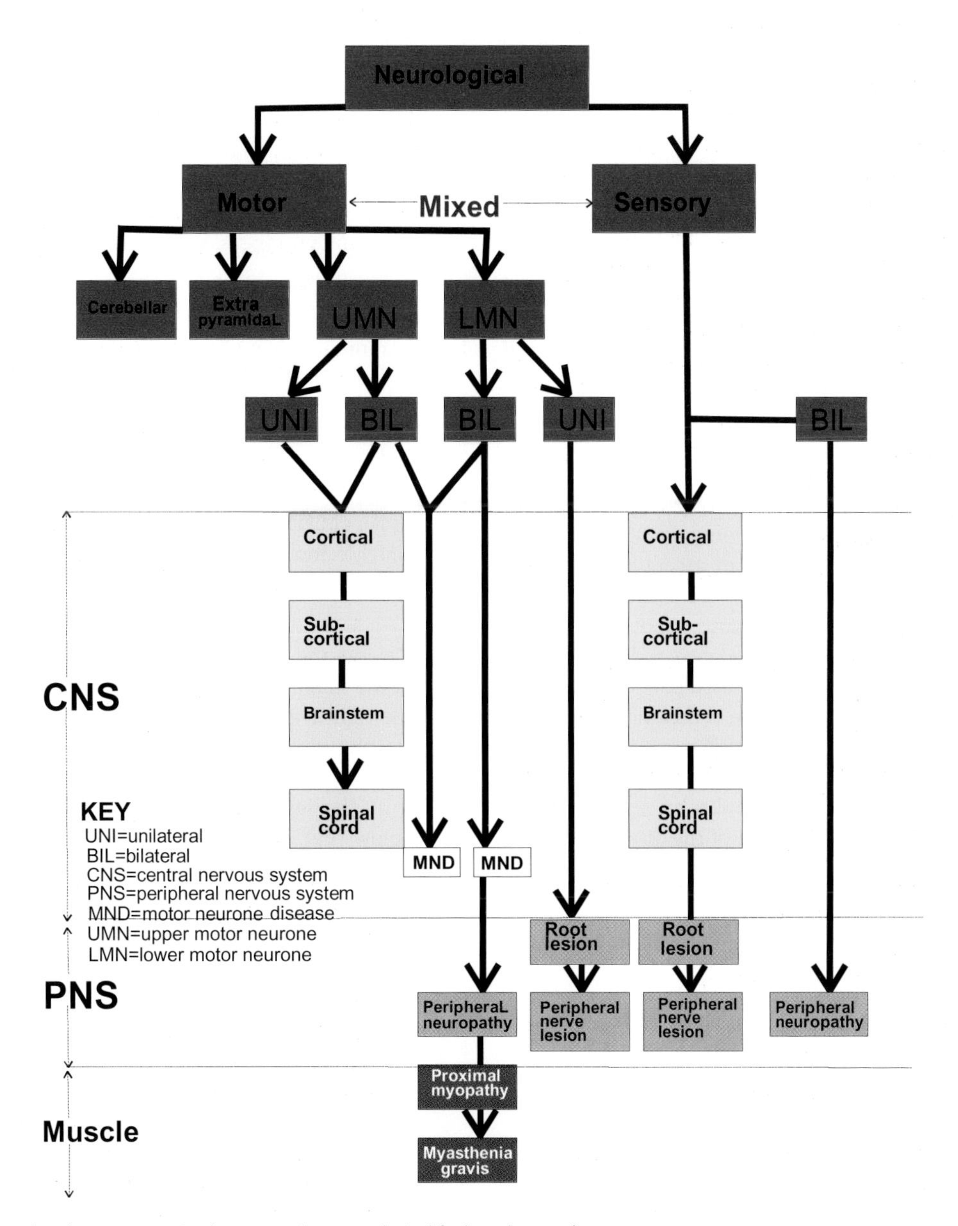

Fig. 10.20 Flowchart summarizing how to analyse neurological findings (see text).

general these descriptions are brief though certain aspects not well described in other textbooks are discussed in some detail

Hereditary polyneuropathies

Hereditary sensory motor neuropathy I is also known as Charcot Marie Tooth disorder or peroneal muscular atrophy; it is inherited as an autosomal dominant and causes a symmetrical polyneuropathy in a glove and stocking distribution. It causes a characteristic distal wasting of muscles of the arms and legs, which slowly progresses up the limbs. In the legs this gives the appearance of an inverted champagne bottle. It is also associated with pes cavus and kyphoscoliosis. The diagnosis is suggested by a family history and the clinical features above and is supported by nerve conduction studies and chromosomal studies. Hereditary sensory motor neuropathy II has the same features as HMSN I but has a slightly delayed onset (third to fifth decades). Hereditary sensory motor neuropathy III or Dejerine–Sottas (*de-je-rin-sot-tas*) syndrome (*Joseph Jules Dejerine (1849–1917), French neurologist, Jules Sottas (1866–1943), French neurologist*) is the recessive form with an early onset in the first decade and could be associated with mental retardation.

Guillain–Barré syndrome

This is an acute inflammatory polyneuropathy. In over two-thirds of patients, a preceding acute viral illness is followed in 1–3 weeks by an ascending paralysis, areflexia with mild sensory involvement. Diagnosis is usually made on the clinical features, supported by nerve conduction studies, showing evidence of demyelination and lumbar puncture showing raised CSF protein. Thirty per cent of patients may require ventilatory support for respiratory paralysis. The prognosis is good with 75–80% recovering without any neurological deficit. Treatment with intravenous immunoglobulin or plasmapharesis commenced early in the course of the disease (within a week) is shown to be effective.

Mononeuropathy

This is where a single nerve trunk is affected leading to LMN weakness and sensory loss specific to the nerve trunk involved. An example of this in the leg is the lateral popliteal nerve palsy (see below).

Mononeuritis multiplex

This is a simultaneous or sequential involvement of isolated nerves or nerve roots over a period of time. Vasculitis is the most common cause of this syndrome and includes multisystem disorders such as systemic

CASE 10.4

Problem. A 57-year-old man was having difficulty walking and felt his right leg seemed stiff on occasion. He also noticed that his left leg felt funny but he could not elaborate further. You suspect a neurological cause and perform a full neurological examination. There are no cranial nerve abnormalities and the jaw jerk was normal. There were no neurological findings in the arms either. In the right leg you find increased tone and seven beats of clonus. There is grade 4/5 power in the leg, with hyper-reflexia and an extensor plantar. You also demonstrate loss of light touch, vibration sense, and proprioception in the right leg. In the left leg, the tone, power, and reflexes are normal except that you cannot elicit a plantar response. There is the loss of pain and temperature sensation in the left leg up to the umbilicus. What is going on?

Discussion. Using the knowledge you have gained from the preceding chapters and the simple stepwise approach just described, you can begin to breakdown what seems to be a complex case.

1. There are both motor and sensory components to the case, so concentrate on the motor side.
2. In the right leg the increased tone, clonus, hyper-reflexia, and extensor plantar point to a UMN lesion (the left leg seems normal from a motor perspective).
3. As it is a unilateral UMN problem you need to observe the pattern of weakness on either side of the mid-line. This looks like a monoparesis of the right leg as the cranial nerves and the arms are not affected. This suggests that the lesion is below the nerve supply of the arms, which puts it at the level of the thoracic spinal cord or below (but not below the L3, L4 as the knee jerks are brisk). As the corticospinal tracts have already crossed in the brainstem, the lesion must be on the same side as the UMN signs, that is, the right half of the thoracic spinal cord (anteriorly).
4. Already you have a good idea where the lesion is likely to be but you still have to explain the sensory features (which appear bizarre at first glance).
5. Start with the right leg. There is the loss of light touch, vibration sense, and proprioception. This

(*continue*)

CASE 10.4 (*continued*)

indicates damage to the dorsal columns. Pain and temperature sensation is normal on this side indicating a dissociated sensory loss, which supports a spinal cord lesion. As the dorsal column fibres do not decussate until high up in the cord, the loss of these modalities will be on the same side as the lesion, that is, the right half of the thoracic cord (posteriorly).

6. The left leg exhibits the loss of pain and temperature sense. Unlike the dorsal columns, the spinothalamic tracts cross within two segments of the spinal cord. Therefore the lesion will be on the right half of the thoracic spinal cord (laterally) also. There is further information here. The sensory loss extends to the umbilicus, which approximates to the T10 level. As the fibres cross within two spinal segments, the true level of the lesion should be around T8 in the spinal cord.

You can see the supporting role the sensory analysis played in this example (the sensory level did help in pin-pointing the lesion further). This case is known as the Brown-Sequard syndrome (*Charles Édouard Brown-Sequard (1817–1894), French neurologist/ physiologist*). It is seen rarely (particularly with the full blown features) because it represents damage to an entire half of the spinal cord, which is not easy to produce naturally. It is useful however as an excellent teaching exercise in matching clinical signs with spinal cord anatomy.

lupus erythmatosis (*loo-pus-eryth-mat-owe-sis*), polyarteritis nodosa (*polly-art-er-eye-tiss-no-dose-a*), Wegener's granulomatosis (*vague-ners-granule-owe-mat-owe-sis*), sarcoidosis, Churg–Strauss syndrome, systemic sclerosis, and other vasculitides (another collective name for disorders that cause clinical symptoms through an inflammatory process of blood vessels).

Lateral popliteal nerve palsy

Also known as common peroneal nerve palsy, this is commonly seen in patients who are bed bound for a long time or in patients with a plaster cast for a fracture of the leg. This is due to the injury of the lateral popliteal nerve around the neck of fibula. When the whole nerve is involved, foot drop ensues due to the weakness of dorsiflexors of the ankle and toes. There is loss of sensation in the whole of the dorsum of the foot. Partial lesions will have less extensive sensory impairment.

Diabetic amyotrophy

This is an asymmetric, femoral neuropathy affecting the thigh muscles causing severe wasting of the anterior thigh, pain, and weakness of knee extension. The knee jerk is absent but sensory impairment is minimal. This condition also reflects poor metabolic control in diabetes and improves with strict glycaemic control.

Duchenne muscular dystrophy

This is an X-linked recessive disorder due to mutation of the 'dystrophin gene'. Pseudo hypertrophy of the calves occur (this means that although the muscles are enlarged they are paradoxically weak) and progressive weakness of the girdle muscles commences early in the first decade leading to waddling gait and Gower's sign (*Sir William Richard Gower (1845–1915), English neurologist*) (when asked to stand from squatting position the patient raises themselves up by climbing up their legs with their hands). Patients may become chair bound in the second decade and develop respiratory failure in the third. Sensory function and reflexes are preserved. The diagnosis is suggested by a family history, serum creatine kinase,electromyography (EMG), and muscle biopsy. Other variants of muscular dystrophy exist including Becker's muscular dystrophy, limb-girdle dystrophy, and fascio-scapulo-humeral dystrophy.

Polymyositis

Polymyositis and dermatomyositis are autoimmune inflammatory conditions affecting the muscles (dermatomyositis is usually reserved for the additional involvement of the skin). There is a proximal muscle weakness affecting the thighs, shoulders, and neck and in addition the muscles can be tender due to the inflammatory process. Problems with swallowing may occur due to pharyngeal striated muscle involvement. Those patients with skin involvement may have a characteristic skin rash around the upper eyelids (described as a heliotrope rash), a vasculitic rash at the fingertips, and occasionally nail fold infarcts. Investigations such an elevated creatine phosphokinase (CPK) level, raised inflammatory markers, EMG, and characteristic muscle biopsy help make the diagnosis.

Finals section

For revision read the examination summary (p. 245) and the keypoints throughout the chapter and do the questions on pp. 267–8. See Tables 10.1 and 10.2 for day-to-day and Finals cases, respectively.

TABLE 10.1 Day-to-day cases

Neurological	Non-neurological
Stroke	Pedal oedema
Parkinson's disease	Paget's disease
Cervical myelopathy	Purpura
Multiple sclerosis	Cellulitis
	Leg ulcers

TABLE 10.2 Finals cases

Neurological	Non-neurological
Day-to-day cases	Day-to-day cases
Cerebellar syndromes	Pre-tibial myxoedema
Motor neurone disease	Necrobiosis lipoidica
	Pyoderma gangrenosum

Key diagnostic clues

The key clues are the same as for the arm. However the single most important aspect of the examination of the legs is the **gait pattern**. Clues to the underlying neurological abnormality (and perhaps the diagnosis itself) may be obtained from watching a patient walk.

Some advice relating to examination problems

General

Use the neurological examination routine for the legs given on p. 245.

The instruction

The examiner may ask you to 'examine the legs neurologically' or just to 'examine the legs'. If you get the second command (which is less specific), stay calm! And begin by scanning the legs for clues. Is there swelling of the ankles or legs suggesting pedal oedema? Is there any deformity of the leg or thigh, which could indicate Paget's disease of the bone. Check the skin surface for more localized lesions, for example, scaly plaque lesions could suggest psoriasis, purply-brown plaques on the anterior surface of the shin would suggest pre-tibial myxoedema, and so on. If no abnormalities are readily apparent (and this quick screen should take seconds only), then progress to a neurological examination. More often these days the examiners will try to point you in the right area in the interests of saving time and will be very specific, for example, 'examine the motor system' or 'perform a sensory examination only'. Occasionally you may get the instruction 'watch this patient walk' or 'comment on this patient's gait' or some variation. So long as you have seen the various types this should not present a problem.

Relax the patient

This goes without saying and the patient should remain relaxed and comfortable throughout your assessment.

Follow-up non-neurological signs

See the relevant section in the Chapter 8. Think how you would do this for some of the cases listed in the 'Finals section' (and perhaps other conditions too).

General look

Do not forget to sneak a peak elsewhere. Check the face and posture and look for evidence of a tremor or involuntary movements in the hands (see p. 228).

Inspection

Your general look can merge into a focused inspection of the legs, looking for wasting, fasciculations, and so on. Make sure that your examiners can see that you are inspecting or they may deduce (wrongly) that you do not know what you are doing.

Analyse as you go

Try to digest the information as you elicit it. This will guide your examination and help you decide on supplementary signs to support your working diagnosis and will aid your presentation as well.

Tone, power, and reflexes

The comments in the relevant section of Chapter 8 are applicable here. Also remember two things:

(1) make sure you can elicit all reflexes proficiently and pay particular attention to the left ankle jerk (see p. 251);

(2) if you cannot elicit reflexes then you must make sure that you try again with reinforcement (see p. 252).

Plantar reflex

Make sure you use some keys or an orange stick (never the bottom of a tendon hammer).

Problem. You are not sure if you have witnessed an extensor plantar.

Solution. if you are unsure, you are allowed to repeat the test. Make sure you focus on the toe and look for the very first deflection. If it is upward it is an extensor plantar. Remember you do not need to explain this in isolation. Are there other signs of a UMN lesion? If there are then this will provide further support for your findings.

Problem. You have demonstrated UMN lesion signs and an extensor plantar but you are unsure whether to elicit other signs such as Gordon's sign, Chaddock's sign, and so on.

Solution. Unlike the arms I would not 'showboat' here. There are many signs you could demonstrate but they will not add anything further to what you already know, that is, that the patient has UMN signs. It is recommended that the cremasteric, anal, or bulbocavernosus reflexes are not demonstrated.

Sensation

Follow the pattern described on p. 263.

Romberg's test

Do not forget to perform this as part of your sensory assessment (unless your examiners stop you). Remember, the patient must be steady before they close their eyes or the test is meaningless!

Gait

So long as you have revised the various patterns this will be straightforward. Remember to make sure that you are close to the patient, so that should they stumble you can catch them. If they fall whilst in your charge, you will fail. Look at the stride length. Is it normal or is it short and shuffling in quality? Is it smooth? Or does the patient stop and start? Do not forget to ask your patient to turn round and walk back after a reasonable interval.

Presentation

Always mention that you would normally perform a full neurological examination and not just the legs in isolation, as there may be clues elsewhere that would help pin-point the source of a lesion. Try to be confident—avoid the words 'seems' or 'might'!

Good luck!

Questions

The more stars, the more important it is to know the answer.

1. What is clonus? **
2. What is Romberg's sign? ***
3. What are the signs of an upper motor neurone lesion? ****
4. What are the signs of a lower motor neurone lesion? ****
5. What features suggest a cerebellar lesion in the legs? ***
6. What is a positive Babinski reflex and what is its significance? ****
7. What is a peripheral neuropathy? **
8. How do you reinforce absent reflexes in the legs? ***
9. What are the causes of a peripheral neuropathy? ***
10. How do you perform reinforcement of the reflexes in the legs? ***
11. What is sensory neglect? **
12. What are the causes of a myopathic gait? ***
13. What is radicular pain? **
14. How do you assess the plantar reflex? ****
15. What is paraesthaesia? **
16. What is allodynia? *
17. What is ataxia? ***
18. What are the affects of an L1 root lesion affecting the right leg? ****
19. What gait would you expect from a patient with Parkinson's disease? ***
20. What is the root value of the knee jerk? ***
21. What is the root value of the ankle jerk? ***
22. How do you perform the cremasteric reflex? **
23. What are the features of neuropathic pain? ***
24. What features do you look for when you are assessing gait? ****
25. Name two conditions associated with pes cavus? **
26. What is a spastic paraparesis? ****
27. What is the root value underlying the extension of the big toe? **
28. Where is the S1 dermatome? **
29. At what level does the spinal cord end? *
30. At what level does the dura mater end? *
31. What is a sensory level and what is its significance? ****
32. What is the Brown-Sequard Syndrome? **

33. What is the cauda equina? **
34. What is a Charcot's joint? ***
35. What neurological sign would you expect to elicit in the legs of a person with a spastic gait? ****
36. Name five drugs that can cause a peripheral neuropathy? ****
37. What is the frequency of tuning fork you should use when testing vibration sense? *
38. If you saw wasting of the legs that resembled 'inverted champagne bottles', what condition would you consider? **
39. What is diabetic amyotrophy? ***
40. Which condition can demonstrate both upper motor neurone and lower motor neurone features in the absence of sensory loss? ***

Score. Give 4 marks for 4 stars, 1 for 1 star, and so on. At the end of the third year, you should be scoring 60-plus and by Finals, 80-plus; 100-plus is very good.

Further reading

As for Chapter 8.

CHAPTER 11

Cranial nerves

Chapter contents

Introduction

The examination of the cranial nerves seems daunting at first sight. It looks complicated and haphazard and does not fit easily into our usual examination routine, that is, to observe, palpate, percuss, and auscultate. Many qualified doctors also find it difficult because the cranial nerve examination is practised much less than those for other systems. The cranial nerves examination is all about good verbal communication and good observational skills. It requires a great deal of active participation from your patient. If your patient cannot understand your commands, for example, if they are drowsy, it is difficult to perform a comprehensive examination. However if your patient is alert and is given clear and precise instructions the examination will be much easier. When reading this chapter, do not try to learn everything at once. Take your time and learn a few sections at a time and when you come to learn about the cranial nerves make sure you understand their individual functions and how to test them before moving on.

Symptoms

Visual loss

Visual loss is a frightening symptom and a careful history needs to be taken to avoid missing potentially treatable lesions that may lead to permanent blindness. Sudden visual loss is also an opththalmological emergency.

Important questions to ask

Was the loss of vision sudden or gradual?

Sudden onset suggests causes such as vitreous haemorrhage or retinal detachment (see later) and vascular causes such as stroke. Transient visual loss can be caused by emboli from arteriosclerotic plaques. Patients will describe a curtain coming down in front of one eye. This usually lasts 20–30 min before the 'curtain' lifts again. This is called amaurosis fugax (*am-more-roe-sis-few-gax*) and is an important symptom as it may signal the possibility of an impending stroke. Visual loss of gradual onset may be caused by cataracts, age-related macular degeneration (ARMD), or primary open-angle glaucoma (*glaw-coma*) (see later). With gradual onset, the loss of vision may be insidious and not recognized until late on in the disease process. This is particularly important in the case of primary open-angle glaucoma because if it is detected early enough, that is, by screening, it can be treated.

What is the nature of the visual loss?

It is important to know what your patient means by loss of vision. For some people this means a loss or blurring of detail (visual acuity). For others this will mean some form of visual field defect, for example, homonymous hemianopia (*hu-mon-ee-muss-hemi-an-owe-pia*) (see later). Others will complain of a loss of central vision (because of diseases affecting the macula of the eye) and others may complain of poor vision at night (nyctolopia (*nick-ta-low-pia*) (see later).

Is one eye or both eyes affected?

Most people will tell you up front whether one eye or both are affected. As a rough rule of thumb, if one eye is suddenly affected the pathology is usually within or around the eye (including the optic nerve). If both eyes are suddenly affected, the visual pathway is usually affected at the optic chiasma (*kai-az-ma*) or distal to the chiasma (see pp. 287–8). This rule is less true for slow visual loss, for example, cataracts or ARMD, which usually develops in both eyes.

Is the eye red or white?

You should be able to observe this directly while you take a history but it is still worth checking that the eye has not been red at some point before their vision was affected. A red eye (in the absence of a subconjunctival haemorrhage—a bleed into the outermost layer of the white of the eye; Fig. 11.1) suggests an inflammatory process involving one of the layers of the eye. This can be due to a range of conditions including bacterial or viral infections (see Fig. 11.2), foreign body, secondary to systemic illnesses such as the seronegative spondyloarthropathies (*spon-dee-low-are-throp-path-ees*) (see Chapter 13), or acute angle closure glaucoma (see later).

Is there pain associated?

Some inflammatory causes of the eye can cause pain of varying severity. This can range from minor discomfort from mild viral conjunctivitis to severe pain if the cornea becomes affected (called keratitis) (*kerra-tight-iss*), which may lead on to frank corneal ulceration. Anterior uveitis

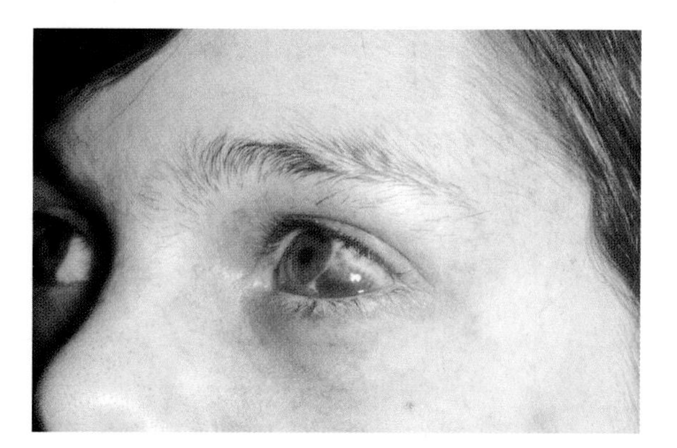

Fig. 11.1 Subconjunctival haemorrhage.

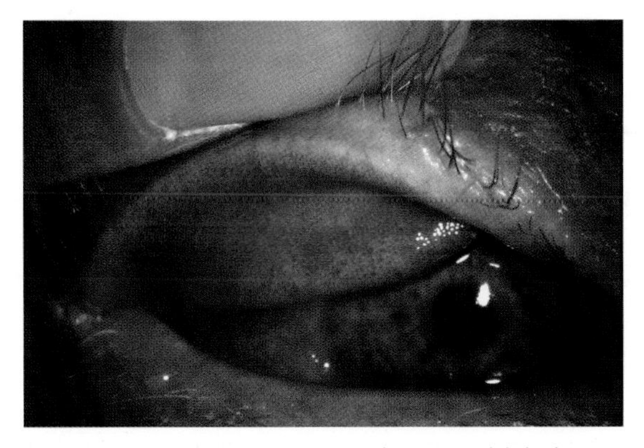

Fig. 11.2 Severe conjunctivitis. Note as the inner eyelid also has a conjunctival lining it is also affected.

(Fig. 11.3) (*you-vee-eye-tis*), also known as iridocyclitis (*i-rid-owe-sigh-cl-eye-tiss*) (inflammation of the iris and ciliary bodies) may become painful particularly when looking at lights (photophobia) and during accommodation, for example, during reading. Acute angle closure glaucoma is an important cause of a painful red eye. This pain can be exquisite in the affected eye and is associated with headache above it, nausea and vomiting, and a reduction in vision. An optic neuritis may cause pain on eye movements.

Has there been any trauma?

Do not assume that patients will volunteer any injury to you. Some events happen so quickly that the patient may only have a vague recollection. Determine what your patient was doing around the time of the visual disturbance. Some occupations are high risk for eye injuries, for example, grinding, turning, and so on, where metal fragments can enter the eye if eye protection is not worn. Even hobbies like squash may pose a danger to the eye. A squash ball is small enough to impact on the globe of the eye to cause a blow-out fracture. The force of impact is transmitted to the orbit of the eye and may be sufficient to 'blow out' its weakest aspect (the floor). There may be blood in the anterior chamber of the eye (hyphaema) (*high-fee-mer*) and swelling around the eye. Later the eye may demonstrate enophthalmos (*ee-nop-thal-moss*) (the eye appears to recede within the socket) and there is an inability to gaze upwards because the eye drops down into the fracture site entrapping the inferior rectus (or inferior oblique) muscles.

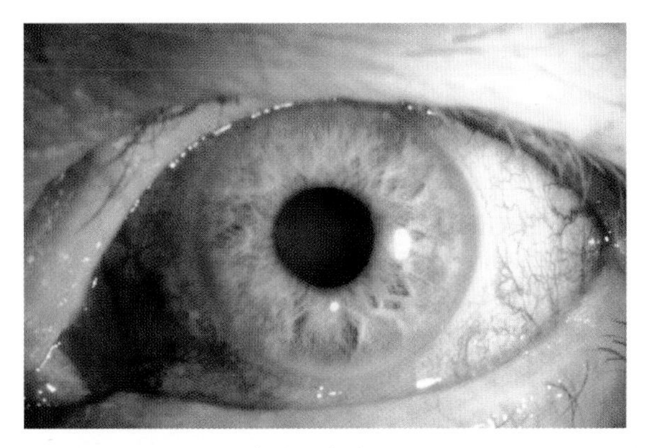

Fig. 11.3 Anterior uveitis (iridocyclitis)

> **Tip**
>
> Any injury to the eye should be assessed by an ophthalmologist.

Are there any associated features?

1. **Floaters.** These are shapeless blobs of varying sizes, which float around in the patient's field of vision. They are usually caused by changes in the **vitreous gel** (this sits behind the lens of the eye and in front of the retina and forms the majority of the volume of the eye). Some people have experienced small faint floaters all their life and these are particularly noticeable when looking against a plain background. If there are new floaters this may represent the vitreous gel separating from the retina (posterior vitreous detachment) and can cause a tear in the retina leading to vitreous haemorrhage or a retinal detachment (see later). This is usually associated with flashing lights. In all cases of new floaters urgent ophthalmological review is required.
2. **Flashing lights.** These suggest traction on the retina. Vitreous or retinal detachment may be the cause. Flashing lights (called photopsia) (*foe-top-sia*) may occur transiently in the build-up to a migraine.
3. **Photophobia.** An aversion to light may be experienced with anterior uveitis. Photophobia may also be experienced in meningitis, encephalitis (*en-keffer-light-iss*), migraine, and with corneal surface problems.
4. **Diplopia.** This is double vision and will be explained fully in the context of eye movements (see p. 298).
5. **Headache and vomiting.** These are non-specific features and may be found in a number of conditions. It may be part of the syndrome of migraine or may develop with space-occupying lesions such as brain tumours or cranial infections like meningitis or encephalitis. It could also be due to acute angle closure glaucoma. If the cause for headache and

vomiting is not obvious, ask if the patient has seen coloured haloes around light sources. This is due to corneal clouding and is highly suggestive of this form of glaucoma.

6. **Nyctalopia.** This is the disturbance of night vision, which is uncommon. It can be due to vitamin A deficiency or may be an early sign of retinitis pigmentosa (*ret-ee-night-iss-pig-ment-toes-ah*)—a genetic condition that initially affects peripheral vision and later leads to blindness (see later).

How does the loss of vision affect you?

Try and gauge the impact of loss of vision on the patient, for example, on work and hobbies as well as everyday life. Even in those cases of irreversible loss there is still plenty that can be done for your patient, for example, visual aids and financial benefits.

Past medical history

This aspect of the history is extremely important as many systemic diseases can affect the eye. One of the most important is diabetes mellitus, which can affect the eye in many ways. All diabetic patients should have some form of ophthalmological assessment at regular intervals. Other conditions that can affect the eye include rheumatoid arthritis—scleritis and episcleritis (inflammation of the deepest and middle layers of the white of the eye, respectively) and seronegative spondyloarthropathy—anterior uveitis.

Drug history

A drug history is always important. Drugs that affect the eye include

(1) **chloroquine (*clo-roe-quin*)**—bull's-eye retina (this is one of the forms of retinopathy produced by chloroquine leading to pigmentation at the centre of the macula surrounded by an area of hypopigmentation; this gives the appearance of a bull's-eye);

(2) **Steroids**—cataracts;

(3) **Ethambutol**-optic neuritis.

Family history

Some conditions can be inherited, for example, optic atrophy, some forms of cataracts, and diabetes mellitus.

Hearing loss

Hearing loss is a debilitating symptom, which can lead to social isolation and depression. Its effects are more pronounced if both ears are affected and the loss is severe. The effects of hearing loss are also determined by the person's stage of life. Severe bilateral hearing loss in a baby will prevent them acquiring normal speech. In an adult hearing loss will interfere with work and social activities.

Keypoints

- Sudden visual loss is an ophthalmological emergency.
- Determine if the eye is white or red, because the causes of visual loss will be different.
- Ask for associated features such as headache, photophobia, and floaters, which could be pointers to the underlying diagnosis.
- Always check a drug history (including illicit drugs).

Important questions to ask

Was the loss of hearing sudden or gradual?

Sudden hearing loss can occur with trauma, for example, a blow over the external auditory meatus (*me-ate-us*) or rapid changes in pressure within the ear canal (called barotrauma) (*barrow-traw-ma*) following an explosion, rapid descent in an aircraft, and so on. Sudden hearing loss is an ear, nose, and throat (ENT) emergency and the patient requires urgent assessment to make sure the cause is treatable. Gradual hearing loss can occur with ageing (sometimes called presbyacusis) (*press-by-a-cue-sis*) or following repeated exposure to loud noise.

Is one ear affected or both?

Most people can cope with hearing loss of any severity in one ear. In fact if the hearing loss is gradual the patient may not realize they have a hearing problem. Sometimes it is the spouse or friends who notice that they have to repeat themselves or that the volume of the television is unusually loud.

Is there associated pain?

Pain in the absence of trauma is usually due to an inflammatory cause. Infections by micro-organisms can inflame the pinna and external auditory meatus (called an otitis (*owe-tight-iss*) externa) or the middle ear (called an otitis media). There are conditions that can cause referred pain to the ear, for example, tonsillitis, but in these conditions hearing is usually unimpaired.

Is there a discharge from the ear?

Otitis externa and otitis media can also produce a discharge. Pain usually precedes the discharge particularly with otitis media because it requires the perforation of the eardrum before the inflammatory contents can escape. Both otitis externa and otitis media can become chronic. Permanent hearing loss is not a problem with otitis externa. By contrast this is a danger with chronic otitis media and this condition should always be referred to a specialist if suspected. In both cases aural discharge can be recurrent or continuous.

Has there been any head injury or a blow over the ear?

In causes of sudden deafness ask about the possibility of trauma, no matter how trivial. A simple slap over the external auditory meatus is capable of generating sufficient pressure to perforate the eardrum.

Do you hear any ringing, whistling, or buzzing in the ears?

Tinnitus is the perception of abnormal noises by the ear. Tinnitus can be as devastating as hearing loss to the sufferer. Ask, 'When are the noises most troublesome?' This is usually at night or in quiet surroundings, particularly when the patient is not distracted by other tasks. Tinnitus is sometimes due to an awareness of the patient's own physiological function, for example, the rushing noise due to blood flow within the ear. Often tinnitus is the marker for hearing loss. Therefore patients with tinnitus should be referred for a hearing assessment.

Tell me about your occupation or hobbies

A patient's occupation (past and present) or their hobbies may be important in the genesis of hearing loss. Any environment that subjects a person to excessive noise over a sustained period of time may cause hearing loss particularly for the higher frequencies (at-risk occupations include those in the aviation industry, road drilling, shipbuilding, motor sports, and musicians (rock/pop and classical) and at-risk hobbies include shooting, listening to loud music, nightclubbing). Certain at-risk jobs should provide ear protection. You should check that these have been provided and that your patient has worn them.

What medications are you on or have you taken?

Certain drugs can cause hearing loss. Usually a person has to be exposed to very high doses intravenously to achieve a toxic level for the cochlear nerve. These drugs are described as ototoxic (*owe-toe-toxic*) and include frusemide, salicylates, and aminoglycoside antibiotics, for example, gentamycin.

How does your hearing loss affect you?

Always try to find out what impact hearing loss has on your patient. A small loss to a telephonist may be more devastating than a greater loss to a retired labourer. Knowing the problems your patients face can guide your strategies in dealing with them, for example, the provision of hearing aids and other assistive devices such as flashing doorbells and lip-reading programmes.

Keypoints

- Deafness is a cause of social isolation and depression.
- Sudden deafness is an ENT emergency.
- Always ask about tinnitus.
- Always ask about regular exposure to noise with occupation, hobbies, or other lifestyle activities.
- Always take a drug history.

Disturbance of smell

Loss of smell

The medical term for the loss of smell is anosmia (*an-oz-me-a*). Hyposmia is a decrease in the ability to appreciate smell. Anosmia is an unpleasant symptom as it decreases our appreciation of food flavours. It also robs the sufferer of a vital warning system, for example, the detection of leaking gas or food going rotten. It is rare for a patient to complain solely of the loss of smell. It is a common accompaniment of upper respiratory ailments such as 'colds' or influenza and is usually recognized as a temporary complication by the sufferer. The most common cause of permanent anosmia is head injury. This is because bundles of primary sensory neurones perforate the cribriform (*crib-ri-form*) plate of the ethmoid (eeth-moid) bone before synapsing with the olfactory bulb. If the brain is subject to an accelerating force (either forwards

TABLE 11.1 Causes of anosmia

Temporary
Upper respiratory tract infection
Allergic rhinitis (*rhine-eye-tiss*), for example, hay fever
Nasal polyps
Permanent
Head injury
Cranial surgery
Tumours of the anterior fossa (at the front of the brain), for example, olfactory groove meningioma (*men-in-jee-owe-ma*)
Drugs or chemicals
Long-term application of nasal spray
Ammonia

or backwards), these fibres can be sheared at this point. The questions you need to ask can be deduced by knowing the causes shown in Table 11.1.

Parosmia

This is sometimes called dysosmia and is the distortion or perversion of the sense of smell. If any environmental reasons for bad smells are ruled out this may be a manifestation of temporal lobe epilepsy (and is a hallucinatory symptom). Uncommonly it can be the aura of a patient with migraine. With a child the possibility of a foreign body up a nostril should always be borne in mind. Patients may also experience parosmia during regeneration of a damaged olfactory nerve.

Keypoints

- The sense of smell combines with taste to produce a wide range of flavours.
- A temporary loss or reduction in the sense of smell and food flavours may occur with upper respiratory tract infections.
- Head injury is the most common cause of anosmia.
- Do not forget drugs as a cause of smell or taste disturbance.

Disturbance of taste

The loss of taste

The medical term for the loss of taste is ageusia (*ay-goo-sia*) (a term not used very often). Hypogeusia is the decrease in the ability to appreciate taste. Many people notice a 'loss of taste' when they have a cold or other upper respiratory tract infection. This highlights the large contribution smell provides for the taste experience. In fact the sense of taste is based on five taste receptors. The classic salt, sweet, sour, and bitter and the recently discovered umami (*oo-mar-me*). Umami is mediated by glutamate (an amino acid) and gives a savoury chicken-like taste. It does not enhance the classic four taste sensations and cannot be synthesized by any combination of sweet, sour, salt, or bitter. The experience of taste is a product of these receptors and smell to produce a flavour, hence it is flavour that is lost when smell is affected. Practically your patient will not make this semantic distinction, therefore always ask,'Has there been a change in your sense of smell also?' Again the questions you need to ask can be deduced by knowing the causes of decreased taste sensation or loss of taste (given in Table 11.2).

TABLE 11.2 Causes of a loss of taste

Facial nerve palsy (in the facial canal proximal to the chorda tympani branch)
Dry mouth (for example, Sjogren's (*show-grens*) syndrome (see p. 391), heavy smoking)
Drugs (antibiotics, anti-cancer chemotherapy, digoxin, angiotensin-converting enzyme inhibitor, and amiodarone)

Headache

A headache is a common symptom and most people have experienced this at sometime in their life. It is important to deduce whether the headache has an innocent or a sinister cause. To do this you need to be familiar with the common causes and how they present (see Table 11.3). You will also need to know the rarer causes and their presentations so you do not miss a potentially treatable condition before it becomes too advanced for treatment. The approach to headache is similar to that of pain elsewhere in the body.

TABLE 11.3 Causes of Headache

Primary
Migraine
Tension headache
Cluster headache
Secondary
Trauma
Referred from eyes, face, sinuses, teeth, and neck
Meningitis or encephalitis
Subarachnoid haemorrhage
Space-occupying lesion*
Drugs
Temporal arteritis
Other medical conditions, for example, hypoglycaemia and infections

* 'Space-occupying lesion' is a non-specific term to describe any lesion in the brain that occupies space. This could be a tumour, abscess, or haematoma (other rarer causes exist). Because the cranium is a closed container any additional swelling will lead to a rise in intracranial pressure and to the symptoms described below. As a general rule space-occupying lesions in the posterior fossa will lead to rapid rises in intracranial pressure as there is very little space for the brain to expand into, whereas tumours in the anterior fossa can grow to relatively large sizes before any rise in pressure causes symptoms. Additional symptoms may be experienced depending on the area of brain affected. A primary cause of headache is where there is no obvious underlying cause for the headache. A secondary cause is where the headache is due to an obvious underlying medical cause.

What to ask

This can be broken into two sections: (1) questions about the headache itself and (2) questions about the potential causes of headache.

Questions about the headache itself

Begin with an open question, 'Tell me about your headache'. This gives your patient an opportunity to give their version of events. However there are key facts you need to establish (if they are not forthcoming in their account).

1. **Where is the headache?** The site of pain can sometimes point you towards a specific condition. Tension headache can be experienced 'like a band' around the head. Migraine tends to be unilateral and temporal arteritis causes tenderness over the temporal arteries in the temple region.
2. **Was the onset sudden or gradual?** Headache of sudden onset is of great concern. If the pain literally comes on in seconds and is severe, 'like being hit by a baseball bat', this could represent a subarachnoid haemorrhage. These patients require urgent investigation. Some variants of migraine can also have a rapid onset. Otherwise most other causes of headaches usually have a gradual onset.
3. **Have you experienced headache like this before?** Recurrent headaches experienced over many years are unlikely to be due to a sinister cause. Causes of recurrent headache include tension headache, migraine, and sinusitis. If headache is recurrent try to get an idea of the frequency of headache. Is it, say, every fortnight or is it daily? Do the headaches occur in a cluster (cluster headaches?—see 'Cranial nerve diseases and investigations' section) or are they related to menstruation (migraine can be triggered by the hormonal changes associated with the menstrual cycle). Also determine whether the frequency of headache has changed. This could represent the development of a space-occupying lesion and therefore requires further investigation. It is now appreciated that migraine and sometimes tension headache can change their character and frequency following regular dosing with medication and become a chronic daily headache. This is called a transformed migraine. The cure for this situation is weaning off the analgesia. This can be difficult to achieve because the patient may experience rebound headache on stopping or reducing their analgesia and will be reluctant to discontinue their medication. They may be convinced that something sinister is going on and that the return of the headache is proof that they need even stronger medication. This process needs to be managed skilfully with firm guidance and counselling.
4. **How long does the headache last?** Most benign causes of headache are short lived, lasting from a few hours to a couple of days. Other headaches are persistent so long as the underlying cause remains active, for example, temporal arteritis or meningitis. Other active disease may not produce a continuous headache but one that is intermittent or that can be aggravated by certain manoeuvres, for example, cerebral tumour worsening with straining, coughing, or sneezing.
5. **How severe is the headache?** This feature can be misleading but still needs to be documented because of the impact on the patient's life. Some benign causes, for example, migraine can cause excruciating pain and prevent the patient from working. Conversely intracerebral tumours may only produce a dull, nagging headache, which can be shrugged off easily.
6. **Can you describe the headache?** The character of the pain is always difficult to describe so you may have to give options. Is the pain burning in nature, sharp, or throbbing? A feeling of diffuse pressure over the top of the head or a band-like constriction may suggest a tension headache. Throbbing pain may suggest a tension headache or migraine. A sharp, shooting (lancinating) pain suggests nerve root irritation or neuralgia. A burning pain may also suggest a neuralgia.
7. **Does the pain come on at a particular time of the day?** A headache that is present on waking or wakes a person from sleep should raise the suspicion of a space-occupying lesion in the brain. This feature is not specific to space-occupying lesions because other headaches such as migraines can also mimic this. A headache that gets worse at the end of the day may be due to a tension headache.
8. **Does anything bring on the pain (precipitating factors)?** Sometimes the cause of the headache is clear cut, for example, following trauma or drug ingestion. Sometimes the precipitant is less obvious, for example, the original stressor in chronic tension headache may have been forgotten over the months. Migraines may be precipitated by stress, fatigue, changes in sleeping habits, menstruation, and alcohol.

9. **Does anything make the pain worse (aggravating factors)?** The headache due to a space-occupying lesion can worsen if the patient bends forwards or if they strain in the toilet. The headache of sinusitus may also worsen if the patient bends forwards. With temporal arteritis, there is tenderness over the temporal arteries at the temples and sometimes over the occiput when the patient combs their hair.
10. **Does anything make the pain better (relieving factors)?** This question is less helpful. Patients with migraine and tension headache find they may get temporary relief if they can get off to sleep. Some people may find a measure of relief with analgesia but run the risk of developing a transformed migraine or rebound headache if they rely heavily on medication (see above).
11. **Do you have any other symptoms (associated factors)?** With migraine, patients may suffer an aura. This tends to be visual, in the form of flashing lights (photopsia) or zig-zag lines (fortification spectra or teichopsia) (*tie-cop-sia*). They may develop blind spots (scotomas) (*sco-toe-maz*) or visual field defects. Most migraine sufferers develop photophobia and nausea (and occasionally vomiting). Patients with meningitis may have associated photophobia and nausea. For symptoms of other conditions see the next section on the potential causes of headache.

Questions about the potential causes of headache

Causes of headache that you should know and their associated features are described below. Please note that a fuller account of these can be found in the 'Cranial nerve diseases and investigations' section.

1. **Migraine.** Unilateral headache (occasionally bilateral), pulsatile in nature, aggravated by exercise or bending, may experience visual aura, for example, zig-zag lines, motor aura, for example, hemiplegia, or sensory aura, for example, hemianaesthesia. The aura usually lasts less than 1 h and is usually followed (but not always) by headache. Also associated with nausea, vomiting, photophobia, phonophobia (aversion to sound), and osmophobia (aversion to smells)
2. **Tension headache.** Usually bilateral headache, 'tight' like a band or a diffuse pressing sensation. Occasionally photophobia or phonophobia (never both together as in migraine).
3. **Cluster headache.** Severe unilateral headache, sometimes burning quality, also ipsilateral (same side) conjunctival injection (red eye), lacrimation, nasal congestion and rhinorrhea (*rhino-rear*) (runny nose), miosis (*my-owe-sis*) (small pupil), and ptosis (*toe-sis*) (drooping eyelid). May have a cluster of attacks with remissions.
4. **Trauma.** Severity of pain usually lessens with time from incident. Can occur weeks to months after event. It can be difficult in late-onset headache or those of prolonged duration to know whether they are truly due to trauma or are a function of an anxiety or depressed state (or seeking compensation). Also associated with dizziness, decreased concentration, anxiety, and depression. Headache may also be as a result of intracranial bleeding. In this situation, clinical features may be due to raised intracranial pressure, that is, nausea, vomiting, focal neurological signs, seizures, and altered conscious level.
5. **Meningitis.** Severe headache, nausea, photophobia, neck stiffness. Other symptoms depend on infecting organism: viral—sore throat, arthralgia, and muscle pain; bacterial—late complications (focal neurological signs and fits, petechial rash). If you suspect meningitis and are faced with a petechial rash (a purply-blue pin-point rash) that does not blanch when a glass tumbler is placed over it or more confluent bruising, this is probably the onset of septicaemia as a result of meningococcal infection. This is a medical emergency and the patient should be given antibiotics immediately (preferably penicillin or cephalosporin).
6. **Encephalitis.** Decreased conscious level, focal or generalized fits, focal neurological signs, neck stiffness.
7. **Subarachnoid haemorrhage.** Severe headache of sudden onset, nausea, photophobia, neck stiffness.
8. **Space-occupying lesion.** Dull headache worse in the morning and with straining, nausea, vomiting, may be focal neurological signs, seizures, personality changes.
9. **Drugs.** A variety of drugs may cause headache, the principal group are the vasodilators, for example, nitrates or calcium channel blockers. Other drugs include caffeine, alcohol, and the contraceptive pill. Associated features will depend on the individual drugs involved but common features are nausea and dizziness. Illicit drugs including cocaine, amphetamine, and cannabis also cause headache. Withdrawal of chronically administered drugs including analgesics, alcohol, and illicit drugs may also cause headache. Associated features in this situation

include sweating, tremor, dizziness, and irritability. A rarer mechanism for drug-induced headache is an aseptic meningitis (an inflammation of the meninges **not** due to an infection). Drugs implicated include non-steroidal anti-inflammatory drugs and intrathecal (*in-tra-thee-cal*) (into the spinal fluid) chemotherapy, for example, vincristine or intravenous immunoglobulin.

10. **Referred pain.** Headache can be referred from eyes, ears, face, sinuses, teeth, and neck. Acute angle closure glaucoma is worthy of mention because its recognition will not only reduce misery but will potentially save vision in the affected eye. Pain is around and above the affected eye and can be severe. Associated features include a red eye, an oval poorly reactive pupil, coloured haloes seen around light sources (due to corneal clouding), nausea, and vomiting.
11. **Temporal arteritis.** Headache localized to temples or occiput, malaise, pain on chewing (jaw claudication), Raynaud's (*ray-nose*) phenomenon of the tongue, visual loss, associated with polymyalgia rheumatica (therefore proximal muscle pain and stiffness) (see p. 389).
12. **Other medical conditions.** Associated features depend on the underlying condition. Hypoglycaemia is worth summarizing—sweating, nausea, dizziness, confusion, aggression, and coma.

Blackouts and syncope

What are they?

A blackout is a colloquial term for a loss of consciousness. Patients sometimes use the word collapse. This word is less specific and embraces patients who fall to the floor with or without loss of consciousness. Neither terms are medical in origin but are in widespread use by the general public. Syncope (*sin-cup-ee*) is a medical term and refers to a sudden transient loss of consciousness and postural tone with spontaneous recovery. The underlying problem is usually within the cardiovascular system.

Keypoints

- Sudden onset of headache (within seconds) suggests a subarachnoid haemorrhage and is a medical emergency.
- The severity of headache is not proportional to the severity of the underlying cause.
- A headache that is present on waking, which worsens with straining, is a space-occupying lesion until proven otherwise.
- A headache with fever, photophobia, and neck stiffness is meningitis until proven otherwise (if a purpuric rash is also present, give antibiotics straightaway as this is an absolute emergency).

What to ask

A blackout can be a challenging symptom for the history taker. The story may be vague, there may be no eyewitness account (a vital component in the investigation of blackouts) and the causes can be wideranging. When asking questions about blackouts, it is worth dividing your enquiry into

(1) questions about the blackout itself;

(2) questions about events leading up to the blackout;

(3) questions about events following the blackout.

Instead of trying to rush to a diagnosis, try and reach it in stages. The answers you receive should allow you to determine which 'system' may be at fault. In a previously fit person the systems that are principally affected are the cardiovascular system, where there is a temporary decrease in the flow of blood to the brain (for example, due to cardiac arrhythmia) and the neurological system, where consciousness is disturbed usually because of epilepsy. The first thing to establish is what your patient means by their terminology. Ask, 'What do you mean by blackout or collapse?' Many patients use these terms interchangeably and they can be used to not only describe loss of consciousness, but dizziness, vertigo, a fall, or even the loss of memory. If the description remains vague you may have to ask a leading question, 'Did you pass out?' Always be on your guard for the uncertain response, 'I don't think so' or 'I might have done'. Take these answers with a pinch of salt. Also try not to get frustrated with your patient. Remember that events can happen extremely quickly. This point highlights the value of an eyewitness account.

Questions about the blackout itself

1. **'How long were you unconscious for?'** At first sight this seems a stupid question but sometimes a helpful bystander may inform them how long they passed out for. Or they may use detective work to deduce how long they were unconscious, for example, I had just put on a CD and when I came round it was still Eminem playing, so it must have been two minutes at the most.' Usually syncope lasts less than a minute. Neurological causes can last several minutes and occasionally hours.

2. **'Have you had blackouts before?'** If they have, try and get an accurate account of how many and how recent. Clearly five blackouts in the space of a week is worrying and needs urgent investigation. One previous attack, 20 years ago (occurring in explicable circumstances, for example, after prolonged standing on the spot (vasovagal syncope)), is less worrying. Establish if they ever had faints at school or in childhood as they may still retain the propensity for syncopal events.
3. **'Are you able to prevent an attack?'** Sometimes patients with syncope recognize the light-headed, pre-syncopal feeling as a warning that they may pass out. If they are able to sit down or lie down quickly they may abort an attack. Patients with epilepsy can never prevent an attack once it begins.

Questions about events leading up to the blackout

1. **'How was your health on the morning of the blackout?'** This establishes a baseline for their health. An older person who is unwell may be at the limit of their ability to compensate so that any additional stress, for example, standing too long or anti-hypertensive treatment may be sufficient to cause syncope.
2. **'What were you doing just before the blackout?'** Loss of consciousness while sitting or lying down is unlikely to be due to syncope. Blacking out following exertion could be due to aortic stenosis. A common scenario is the patient who has been standing for long periods particularly in a warm environment. These are essential prerequisites for vasovagal syncope.
3. **'Did you have any chest pain or palpitations before the blackout?'** This question probes the possibility of a cardiovascular cause for the blackout, for example, myocardial infarction or arrhythmias. If the answer is 'yes' then further questions need to be asked to refine the diagnosis (see Chapter 4).
4. **'Did you have pain anywhere else?'** This question is a check for other possible causes, for example, headache—subarachnoid haemorrhage? stroke? hypoglycaemia?
5. **'Did you have any unusual feelings or symptoms before blacking out?'** This question is important. A light-headed feeling, a hot or cold feeling rising up the body (or down) accompanied by nausea, sweating, and occasionally ringing in the ears could be the result of syncope. More unusual symptoms such as a strange feeling, taste, smell, or nausea (often difficult to describe) prior to the blackout may be the aura preceding an epileptic fit. Patients with known epilepsy learn to recognize their aura as a warning of an impending fit.
6. **'What was the last thing you remember before blacking out?'** This gives your patient another opportunity to recall any of the above.

Questions about events following the blackout

1. **'What is the first thing you remember when you came round?'** This is another important question. If they remember being on the floor and were instantly aware of their surroundings, this would suggest a cardiovascular cause leading to a syncopal attack. However, if the first thing they remember is coming round in the ambulance or hospital (despite eyewitness accounts of the patient being conscious), this would strongly favour epilepsy as a possible cause. Following a seizure, epileptics are frequently confused and often have no recollection of events for minutes, hours, and occasionally days afterwards. This is described as the post-ictal (*ick-tal*) state.
2. **'Did you injure yourself?'** People who have epileptic seizures lose control of their limbs and can fall to the floor unprotected and sustain injuries. Also ask, 'Did you bite your tongue?' This injury may suggest the possibility of epilepsy (although it can occur with other forms of loss of consciousness if the tongue is caught accidently in the teeth).
3. **'Did you wet yourself?'** This is an embarrassing question but if your patient has lost bladder control this is strongly suggestive of epilepsy. However be wary of older patients or patients with existing continence problems as they may lose bladder control regardless of the reason for losing consciousness.

Do not forget other aspects of your history, which may give supporting evidence.

Past medical history

Ask the patient if they have epilepsy. It is surprising how some patients do not volunteer this up front. Also check if they have diabetes. A prolonged episode of hypoglycaemia can lead to unconsciousness (therefore a blood sugar level should always be checked on any unconsious patient). Also check if they have had any previous neurosurgery as seizures may be a complication of this surgery.

Drug history

Check if the patient is on anti-convulsant medication and if it has been taken regularly. Are they on anti-hypertensive, anti-anginal, or anti-Parkinson's medication as they can lead to postural hypotension. Tricyclic anti-depressant drugs can lower the seizure threshold in susceptible people, leading to fits.

Family history

Ask if there is a family history of epilepsy or heart disease.

Social history

Check especially for alcohol consumption. Alcoholics may drink until they are stuperose and may still deny that they have a problem (often leading to protracted and fruitless investigations). They may also develop seizures if they drink excessively in a session or paradoxically if they abstain from drinking. Also check if they drive. If they do drive they must be told **not** to drive until the cause of their blackout has been determined. Those diagnosed with epilepsy must be seizure free for 1 year before they can resume driving. If you are lucky enough to interview an eyewitness, it is useful to ask many of the questions you asked the patient. This allows you to gauge which aspects of the history are reliable. An eyewitness account is even more important if your patient is confused. A description of the blackout and events just before and after are the most valuable aspect of their account. Ask the following.

1. **'Did the patient become pale prior to losing consciousness?'** Pallor suggests a cardiovascular cause.
2. **'Did they shout or cry out?'** In epilepsy there is often an involuntary shout or groan during the tonic phase (see 'Cranial nerve diseases and investigations' section), before the patient falls to the floor. Care must be used when interpreting this observation because sometimes a person may cry out when they stumble or trip. Therefore make sure that the witness is sure that an accidental fall did not occur before ascribing the shout to epilepsy.
3. **'Did they fall without protecting themselves?'** When someone trips they automatically attempt to break their fall with their arms. With epilepsy because all voluntary muscle control is absent, patients fail to protect themselves when they fall to the ground (often leading to injury).
4. **'Did they lower themselves to the floor?'** Patients with syncope can recognize they are about to pass out and try to get on to the floor before they fall to the floor. Patients with abnormal illness behaviour or malingerers also get themselves on to the floor (often exhibiting strange movements when on the floor to mimic a fit). Have an index of suspicion for this type of patient if they give a story of multiple blackouts without injury.
5. **'Did they go rigid and then start jerking their limbs?'** This is the classical description of a seizure and is highly suggestive of epilepsy. However even with this description the diagnosis may still not be clear cut. Some people who hit their head or who become temporarily anoxic (lack of oxygen) can also develop seizures, which are not due to epilepsy.
6. **'How long were they unconscious?'** See above.
7. **'Were they confused when they came round, if so how long did this last?'** The greater the duration of confusion the greater the chances are that you are dealing with epilepsy.

Do not be alarmed if the diagnosis is not clear following your history (and examination). This is common. Try and determine whether the cause is cardiovascular or neurological (usually epilepsy) in nature. This is important, as this will guide your subsequent investigations. Table 11.4 will help you to make the distinction. If this was not difficult enough, many of the criteria that help to differentiate a cardiovascular cause from a neurological one are blurred when dealing with the elderly and these are also highlighted in Table 11.4. Be flexible and be prepared to change your working diagnosis as more information is gathered on many occasions. Above all, remember that even the experts get it wrong. People have been wrongly labelled as epileptics or have had the diagnosis overlooked by neurologists. This highlights the difficulty of this particular symptom and why a detailed assessment is vital. Therefore be meticulous and patient and be prepared to see these patients on many occasions before the vital clue is unearthed.

Dizziness

What is it?

Dizziness is a common description that people use to describe a variety of symptoms. These include light-headedness, wooziness, vertigo, feeling unsteady, confusion, and anxiety. Dizziness is rarely life threatening, especially if it is infrequent and short lived, for example, lasting a few seconds only. The true significance of dizziness lies in its underlying cause. A patient who is ill, for example, with an infection, may report dizziness when they exert themselves. This will be more noticeable if they have been bed bound for long periods. Dizziness in this context does not require investigation unless it becomes prolonged. Your history should identify patients who are at risk of blackouts. When dizzi-

TABLE 11.4 Contrasting symptoms of cardiovascular and neurological causes of blackout with modifications for the older patient. Adapted from **Table 3** (p.21), *Epilepsy in elderly people* by Raymond Tallis (1995), with permission from Martin Dunitz.

Feature	Usual distinction		Modification in older patients
	Faints	Fits	
Posture	Usually occur in the upright position	Not position dependent	Faints in older people are not position dependent because they are often due to position-ndependent pathology
Onset	Gradual	Sudden	Loss of consciousness may be quite abrupt in syncope in an older person; partial complex seizures may have a gradual onset
Injury	Rare	More common	A syncopal attack may be associated with significant soft tissue or bony injury in an older person
Incontinence	Rare	Common	An individual prone to incontinence may be wet during a faint; partial seizures will not usually be associated with incontinence
Recovery	Rapid	Slow	A fit may take the form of a brief ('temporal lobe') absence; a faint associated with a serious arrhythmia may be prolonged
Post-event confusion	Little	Marked	A prolonged hypoxic episode due to a faint may be associated with prolonged post-event confusion
Frequency	Usually infrequent with a clear precipitating cause	May be frequent and usually without a precipitating cause	Faints associated with cardiac arrhythmias, low cardiac output, postural hypotension, or carotid sinus sensitivity may be very frequent

Keypoints

- Always determine what your patient means by a blackout.
- Always try and get an eyewitness account of the blackout.
- Determine what the patient's health was like leading up to the blackout.
- Ask if there were any symptoms such as chest pain or palpitations before the event.
- If the patient bit their tongue and was incontinent and confused after the blackout, this is strongly suggestive of epilepsy.
- If the blackouts happen while the patient is standing and some events prevented by sitting or lying, this is strongly suggestive of syncope.

ness is the prelude to a blackout it is called pre-syncope (*pre-sin-cup-ee*).

Causes

See Table 11.5.

What to ask

First ask, 'What do you mean by dizziness?' The answer to this is crucial, as it will determine your next sequence of questions. Be prepared to ask supplementary questions to refine your patient's answer, for example, 'Is it a light-headed feeling?' (syncope? hypoglycaemia?), 'Did the room spin round?' (vertigo?), or 'Do you feel your balance is poor?'(ataxia?). Then ask, 'Did you feel that you were going to pass out?' If the answer to this is 'yes', this increases the chance of the patient's event being pre-syncopal (beware that this is subjective and someone who is very anxious may swear blindly that they were even going to die). Also ask, 'Were you able to stop yourself passing out?' Many people will attempt to sit or lie down during a dizzy episode and this may abort an attack if it is due to reduced blood flow to the brain. Now ask, 'What was your health like just before the attack?' (this establishes a baseline for their health), 'What were you doing just before the dizzy episode?', 'Did you have any chest pains or palpitations?', 'Did you have any pains elsewhere?', and 'Did you have any other symptoms?' The relevance of these questions is explained in the blackout section.

Other worrying symptoms that suggest the need for further investigation include

TABLE 11.5 Causes of dizziness

Physiological
Warm environment*
Over-exertion*
Anxiety
Hyperventilation
Cardiovascular
Low cardiac output*
Congestive heart failure*
Myocardial infarction*
Cardiac arrhythmia*
Vasovagal syncope*
Postural hypotension*
Neurological
Transient ischaemic attack†
Vertigo
Acute labyrinthitis
Ménière's syndrome
Benign positional vertigo
Epilepsy*
Endocrine
Hypoglycaemia*
Addison's disease*
Myxoedema
Thyrotoxicosis
Anaemia
(All causes)
Hypoxia
Respiratory disease
Cardiovascular disease

* Also causes blackouts.

† Only causes blackouts if posterior circulation transient ischaemic attack.

- blackouts (see p. 277)
- diplopia or blurred vision
- hearing loss
- dysphasia (a disorder of language)
- limb weakness

Keypoints

- Always determine what your patient means by dizziness.
- Discover what their health was like before the attack.
- Ask if there were any other symptoms associated with the attack, for example, chest pain or palpitations.
- Ask if they have ever lost consciousness or felt that they were about to lose consciousness.
- Check what medications they take.
- Worrying features that warrant further investigations include blackouts, focal neurological signs, and chest pain or palpitations.

- sensory abnormalities
- chest pain or palpitations.

Vertigo

What is it?

This is the false perception (hallucination) of movement. The patient feels the environment is spinning or swaying, when this is clearly not the case. Any person can experience vertigo by spinning round rapidly on the spot. This sets up a rotational current in the fluid of the semicircular canals (SCCs), which in turn stimulates the hair cells within the current. This informs the brain that the body is spinning. However when you stop, the fluid within the canals still has momentum and will continue to stimulate the hair cells fooling the brain into thinking the environment is still rotating. Disease of the 'vestibular system' can also fool the brain into thinking that the environment is spinning. The resultant vertigo can be so severe that the patient can fall to the floor. They may also suffer with nausea and may vomit.

Causes

The causes of vertigo are

- acute labyrinthitis
- benign paroxysmal positional vertigo (BPPV)
- Ménière's (*many-airs*) syndrome (*Prosper Ménière (1799–1862), French ENT surgeon*)
- acoustic neuroma (*new-roma*).

A description of the above can be found in the 'Cranial nerve diseases and investigations' section later.

What to ask

The majority of people will complain of dizziness rather than vertigo. Therefore you will only establish that true vertigo exists by probing what they mean by dizziness. If the answer is vague then you may have to ask the leading question, 'Does the room and its contents spin around?' Also ask the following supplementary questions.

1. 'Do you feel sickly?'
2. 'Have you vomited?'
3. 'Are you able to walk around during an attack?'
4. 'Has your hearing been affected?' (Ménière's syndrome?)
5. 'Have you ever heard a ringing or buzzing sound in the ears?' (Ménière's syndrome?)
6. 'Does it occur when you change your position?' (BPPV?)

Keypoints

- Vertigo is the hallucination of movement.
- With true vertigo the patient will be unable to walk and will fall to the ground.
- Vertigo is usually accompanied by nausea and sometimes vomiting.
- Always ask about hearing impairment and tinnitus when faced with vertigo.

TABLE 11.6 The functions of the cranial nerves

(I) Olfactory nerve	Sense of smell
(II) Optic nerve	Visual acuity, visual fields, colour vision, and pupillary light and accommodation reflex (sensory part)
(III) Oculomotor nerve	Eye movements and pupillary light and accommodation reflex (motor part)
(IV) Trochlear (*trock-leer*) nerve	Eye movements
(V) Trigeminal (*try-jemmy-nal*) nerve	Facial sensation, muscles of mastication, and corneal reflex (sensory part)
(VI) Abducens nerve	Eye movements
(VII) Facial nerve	Facial muscles, taste to the anterior two-thirds of the tongue, stapedius muscle, and corneal reflex (motor part)
(VIII) Vestibulocochlear (*vest-tib-you-low-cock-leer*) nerve	Hearing and balance
(IX) Glossopharyngeal (*gloss-owe-fa-wren-jeel*)nerve	Sensation of palate and pharynx and the gag reflex (sensory part)
(X) Vagus (*vague-us*) nerve	Palatal and pharyngeal muscles, sensation of the respiratory system, and the gag reflex (motor part)
(XI) Accessory nerve	Sternomastoid and trapezius muscles
(XII) Hypoglossal nerve	Motor supply of the tongue

The importance of examining the cranial nerves

There are twelve cranial nerves each arising from the brainstem. They provide important motor and sensory function to the head and neck including the eyes, ears, and some internal organs (Table 11.6). Damage to any one of them will cause motor or sensory loss to the areas supplied. In addition the special senses such as sight, hearing, smell, and taste can also be affected. Knowledge of the function of each nerve is therefore vital to enable you to deduce any abnormality you may encounter. Although there are twelve separate nerves, their functions overlap. When examining the nerves at least for the first few attempts it is easier to think of them as individual nerves and perform the relevant examination. This will ensure none are missed out. It is actually a bit more complicated than this because each nerve may have more than one test and not all parts of each nerve can or will be tested. With more experience it will become smoother and you and the patient will move around less. Finally, try to think ahead all the time, whilst doing one test you should be thinking about the next thing you are going to say or do to the patient. Eventually examining the cranial nerves will become second nature and your thoughts will be focused on picking up the abnormality!

Examination of the cranial nerves summary

1. Getting prepared.
2. Introduce yourself to the patient.
3. Get the patient in position.
4. Whilst doing 2–3, be having a 'general look'.
5. Ask if there is any change in their sense of smell (I tested) or taste (I and VII tested) (DF 2/10).

6. Check visual acuity (II tested) (DF 6/10), assess the visual fields (II tested) (DF 7/10), test colour vision, test the pupillary light and accommodation reflexes (II and parasympathetic III tested), and perform fundoscopy (II tested) (DF 9/10).
7. Inspect for ptosis and a squint and check eye movements: look for nystagmus and ask about diplopia (III, IV, and VI tested).
8. Test facial sensation (V tested), assess the muscles of mastication (V tested), test corneal reflex (V tested), and assess the jaw jerk reflex (V tested).
9. Assess the muscles of facial movement (VII tested).
10. Assess hearing (VIII tested) and perform Weber's and Rinné's tests (VIII tested).
11. Assess movement of the soft palate (IX and X tested) and assess sensation of the soft palate (IX and X tested).
12. Assess the trapezius and sternomastoid muscles (XI tested).
13. Assess the tongue and tongue movements (XII tested).
14. Now you have finished make sure the patient is comfortable.
15. Wash your hands.
16. Presentation.

Examination of the cranial nerves in detail

1. Getting prepared.

You will need to collect your equipment to take to the bedside. For a complete examination of the cranial nerves you will need the following:

- 'wisp' of cotton wool
- unused neurology pin
- ophthalmoscope
- tuning fork (256 or 516 Hz)
- red hat pin
- tongue depressor
- bedside Snellen chart *(Herman Snellen (1834–1908), Dutch ophthalmologist)*
- reading material.

2. Introduce yourself to the patient.

Put out your hand to shake the patient's hand. Say something like, 'Hello I'm John Hughlings-Jackson, a first-year student. Do you mind if I examine your face, eyes and ears?'

3. Get the patient in position.

This examination is almost unique in that it is best performed out of bed, with you and your patient sitting on a chair at equal heights and with their face almost at arm's length from you (Fig. 11.4). If your patient is too frail, it is best to leave them in bed.

4. Whilst doing 2–3, be having a 'general look'.

Whilst introducing yourself and getting into position be looking around the bedside for any clues, for example, a hearing aid or a pair of glasses. Look at the patient. Do they seem distressed or in pain or are they comfortable? Inspect the patient's face. Is there any rash (systemic lupus erythmatosus (SLE)?—see p. 391), facial asymmetry (VIIth nerve palsy?—see later), or eyelid or pupil abnormality (see later)? Does the mouth droop or the voice sound unusual when they respond to your introduction (see pp. 215–16, 315 and later)? Any abnormality will give you a point of focus for your examination.

Olfactory nerve (cranial nerve I)

5. Ask if there is any change in their sense of smell (I tested) or taste (I and VII tested) (DF 2/10).

The olfactory nerve is responsible for the sense of smell. In the clinical setting, the sense of smell is rarely tested objectively (there are bottles with standard smells that exist for this purpose but the author has yet to see them used). Practically this nerve is assessed by a crude screening question, 'Do you have any problems with your sense of smell?' If your patient says 'no', then it is unlikely they have anything wrong with this particular nerve (the exception would be a unilateral loss of smell which could be compensated by the other nostril). 'If they say 'yes', make sure you ask this supplementary question, 'Do you have a cold or blocked nose at the moment?' If they say 'yes', this simple question will stop you going off on an unfruitful tangent. If they do not have a cold you will have to question them further to find the cause of their lack of smell (see p. 273). You can go on to confirm their lack of smell by testing it with some strong recognizable smells, for example, orange or coffee. Get your patient to close their eyes and make them occlude one nostril by pressing it firmly from the outside with a finger (a finger up the nostril looks uncouth and may unearth untold horrors!). Now get them to take a sniff and to try and identify the aroma. Then occlude the other nostril and repeat the test. If any abnormality is found the nostrils should be inspected for foreign bodies or polyps. Ideally experts should perform this, that is, ENT specialists.

Keypoints

- Ask if there is any change in the sense of smell or taste.
- Use a range of familiar scents if you are going to test the sense of smell by the bedside.
- Always test each nostril separately (by occluding the other nostril with a finger).

When you ask your screening question for smell, it is timely to ask about taste also (VII nerve). As taste is intimately related to smell, if smell is affected it is likely that taste will be as well (as anyone who has had a blocked nose can testify). If however the sense of smell is unaffected but taste is, then you will need to enquire further to see if you can determine a possible cause for the loss of taste (see p. 274).

Optic nerve (cranial nerve II)

6. Check visual acuity (II tested) (DF 6/10), assess the visual fields (II tested) (DF 7/10), test colour vision, test the pupillary light and accommodation reflexes (II and parasympathetic III tested), and perform fundoscopy (II tested) (DF 9_/10).

The optic nerve is responsible for vision. Begin by asking if the patient has any problems with their eyesight: 'Do you wear glasses or contact lenses?' and 'Are you short or long sighted?' This may provide some initial clues and enables you to make allowances for long-standing problems. If your patient is wearing spectacles ask them politely 'Could you take off your glasses, sir?' Inspect the eyebrows, eyelids, sclera, and pupils. Is there any difference between the eyes? Look specifically for drooping eyelids (ptosis—see later), any deviation of the eyes (strabismus or squint, see later), unequal pupils, or a prosthetic eye. Learning how to spot a prosthetic eye is not usually taught but it is worth knowing so you do not end up with egg on your face. Sometimes the colour of the prosthetic eye is a brilliant white compared with the normal sclera. It sometimes has a shinier appearance and fails to move in any direction (some modern prosthesis can exhibit limited movement but this still looks unrealistic). It is simplest to examine the optic nerve in five stages: visual acuity, visual fields, colour vision, pupil light and accommodation reflexes, and fundoscopy.

Visual acuity

What is it?

This is the ability of the eye to discriminate fine detail·

How to examine

Most people have had their eyesight checked and so should be familiar with the technique. Ideally a Snellen chart is used at 6 m. This is cumbersome in the bedside setting so a 3 m 'end-of-the-bed' version is available. Make sure the patient is wearing their distance glasses (it is so embarrassing to diagnose a severe defect only for the patient to pipe up 'Of course, if I was wearing my glasses I could have read it, no problem!'). The Snellen chart is made up of letters of decreasing size as you read down the chart. Each line is of a standard size so that the vision of your patient can be compared to that of a population of people with healthy sight. You must test one eye at a time. Simply asking the patient to close one eye is inadequate. Some patients find this difficult and even if they succeed it can alter the vision of the eye under test. Ideally an occluder should be used but most people ask the patient to cover their eye with a hand and check they are not cheating,

Tip

Double check that those patients who do wear glasses have fully covered their eye

Say to your patient, 'Can you cover your right eye with your right hand and read the top letter for me. Carry on reading down the chart.' Even when the patient wants to give up, encourage them to continue. The aim is to get your patient to read down the chart until they are unable to read the letters on a particular line. This is the limit of their visual acuity and you should note which line this is. The lines are numbered, usually 60 at the top down to 5 or 6 at the smallest letters at the bottom. You should find this limit for the other eye too. The visual acuity for each eye is represented by a fraction. The top figure represents how far your patient should be away from the Snellen chart when reading it. It is measured in metres and is usually 6. The bottom figure represents the lowest line the patient can read. Most charts label the lines, from top to bottom, 60, 36, 24, 18, 12, 8, 6, and 5. These figures are chosen because most people should be able to read the top line at 60 m, the next line at 36 m, and so on. Therefore people with normal vision can read at least the 6 line (often when their vision is corrected with glasses) and therefore have 6/6 vision. You may have heard the term 20/20 vision—this is the equivalent when the distance is measured in feet rather than metres. If your patient can only read the top line their vision is represented as 6/60. This means they can read at 6 m what a healthy person can read at 60 m. If the patient is unable to read the top letter (which is very poor sight) move the chart to 3 m (if they can read it here their vision is 3/60) or even 1 m. If the patient still has difficulty reading the first line, see if they can count fingers at 1 m, recognize hand movements, or finally, perceive light.

Tip

If you do not possess a standardized visual chart, you can assess vision crudely by getting the patient to read any material close by, for example, a newspaper or your name badge. This will identify any gross visual disturbance or disparity between the eyes. Again check to see if they normally wear reading glasses. If they cannot see any reasonably sized print, see if they can count fingers held up in front of them.

Visual fields

What are they?

When you look at an object, you see not only your point of interest with good quality colour vision (by virtue of the macula, an area of the retina rich in cones, which are the colour-sensitive photo-receptor^s) but you are also aware of surrounding items, for example, as you read this text you may be aware of the immediate environment, such as the desk the book may be resting on. The rest of the retina supplies this 'peripheral' vision by viture of mainly rods, which are the non-colour sensitive photo-receptors and which give a poorer image quality. Visual fields examination represents a mapping out of the patient's peripheral vision and the aim is to discover any areas of visual loss within them.

How to examine

The bedside method of testing visual fields is called the confrontation test. Basically compare your visual fields (which are hopefully normal) with your patient's. To do this the examination position is critical (see Fig. 11.4). The patient may already have their left eye covered with their left hand following their visual acuity assessment. If so, you should cover your right eye with your right hand. To make a direct comparison between you and your patient's visual fields it is essential that your face is on the same level and about 1 m apart (like looking in a mirror). Say, 'I want you to look directly into my left eye and I want you to keep your head and eyes still at all times.' You want your patient to look straight ahead while you bring in your visual source from the periphery. Wiggling your index finger makes a crude but acceptable target. To be more accurate you could use a light source, counting fingers, or a white or better still red neurological hat pin to assess the visual fields. Make sure your target is equidistant between you and the patient. The length of your arms will limit the extent of their visual fields that you can test. Say to your patient, 'Tell me when you can see my finger moving.' When the patient says 'now' you can confirm your findings by stopping and starting your finger movements, 'Are my fingers still moving?' It is traditional to examine the visual fields in four quadrants: upper temporal, upper nasal, lower temporal, and lower nasal (Fig. 11.5). You should bring your finger in from the extremity of each quadrant as a bare minimum. Your aim is to map out as much of the visual fields as is possible.

Once you have checked out the field of the patient's right eye. Say to your patient, 'Uncover your left eye, sir and now cover your right eye with your right hand.' This time you will cover your left eye with your left hand and ask the patient to look at your right eye. Now map out the field for the other eye. Remember your fingers are crude targets and may miss a subtle defect or not define a defect very well, so after using fingers as

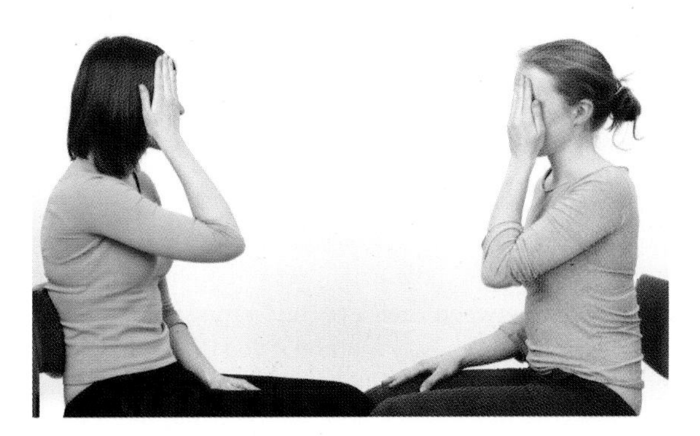

Fig. 11.4 Position for testing visual fields.

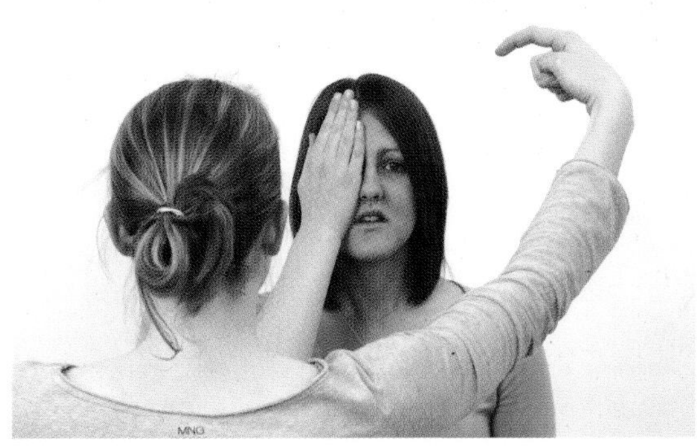

Fig. 11.5 Testing the visual fields by confrontation. Bring the target in from the periphery.

> **Tip**
>
> You may find it difficult to test the nasal fields without swapping the hand that covers your own eye, that is, if your right hand is covering your right eye, you will be using your left hand as the target. This will feel natural until you reach your nasal fields where your inclination will be to force your left arm across your body. Rather than get into this clumsy position, simply cover your right eye with your left hand and use your right hand as the target.

a target use your red neurological pin. Compression on the optic nerve or chiasma may manifest as a duller colour red called 'red desaturation'. Also use the neurological pin to map out the blind spot. The blind spot is a physiological scotoma (see later) and corresponds to the optic disc (where there are no photoreceptors as this is the exit point for the optic nerve). Using your neurological pin, move it slowly in from the temporal side of the eye being tested level with the eye. Your patient should continue to look at your eye as before. They should be aware of the red tip of the pin as it moves slowly inwards until a point is reached where the tip vanishes. If you move the pin further inwards, the tip should reappear again. This 'vanishing' point is only momentary and can be easily missed. Try this on yourself to see how small this point is. Just focus on a point in the distance and bring in a target from the temporal side of the eye you are testing. Make sure that your other eye is closed because the fields of both eyes overlap. This will give you a feeling for what is 'normal'. If however you can move the pin around in a larger area around the blind spot with the tip remaining invisible then this may be an enlarged blind spot and is a feature of papilloedema (*pap-ill-ee-deema*) (see later).

> **Tip**
>
> Practise these manoeuvres on yourself first until you feel confident to perform them on a patient.

> **Tip**
>
> Inevitably during many visual field assessments you will find patients turning their heads or gazing directly at your fingers. If this happens don't become exasperated, just keep reinforcing the command, 'No sir! Keep your head still and just look straight into my eyes.'

Abnormal findings

There is a range of deficits you may pick up from total blindness in one eye to small areas of visual loss (called scotomas). Sometimes the pattern of visual loss can give you a clue to the location of a lesion (see Fig 11.6). It is useful to know the following definitions.

1. **Hemianopia.** This is the loss of one half of a field of vision.
2. **Homonymous hemianopia.** This is the loss of the same half of the visual field in each eye, for example, the left half of the left and right eyes (see Fig. 11.6).
3. **Quadrantinopia (*quad-ran-tin-owe-pia*).** This is the loss of one-quarter of a field of vision.

When interpreting schematic representations of visual fields you need to remember that the image is inverted on the retina. Light rays from the top of an object will be the bottom-most point of the image on the retina. Also light from the temporal half of a field will strike the nasal portion of the retina and light from the nasal half of a field will strike the temporal portion of the retina. The other feature to remember is that nerve fibres from the left and right temporal retinae do not cross the mid-line at the optic chiasma and therefore terminate in the ipsilateral occipital cortex. The fibres from the nasal retinae do cross the mid-line at the optic chiasma and therefore end in the contralateral occipital cortex (see Fig. 11.6).

Colour vision

What is it?

This is a function of our cone photoreceptors .We have three types, which are sensitive to either red, green, or blue wavelengths of light. Colour vision defects can either be congenital or acquired. Congenital defects can occur because of the absence of all colour photoreceptors (monochromatism—very rare), absence of one or more of our three types of cone photoreceptors (rare), or an error of one of the cone types to be sensitive to the correct wavelength of light (common in males). Acquired colour defects are usually a function of optic nerve compromise such as compression by an optic nerve tumour or demyelination in multiple sclerosis and can be a relatively early phenomenon.

How to examine

Colour vision can be measured subjectively, for example, by comparing how bright your patients rate your red hat pin between their eyes and rating both colours out of 10. This is an easy method if you do not have any other method to hand but it is not very accurate because it is quite crude and assumes that one eye is

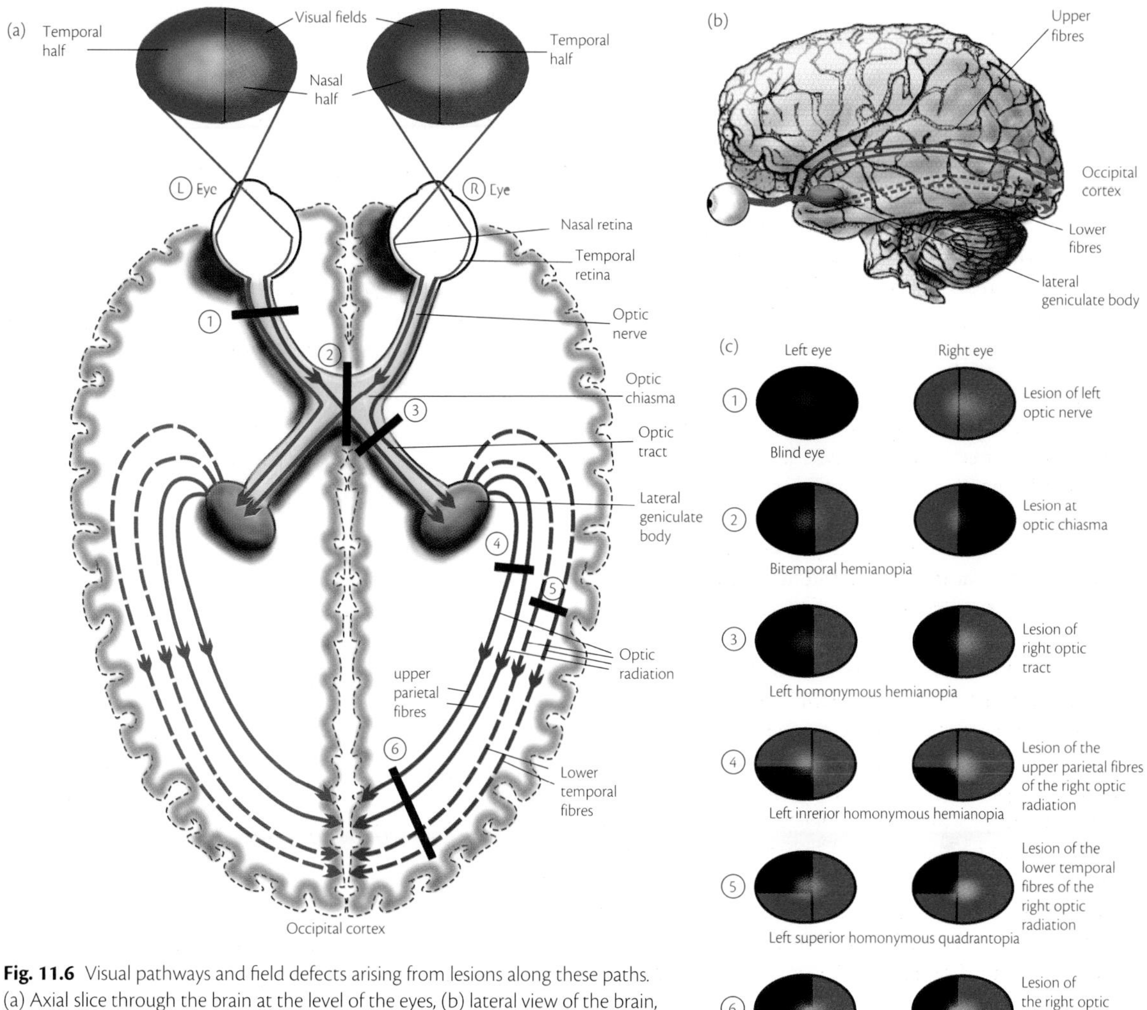

Fig. 11.6 Visual pathways and field defects arising from lesions along these paths. (a) Axial slice through the brain at the level of the eyes, (b) lateral view of the brain, (c) visual defects associated with lesions indicated. Nerve impulses travel down the optic nerves (the nasal fibres crossing at the chiasma) before travelling along the optic tracts to relay in the lateral geniculate bodies. The impulses then travel along the optic radiation to terminate in the occipital cortex. Ultimately the right occipital cortex is responsible for the left half of the visual fields and the left occipital cortex is responsible for the right. The brain is able to synthesize the visual stimuli and correct the inversion of the images to produce meaningful vision.

normal! There are a number of standardized tests to objectively test colour vision though. The most common one is the Ishiara plates. These were designed to test for congenital colour defects but many people use them for acquired defects too. The 'plates' or pages of the book are made up of patterns of dots, which are different colours but have the same brightness. The dots form a square pattern on the page, and has a number hidden within it. A person with normal vision should be able to read the numbers quickly and easily. However depending on the type of colour vision defect different numbers or no numbers at all may be seen.

Pupillary light and accommodation reflexes

Pupillary light reflex: what is it?

This is the constriction of the pupil when a light is shone in the eye and helps to limit the amount of light entering the eyes in bright conditions. In normal circumstances both pupils will constrict when light is shone in one eye. Therefore the reflex is described as direct in the eye being illuminated and consensual in the other eye. On shining a light into someone's eyes, the nerve impulse travels up the optic nerve (cranial nerve II), relaying in the brainstem before passing down the parasympathetic branch of the oculomotor nerve (cranial nerve III). This causes the pupil of that eye to constrict through the sphincter pupillae muscle (direct reflex). Impulses also pass to the oculomotor nerve of the other eye, leading to constriction of that pupil also (consensual reflex). See Fig. 11.7.

Pupillary light reflex: how to examine

First inspect each pupil and make sure that they are equal in size and that they are round and regular. Any asymmetry in pupil size or shape needs to be explained (see later). A small difference in pupil size of about a millimeter is acceptable and may be physiological, especially if this relationship is maintained both in bright and poor illumination and is variable between eyes. Pupils that are constricted are called miotic (the process of constriction is called miosis) and pupils that are dilated are called mydriatic (*mid-dree-attic*) (the process of dilatation is called mydriasis (*mid-dree-ay-sis*)). Healthy pupils will be constricted in bright sunshine and dilated in poor light. Despite this range in size they should still display the direct and consensual reflex (although it is much harder to spot the change in size when the pupils are small to begin with). Warn your patient, 'I am going to shine a light into your eyes ... it will be a little bright.' Your pen torch should be brought in from the side of the face and shone in the same eye on two successive occasions (shine the light for no more than a split second). The first time, look at the same pupil for the direct reflex and the second time look into the other pupil for a consensual response. It is sometimes taught to put a hand vertically from the nose to the forehead (to stop some light shining in both eyes), but this technique looks clumsy and is unnecessary. Now do the same to the other eye. You should have used your torch on four separate occasions.

Tip

It can be difficult to spot the constriction if the pupils are small to begin with. If this is the case try to reduce background light as much as possible, for example, closing blinds or switching off the bedside lamp. Or take your patient to somewhere dimly lit and try again.

Pupillary accommodation reflex: what is it?

When you look into the distance and then switch your focus to an object close to your eyes, the adjustment process is called accommodation. During this process your eyes turn inward marginally (converge) and the pupils constrict to limit the light received to the approximate area of interest. As before the impulse travels up the optic nerve and relays in the brainstem, before returning down the oculomotor nerve to constrict the pupil.

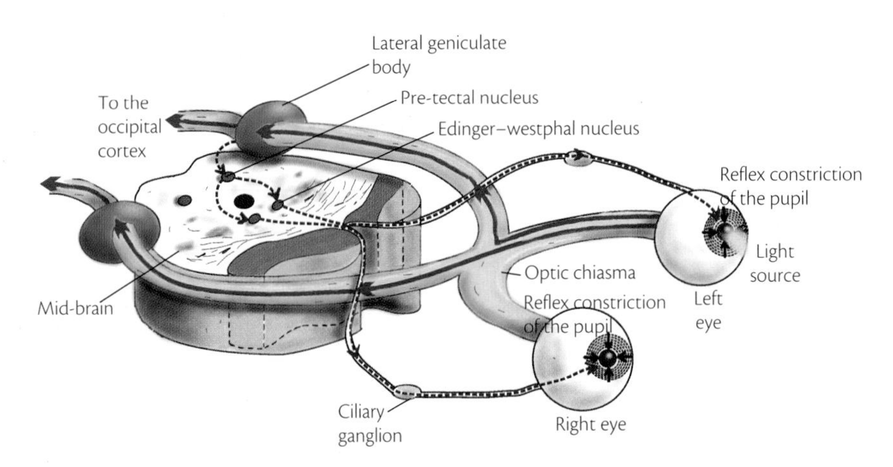

Fig. 11.7 Pathways associated with the pupillary light reflex. A light shone into the left eye leads to nerve impulses conducted in the normal way along the optic chiasma to the lateral geniculate body (some impulses continue to the occipital cortex). The brightness of the light triggers impulses along another (reflex) pathway leading to the pre-tectal nucleus and then to both Edinger-Westphal nuclei (The parasympathetic nucleus of the 3rd nerve). Further impulses travel via the ciliary ganglion to the sphincter pupillae muscle of both eyes which contract in response to limit the light entering the eyes.

Pupillary accommodation reflex: how to examine

Choose a distant point that is at least 6 m away (ideally the further away the better). It is better to give the patient an object to focus on rather than just telling them to gawp into the distance. Say something like, 'Look at the number one on the clock on the far wall.' Observe the size of the pupils and wait until you are certain they are focusing on the distant object. Have your near target, preferably a very small picture or a small letter (because they will stimulate accommodation better, however many use their index finger) close to your patient's face (at a distance of about 15 cm) and then quickly ask them to look at your finger. Observe the pupils and see if they constrict as they focus on your finger. Be careful to get a good look at both pupils because in some conditions the pupils will remain constricted for some time and so you will not be able to repeat the test. The reaction is often very minimal so it can be easily missed! This test was important in the days when syphilis was rife when patients sometimes exhibited Argyll-Robertson (*are-guile-robert-son*) pupils (*Douglas Moray Cooper Lamb Argyll-Robertson (1837–1909), Scottish ophthalmologist*). In this condition the pupils are small and irregular and the key feature is that they do not react to light but constrict with accommodation. Nowadays this is rarely seen, although it can occur in some people with diabetes.

(a)

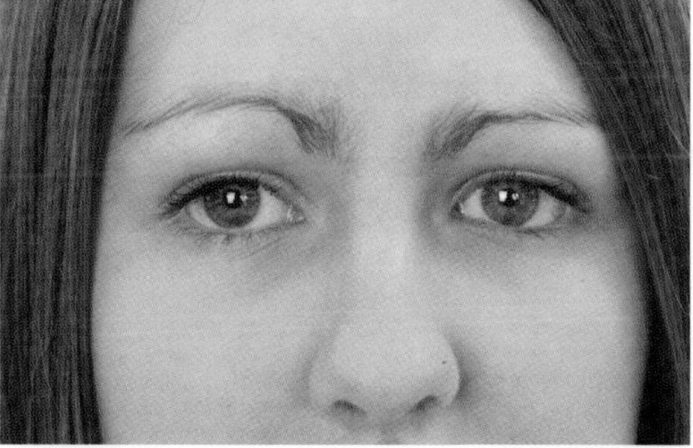

(b)

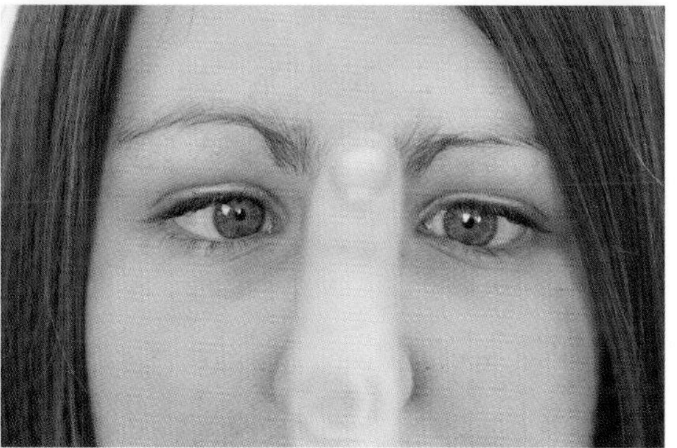

Fig. 11.8 Testing the accommodation reflex. (a) Looking into the distance, (b) focusing on finger: note the convergence of the eyes and constriction of the pupils.

Tip

Choose somewhere slightly elevated for the distant point and keep your finger slightly above the level of the patient's eyes when you ask them to focus on it. This prevents the upper eyelid from obscuring your view of the pupils (see Fig. 11.8).

Abnormal findings

1. **Pin-point pupils.** See Fig. 11.9. Caused by bilateral instillation of miotic eye drops, for example, pilocarpine (*pile-owe-carp-een*), opiate overdose, brainstem stroke (pontine), bilateral Horner's syndrome (*Johann Friedrich Horner (1831–1886), Swiss ophthalmologist*), and old age.
2. **Dilated pupils.** See Fig. 11.10. Caused by bilateral instillation of mydriatic eye drops, for example, tropicamide (*trow-pick-amide*), fear or anger, drug overdose, for example, anti-cholinergic drugs, and brainstem stroke (mid-brain).
3. **Unilateral miosis.** See Fig. 11.11. Caused by miotic eye drops in the affected eye, Horner's syndrome, and Holmes–Adie (*homes-ay-dee*) pupil (*Sir Gordon Holmes (1876–1965), English neurologist, William John Adie (1886–1935), Australian-born British physician*).

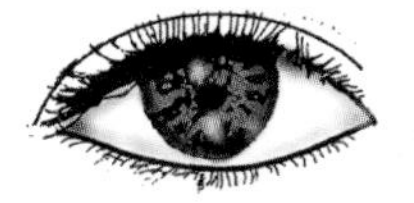
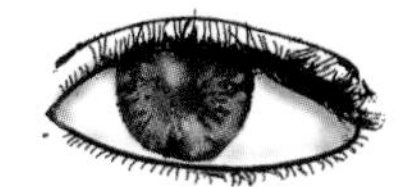

Fig. 11.9 Bilateral miosis.

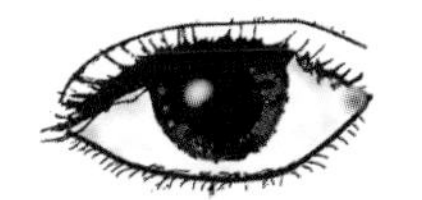
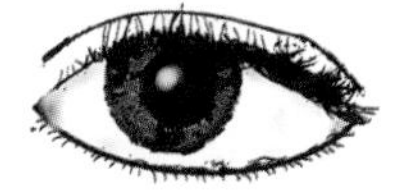

Fig. 11.10 Bilateral mydriasis.

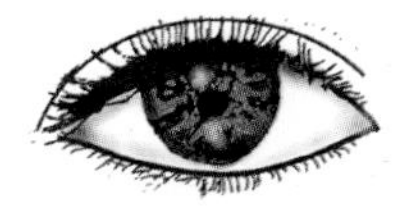
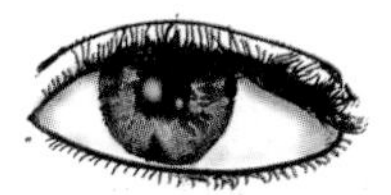

Fig. 11.11 Unilateral miosis of the right eye.

4. **Fixed oval pupil (not reactive to light or accommodation).** Caused by acute untreated glaucoma.
5. **Grossly irregular pupil (not reactive to light or accommodation).** Caused by previous trauma and adhesions of the iris to the lens, which occurs in irits (called posterior synechiae (*sign-ee-key-eye*)).
6. **Unilateral mydriasis.** See Fig. 11.12. Caused by mydriatic eye drops in the affected eye and IIIrd nerve palsy.
7. **Argyll-Robertson pupils.** Small irregular pupils (not reactive to light but react to accommodation). Caused by syphilis and diabetes mellitus.
8. **Marcus Gunn pupil (relative afferent pupillary defect (RAPD)).** (*R. Marcus Gunn (1850–1909), Scottish ophthalmologist.*) This is due to either damage of the optic nerve, for example, due to retrobulbar neuritis secondary to multiple sclerosis or massive retinal damage, for example, a retinal detachment. A RAPD can be demonstrated by the swinging light test. First shine a very bright light in one eye from the side for 3 s. If this eye is normal, both pupils will constrict briskly. Quickly swing the light over to the other eye. If the second eye is affected the pupil is seen to dilate rather than constrict. This is because the change in stimulus to the second eye has changed from the powerful direct reflex coming from the normal first eye and is now much weaker because it is coming from the damaged afferent pathway from the second eye. After 3 s quickly swing the light back to the first eye and now note both pupils will constrict again. You can keep swinging between the eyes to check your findings. To make yourself look slick, perform this test following testing the direct and consensual pupil reactions.

Tip

When faced with pupillary abnormalities also check for drooping eyelids (ptosis—see later). The presence of ptosis will exclude many causes but not a IIIrd nerve palsy or Horner's syndrome.

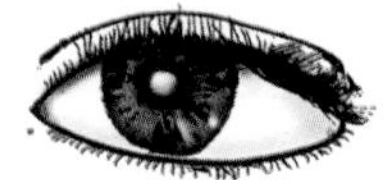

Fig. 11.12 Unilateral mydriasis of the right eye.

Fundoscopy

What is it?

The fundus (*fun-duss*) in this context is synonymous with the retina. Fundoscopy is the examination of the retina and the structures that enter and leave it using an instrument called an ophthalmoscope (sometimes the technique is called ophthalomoscopy but this is rather a mouthful). In reality, when you become skilled at performing fundoscopy you can inspect other structures of the eye including the lens and abnormalities in the vitreous humour.

How to examine

Everyone who has tried fundoscopy knows how difficult it is to perform. There are four stages that you have to master before you can become proficient at this procedure:

(1) being familiar with the ophthalmoscope (see Fig. 11.13);

(2) being familiar with using the ophthalmoscope on a patient;

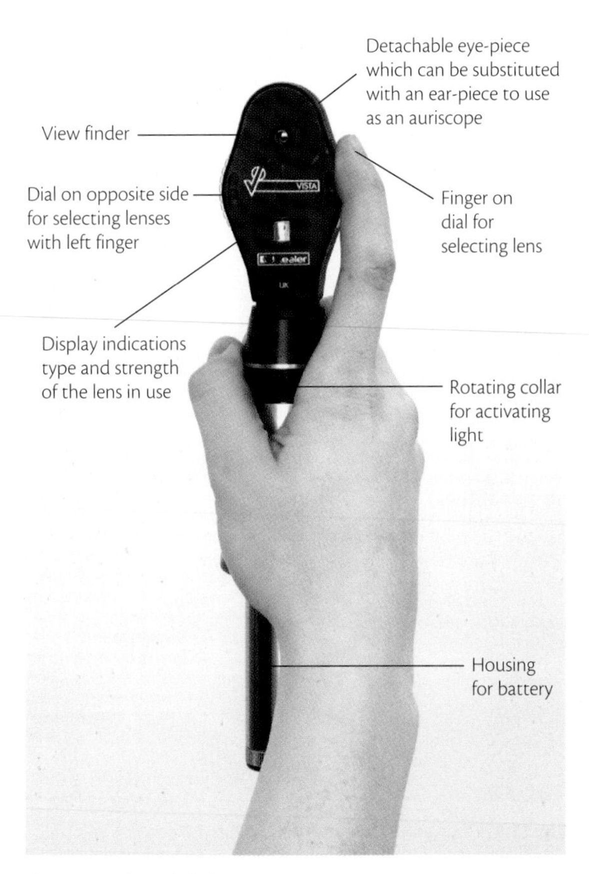

Fig. 11.13 The ophthalmoscope.

(3) being familiar with the normal fundus;

(4) learning what different abnormalities can affect the fundus.

1. First, familiarize yourself with the controls of the ophthalmoscope. There is usually a dial, which can be turned by the index finger of either hand depending on which eye you are examining. The dial alters the lenses within the instrument. These range from positive lenses (these may have red numbers and are used to focus your view in long-sighted (hypermetropic) patients) to negative lenses (these may have black numbers and are used to focus your view in short-sighted (myopic) patients). Some models of ophthalmoscopes use red numbers for negative lenses and black for positive lenses, so be wary. There is also a switch to activate the light. On most models you will press in a switch and rotate a collar or the base of the ophthalmoscope to turn the light on. There may also be controls to alter the size, strength, and colour of the beam. A small beam is used when looking through a small pupil in order to minimize reflections, but the larger the beam the better in a dilated patient. The green light or 'red free' is used to increase contrast when looking at red things on the retina. Small haemorrhages are therefore easier to see.

2. Now it is time to try and use the instrument on a patient. See Fig. 11.14. To best see the fundus, your patient's pupils should be adequately dilated. The best method for achieving this is with short-acting eye drops. Unfortunately unless you are in a specialist eye clinic, it is more likely that your patient will not have this done. The next best thing is to find a room that can be darkened sufficiently to allow your patient's pupils to dilate—the pupils will constrict when you shine your light in though! If your patient wears glasses, these must be removed. If you wear glasses however, it is perfectly acceptable for you to leave them on (as it reduces the need to correct for both your own vision and the patient's with the opthalmoscope).

To look in the patient's right eye hold the ophthalmoscope in your right hand and use your right eye. You will have to examine from the right hand side of the patient. Similarly, for the patient's left eye, use your left eye and left hand and examine from the left-hand side of the patient. You have to get very close to your patient so make sure you have had a shower and not eaten garlic the previous night! Now hold your ophthalmoscope steady and peer through its aperture. Some people emphasize that your redundant eye should remain open. As you improve you will be able to do this but in the early stages it is easier to keep the eye shut.

Get your patient to look slightly upwards for two reasons: first, so their eyelids do not obscure the pupils (you may have to use the thumb of your other hand to gently pull the upper eyelid out of the way) and second, so that when you move in from the side you 'hit' the optic disc almost immediately (the optic disc is an important reference point—see later). Say to your patient, 'Look straight ahead please, where the ceiling joins the wall, try and concentrate on that spot even if I get in the way.' While you have the patient at arm's length elicit the red reflex in both eyes. You should see a red reflection just like the red eyes on an amateur photograph. An absent or reduced reflex implies an

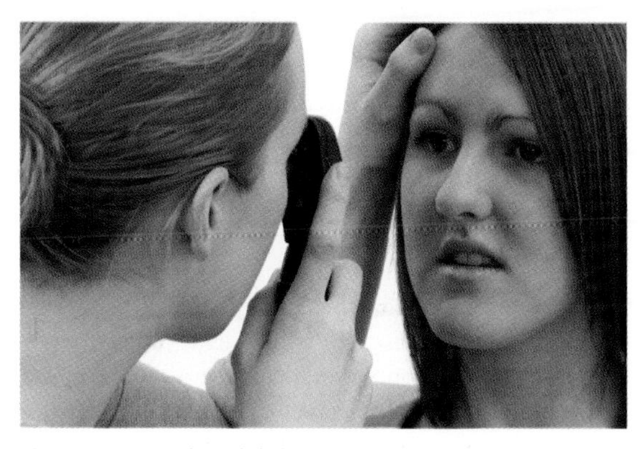

Fig. 11.14 Using the ophthalmoscope.

> **Tip**
>
> It can be difficult to tell if the light has been activated so point the ophthalmoscope towards your palm and look for a small circle of light. When you have finished using the ophthalmoscope it is even more important to check that it has been switched off completely. So point it at your palm again and make sure the light has gone. This is because it is very easy to leave it on and drain the batteries, leaving the ward without a functioning opthalmoscope (it is amazing how some wards do not even have a stock of spare batteries).

> **Tip**
>
> Practise getting the feel of the ophthalmoscope and use it with both hands. Get used to turning the dials with the index finger of either hand, before trying it on a patient.

opacity somewhere in the path of the retina. The most commone cause is a cataract. Move in slowly until you see the retina. Focus the ophthalmoscope by using the negative lenses if the patient is short sighted and the positive lenses if the patient is long sighted.

Now identify the optic disc. The optic disc represents the exit point of the nerve fibres from the retina to become the optic nerve. Once in focus, comment upon its three Cs: the colour· the contour, and the cup. The colour of the optic disc is usually a light pinky-orange. If there is optic atrophy (see later) the disc becomes a pale yellow colour. Papilloedema (see later) produces a reddy-pink disc. The contour of the disc is usually well defined. With papilloedema the margin of the whole disc becomes indistinct and blurred (see diagram). The optic cup is the small oval aperture within the optic disc, which transmits the blood vessels to the retina. The diameter of the cup is normally small compared to that of the optic disc (see Fig. 11.5). If there is ischaemia of the optic nerve or if there is glaucoma (a condition with raised intraocular pressure (IOP) and a damaged optic nerve causing visual field defects) there is loss of the nerve fibres and this leads to an increase in the cup diameter relative to the optic disc, a process called 'cupping'. Determining what constitutes 'glaucomatous cupping' is subjective and has led to disagreement. For the non-ophthalmologist if there is any doubt send your patient to an expert for further evaluation.

There are four 'arcades' of arteries and veins radiating from the optic disc, each extending into the superior and inferior temporal and the superior and inferior nasal quadrants. Follow each in turn, noting the appearance of the vessels and the surrounding retina. Now get the patient to look up, down , left, and right to see the peripheries of the retina. Some signs such as pigmentation in retinitis pigmentosa may only be seen when looked for in the peripheries. This will give you a good systematic method of reviewing the fundus. Some advocate asking the patient to look into the four different directions, however this causes the pupil to move and may disorientate you. Now say to your patient, 'Look directly into the light for me ... I know it is difficult.' This will enable you to assess the macula. You may have to refocus the ophthalmoscope. Finally, 'rack back' through the positive lenses and review the more anterior structures of the eye. These include the vitreous for floaters and even the iris.

3. See Fig. 11.15. The only way to appreciate what a normal fundus looks like is to see as many as you can. It is worth looking at ophthalmology atlases, which will show you the variety of normal fundi that exist.

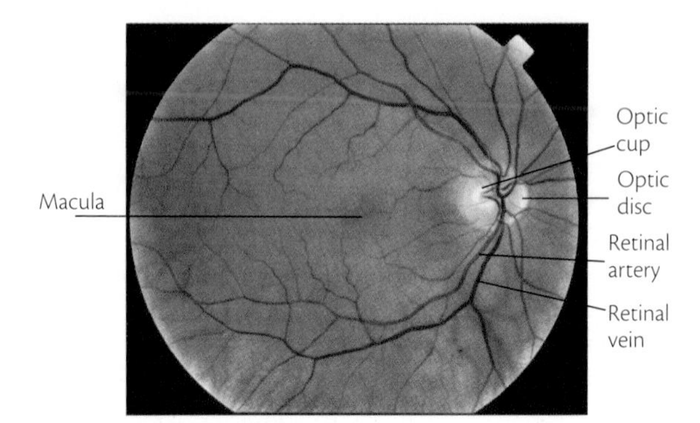

Fig. 11.15 Normal fundus.

4. Similarly the best way to learn about pathology is to study the appearances in an ophthalmology atlas and take any opportunity you can to see these in real patients if you hear about them. Ophthalmology clinics and diabetic eye clinics are the best places to see common abnormalities. Figs 11.16 and 11.17 show the appearances of important abnormalities you should be conversant with.

Papilloedema

Papilloedema refers to the appearance of the fundus in response to raised intracranial pressure. As a consequence of this pressure the eye goes through a sequence of changes.

(a)

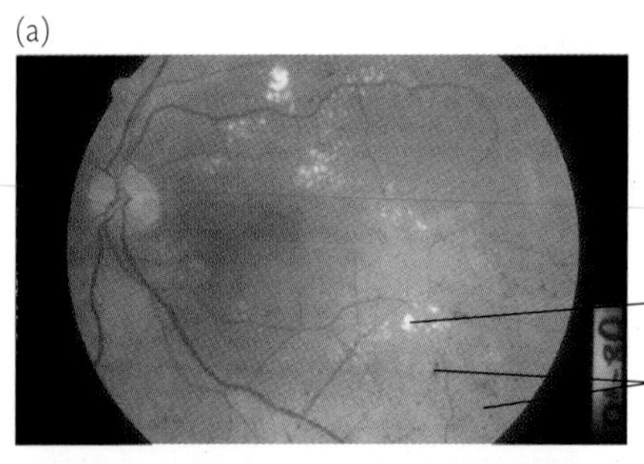

(b)

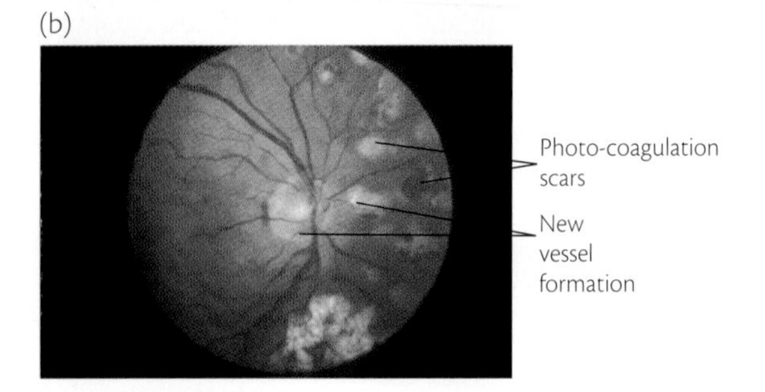

Fig. 11.16 Diabetic retinopathy. (a) Background retinopathy, (b) proliferative retinopathy.

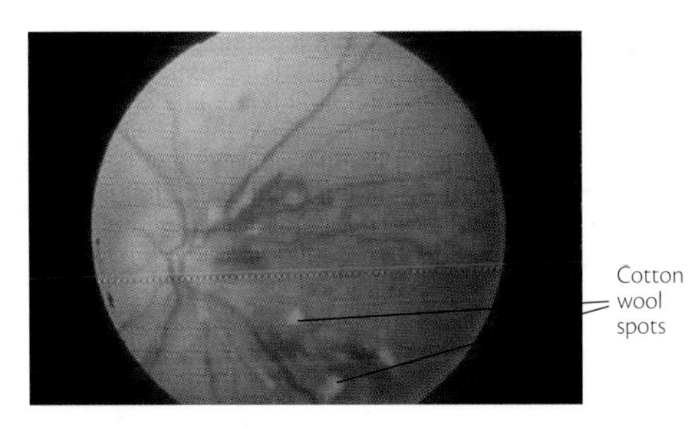

Fig. 11.17 Hypertensive retinopathy showing cotton wool spots.

1. Initially there is a loss of venous pulsation and the veins may become more dilated and tortuous. Not many clinicians have the expertise to spot these early changes.
2. Then the optic cup becomes pinker and indistinct.
3. The contour of the optic disc becomes blurred and vessels seem to disappear at the margins of the disc, rather than running straight into the optic cup.
4. The whole of the optic disc becomes pink and swollen.
5. Other changes may be seen depending on the underlying cause, for example, malignant hypertension—flame-shaped haemorrhages radiating from the optic disc.

The causes of papilloedema are

(1) raised intracranial pressure;

(2) space-occupying lesion, for example, cerebral tumour, intracranial haematoma, or cerebral abscess;

(3) malignant hypertension (see Fig. 11.18);

(4) benign intracranial hypertension (BIH);

(5) severe hypercapnia (*high-per-cap-knee-a*);

(6) complication of meningitis;

(7) central retinal vein thrombosis (see Fig. 11.19).

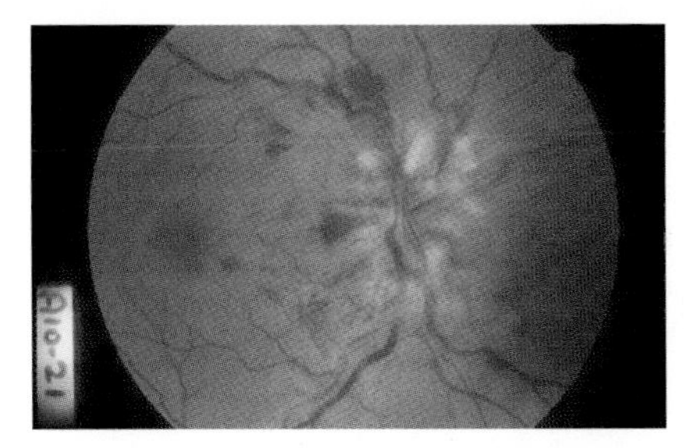

Fig. 11.18 Papilloedema secondary to malignant hypertension.Note the veins seem to disappear on approaching the optic disc or loop over the swollen margin. Also note the flame shaped haemorrhages.

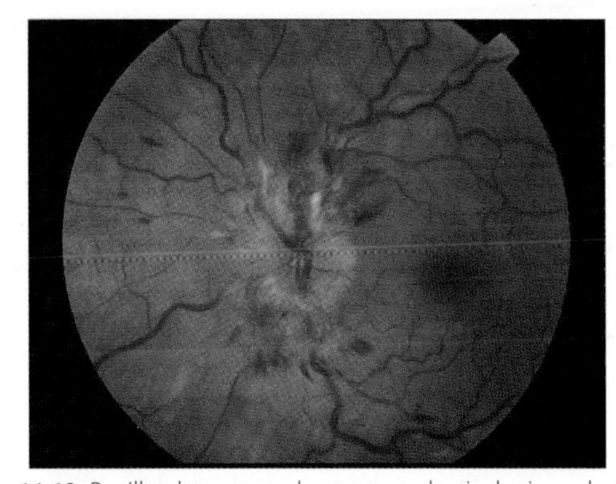

Fig. 11.19 Papilloedema secondary to central retinal vein occlusion. Note similar appearance of the optic disc,. However, haemorrhages are scattered more widely than in malignant hypertension.

The presence of papilloedema indicates the need for further investigation. It is also a cautionary sign when considering a lumbar puncture. If a lumbar puncture is performed in the presence of raised intracranial pressure there is the risk of 'coning', where the brainstem is forced down through the foramen magnum with lethal consequences. A computed tomography (CT) scan **must** be performed prior to the consideration of a lumbar puncture in the presence of papilloedema. However the absence of papilloedema does not rule out the possibility of raised intracranial pressure (because the eye changes may lag behind the onset of raised pressure). Therefore do not perform a lumbar puncture if the history suggests the possibility of raised intracranial pressure even if the discs are normal.

CASE 11.1

Problem. You are performing fundoscopy and are struggling to see any landmarks in the fundus. Why is this?

Discussion. Initially your technique may be to blame as you get used to use the ophthalmoscope. Many people have difficulty using their non-dominant eye while holding the instrument with their non-dominant hand. Only practice will solve this. However the biggest stumbling block to visualizing the fundus is constricted pupils. Most people attempt to view the fundus in broad daylight and are destined to fail. The pupils need dilating with short-acting eye drops like tropicamide. The next best thing is a room that can be made dark enough to allow the pupil to dilate sufficiently.

Keypoints

- With any visual disturbance always check visual acuity with a standardized assessment chart, for example, Snellen chart.
- With any visual disturbance always check the visual fields.
- If the pupils are not equal in size this must be explained.
- Always observe the response of the pupils to light and accommodation.
- Fundoscopy is a vital technique and must be mastered.
- Only perform fundoscopy with the pupils properly dilated either with short-acting dilating eye drops or a sufficiently darkened room otherwise you are doomed to fail.
- Make sure that you are familiar with the range of normal fundi that can be found.
- Make sure that you are familiar with the appearances of common diseases you are likely to see in everyday practice.
- A swollen optic disc is an indicator of raised intracranial pressure.
- Do not perform a lumbar puncture in the presence of papilloedema without a normal CT scan to check it is safe to do so.
- Do not perform a lumbar puncture without a CT scan if the history suggests raised intracranial pressure even if the optic discs are normal.

Oculomotor (III), trochlear (IV), and abducens (VI) nerves

7. Inspect for ptosis and a squint and check eye movements: look for nystagmus and ask about diplopia (III, IV, and VI tested).

Inspect for ptosis

What is it?

Ptosis is the medical term for a drooping eyelid. Normally with ptosis, the lower margin of the eyelid passes just below the upper border of the pupil when a person is awake. The lid can droop sufficiently to encroach on the visual axis. At this point the lid will interfere with the patient's upper field of vision.

Significance

The levator palpebrae (*le-vay-tor-pal-pe-bray*) is the main muscle that elevates the eyelid and is supplied by the IIIrd cranial nerve. Mullers muscle also helps lift the eyelid to a small degree and is supplied by the sympathetic system. This is why the eyes appear more open when the body is in a frightened state and why a complete lesion of the IIIrd cranial nerve produces a complete ptosis whereas a lesion of the sympathetic system (Horner's system, see pp. 89, 410) produces a partial (small) ptosis.

TABLE 11.7 Causes of Ptosis

Myogenic	Horner's syndrome, IIIrd nerve palsy, and chronic progressive external ophthalmoplegia*
Neurogenic	Myasthenia gravis, mytonia dystrophica
Tendon	Involutional (= old age)
Others	Trauma, infection, inflammation, tumours, and congenital

* See main text for details.

Causes

Causes of ptosis are given in Table 11.7. They are easy to remember if you think of the different anatomical structures requires to lift the eyelid, that is, the nerves, muscles, tendon, and of course the 'other' group as well. It is important to remember some causes of pseudo ptosis, that is, cases that look like ptosis but are not really. These include the fellow eyelid being retracted, for example, in thyroid eye disease or the globe being sunken in enophthalmos, for example, after a blow-out fracture of the orbit.

What to look for

A complete ptosis is obvious. Mild degrees of ptosis can be easily missed. Make sure that your patient is looking directly ahead and focus on the eyelids (if they are looking up or down the appearance of the eyelids will be misleading). Does one seem to droop more than the other? If it does quickly check there is no obvious infection or swelling there. Also quickly check pupil size. A tiny pupil (miotic) may suggest a Horner's syndrome and a large pupil (mydriatic) that does not react to light suggests a IIIrd nerve lesion. Bilateral ptosis, which is mild, is very hard to spot. However if you notice both eyelids encroaching on the visual axis, this is abnormal. See Figs 11.20–11.22.

Inspect for a squint

What is it?

The eyes are normally aligned in parallel and move together as a unit. A squint (medical term strabismus) (*stra-biz-muss*) is where one of the eyes deviates from the

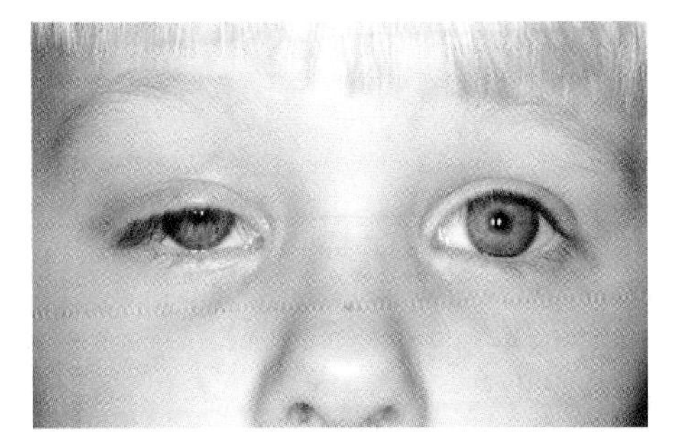

Fig. 11.20 Congenital ptosis. Note the right pupil is of comparable size to the left.

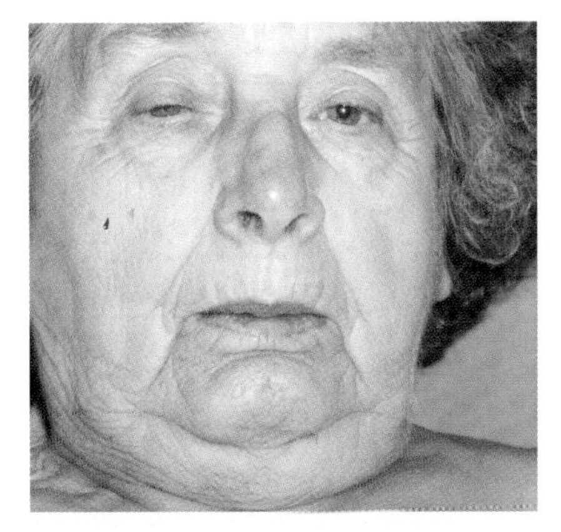

Fig. 11.21 Bilateral ptosis due to myasthenia gravis. Ptosis improved with injection of cholinesterase inhibitor.

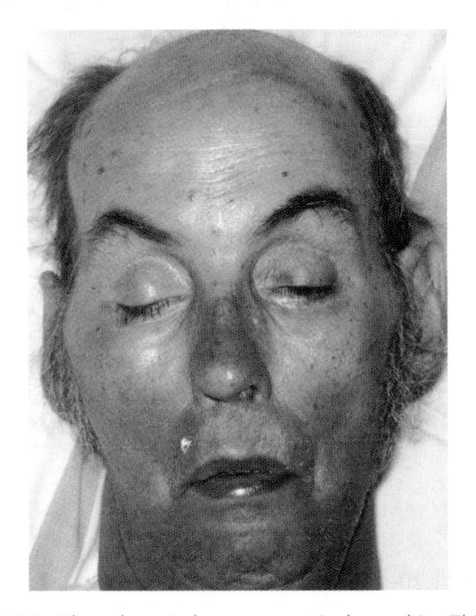

Fig. 11.22 Bilateral ptosis due to myotonia dystrophica. This patient has the typical facies of the condition. There is the 'hollowing out' of the temples because of wasting of the temporalis muscles. There is also wasting of the masseters of the cheeks and of the sternomastoids also. As this is a myopathic cause he is unable to wrinkle his forehead to improve his ptosis.

Tip

With most forms of ptosis the patient compensates by contracting their frontalis (*front-ay-lis*) muscle (the muscle that makes the forehead wrinkle) to produce a modest elevation of the eyelids. The exceptions to this rule are the myopathic causes of ptosis where this muscle may also be affected.

Tip

If the ptosis is sufficient to compromise the upper field of vision, the patient may tilt their head backward to improve their field of vision.

parallel. If the affected eye turns inward this is called a convergent squint. If the affected eye turns outwards this is called a divergent squint. Squints can be further classified as concomitant or paralytic. A concomitant squint is where the deviation remains constant whichever direction the person looks. It is termed incomitant if this is not the case. A paralytic squint is where the affected eye has a weakened extra-ocular muscle. The angle of deviation is maximal when looking in the direction of action of the paralysed muscle.

Significance

Concomitant squints are usually found from childhood onwards and may be congenital or due to refractive errors. The developing brain suppresses the image from the affected eye, preventing diplopia. If this suppression occurs during a child's critical development period, which is up to about the age of 8 years, the eye may never develop to be as strong as the other, that is, it will produce amblyopia (*am-blee-owe-pia*) (otherwise known as a 'lazy eye'). Refractive errors need to be corrected with spectacles. Amblyopia is usually treated by covering the good eye, in a bid to force the use of the lazy eye. This form of squint therefore must be rectified before the image from the affected eye is irreversibly suppressed. Paralytic squints are usually due to lesions of the IIIrd or VIth nerve (the squint due to the IVth nerve is subtle). Patients with paralytic squints need further evaluation to find an underlying cause (see later).

Check eye movements: look for nystagmus and ask about diplopia

All three cranial nerves supply the extra-ocular muscles and are responsible for the smooth and co-ordinated movement of the eyes (this is conjugate eye move-

Fig. 11.23 Nystagmus of the left eye on looking to the left.

ment). Problems with any of these nerves will impair eye movements and lead to double vision.

Nystagmus: what is it?

See Fig. 11.23. This is the involuntary, repetitive oscillation of one or both eyes. Each oscillation can be of equal rate where the nystagmus (*nis-stag-muss*) is called pendular, or there can be a fast and a slow phase when it is termed jerky. With jerky nystagmus the direction of nystagmus is determined by the direction of the fast phase, for example, if the eye flicks out quickly to the right and slowly returns to the left, the direction of nystagmus is to the right. Nystagmus is usually in the horizontal plane but occasionally can occur in the vertical plane (where you should be suspicious of a brainstem lesion). It can also be rotatory usually due to vestibular lesions). If nystagmus is severe it can be observed at rest. Otherwise it has to be provoked by eye movements (the basis of clinical testing below).

Nystagmus: significance

Nystagmus is a problem maintaining the posture of the eye or conjugate eye movements. The problem can be anywhere along a pathway that includes the eye itself, the vestibular system, the cerebellum, the brainstem, and their complex interconnections. Paradoxically it is not the fast phase of nystagmus that is abnormal. Rather it is the slow phase, which represents the aberrant drift of the eye away from the visual source and the fast phase is the compensatory flick back to the target.

Nystagmus: causes

The causes of nystagmus are

- physiological (optokinetic nystagmus, end-point nystagmus, and vestibular stimulation)
- congenital
- visual impairment
- vestibular disease (BPPV)
- central lesions
- cerebellar disease.

1. **Physiological.** These are normal responses of the eye to various stimuli. Optokinetic nystagmus is the jerky nystagmus that can sometimes occur when tracking a fast-moving target, for example, watching scenery going by in a car. End-point nystagmus is the jerky nystagmus that can occur at the extremes of gaze. Vestibular stimulation will occur if a person spins repeatedly. They become dizzy and may exhibit jerky or rotational nystagmus. Vestibular stimulation can also occur by introducing cold water into the ear canal. This is called caloric testing and is a recognized test of labyrinthine function.
2. **Congenital.** This is present at or soon after birth. The nystagmus is usually seen in all directions of gaze and is pendular in nature. It is often familial and has no other serious consequences.
3. **Visual impairment.** People with severe visual impairment have difficulty fixing on a target; the eye roves around and the associated nystagmus is pendular in nature.
4. **Vestibular disease**. The vestibular system is concerned with maintaining balance. Lesions affecting its peripheral apparatus, for example, SCCs, can cause a jerky or rotational nystagmus. The direction of nystagmus is away from the affected side. Associated diseases that affect this apparatus include viral labyrinthitis and Ménière's syndrome. Associated symptoms may include vertigo, tinnitus, and deafness. These forms of nystagmus tend to be self-limiting.
5. **Central lesions.** A central lesion in this context means a problem in the central nervous system (or brain essentially). The areas that are affected are usually the posterior fossa (an area of the brain that houses the cerebellum) or the brainstem. A tumour, demyelinating diseases such as multiple sclerosis, or a stroke affecting these areas can cause vertigo and nystagmus (which may behave like benign positional vertigo). The difference with central lesions is that there is no delay before the onset of nystagmus, it is not fatiguable, and head movements in any direction can provoke it (see 'Hallpike-Dix manoeuvre' section).
6. **Cerebellar disease.** The cerebellum is also concerned with balance and the co-ordination of movement. Lesions of the cerebellum lead to ataxia (unsteadiness) and a jerky nystagmus with the direction towards the affected side. A wide range of diseases can affect the cerebellum including tumours, multiple sclerosis, stroke, alcohol, inherited disease, and degenerative disorders. To examine, hold your finger about 1 m away from the patient. Ensure your patient

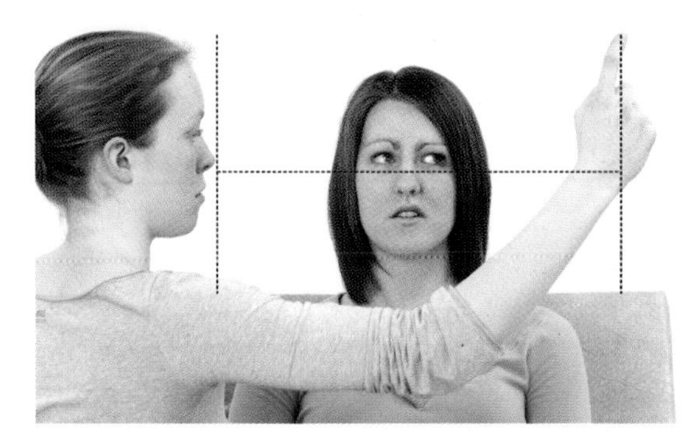

Fig. 11.24 Testing eye movements for diplopia and nystagmus.

does not turn their head as they follow your finger. Say, 'I would like you to keep your head still and to follow my finger by moving your eyes only' (also add, 'Please tell me if you see double at any time' (see later)). Now slowly move your finger through a 'H' configuration. It does not matter which part of the 'H' you start on, so long as you trace along its entirety (see Fig. 11.24). Move you finger smoothly to each extreme of your 'H' configuration. You will have to judge how far you move your finger but it should only be to a point where your patient's eyes can comfortably view it without straining or moving their head. As the eyes move look for any abnormal oscillation of the eyes. If nystagmus is present determine whether it is jerky, pendular, or rotational and if it is jerky, work out its direction. You will not be able to deduce the significance of the nystagmus solely on the basis of eye movements. You will need a history and full neurological examination to enable you to do so. Also nystagmus may be more complex than has been described. Some conditions can affect more than one organ or neural pathway producing a hybrid nystagmus, for example, an acoustic neuroma can affect

CASE 11.2

Problem. A 43-year-old woman presents to an acute admissions unit with a sudden onset of vertigo. The room spins around a vertical axis and is associated with nausea. She has no deafness or tinnitus. You check her eye movements and you notice nystagmus to the left in all directions of gaze. What is the diagnosis?

Discussion. This story sounds typical of an attack of acute labyrinthitis. There is a sudden onset of true vertigo without tinnitus or deafness, which distinguishes it from Ménière's syndrome. With vestibular disease the direction of nystagmus is away from the affected side, in this case the affected organ is the right labyrinth.

CASE 11.3

Problem. You see a 36-year-old man who is a known epileptic. He is on phenytoin and has been well controlled since his dose was increased 6 weeks prior to presentation. He now feels unsteady on his feet and groggy. The consultant asks you to examine his eye movements and you notice nystagmus in both directions of gaze. What is the cause of the nystagmus?

Discussion. The cause is phenytoin toxicity. Phenytoin has a narrow therapeutic range and small increases in dosage can rapidly lead to toxicity. Symptoms and signs include dizziness, ataxia, tremor, and nystagmus. In this case, an increase in dose occurred 6 weeks ago. It is also worth checking if any new medications have been added because some drugs can interfere with the metabolism of phenytoin. Blood needs to be taken for a phenytoin level to confirm a high plasma level and the dose reduced accordingly.

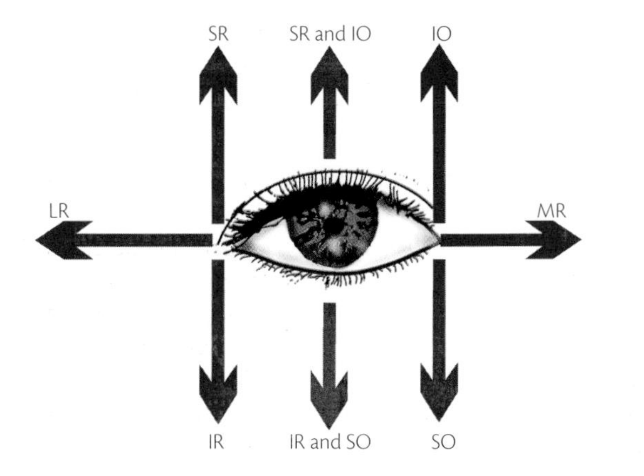

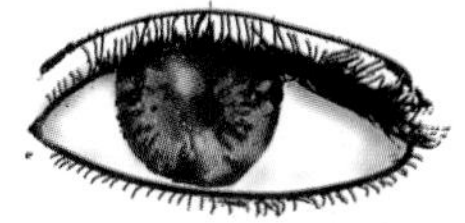

Fig. 11.25 The direction of action of the eye muscles. MR, medial rectus; LR, lateral rectus; SR, superior rectus; IR, inferior rectus; IO, inferior oblique; SO, superior oblique.

the vestibular nerve causing nystagmus and as it grows it can also compress the brainstem and affect central vestibular or cerebellar pathways.

Diplopia: what is it?

This is the resultant double vision caused (usually) by extra-ocular muscle dysfunction.

Diplopia: significance

Commonly this is because of damage to the nerve supply to the extra-ocular muscles, that is, the IIIrd, IVth, and VIth nerves. Other mechanisms are discussed later. Normally, eye movements are controlled by six extra-ocular muscles working together in pairs (see Fig. 11.25). Remembering their function is relatively easy as their name reflects their actions (with notable exceptions), for example,

(1) superior rectus—elevates the eye superiorly;

(2) inferior rectus—depresses the eye inferiorly;

(3) lateral rectus—pulls the eye laterally (called abduction);

(4) medial rectus—pulls the eye medially (called adduction.)

The exceptions are the 'obliques,' which have complex paths prior to their insertion on to the globe of the eye, such that their actions are opposite to that suggested by their name:

(1) inferior oblique—elevates the eye;

(2) superior oblique—depresses the eye.

As the Fig. 11.25 points out, eye elevation and depression are more complicated. The superior and inferior recti muscles have their greatest effect when the eye is abducted. The superior and inferior oblique muscles have their greatest effect when the eye is adducted. When the eye is mid-way between abduction and adduction, the superior rectus and inferior oblique combine to elevate the eye and the inferior rectus and the superior oblique combine to depress the eye. Note that some of the extra-ocular muscles also have rotational effects but you do not need to know these (a technique for identifying a IVth nerve palsy in the presence of a IIIrd nerve lesion uses this principle) see p. 301.

Neural centres in the brainstem and cerebral cortex co-ordinate eye movements so that light from an object will fall on corresponding points of the retina of each eye (usually the macula). This binocular input allows the brain to build up a three-dimensional picture of the environment. If however one of the extra-ocular muscles is weak, the corresponding light rays from an object will strike a different and more peripheral portion of the retina of the affected eye leading to a fainter double image (see Fig. 11.26).

There are three important things to remember about diplopia as they will help in locating the affected eye.

1. The greatest separation of images occurs when the eye is trying to look in the direction of action of the weakened muscle, for example, if the lateral rectus is weak, the greatest separation of the image occurs when the eye tries to abduct.
2. The outer image is always the false image.
3. The affected eye always produces the false image.

Diplopia: how to examine

The aim of examination is to stress the extra-ocular muscles and to observe for any failure of eye move-

CASE 11.4

Problem. A 59-year-old man presents with a 4-week history of headache, which is worse in the morning and associated with nausea. He is also unsteady on his feet and finds himself lurching to the right. He had fallen on the morning of presentation and felt he needed to be checked over. You examine him and notice he is thin and anxious with tar staining of the fingers of his right hand. He has papilloedema on fundoscopy and has nystagmus on looking to the right. You perform a full neurological examination and discover that he has an intention tremor of his right hand and exhibits past pointing with it. He has a wide-based gait and tends to stagger to the right especially when he turns around. What is the diagnosis?

Discussion. His story is worrying. The neurological signs you have unearthed suggest two problems. The headache, which is worse in the morning and the papilloedema point towards raised intracranial pressure. The nystagmus to the right, the intention tremor, the past-pointing of the right hand, and his staggering to the right, suggest a lesion in the right cerebellar hemisphere. There is a strong possibility that the gradual progression of symptoms is produced by a tumour. Primary tumours are rare in adults and it is more likely that this represents secondary spread. A further clue in the history is that he has tar staining of his fingers. It is likely that he is (or was) a heavy smoker and this could represent a bronchial carcinoma with metastases to the right cerebellar hemisphere (or a paraneoplastic syndrome). This man needs a CT/magnetic resonance imaging (MRI) scan of the brain as well as a chest X-ray.

ment in any direction. Use the same method as you have been taught for eliciting nystagmus.

> **Tip**
>
> As you get proficient you will be able to look for nystagmus and a failure of eye movement at the same time.

If eye movements are normal both eyes should track your finger smoothly to the extremes of your 'H' configuration (without evidence of nystagmus). However you must always ask, 'Did you have double vision at any point?' Occasionally a weakness of the ocular muscle is subtle enough to go unnoticed during testing. If this occurs the cover test can identify which eye is at fault. Identify at which point the patient saw double and repeat the movement of your finger in that direction. Say, 'Tell me when the two images are farthest apart.' Having identified this point you need to cover each eye in turn in a bid to extinguish the false image. Say, 'Concentrate on both images. One should be clear and distinct and the other should be fainter.' Get them to point to both images in the air as a check. The fainter image should be the outer one. Then warn your patient that you are about to cover each eye in turn and you would like them to tell you when the fainter (false) image disappears. The covered eye that is responsible for the disappearance of the false image is the affected eye. Note the direction the eye is looking in so you can determine the affected muscle.

> **Tip**
>
> If you see any deviation in eye movement and the patient does **not** experience diplopia, this usually means that the patient is blind in one eye.

A detailed knowledge of the anatomical courses of all the cranial nerves is not essential but it does help in the understanding of where and why these nerves are vulnerable to damage. You do need to have a grasp of the function of these nerves so you can work out which nerve is at fault.

IIIrd nerve palsy

See Fig. 11.27.

1. **Functions of the IIIrd cranial nerve.** Elevates the eyelids (via the levator palpebrae), constricts the pupil (via the sphincter pupillae muscle of the iris), and innervates the superior rectus, inferior rectus, and medial rectus muscles.
2. **Features of a IIIrd nerve palsy.** A combination of inspection and examination is needed to diagnose a IIIrd nerve palsy.
   1. Ptosis of the affected eye (paralysis of levator palpebrae).
   2. If you elevate the eyelid you may notice two features:

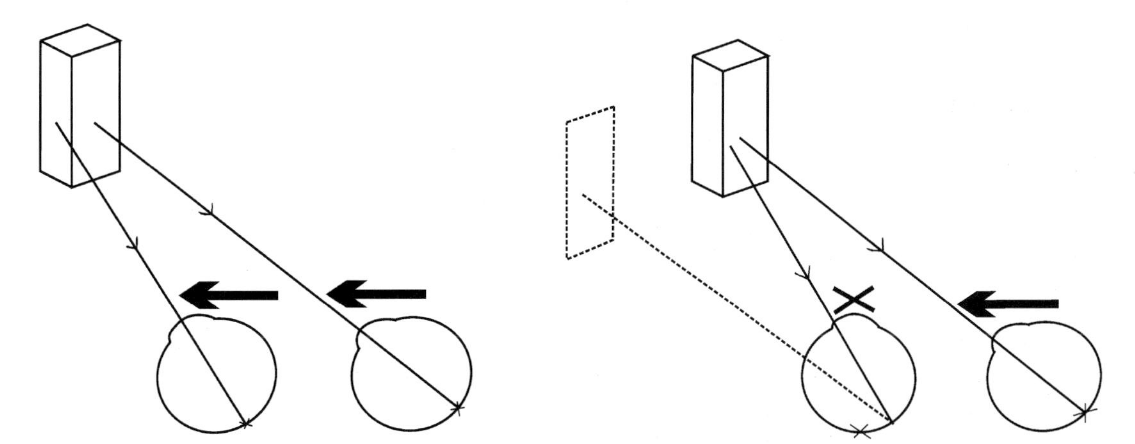

Fig. 11.26 The mechanism of diplopia due to the paralysis of the left lateral rectus muscle. The eyes work as a functional pair: (a) both eyes look to the left to view an object. Each eye moves together to allow focussing of the image on each macula allowing the object to be seen with the greatest clarity. Note the slightly different (but overlapping) aspects of the object seen with each eye leading to a 3D view (the depth perception associated with stereoscopic vision). (b) With a left 6th nerve palsy the left eye is unable to look to the left (abduct). Light from the object is only able to strike the periphery of the retina where there are fewer photoreceptors. As the brain is used to the eyes working in tandem, it will extrapolate where it believes the light rays would originate from if the eye was moving normally. Hence a second *false* outer image. As the density of photoreceptors is less than at the macula this false image is also fainter. Finally there is a loss of depth perception because of overlap of the visual fields.

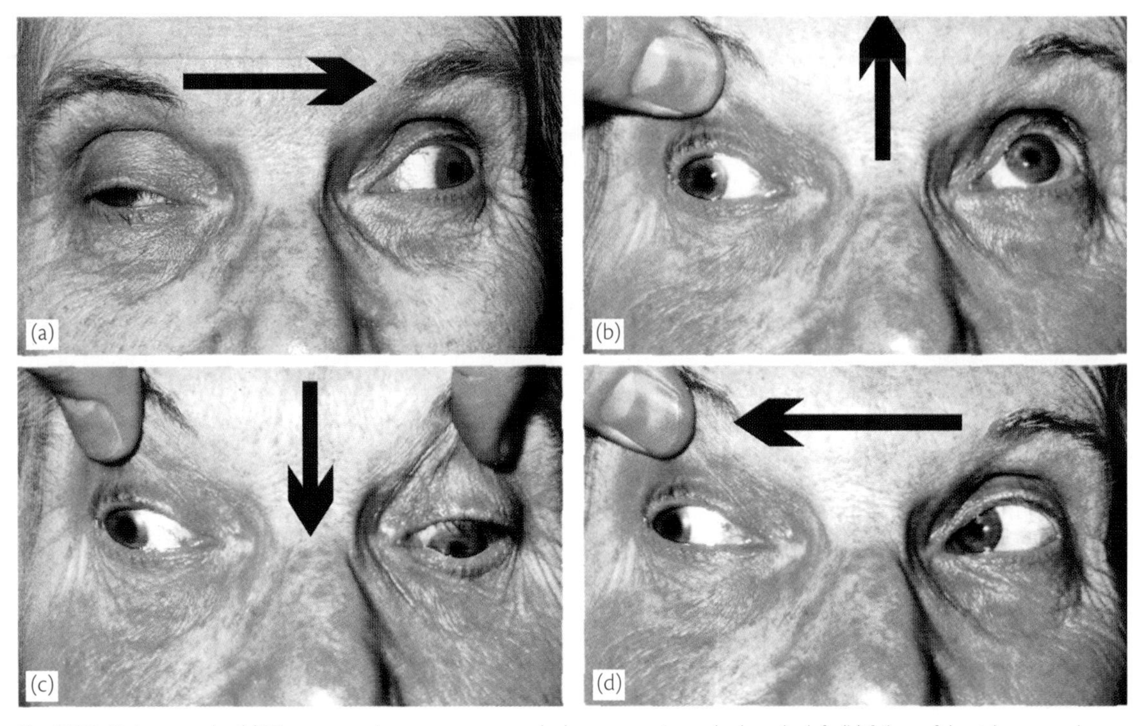

Fig. 11.27 IIIrd nerve palsy. (a) Divergent squint more pronounced when attempting to look to the left, (b) failure of the right eye to elevate, (c) failure of down-gaze in the right eye, (d) successful abduction of the right eye indicating functioning lateral rectus (and VIth nerve). Reprinted from **Fig. 14.38(a)–(d)** (p. 14.13), *Atlas of Clinical Neurology* (2nd edn), by G. David Perkin, Fred Hochberg, and Douglas C. Miller (1993), Mosby Publications, with permission from Elsevier.

   (1) dilated pupil (paralysis of sphincter pupillae);
   (2) the position of the eye is depressed and abducted (down and out) because of the unopposed actions of the superior oblique and the lateral rectus muscles, that is, a divergent squint.

3. Very little eye movement occurs and diplopia is evident in nearly all directions of gaze.

When all the above criteria are present this is known as a complete IIIrd nerve palsy.

Sometimes you may only get a partial ptosis and an unaffected pupil. This used to be called an incomplete or partial IIIrd nerve palsy. Now it is called a IIIrd nerve palsy with pupillary sparing.

> **Tip**
>
> The pupillary fibres run on the outside of the IIIrd nerve where they are vulnerable to compression. Therefore if the pupil is involved in a IIIrd nerve palsy consider a compressive lesion such as a posterior communicating artery aneurysm. If the pupil is spared consider a vasculitic cause or diabetes mellitis.

> **Tip**
>
> To check if the IVth nerve is intact in the presence of a IIIrd nerve palsy, observe the eye as you move your finger down. The affected eye will already be in a depressed position. If the IVth nerve is intact the eye will rotate inwards in response.

3. **Causes.** Posterior communicating artery aneurysm, multiple sclerosis, brainstem infarct, brainstem neoplasm, raised intracranial pressure, diabetes mellitus, and hypertension.

IVth nerve palsy

1. **Function of the IVth cranial nerve.** The only function of the IVth nerve is to supply the superior oblique muscle (which depresses the eye in the adducted position).
2. **Features of a IVth nerve palsy.** A IVth nerve palsy is unusual.

1. The patient may have a slight tilt of their head away from the affected eye as a compensatory manoeuvre to minimize the diplopia (the weak superior oblique enables the unopposed superior rectus to slightly elevate the eye. There is also a slight outward rotation of the eye. The subtle tilt of the head helps to realign the images from both eyes).
2. Diplopia is noted when the eye is made to look down and away from the affected eye and the images will be one above the other. The patient will have difficulty reading and walking downstairs because these activities rely on the superior oblique muscle.

3. **Causes.** Trauma, multiple sclerosis, infarct, and neoplasm of the brain stem.

VIth nerve palsy

See Fig. 11.28.

1. **Function of the VIth cranial nerve.** The only function of the VIth nerve is to supply the lateral rectus muscle (which abducts the eye).
2. **Features**
   1. The affected eye will be pulled inward because of the unopposed action of the medial rectus muscle (this appearance is called a convergent squint).
   2. There may be voluntary ptosis as the patient attempts to suppress the diplopia (to check for this pseudoptosis, gently close the eyelid of the unaffected eye and the patient should open the lid of the affected eye to see).
   3. Diplopia will occur in nearly all directions of gaze (except adduction of the eye). It will be maximal when there is attempted abduction of the eye and the images will be side by side.
3. **Causes.** Multiple sclerosis, brainstem infarct, brainstem neoplasm, mononeuritis multiplex (see p. 264), and raised intracranial pressure.

Other causes of ocular palsies

Occasionally you may be faced with ophthalmoplegia that does not follow the normal rules, that is, it does not have the characteristics you would expect in a IIIrd, IVth, or VIth nerve palsy. For example, you discover a superior rectus and a lateral rectus palsy in the same patient. A IIIrd nerve palsy never selectively affects one muscle group. All the muscles it supplies (superior, medial, and inferior recti) will show signs of weakness. This together with a VIth nerve palsy makes for an unlikely combination. Other causes of ocular palsies, which need to be considered, are

- disease of the orbit, for example, blow-out fracture
- proptosis
- extra-ocular muscle infiltration, for example, thyroid eye disease
- extra-ocular muscle weakness, for example, myasthenia gravis
- chronic progressive external ophthalmoplegia (CPEO).
- lesion of higher pathways, for example, internuclear ophthalmoplegia (INO).

1. **Disease of the orbit.** As described earlier, a blow-out fracture of the floor of the orbit will allow the eye to recede into the socket. There may be entrapment of the inferior rectus or inferior oblique impairing their function. Proptosis can put the extra-ocular muscles at a mechanical disadvantage.
2. **Extra-ocular muscle infiltration.** Thyroid eye disease can cause ophthalmoplegia either because of exophthalmos or infiltration of the muscles. The superior rectus and lateral rectus muscles are the

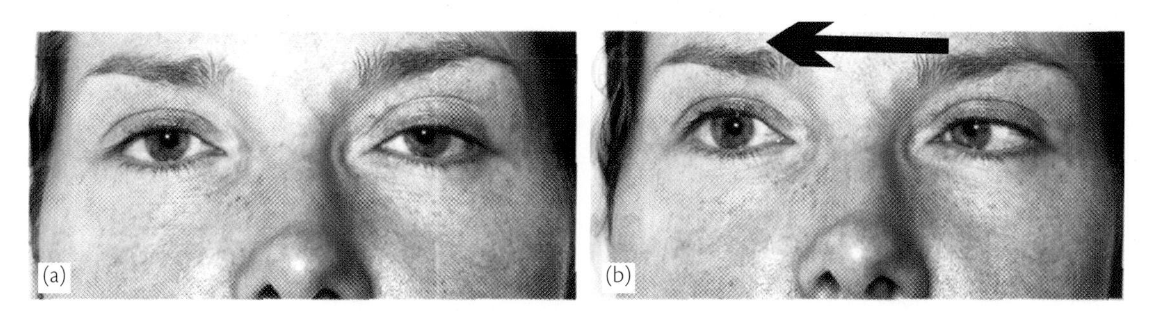

Fig. 11.28 VIth nerve palsy. (a) Mild convergent squint, (b) failure of the right eye to abduct. Reprinted from **Fig. 14.38(a)** and **(b)** (p. 11.4), *Atlas of Clinical Neurology* (2nd edn), by G. David Perkin, Fred Hochberg, and Douglas C. Miller (1993), Mosby Publications, with permission from Elsevier.

most commonly affected and the infiltration will gradually lead to progressive weakness. In chronic cases fibrosis can tether the muscle altogether.

3. **Extra-ocular muscle weakness.** Myasthenia gravis is a disorder of the neuromuscular junction (see Fig. 11.21). It leads to the depletion of the neurotransmitter acetylcholine preventing the transmission of the nerve impulse in skeletal muscle. There is a variable ptosis and ophthalmoplegia. Muscular weakness is worse with repeated activity and becomes more noticeable towards the end of the day.
4. **CPEO.** Historically called ocular myopathy, this is a progressive paralysis of the extra-ocular muscles. There is usually a bilateral progressive ptosis followed later by extra-ocular muscle weakness. This is the most common presentation of the mitochondrial myopathies. Mitochondria are the energy-producing powerhouses of cells. In these groups of conditions mutations in the mitochondria lead to deficient energy production. The age of onset and other features depend on the type of mutation.
5. **INO.** To enable both eyes to move as a co-ordinated unit, they need to be interconnected. This is achieved through the median longitudinal fasciculus. Among other functions this connects the VI nerve of one eye (controlling the lateral rectus) to the IIIrd nerve of the other eye (controlling the medial rectus). If there is damage to this pathway it disrupts conjugate movement in the horizontal plane. This usually manifests as nystagmus in the abducting eye and a failure of adduction of the other eye. However if the direction of gaze is reversed, the eye that failed to adduct can abduct fully and now has nystagmus. The other eye is unable to adduct. INO is unusual and occurs most often in multiple sclerosis. It may also occur with brainstem infarct, trauma, or syringobulbia.

Monocular diplopia

The final point about diplopia is that it can occur as a result of disease in one eye and is called monocular diplopia. It used to be taught that if diplopia persisted when one eye was covered, then it was likely that the patient was hysterical or malingering. Although these diagnoses must be borne in mind, it is now appreciated that monocular diplopia can be due to cataracts, scarring of the cornea, pathology of the iris, or vitreous or aqueous humor. These conditions can refract and split the light rays from an object to form a double image.

Keypoints

- With jerky nystagmus the direction of the fast phase of nystagmus represents the direction of nystagmus.
- With diplopia there are three important facts to remember:
- the greatest separation of images occurs when the eye tries to look in the direction of the paralysed muscle
- the outer image is always the false image
- the affected eye always produces the false image.
- A IIIrd nerve palsy causes ptosis, an eye that looks down and out (a divergent squint), sometimes a dilated pupil, and eye movements that are very restricted.
- A IVth nerve palsy causes diplopia when the patient reads or walks downstairs.
- A VIth nerve palsy causes a convergent squint and a failure of abduction of the eye.

Trigeminal nerve (cranial nerve V)

8. Test facial sensation (V tested), assess the muscles of mastication (V tested), test corneal reflex (V tested), and assess the jaw jerk reflex (V tested).

The trigeminal nerve is the largest cranial nerve and has three large branches, the ophthalmic branch, the maxillary branch, and the mandibular branch. Through these branches it provides sensation to the face and front half of the head, sensation to the mucous membranes and sinuses, and the motor supply to the muscles of mastication.

Test facial sensation

All three branches of the trigeminal nerve carry sensory fibres from the face and head. The areas they serve are represented in Fig. 11.29. Sensory abnormalities are more common than motor abnormalities in lesions of the trigeminal nerve.

Take a piece of cotton wool and roll part of it in your fingers to form a 'wisp'. Say to your patient, 'Close your eyes please and say "yes" if you can feel me touching you. Does it feel like you would expect cotton wool to?' This qualification is important with all modalities of sensory testing because the stimulus may be felt but may have a completely different quality, for example, it could feel like pins and needles or be experienced as

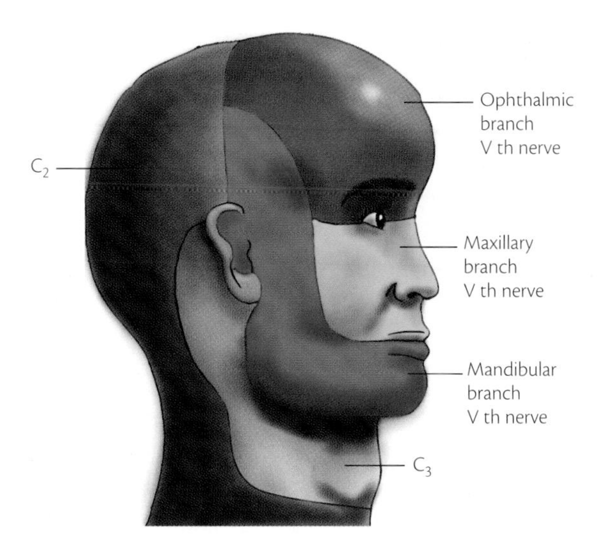

Fig. 11.29 The sensory divisions of the head and neck.

pain with some neurological problems. Only dab once, so that you test light touch sensation. Compare each side, maxillary branch to maxillary branch, mandibular branch to mandibular branch, and so on. If you find an abnormal area you must test the area in detail and try and work out its limits. Now check pain sensation by repeating your testing but this time with your neuropins. Say to your patient, 'Close your eyes and tell me if this feels sharp or blunt.' You can also check temperature sensation very crudely by using the cold tines of a tuning fork. This is a useful exercise if you are not sure whether pain sensation is impaired (some patients' responses can be inconsistent). If it is impaired the cold tuning fork is often perceived as warm.

Assess the muscles of mastication

For the uninitiated these are the muscles that are responsible for chewing (and not for controlling your right wrist). The main muscles are the masseters (*mass-itters*) (cheeks) and the temporalis (*temp-or-ale-iss*) muscles (temples), both responsible for clenching the teeth together and the pterygoids (*terry-goids*), which move the jaw from side to side. A quick inspection of the face is useful, looking for wasting of the temporalis muscle. If this muscle is wasted it leads to a 'hollowing out' of the temples. Otherwise the rest of the examination relies on you palpating the muscles. Say to your patient, 'Clench your teeth for me'. Feel for the masseter by pressing on the cheeks either side of the mouth. While the teeth are still clenched, also feel for the temporalis by placing your fingertips on either temple. Get the patient to relax and feel the tension disappear from the temples. Also get the patient to open their jaw against resistance. Use your thumb applied to the under-surface of the jaw to apply the resistive force. Practise on yourself and other patients to learn how much force the jaw can overcome. In patients with a motor weakness it takes little force to keep the mouth from opening and sometimes the jaw can slew to one side (if there is a weakness of the pterygoids on that side). Finally, place an index finger on one side of the jaw and ask your patient to push their jaw against it. This tests the pterygoid muscles directly. Now do the same on the other side. Using this technique you may pick up a subtle weakness on one side that might not be obvious on direct observation.

Test corneal reflex

What is it?

The corneal reflex is a useful protective mechanism for the eyes. When either cornea is touched, it results in the reflex blinking of both eyes. The sensory impulse is conducted by the trigeminal nerve (afferent limb) and the motor response occurs via the facial nerve (efferent limb). This is an important reflex to test (although it is often overlooked) because it can be the earliest sign of a Vth nerve palsy, for example, due to an acoustic neuroma.

How to examine

Say to your patient, 'I am going to dab this piece of cotton wool on to your eye; it may feel a little uncomfortable. Look straight ahead for me and keep your eyes wide open.' With the patient looking forward bring the wisp of cotton wool in from the side of the face and gently dab the cornea (see Fig. 11.30). Aim for the transparent area at the front of the eye and not the white sclera. You **must** approach from the side, or your patient will blink because of the visual threat. If you touch the eyelids the patient will also blink and your

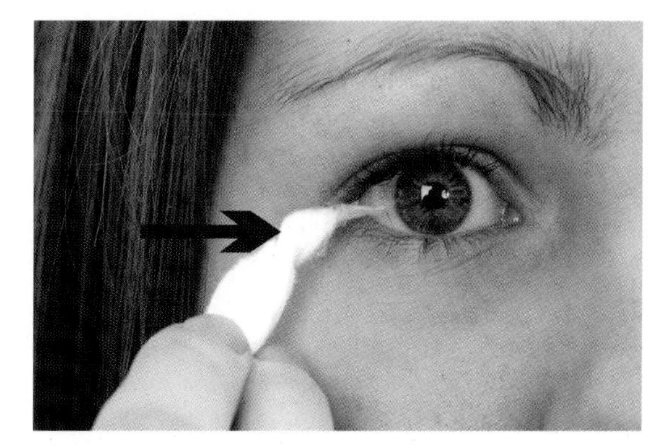

Fig. 11.30 Eliciting the corneal reflex.

examination will be invalid again. The best method is a bold and swift movement in from the side with the cotton wool (avoiding the eyelids). As you near the cornea slow your movement so that you apply the slightest touch on the cornea. Then remove the cotton wool rapidly before the patient has a chance to blink. Check that both eyelids blink appropriately before testing the other eye. If the corneal sensation is impaired, when you touch the cornea, there will be no blinking (blinking may also be impaired if there is a lower motor neurone VIIth nerve palsy but this will be more obvious). The final thing to note is that most people have an automatic rate of blinking. So you have to time your dab in between this regular rate so that your movement and the patient's blinking do not coincide.

Assess the jaw jerk reflex

What is it?

The jaw jerk is like any other reflex elicited in the body, except the muscle involved is the masseter muscle. The stretch stimulus provided by the tendon hammer is detected by the proprioceptive end-organs in the muscle and is conducted via the sensory fibres of the trigeminal nerve. After negotiating the reflex arc, the impulse is conducted down the motor fibres of the same nerve back to the masseter muscle.

Significance

It has some minor clinical value in locating a lesion within the central nervous system. If an abnormal reflex is obtained it indicates that the lesion is above the pons of the brainstem. The reflex can only be elicited in the presence of bilateral upper motor neurone lesions, for example, bilateral cortical infarcts. Its value is in excluding spinal cord compression as a cause of bilateral upper motor neurone signs in the arms and legs. The utility of this test has been diminished because of the availability of CT and MRI scans that can readily image the brain and upper cervical cord.

How to examine

See Fig. 11.31. This test can look quite brutal and may frighten your patient. You need to reassure them beforehand. Say to them, 'Relax now, open your mouth, and let your jaw hang loose. Don't open it wide, just let it sag open. Now I'm going to tap very gently with this tendon hammer on to my finger ... it won't hurt.' The normal response is for the jaw to flick down a short distance. If there is a bilateral upper motor neurone lesion the reflex will be brisk. When you see it for the first time a brisk jaw jerk will be unmistakable. The jaw bounces down as if it was on a piece of elastic and the jaw may close altogether. Sometimes you can see a wave of contraction at the sides of the jaw. Although the reflex is described as brisk, its duration of action is slightly longer than a normal one. The term an exaggerated reflex is probably a more accurate one.

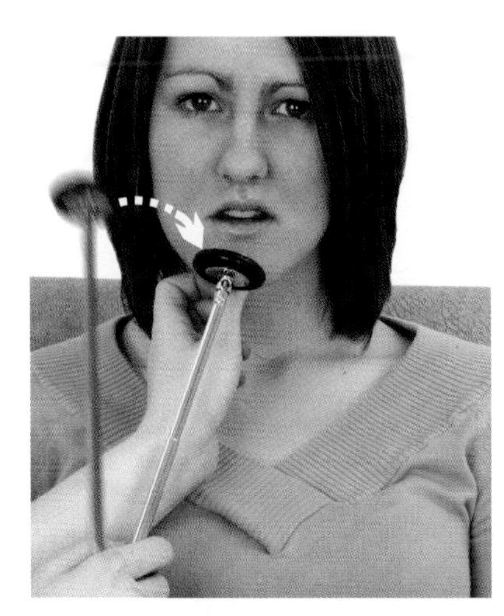

Fig. 11.31 Demonstrating the jaw jerk.

Keypoints

- The corneal reflex may be the earliest sign of a Vth nerve palsy.
- Always approach from the side when testing the corneal reflex and make sure you touch the cornea and not the sclera.
- Sensory dysfunction of the Vth nerve is more common than motor dysfunction.
- The jaw jerk is of limited value and is only abnormally brisk in the presence of bilateral upper motor neurone lesions.

Facial nerve (cranial nerve VII)

9. Assess the muscles of facial movement (VII tested).

The facial nerve supplies the muscles of facial expression. It also has other specialist functions, which are useful to know as they may help pin-point where an abnormality is (in a lower motor neurone lesion only). The VIIth nerve is one of the most common cranial nerves to be affected by disease (deafness and blindness are usually due to disease of the sensory organs rather than the cranial nerves themselves). It is worth knowing the neuroanatomy of this particular nerve to understand the variety of features associated with its dysfunction (see Fig. 11.32). The lower motor neurone of the facial nerve arises in the pons (part

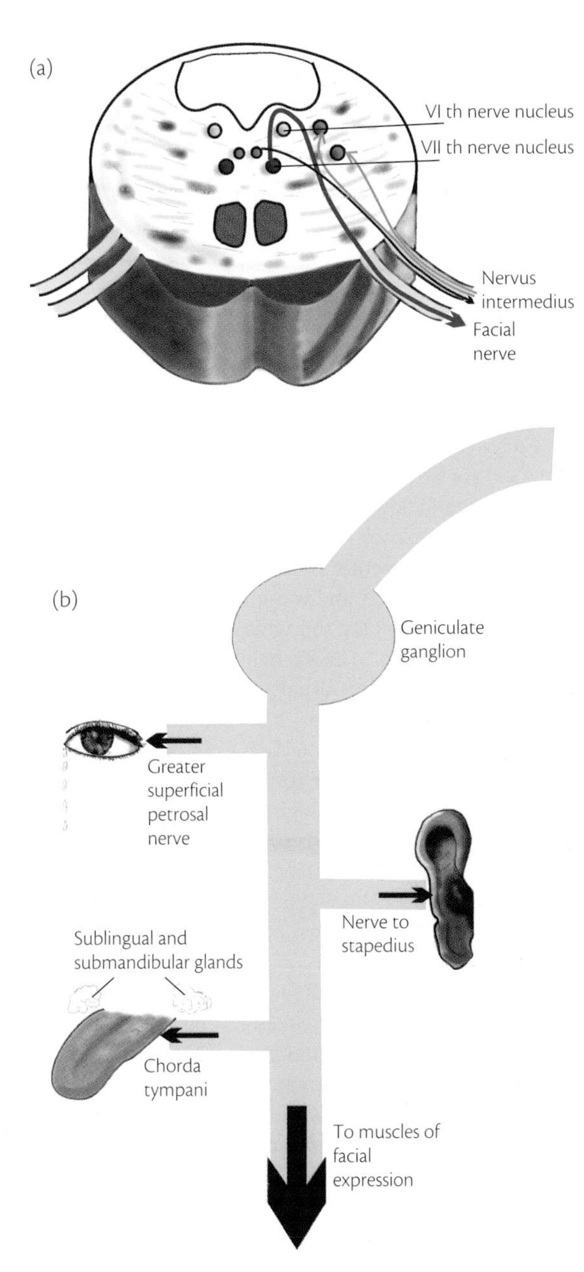

Fig. 11.32 Neuroanatomy of the VIIth nerve in the brainstem and its subsequent branches. (a) Brainstem at the level of the pons showing the facial nerve nucleus and surrounding structures, (b) branches of the facial nerve.

of the brainstem). The axon winds around the VIth nerve nucleus before leaving the lateral aspect of the brainstem. At this point it joins the nervus intermedius (*nerv-ous-inter-me-de-us*), the specialized part of the facial nerve that carries taste fibres, as well as fibres that stimulate lacrymation (tearing of the eye) and salivation. The facial nerve crosses the cerebellopontine angle with the vestibulocochlear nerve (VIIIth nerve) and both enter the internal auditory canal (where the VIIIth nerve supplies the ear and balance organs). The facial nerve travels in the facial canal and relays in the geniculate ganglion (*jen-nick-you-let*) before giving off three branches.

1. The greater superficial petrosal (*pet-rose-al*) nerve. This supplies the lacrymal gland and salivary glands to produce tears and saliva.
2. The nerve to stapedius (*sta-pee-dee-us*). This supplies the tiny stapedius muscle, which contracts in the presence of loud noises to dampen the movement of the stapes at the cochlea.
3. The chorda tympani nerve. This supplies taste sensation to the anterior two-thirds of the tongue.

The facial nerve then exits the skull through the stylomastoid foramen and runs in the substance of the parotid gland, dividing into a number of branches that supply the muscles of the face.

How to examine

Inspection will often lead you towards the diagnosis. Discovering a unilateral VIIth nerve palsy is the easy part. There will be obvious asymmetry of the face with drooping of the corner of the mouth on the affected side and flattening of the nasolabial (*nay-zo-lay-be-al*) groove (the skin crease linking nose and the corner of the mouth on either side, which accentuates when you smile). You will be expected to work out if it is an upper motor neurone lesion, that is, the nerves from the cortex supplying the facial nerve or a lower motor neurone lesion, that is, the facial nerve itself. The upper half of the face (the frontalis and orbicularis oculi (*orb-ick-you-lar-iss-ock-you-lie*) muscles) has dual innervation from both the left and the right side of the cerebral cortex. However, the lower half of the face is innervated from the contralateral cortex only (see Fig. 11.33).

Upper motor neurone VII lesion

If there is an abnormality of the right cerebral cortex, for example, due to a stroke, the upper half of the left side of the face will still receive impulses from the left cerebral cortex via the left facial nerve and will appear normal. However, the lower half of the face does not have this dual innervation and weakness at this level will be evident.

Lower motor neurone VII lesion

In contrast to this, if the right facial nerve is affected by, for example, a Bell's palsy (*Sir Charles Bell (1774–1842),*

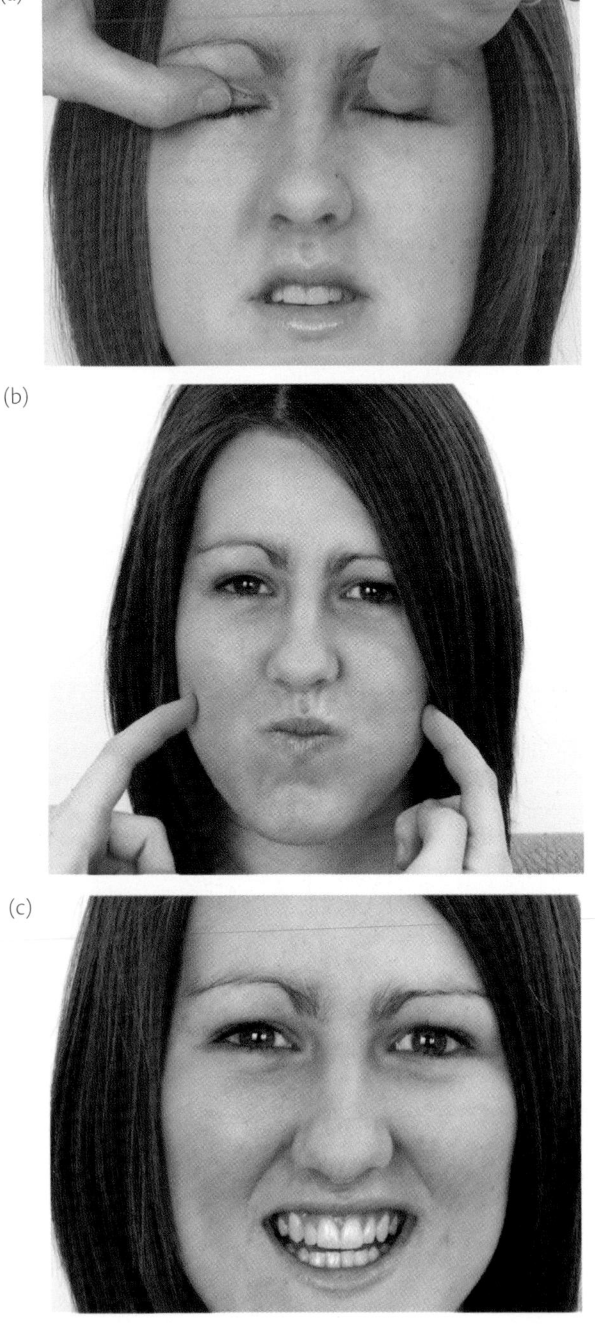

Fig. 11.33 Testing the facial nerve: (a) screwing the eyes up tight, (b) blowing the cheeks out, and (c) showing the teeth.

Scottish surgeon) (see later), both the upper and lower half of the face will be affected because the final common pathway, which delivers the motor impulses to the facial muscles, is disrupted. See Fig. 11.34.

It is easiest to work down the face testing the muscle groups as you go. Say to your patient, 'raise your eyebrows' (frontalis muscle); you may have to demonstrate this yourself so they know what you want. Some patients find this difficult to do and if this is the case ask them to follow your finger upwards with their eyes while keeping their head still. As they strain to follow your finger above their natural horizontal gaze, the forehead will automatically wrinkle (unless there is a lower motor neurone lesion on one side of the face). Now say, 'Close your eyes tight and stop me opening them' (orbicularis oculi muscle). A normal person will be able bury their eyelashes tightly under the lower lid. Now place both your thumbs on each eyelid and gently attempt to open them. If the muscles are strong this can be quite difficult to do. However a mild 'lower motor' weakness on one side will allow you to peel back the eyelid easily with your thumb. In a severe, lower motor neurone palsy, the eyelid may fail to close altogether and you may see the eyeball turning upwards to display the white sclera (this is called Bell's phenomenon). The eyeball turning upwards is a normal process but it is usually hidden behind a closed eyelid. If the eyelid does not close then the eye is in danger. The eyelid provides protection from dirt and grit and if this barrier is missing the cornea can become ulcerated and infected. If the risk is high, doctors may sew part of the upper and lower eyelids together to protect the eye (this operation is called a tarsorrhaphy (*tar-sorra-fee*)). Now say to your patient, 'Blow your cheeks out (buccinator (*buck-sin-ate-ter*) muscle). Press both cheeks with your fingers and make sure the tension feels roughly the same on either side. A difference will suggest a lesion on the weaker side. Say, 'Show me your teeth' (orbicularis oris muscle). You may have seen drooping of the corner of the mouth on initial inspection and this manoeuvre should exaggerate any weakness. Normally you should get a complete view of their teeth but a weakness on one side will lead to those teeth being obscured by the paralysed lips. Be on the look out for those older patients with a sense of humour who when you say, 'show me your teeth' will point to their dentures in a denture pot.

Tip

Do not get your patient to smile as a test of facial expression. This is because the descending pathways used to express emotions are different to the upper motor neurones that are under voluntary control. As a result the patient may be able to smile spontaneously and give the false impression that there is no weakness.

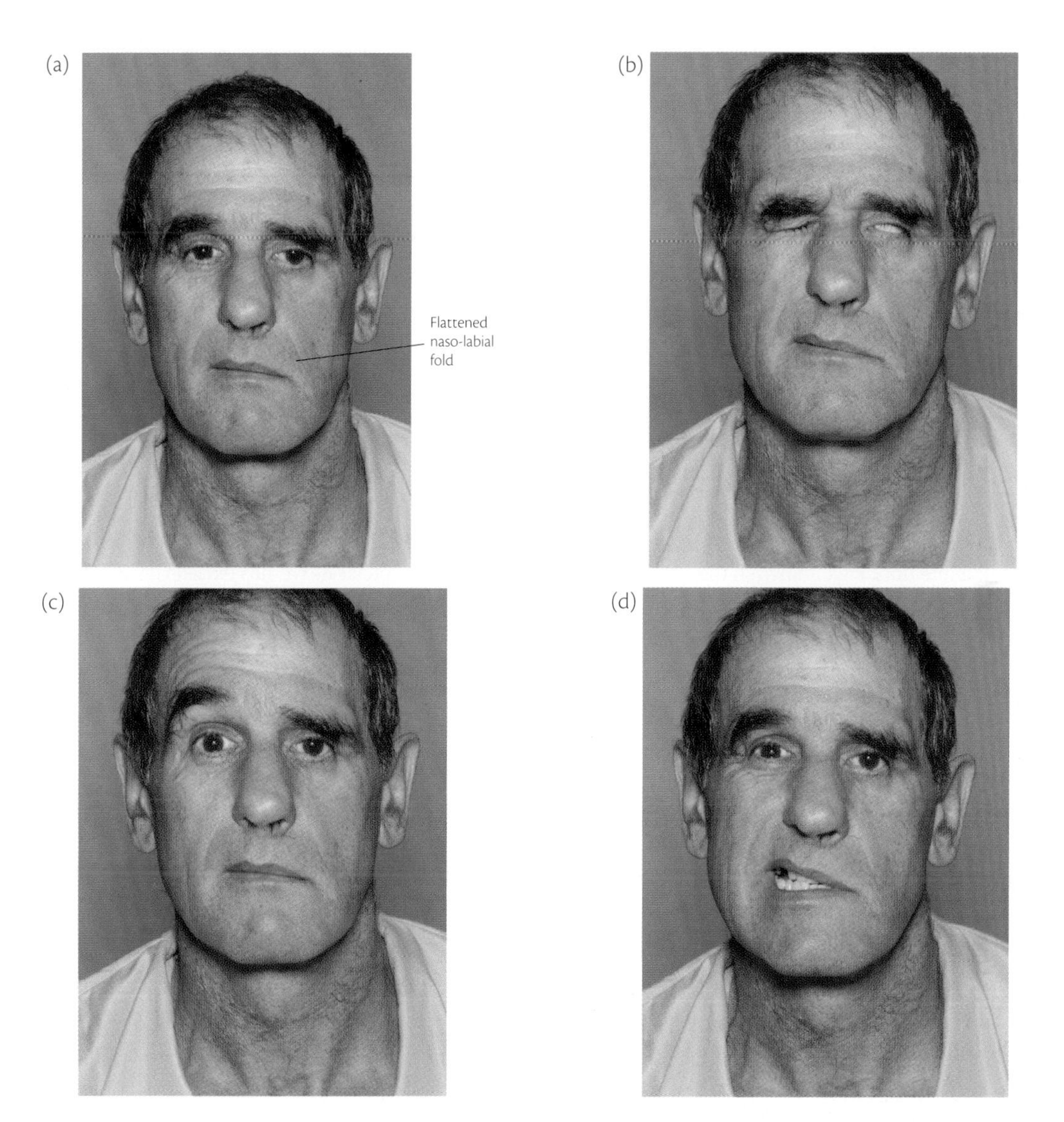

Fig. 11.34 A left lower motor neurone facial nerve lesion. (a) The patient at rest. Note the drooping of the lips on the left and flattening of the nasolabial fold. (b) Screwing the eyes up tight: note Bell's phenomenon on the left. (c) Raising the eyebrows: the patient is unable to raise the eyebrow on the left side with lack of wrinkling of the frontalis muscle on that side. This confirms that this is a lower motor neurone lesion rather than an upper motor neurone lesion. (d) Showing the teeth: there is lack of movement of the mouth on the left.

> **Tip**
>
> Occasionally you may get caught out by a patient with bilateral facial nerve palsies (see later) as there will be no asymmetry of the face. The key to spotting this condition is to observe that there is very little movement of the facial muscles when you get them to run through the above regime.

Abnormal findings

It is worth considering the sites in the nervous system where the facial nerve is vulnerable to injury. The following sequences illustrate these, see also Fig. 11.32.

1. Upper motor neurone lesion

- contralateral facial nerve palsy
- only lower face affected because of dual innervation of the upper face
- also possible contralateral hemiplegia.

Causes

- stroke
- tumour
- multiple sclerosis.

2. Lower motor neurone lesion

The pattern of other cranial nerve involvement plus other clinical features may give further clue to the location of the lesion.

2a. The pons

- ipsilateral facial nerve palsy
- ipsilateral VIth nerve palsy
- (both the VIth and VIIth nerve are at the same level in the pons)
- contralateral hemiplegia (the corticospinal tracts do not cross the mid-line until lower down in the medulla.

Causes

- stroke
- tumour
- multiple sclerosis.

2b. Cerebellopontine angle

- ipsilateral facial nerve palsy
- ipsilateral VIIIth nerve palsy
- ipsilateral Vth nerve palsy
- ipsilateral cerebellar signs
- (possibly IXth, Xth, and XIth palsy also)
- in addition the facial nerve palsy at this level will lead to dysfunction of the three major branches
- the greater superficial petrosal nerve—leads to a loss of lacrimation and salivation
- the nerve to stapedius—leads to hyperacusis (*high-per-a-cue-sis*) (this is the unpleasant exaggeration of normal sound due to the lack of damping that is normally produced by the contraction of the stapedius muscle)
- the chorda tympani nerve—leads to loss of taste over the anterior two-thirds of the tongue.

Causes

- acoustic neuroma (see later)
- meningioma.

2c. Facial canal

- no other cranial nerves involved at this level
- the location of the lesion within the facial canal will dictate the clinical symptoms. The three branches described in **2b** come off the facial nerve in the order written. Therefore a lesion after the greater superficial petrosal nerve but before the nerve to stapedius will spare lacrimation and salivation but will still lead to hyperacusis.

Causes

- Bell's palsy (see later)
- Ramsay-Hunt syndrome (*J. Ramsay-Hunt (1874–1937), American neurologist*) (see later)
- fracture of the skull base
- spread from otitis media.

2d. Distal to stylomastoid foramen

- at this point the facial nerve has exited the skull and is travelling through the substance of the parotid gland dividing into its final branches to supply the facial muscles. Some of the facial muscles may be spared depending on which branches have been affected.

Causes

- cancer of the parotid gland
- surgery to the parotid gland
- sarcoidosis.

3. Bilateral facial nerve palsies

- bilateral strokes (cause of upper motor neurone lesions)
- multiple sclerosis (cause of upper motor neurone lesions)
- myasthenia gravis
- muscular dystrophy (some forms, for example, facio-scapulo-humeral dystrophy)
- Guillain–Barré syndrome
- sarcoidosis
- bilateral Bell's palsy.

Vestibulocochlear nerve (cranial nerve VIII)

10. Assess hearing (VIII tested) and perform Weber's and Rinné's tests (VIII tested).

The vestibulocochlear nerve is responsible for hearing and balance although it is only the auditory aspect of the nerve that is routinely tested.

Keypoints

- You must determine whether a facial nerve lesion is upper motor neurone or lower motor neurone in origin.
- The forehead has bilateral cortical representation and is only paralysed if there is a lower motor lesion or bilateral upper motor lesions.
- A facial nerve palsy of lower motor neurone type may render the ipsilateral eye unprotected.
- Smiling is a misleading test of the facial nerve.
- Beware of missing bilateral facial nerve palsies.

Assess hearing

It is only possible to make a crude assessment of hearing during the cranial nerve examination. There may be clues before you start your assessment. Your patient may have a hearing aid or you may notice that you have to repeat your questions or instructions many times. Some doctors advocate occluding one ear and asking the patient to identify a ticking watch or fingers being rubbed together. Another more sensitive approach involves whispering numbers into either ear. This has the advantage that you can vary the volume you use to state the numbers. Say to your patient, 'I am going to rub your earlobe and I want you to repeat the numbers I whisper to you.' It is important that you rub the earlobe of the ear that is **not** being tested. This creates a noise that 'masks' this ear and prevents it from assisting the ear under test. If the patient does have a hearing impairment and the other ear is not masked, this ear may pick up the sounds and lead to the false impression that hearing in the tested ear is unaffected.

Now whisper random numbers into the patient's ear, while rubbing the other ear. Most people will be able to repeat your numbers back. If the patient cannot hear you, then raise the volume of your voice. This suggests some hearing impairment. If you have to shout into the ear, you will draw the correct conclusion. If you suspect hearing loss you should go on to perform Weber's (*web-bers*) and Rinné's (*rin-ayz*) tests to differentiate between conductive and sensorineural deafness.

Conductive deafness

What is it?

This is the inability of the outer and middle ear to conduct sound to the inner ear. This can be due to disease anywhere from the external auditory meatus to the stapes (also called the stirrup, one of the tiny 'ossicle' bones of the ear that articulates with the oval window of the cochlea, see Fig. 11.35).

Causes

The causes of conductive deafness are

- otitis externa
- otitis media
- Paget's disease (affecting the ossicles)
- perforated ear drum.

Sensorineural deafness

What is it?

This is due to damage to the cochlear (the sense organ, which is a shell-like apparatus that converts acoustic vibration into neural impulses) or to the cochlear nerve, which together with the vestibular nerve conducts sensory input to the brain as the vestibulocochlear nerve.

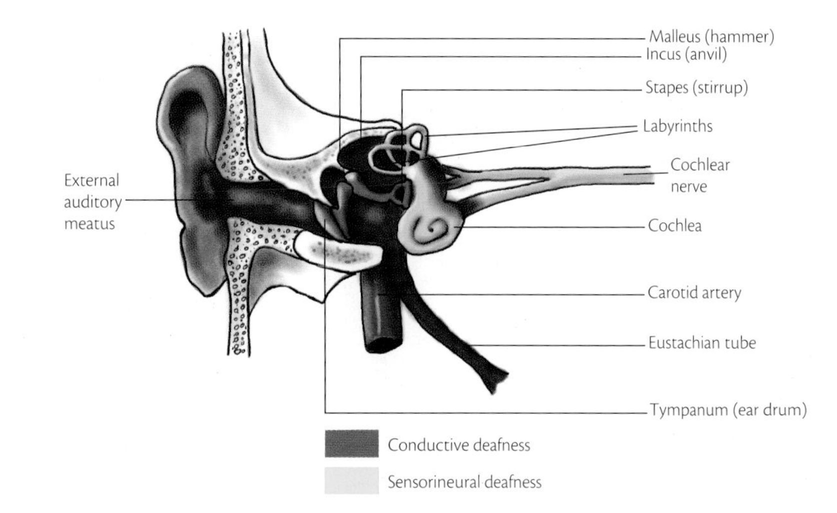

Fig. 11.35 The anatomy of the ear and the apparatus involved in conductive and sensorineural deafness.

Causes

The causes of sensorineural deafness are

- presbycusis (due to ageing)
- noise-induced deafness
- ototoxicity due to drugs, for example, high-dose frusemide or gentamycin.

Perform Weber's and Rinné's tests

Weber's test

Weber's test (*F. E. Weber-Liel (1832–1891), German otologist*) is sometimes described as a lateralizing test, that is, it is used to determine which ear is affected (in practice it is not as clear cut as this as you need information from Rinné's test to help with this). You need a 512 Hz tuning fork, which is smaller than the ones normally lying about the wards. Vibrate the tuning fork and place it in the middle of the patient's forehead. Ask, 'Can you hear the noise? Does it sound the same in both ears or can you hear it louder in one than the other?' If your patient has healthy hearing, they should hear the noise equally in both ears. If they hear the noise louder in one ear, this either means there is a conduction deafness in the ear perceiving the louder sound or there is a sensorineural deafness in the other ear (see Figs 11.36 and 11.37). To help distinguish between the two possibilities you need to perform Rinné's test. One further point to note is that the tuning fork can be heard equally by both ears in the presence of hearing impairment. In this case, hearing loss will be approximately equal for each ear.

Rinné's test

See Fig. 11.38. Rinné's test (*Friedrich Heinrich Adolf Rinné (1819–1868), German ENT surgeon*) relies on the principle that in the healthy individual, air conduction is better than bone conduction. If this is the case it is described

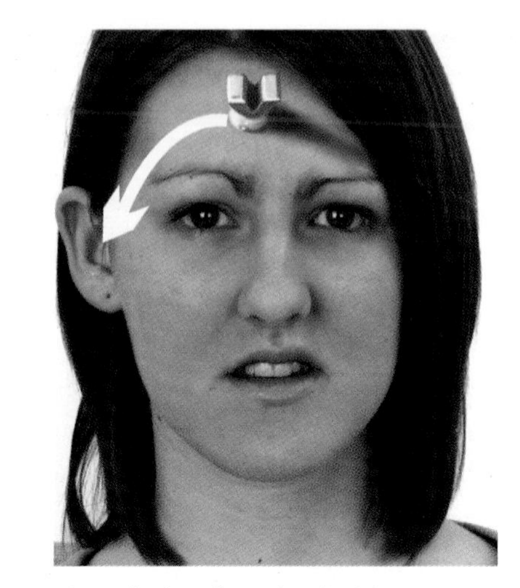

Fig. 11.37 Lateralization of sound to the right ear.

(a)

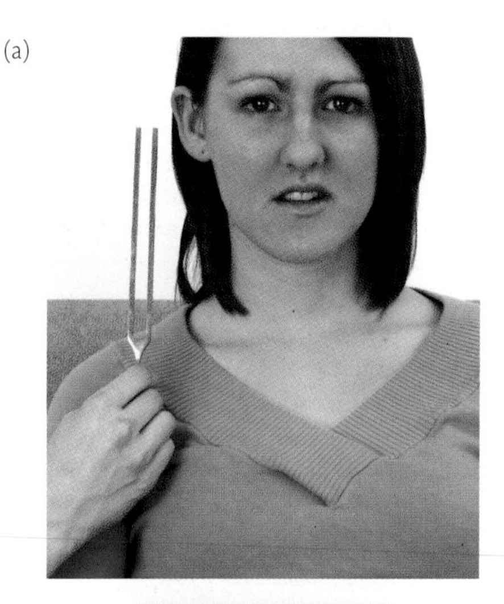

(b)

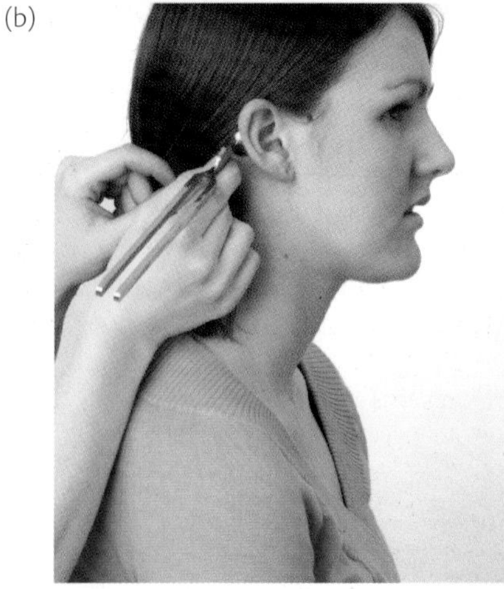

Fig. 11.38 Rinné's test: (a) air conduction, (b) bone conduction.

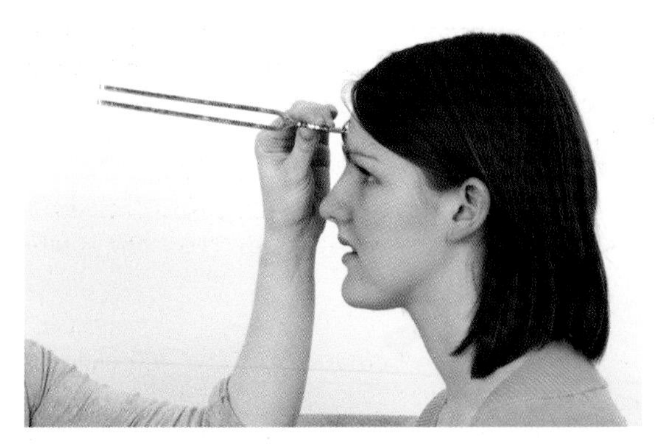

Fig. 11.36 Weber's test.

Tip

Another way of performing this test is to set the tuning fork vibrating and put the tines in front of the ear. Then using the same force set the tuning fork vibrating again and this time place it on the mastoid process; ask the patient which was louder. The interpretation remains the same as above.

Tip

Never diagnose hearing impairment until you have checked the ear for wax. Most opthalmoscopes are multi-purpose and can be used as an otoscope (*owe-ta-scope*) (sometimes called an auriscope). The head screws off and you can put on the otoscopic attachment. This allows you to clip on earpieces of different sizes. Switch the light on in the normal ear and carefully introduce the earpiece into the auditory canal of the ear. With your free hand you need to pull the ear firmly upwards and backwards (much the same position that teachers used to pull the ear of a naughty child, before it was outlawed). This straightens out the auditory canal and allows you to get a good view of the eardrum. If this view however is obstructed by a lot of brown gunky stuff, your patient has a lot of earwax. This needs removing before the ears can be tested formally.

CASE 11.5

Problem. You examine a middle-aged man who has been complaining of pain in the left ear for a fortnight. He has noticed the hearing has deteriorated in that ear and you confirm this clinically by whispering various numbers into each ear. You perform Weber's and Rinné's tests. With Weber's test the sound from the tuning fork is heard loudest in the left ear and the Rinné's test is negative in that ear. Can you explain this?

Discussion. This case is straightforward. The patient has already indicated that the problem is with his left ear and you have confirmed that the hearing is impaired. Weber's test indicates that either there is a conductive hearing loss in the left ear or a sensorineural hearing loss in the right ear. A negative Rinné's test is where bone conduction is better than air conduction. Therefore a negative Rinné's test in the left ear confirms a conductive hearing loss in the left ear. This man needs his ear examined with an otoscope for signs of an otitis media.

CASE 11.6

Problem. You examine an elderly woman who has been described as 'hard of hearing' by her son. She says she is not bad when speaking 'one on one' in a quiet room but struggles with conversation if there is a lot of background noise. Her eardrums are normal on otoscopic examination and you perform Rinné's and Weber's tests. She hears the tuning fork directly in front of her and both ears are Rinné positive. Explain the results.

Discussion. This case is tricky. The history suggests the patient has some hearing impairment but superficially she performs normally with the tuning fork tests. However you must remember that a positive Rinné's test can either indicate normal hearing or sensorineural hearing loss. It is therefore possible that this woman has bilateral sensorineural hearing loss, which is roughly equal in both ears, leading to a Weber's test that is heard equally in both ears. An audiogram is needed to assess the hearing more accurately before any strategies such as hearing aids can be employed.

as a positive Rinné's test. Find the mastoid process. This is the bony prominence just behind the ear. Set the tuning fork vibrating and place the base on this spot. Say to your patient, 'Tell me when you can no longer hear the tuning fork.' When your patient indicates that they can no longer hear the tuning fork, move the tuning fork so that the end of the prongs are just by the entrance to the ear. Ask them, 'Can you hear it now?' The healthy patient should hear it. If the patient does not hear the tuning fork this implies a conduction defect in that ear. This is described as a negative Rinné's test. If the patient has a sensorineural deficit in the tested ear you will elicit a positive Rinné's test (so long as the hearing loss is not so bad that they cannot hear the tuning fork). Any hearing deficit that you find needs to be assessed more fully by an audiological department.

Glossopharyngeal (IX) and vagus (X) nerves

11. Assess movement of the soft palate (IX and X tested) and assess sensation of the soft palate (IX and X tested).

As lesions of the IXth and Xth nerves rarely occur in isolation they will be considered together. I will only discuss those functions that are routinely tested. The glossopharyngeal nerve (IX) is a mixed nerve with motor, sensory, and some parasympathetic activity. It

> **Keypoints**
>
> - Determine whether hearing loss is conductive or sensorineural.
> - Conductive deafness may be reversible whereas sensorineural deafness is usually irreversible.
> - Make sure that wax has been removed from the ear before referring for a formal hearing assessment.
> - Rinné's test helps to determine whether hearing loss is conductive or sensorineural in nature.
> - Weber's test helps to determine which ear is the affected ear.

carries sensory input from the palate and the pharynx and taste from the posterior third of the tongue. It provides the afferent limb of the gag reflex. The vagus nerve (X) is also a mixed nerve with motor, sensory, and parasympathetic activity. It provides the motor supply to the pharynx, soft palate, and larynx and provides the efferent limb of the gag reflex.

Assess movement of the soft palate

Say to your patient, 'Can you open your mouth please, sir.' Now shine a torch into the back of the mouth and look at the soft palate. Be familiar with what a normal soft palate looks like. It should be symmetrical and divided roughly into two by the fleshy uvula that dangles down (see Fig. 11.39). The patient's tongue may obscure your view. If this happens you will need to use a tongue depressor (see Fig. 11.39). Say, 'I'm just going to press down on your tongue with this stick. It might be a little uncomfortable.' For this reason it is best not to dilly dally once it is in the mouth. Check for asymmetry. Now ask your patient to say 'aaah!' The soft palate should elevate and the uvula should stay central. If there is unilateral weakness of the soft palate the uvula is pulled away from the weakened side.

Assess sensation of the soft palate

With the mouth still open say to your patient, 'I am just going to touch the back of your mouth gently with this stick, let me know if you can feel it.' Using your orange stick gently touch the back of the palate, withdraw your stick, and wait for your patient's response. Now touch the opposite side and ask your patient to compare the two sides. It is very easy to trigger the gag reflex doing this. If you do, apologize to your patient.

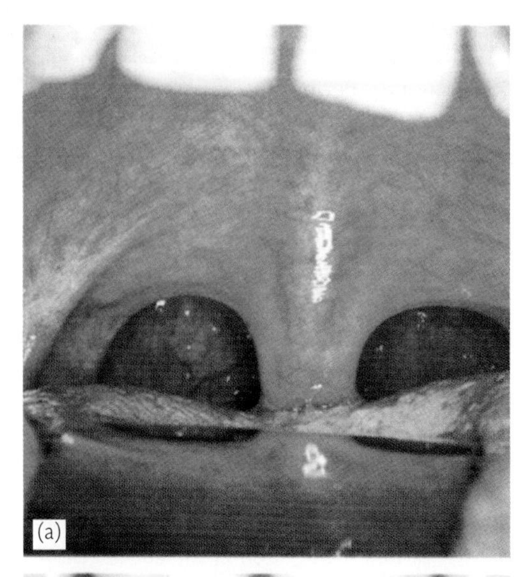

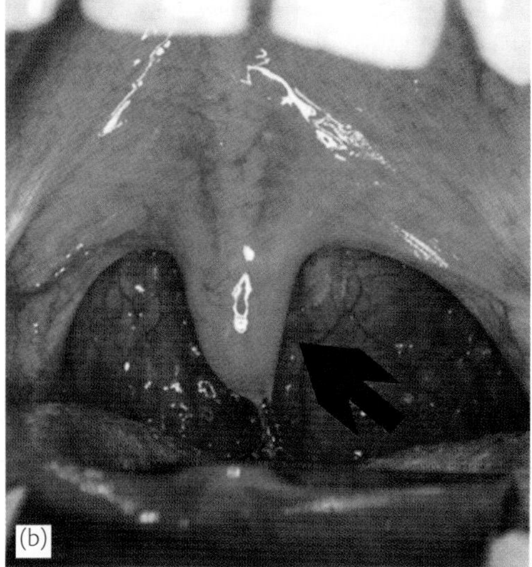

Fig. 11.39 Xth nerve palsy. (a) uvula in the midline, (b) on elevation the uvula moves away from the weaker side. Reprinted from **Fig. 14.63(a)** and **(b)** (p. 14.22), *Atlas of Clinical Neurology* (2nd edn), by G. David Perkin, Fred Hochberg, and Douglas C. Miller (1993), Mosby Publications, with permission from Elsevier.

Gag reflex

What is it?

If the posterior wall of the pharynx is stimulated, there follows a choking or gagging response as the pharynx constricts and elevates as a protective measure.

How to examine

This is an unpleasant reflex to elicit for the patient. Say something like, ' ... and now I'm just going to touch the back of your throat very briefly. I am afraid it might cause a choking sensation, but it needs to be done and will be over quickly … well done.' Use your tongue depressor and gently touch the back of the throat on one side. In the normal circumstance the patient will gag. Both sides of the throat need to be tested although it can be very difficult to cajole your patient into having it done a second time. A brief apology afterwards might convince them you are not a sadist. If a gag reflex is not elicited you need to ask the patient if they felt the tongue depressor touch the back of the throat. If they did not, it suggests that the afferent limb of the reflex (IXth nerve) is affected (or possibly the IXth and Xth nerves together). If they felt the stimulus it suggests that only the efferent limb is affected (Xth nerve).

It is important to note that an absent gag reflex can be found in normal people. It is only if the reflex is absent unilaterally or if the patient presents with symptoms, for example, dysphagia, aspiration of fluids into the lung, and so on that this finding will be significant.

Accessory nerve (XI)

12. Assess the trapezius and sternomastoid muscles (XI tested).

This nerve innervates trapezius and sternomastoid (full name—sternocleidomastoid) muscles together with a contribution from the spinal cord.

Tip

As the gag reflex is an unpleasant test, eliciting the gag reflex should not be part of the normal examination routine. Only perform it if your patient has relevant symptoms such as dysphagia, nasal regurgitation of fluids, or dysphonia.

Keypoints

- Lesions of the lower cranial nerves rarely occur in isolation.
- The soft palate elevates **away** from the weakened side.
- The glossopharyngeal nerve supplies the afferent limb of the gag reflex and the vagus nerve supplies the efferent limb.
- An absent gag reflex can be a normal variant.
- A gag reflex that is absent unilaterally or is absent bilaterally with symptoms such as dysphagia, dysphonia, or aspiration is abnormal.

Trapezius

Say to your patient, 'Shrug your shoulders.' Show the patient how to do it and then watch for asymmetry. Get them to repeat the movement but this time say, 'Stop me pressing your shoulders down'. Place both your hands on their shoulder and press down. Feel if there is any gross difference in muscle power on each side.

Sternomastoid

Say to your patient, 'Turn your head to the right.' Again demonstrate how to do this so that the head is looking over the shoulder. Then say 'Keep your head in that position and stop me pushing it back to the middle.' Gently push your hand against the patient's jaw and increase the pressure gently (see Fig. 11.40). Also palpate the belly of the left sternomastoid muscle as it contracts. Then say, 'If you could turn your head to the left side now,' and now test the other side remembering to palpate the right sternomastoid muscle.

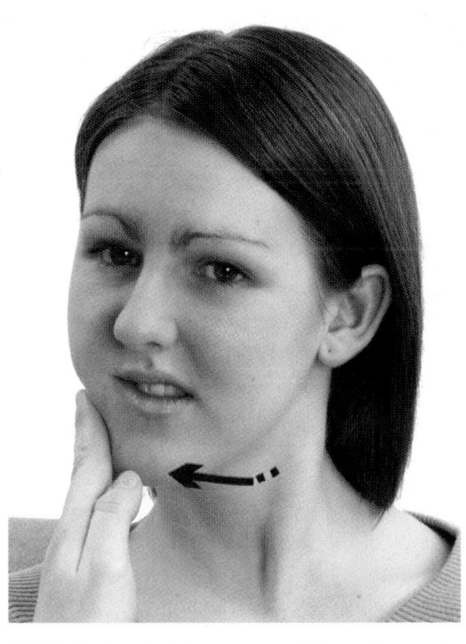

Fig. 11.40 Testing the left sternomastoid muscle: note the contraction.

Keypoints

- Observe the neck and shoulders and make sure they are symmetrical.
- Assess the power in the sternomastoid and trapezius muscles.

Hypoglossal nerve (XII)

13. Assess the tongue and tongue movements (XII tested).

This is the motor nerve supplying the intrinsic muscles of the tongue. Like the facial nerve, each hypoglossal nerve has bilateral cortical representation. Therefore a unilateral supranuclear lesion will not have any discernible effect on tongue function. Bilateral cortical infarcts will produce a 'spastic tongue', which has limited movement and cannot be protruded from the mouth. This is part of the syndrome of pseudobulbar palsy (see later). A unilateral lesion of the XIIth nerve (lower motor neurone) will produce wasting of the tongue, with possible fasciculations on the side of the lesion.

Say to your patient,'Open your mouth.' Look at the patient's tongue. Is it wasted and fasiculating (bulbar palsy?—see below). Now assess the tongue movements. Ask, 'Can you put your tongue out for me ... and move it from side to side.' If there is a unilateral weakness of the tongue it will deviate to the weaker side with protrusion (see Fig. 11.41). If any doubt remains, also say to your patient, 'Push out your cheek with the tip of your tongue.' Using this method you can use your index finger to press the cheek to gauge the amount of force the patient can generate with the tongue and compare both sides.

Tip

When you get slick at examining the cranial nerves you will assess the tongue while you are assessing the soft palate with the patient's mouth open.

Jugular foramen syndrome

Isolated lesions of the lower cranial nerves rarely occur. Instead a group may be affected, often in recognizable combinations, for example, the jugular foramen syndrome. This is the unilateral combination of IXth, Xth, and XIth cranial nerve lesions. A right-sided lesion will cause the soft palate to elevate and pull the uvula across to the left. There will be loss of taste and sensation to the posterior third of the tongue and pharynx and a decreased gag reflex on the right. The right shoulder may droop lower than its opposite counterpart and there will be difficulty shrugging it. Also there will be an inability to turn the head to the left.

Cause

Tumour of the skull base, for example, meningioma.

Bulbar palsy

The pons and medulla of the brainstem are sometimes referred to as the bulb because of their anatomical appearance. A bulbar palsy is the term reserved for bilateral dysfunction of the lower cranial nerves IX, X, and XII. The tongue is wasted, flaccid, fasciculates, and lacks movement. The patient will suffer with dysphagia, which is worse with liquids, which regurgitate up the nose. They will also have speech that lacks volume (dysphonia) and is indistinct. Because of difficulty swallowing liquid, saliva pools in the mouth and periodically the patient will pause to swallow it.

Causes

The causes of bulbar palsy are

- motor neurone disease
- Guillain–Barré syndrome
- polio.

Pseudobulbar palsy

This is due to bilateral upper motor neurone lesions. The tongue is spastic and cannot be moved rapidly from side to side. There is dysphagia with nasal regurgitation of liquids. Saliva cannot be swallowed and may drool from the mouth. The speech is high pitched and monotonous (has been likened to Donald Duck speech). There will usually be evidence of bilateral hemiparesis with bilateral extensor plantars and the jaw jerk will be brisk. The patient may exhibit emotionalism and may cry or laugh inappropriately.

Causes

- bilateral strokes
- multiple sclerosis.

Keypoints

- The tongue will deviate **towards** the weakened side.
- A bulbar palsy occurs with a bilateral lower motor neurone lesion.
- A bulbar palsy causes a wasted fasciculating tongue with dysphagia (nasal regurgitation of liquids) and an indistinct low volume speech.
- A pseudobulbar palsy causes a 'spastic' poorly moving tongue with dysphagia (nasal regurgitation of liquids), a high-pitched monotonous speech, drooling, and a brisk jaw jerk

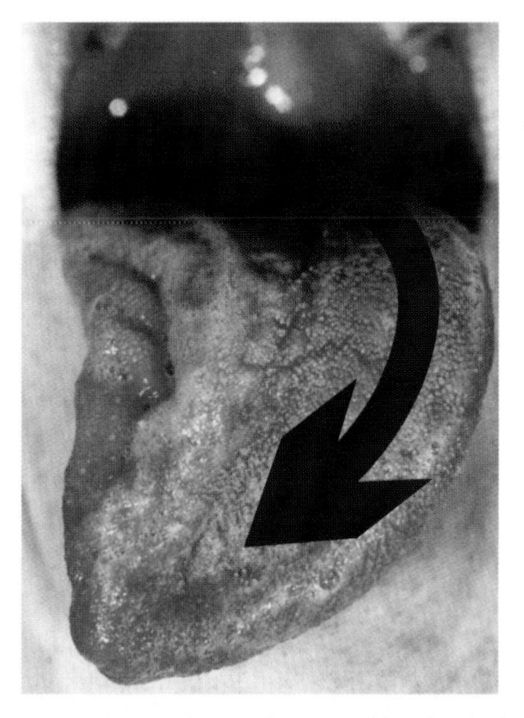

Fig. 11.41 XIIth nerve palsy. Note the wasting of the right side of the tongue with deviation towards this weakened side. Reprinted from **Fig. 14.67** (p. 14.23), *Atlas of Clinical Neurology* (2nd edn), by G. David Perkin, Fred Hochberg, and Douglas C. Miller (1993), Mosby Publications, with permission from Elsevier.

14. Now you have finished make sure the patient is comfortable.

As with all examinations it is etiquette to make sure the patient is both comfortable and returned to their original position after the examination. Thank them for their help.

Wash your hands

15. Wash your hands.

Don't bug your patients.

Presentation of findings

16. Presentation.

If you have elicited an abnormality then the presentation of the cranial nerves is quite simple. As with all presentations it is best to present your positive findings first, followed by any important negative ones. This however should only be done if you are quite sure of the abnormalities. It is even more impressive if you can give a diagnosis or a differential before you are asked. For example, 'The patient has a left lower motor neurone facial weakness as demonstrated by asymmetry of the face and weakness of the left facial muscles including the forehead. There were vesicles in the external auditory meatus. There were no other abnormalities of the eighth or ninth cranial nerves.' The diagnosis is Ramsay-Hunt syndrome affecting the left VIIth nerve only.

Other signs

Kernig's sign

Kernig's sign (*Vladimir Kernig (1840–1917), Russian physician*) is one of the classical tests for meningism (*men-in-jism*) (see Fig. 11.42). With the patient lying on their back, flex their hip to 90° as well as their knee. Then slowly extend the knee as far as you can. With meningism, you will be unable to extend the knee beyond 135° without eliciting pain and resistance. Some patients who are not very lim-

(a)

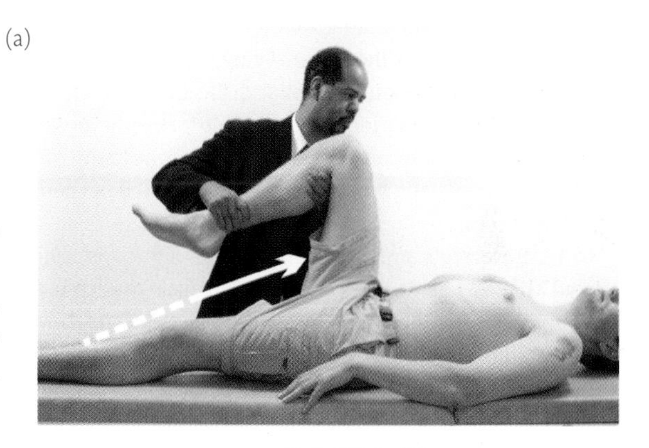

(b)

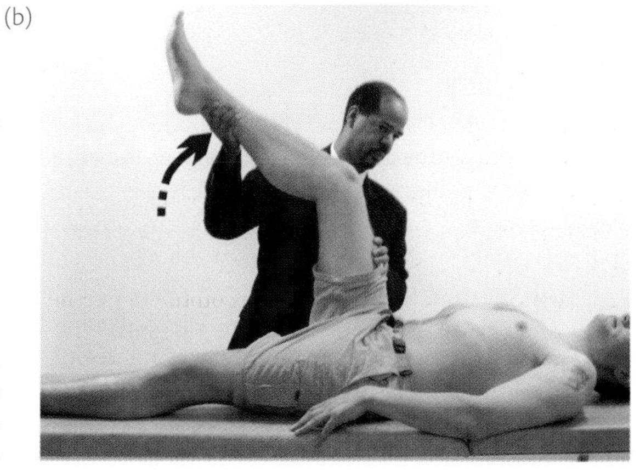

Fig. 11.42 Eliciting Kernig's sign.

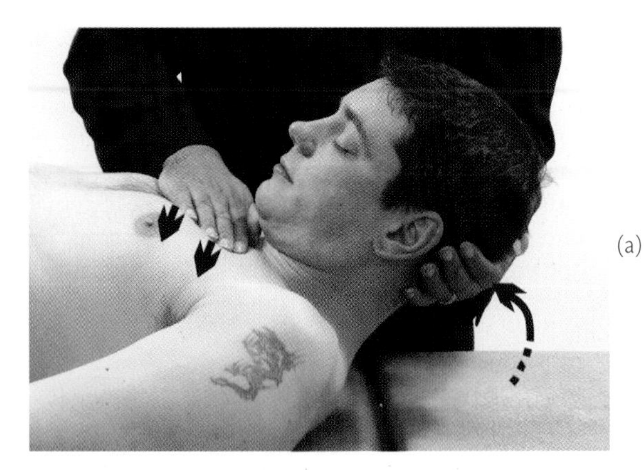

Fig. 11.43 Brudzinski's sign (see text).

ber may also experience difficulty extending their knee fully. However you should be able to coax them beyond 135° and there is no pain associated.

Brudzinski's sign

Brudzinski's *(brew-zin-skiz)* sign *(Jósef Brudzinski (1874–1917), Polish physician)* is another test of meningism (see Fig. 11.43). Again with the patient lying supine, place one hand behind the patient's head and the other on their chest. Then lift the patient's head while pressing down firmly on the chest to prevent the patient from rising off the bed. If the patient has meningism they will flex their hips and knees.

In both Kernig's sign and Brudzinski's sign it is suggested that the signs are produced because the motor nerve roots are irritated as they are put on stretch as they pass through the inflamed meninges. Although both signs are regarded as classical, their sensitivity is very poor. They will be negative in many cases that will go on to be proven meningitis.

Nuchal rigidity

This manoeuvre is what most clinicians understand by eliciting neck stiffness. Both hands are placed behind the head in a cradling fashion. The neck is then gently flexed forwards. If the patient has meningism, they will find this painful and will actively resist the movement.

The diagnosis of meningitis demands clinical judgement and experience certainly helps. This judgement will be based on the history and examination. An experienced clinician may still perform a lumbar puncture even in the absence of Kernig's sign, Brudzinski's sign, or neck stiffness if they believe the clinical situation demands it.

Hallpike-Dix manoeuvre

This manoeuvre is used in the investigation of vertigo (see Fig. 11.44). It is principally used to diagnose BPPV but it may unearth other disease as well. First check that your patient does not have neck problems prior to

(a)

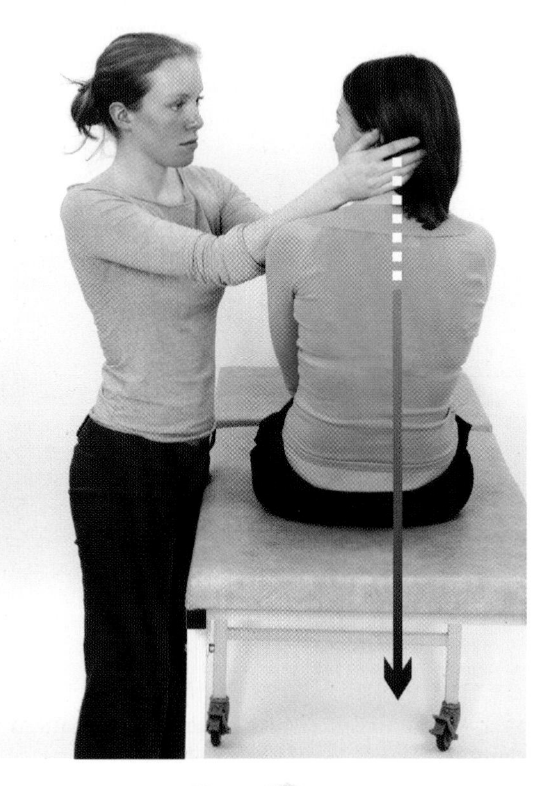

(b)

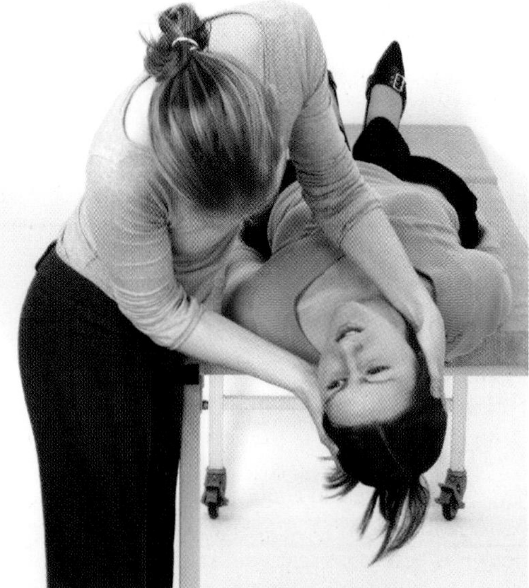

Fig. 11.44 The Hallpike-Dix manoeuvre (see text).

testing. Now sit your patient on a couch. Your aim is to get the patient to lie down on the couch so that their head and neck will dangle over the top of the couch. Either sit them on the couch and estimate where they need to be to enable you to do this or you can go through a 'dry run' by getting them in the required position and then get them to sit up from there (be aware that you may stimulate vertigo while doing this). Now grasp the head and turn it 45° to one side. Warn your patient that you are going to lower them over the edge of the couch and it may set off their vertigo. If the vertigo occurs, tell them to keep their eyes open if at all possible and not to try to sit up (all natural reactions to the vertigo). Then briskly push the patient backward until they are lying flat and continue to lower their head until it is about 30° below the level of the couch. Observe their eyes and be prepared to wait up to 10 s before anything happens. If they have BPPV, after a latent period nystagmus may develop along with vertigo. The nystagmus is usually rotary, with the top part of the cornea rotating downward towards the affected ear. This is usually short lived, lasting no more than 20 s. If the patient sits up, they may experience milder vertigo and nystagmus can be seen but in the opposite direction to what was previously seen (see p. 324 for explanation). If you repeat the test, vertigo and nystagmus may return but the duration will be less. After two to three repetitions this reaction will no longer be elicited and the nystagmus is termed fatiguable. If you do not elicit any reaction the first time, turn the patient's head 45° to the other side and repeat the manoeuvre. Sometimes with brainstem lesions, nystagmus may also be provoked with this test. In these cases there is usually no latent period before the onset of nystagmus and it does not fatigue with testing.

Primitive reflexes

Primitive reflexes are a collection of reflexes that are present during babyhood but are eventually suppressed by the increasing activity of the frontal lobes. Damage to the frontal lobes may lead to the re-emergence of these reflexes.

1. **Snout/pout reflex.** This can be elicited by tapping the lips very gently with a tendon hammer. The test is positive if the lips pout in response.
2. **Rooting reflex.** If the upper lip is stroked on either lateral extremity, the patient will move their mouth towards the finger (like a baby searching for a nipple).
3. **Palmomental (*palm-owe-mental*) reflex.** Stroke the palm of one hand while looking at the lower lip and jaw on the same side of the face. An abnormal response is a contraction of the ipsilateral mentalis (*men-tail-iss*) muscle of the lower lip.

The utility of these reflexes is limited. They remain impressive signs to delight your colleagues with.

> **Tip**
>
> If you perform this test in the ward setting, you will have to lay your patient across the bed to allow their head and neck to dangle over the edge. In this situation you will have to go behind the patient and support their head as you lie them down on the bed. Once you lower their head to 30° below the level of the bed you will be able to see their eyes and observe whether they have nystagmus.

Cranial nerve diseases and investigations

In the earlier parts of this chapter, various medical conditions have been mentioned. In this section I now describe these. In general these descriptions are brief though certain aspects not well described in other textbooks are discussed in some detail

Epilepsy

To the lay public, epilepsy conjures up an unconscious person who convulses, jerking all four limbs rhythmically. Some believe people with epilepsy are likely to be mentally impaired or become that way as a result of a fit. The latter assertion is clearly untrue as the majority of people with epilepsy are of normal intelligence. The classical 'grand-mal' seizure is just one way in which an epileptic person might present and the definitions of epilepsy and seizures will give clues as to why this might be.

Epilepsy: what is it?

This is a pathological state where a person has a continuing susceptibility to seizures.

Seizures: what are they?

This is the physical manifestation of paroxysmal, uncontrolled discharges of neuronal activity occurring anywhere in the brain. Therefore a seizure can produce a variety of clinical presentations depending on the area of brain affected.

Classification

What follows represents a simplified classification based on the international league of epilepsy recommendations. Seizures can be generalized or partial (local).

Generalized seizures

A generalized seizure is where the electrical discharge spreads to both cerebral hemispheres simultaneously. Consciousness is impaired and there may or may not be convulsions evident. If this occurs from the outset, the seizure is termed primary generalized. Generalized seizures may be atonic, tonic, clonic, tonic–clonic, myoclonic, or absences. With atonic seizures, the person loses control of all voluntary muscles and falls to the floor. With tonic seizures these muscles contract leading to rigidity. Again the patient will fall to the floor because they are unable to make any postural corrections. With clonic seizures the person exhibits jerking of the limbs and trunk as the muscles contract and relax alternately. With tonic–clonic seizures this clonic phase will follow the period of tonic contraction. Tonic–clonic seizures are what the lay public recognize as fits and what used to be termed grand-mal seizures. Myoclonic seizures are seizures that are described as rhythmical, shock-like jerking movements that are less coarse and violent than clonic seizures. An absence seizure is a non-convulsive episode usually seen in childhood and is synonymous with 'petit-mal' seizure. This usually manifests as a period of vacant staring often attributed to day-dreaming and is usually short-lived.

Partial seizures

Partial seizures (also called focal seizures) are those where the electrical activity is confined to a focal area of the brain. Partial seizures are further subdivided into simple and complex partial seizures. Simple partial seizures are those where consciousness is not affected and complex partial seizures are those where consciousness is impaired. Simple partial seizures produce effects depending on which area of the brain is affected. This could be motor, sensory, autonomic, disturbed memory, speech abnormality, and so on. The electrical disturbance may spread and consciousness may become impaired, that is, the seizure becomes a complex partial one. If this disturbance spreads to both hemispheres then it will become a secondary generalized seizure. One particularly dramatic demonstration of this spread of activity is the 'Jacksonian (*jack-sew-knee-an*) march' (John Hughlings-Jackson (1835–1911), UK neurologist). This is a focal seizure, which has progressive motor effects. It may start with the twitching of a hand before spreading up the arm to the trunk and lower leg. This form of seizure is uncommon. A complex partial seizure may commence from the outset or develop from a simple partial seizure. Many of these seizures originate in the temporal lobe and the phenomenon was therefore named temporal lobe epilepsy.

Presentation

A generalized seizure, whether primary or secondary, will present in the same manner. In a typical tonic–clonic seizure, the first phase is the tonic phase. All the muscles of the body contract and the body goes rigid. At this stage the patient may give out a cry as the contraction of the respiratory muscles forces air out of the larynx. In the tonic stage the person falls rigidly to the ground with the possibility of injury. The contraction of other muscle groups can lead to tongue biting and urinary and possibly faecal incontinence. During this phase there is no flow of oxygen into the lungs and the patient becomes rapidly cyanosed (this is the presentation for pure tonic seizures before recovery). This may last up to a minute before the clonic phase supervenes. There follows rhythmic jerking of the limbs and trunk, which may last several minutes. 'Frothing at the mouth' may be caused by the convulsing jaws churning up saliva that has pooled in the mouth (a purely clonic fit will exhibit these features only). A period of unconsciousness follows before recovery. When they recover from a fit an epileptic person is usually confused for a variable length of time, called the post-ictal period ('ictal' means fit). For some elderly patients this can last several hours or even days (the possibility of epilepsy should always be considered in older patients with recurrent confusional states that evade diagnosis). Occasionally a series of seizures may follow each other concurrently (called status epilepticus) and this is a medical emergency. The patient is in danger of dying of cardiorespiratory failure and prompt treatment is therefore required. Some patients may experience an aura prior to a convulsion. This may be a smell, taste, or strange indefinable feeling. These auras represent simple partial seizures experienced as a prelude to a secondary generalized seizure. Some recognize their auras as harbingers of a fit and attempt to get to a place of safety before the onset of the seizure.

Simple partial seizures produce clear-cut symptoms depending on the area of the brain affected. It may not always be easy to attribute the more unusual manifestations of these seizures to epilepsy, for example, recurrent disturbance of mood, strange sensations, and so on unless the possibility is borne in mind. Complex partial seizures involve impairment of consciousness, which may be partial, so that the patient has some awareness of events happening around them. Things may seem unreal (a situation called jamais-vu (*jam-ay-voo*)) or there may be a sense of experiencing events over again (called déjà vu (*day-jah-voo*)). The patient may also experience hallucinations, which may involve any sense including visual, taste, or smell. Even with the total loss of conscious control, the patient may still be able to exhibit complex behaviour patterns without memory (called automatism). Following a seizure the patient may feel exhausted and confused and they may have a headache.

Causes

There are many causes of epilepsy, ranging from genetic syndromes, which are inherited, to acquired causes such as trauma or stroke. In addition there are circumstances where illness or anti-social behaviour can lead to seizures without the patient being epileptic, for example, electrolyte imbalance or alcohol or drug misuse. In some cases the cause of epilepsy is unknown and is called idiopathic epilepsy. What is increasingly clear is that with the refinement of diagnostic tools such as CT or MRI scanning, structural lesions have been found in cases that would have been labelled idiopathic in the past. The final point to make is that certain causes of seizures predominate at different stages of life (see Table 11.8).

TABLE 11.8 Causes of epilepsy

Children
Genetic syndromes
Birth injury, for example, anoxia or infection
Head injury
Adults
Head injury
Stroke
Alcohol or drug misuse
Meningitis or encephalitis
Metabolic
Elderly people
Stroke
Neurodegenerative, for example, Alzheimer's disease
Cerebral tumours
Head injury

None of the groups are mutually exclusive, therefore causes that are common in the elderly group can occur, albeit rarely, in the childhood group, for example, cerebral tumours.

Some epileptic people can find their seizures precipitated by stress, anorexia, alcohol, or lack of sleep. Some can have epilepsy triggered by flickering lights and even music (sometimes called reflex epilepsy). Those controlled on anti-convulsants may find they lose control because the addition of drugs can interfere with the metabolism of the drug and lead to inadequate drug levels.

Treatment

The treatment of epilepsy is beyond the scope of this book. It involves the specialized knowledge of different age groups, that is, children, adults, and elderly people, plus dealing with circumstances such as the treatment of women in pregnancy. Certain principles need to be followed including those given below.

1. Identify an underlying cause and remove or modify the cause if possible.
2. If the cause cannot be cured the patient will need stabilizing with anti-convulsant therapy.
3. The patient will also need educating about epilepsy and how to live with it.
4. Families and carers also need education.
5. Driving is an issue and patients cannot drive in the UK until they are seizure free for a year.

Age-related macular degeneration

This is a progressive deterioration of vision as a result of degeneration occurring at the macula. It is called age-related' because it is rare before the age of 50 years. It is one of the most common causes of visual loss in the elderly population in the western world. Because the macula is affected it is central vision that is progressively lost, making detail harder to discriminate. Surviving peripheral vision allows the patient to negotiate their environment until late on in the disease process. It is thought that the disease is due to the deposition of waste debris called drusen, although how this contributes to the pathogenesis is not clear. There are two types of ARMD, atrophic (or dry) ARMD and exudative (or wet) ARMD. Atrophic ARMD is the most common form and drusen promotes the atrophy of photoreceptors and related structures. Exudative ARMD is triggered by new vessel formation of the choroids (*coh-roids*). Fluid leaks from these vessels, which leads to the distortion of the resulting image.

Glaucoma

Glaucoma is a disorder of the optic nerve, which is usually (but not always) associated with raised IOP. There is eventual ischaemia of the optic nerve head with damage to nerve fibres leading to visual loss. This process produces optic cupping and in chronic cases, optic atrophy. A level of 21 mm Hg is used as a cut-off above which the clinical likelihood of glaucoma is substantially increased. However there are people who develop glaucomatous changes at levels below this value and conversely there are people who have elevated IOP with no evidence of glaucoma. Intraocular pressure is a function of the flow of aqueous fluid within the eye. This is manufactured from the ciliary bodies and circulates within the eye, before draining through a trabecular meshwork at the angle of the anterior chamber. The fluid is then removed by the canal of Schlemm (*Friedrich Schlemm (1795–1858), German anatomist*), which drains into the episcleral veins. Any interruption of this drainage system can lead to glaucoma.

Primary open-angle glaucoma (chronic simple glaucoma)

This is an insidious condition, because the rise in IOP is gradual and the patient can compensate for any loss of vision in the early stages. The IOPs are usually over 21 mm Hg. As the name suggests the angle is open and it is unclear why the drainage gets blocked. It is not usually seen before the age of 40 years and it is common in the sixth decade. It is more common among Afro-Caribbean people and the myopic (short-sighted) eye is more susceptible. The eye is white, vision deteriorates gradually, and there may be a subtle arcuate scotoma. The optic disc is cupped. Treatment is with a range of eye drops that can be used separately or in combination, for example, β-blockers, pilocarpine, and carbonic anhydrase inhibitors

Primary close-angle glaucoma (acute close angle glaucoma)

This is a dramatic condition and symptoms can develop rapidly over a few hours. This is an ophthalmological emergency and if not treated can lead to permanent visual loss. It is more common in people with a shallow anterior chamber, which can predispose to the blockage of the angle by the iris. The hypermetropic (long-sighted) eye is more vulnerable to this complication. Again this form of glaucoma is rare before 40 years and is more common in the sixth decade. Caucasians are more at risk than black people and women more than men. Why this blockade occurs is not fully understood but it seems to be maximal when the pupil is dilated (so it is more common at times of poor light). There is a rapid rise in IOP, which can be in the region of 50–100 mm Hg. This leads to corneal clouding, which can produce rainbow-coloured haloes around light sources (these haloes may occur weeks before a full attack). There is a rapid loss of visual acuity and the eye is red because of injection of the ciliary blood vessels around the cornea. There is also pain in and around the eye, headache above the affected eye, and possibly nausea, vomiting, and photophobia. The pupil is semi-dilated, oval, and fixed and it therefore fails to react to light or accommodation. Treatment is pain relief and anti-emetics, eye-drops such as pilocarpine or carbonic anhydrase inhibitors, and a peripheral iridectomy (an incision into the iris to facilitate drainage of the aqueous fluid—this can be done surgically or by laser). The other eye is usually done as a precaution because the other eye often becomes affected weeks later.

Cataracts

Cataracts are any opacity found in the lens of the eye. The crystalline lens is transparent and is an important structure in fine tuning the focusing of images on the retina (called accommodation). Any opacity in the lens has the potential for obscuring vision. Types of cataracts include

- developmental cataracts
- congenital cataracts
- cataracts associated with eye disease
- cataracts associated with systemic disease
- age-related cataracts.

Developmental cataracts

These are tiny opacities in the lens, which are incidental findings because they do not interfere with vision. They can be whitish or bluish dots or finger-like projections and are seen in the periphery of the lens.

Congenital cataracts

These tend to be rare nowadays. Some may be idiopathic but others may be the result of intrauterine infections or as a consequence of maternal disease, for example, rubella (german measles), syphilis, or Down's syndrome.

Cataracts associated with eye disease

Cataracts may occur as a result of

- trauma (both penetrating or non-penetrating eye injury)
- iritis or keratitis
- radiation injury.

Cataracts associated with systemic disease

There are a number of conditions that are associated with cataracts:

- diabetes mellitus—similar to age-related cataracts but develop earlier
- steroid treatment—may develop posterior subcapsular cataracts
- hypoparathyroidism (See p. 352)
- dystrophica myotonica (see p. 221, Fig. 11.22).

Age-related cataracts

These occur as a consequence of ageing and are a slow progressive cause of blindness. They may also cause glare in bright lights, dark fixed spots in the field of vision, and occasionally monocular diplopia. There are three main types:

- nuclear sclerosis
- posterior subcapsular cataract
- cuneiform (*cue-knee-form*).

Nuclear sclerosis

This is a very slow, progressive hardening and yellowing of the lens. The lens is less pliant and is therefore less able to respond for close vision. Short-sighted patients may sometimes be able to give up their reading glasses as a result.

Posterior subcapsular cataract

This cataract is rapidly progressive and occurs in the cortex of the lens. It often obstructs central vision early and therefore requires early intervention. It can be seen with steroid treatment.

Cuneiform

This cataract is slowly progressive with finger-like opacities appearing at the periphery of the lens and radiating inwards like the spokes of a wheel. They only affect vision when they encroach into the centre of the lens.

All three types of cataract can lead to a 'mature cataract', given time and no treatment. In this situation the whole of the lens is opacified. Treatment for cataracts involves the surgical removal of the cataract and the implantation of an intraocular lens.

Retinal detachment

This is where the retina separates from its underlying pigment epithelial layer. Patients complain of floaters and may experience flashing lights as the result of traction on the retina. At some point afterwards the patient will describe a shadow or curtain extending over their field of vision. If the macula is involved, the visual acuity will be dramatically reduced. This occurs commonly in trauma, for example, in boxers and in people who are very short sighted. The treatment is surgical and involves the repair of the retina together with the sealing of any retinal tear or break.

Vitreous haemorrhage

This is bleeding into the vitreous humour of the eye. The most common reason is bleeding from abnormal new vessels on the retina (the most common cause is diabetes mellitus). This complication is the reason for the constant surveillance of diabetic fundi and any new vessels seen are treated with laser therapy. Patients complain of floaters in their vision and visual acuity may be affected if the haemorrhage is large. Flashing lights suggest retinal traction and may be the prelude to vitreous detachment as the blood organizes, fibroses, and then contracts.

Retinitis pigmentosa

See Fig. 11.45. This is the syndrome of night blindness, constriction of the peripheral fields of vision, and a characteristic appearance of the retina, which is a dark spiculated/reticulate pigmentation seen at the periphery of the retina. The first symptom is usually night blindness, then as the disease progresses, there is constriction of the visual fields until there is tunnel vision. In many cases the disease is inherited and it can follow any pattern of inheritance, that is, autosomal dominant, autosomal recessive, or linked to the X chromosome (X-linked). It may also be associated with rare metabolic disorders such as abetalipoproteinaemia (*ay-beater-lie-poe-pro-teen-ee-mia*), Refsum's (*ref-sums*) disease (*S. Refsum, Norwegian physician*), Laurence–Moon–Biedl syndrome (*J. Z. Laurence (1830– 1874), British ophthalmologist, R. C. Moon (1844–1914), American ophthalmologist, A. Biedl (1869–1933), Czechoslovakian physician*).

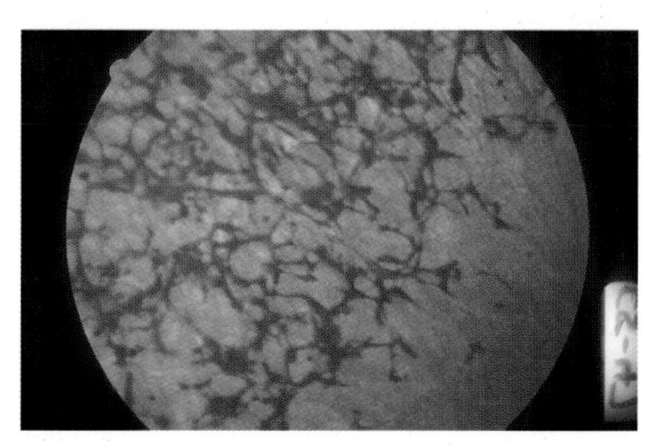

Fig. 11.45 Retinitis pigmentosa.

Optic atrophy

This is the irreversible degeneration of the optic nerve head and associated fibres leading to visual loss and a pale optic disc. There are a variety of causes of optic atrophy. Hereditary causes can be autosomal dominant (usually milder disease) or autosomal recessive. One particular form, Leber's *(leb-buzz)* optic atrophy *(Theodor von Leber (1840–1917), German ophthalmologist)*, may be X-linked because it predominantly affects males. It usually presents around the age of 20–30 years. Acquired causes include

- compression of the optic nerve, for example, pituitary tumours
- central retinal artery occlusion
- trauma
- optic neuritis (see below)
- toxins, for example, alcohol or tobacco
- retinal degeneration, for example, due to retinitis pigmentosa.

The only hope for treatment is to intervene early in those cases with an underlying cause before irreversible visual loss.

Optic neuritis

This is the inflammation of the optic disc and optic nerve and the most common cause in the UK is multiple sclerosis. If the optic disc is affected this is called papillitis *(pap-ill-light-iss)* and this produces changes that can be seen on fundoscopy. If the optic nerve is affected this is sometimes called retrobulbar neuritis inferring that the inflammation is behind the optic disc and as a result produces no visible changes on fundoscopy. Papillitis is the resultant swelling of the optic disc due to inflammation and the appearance on fundoscopy is indistiguishable from that of papilloedema. The term papilloedema should only be used if the cause is clearly due to raised intracranial pressure. The features that help distinguish papillitis from papilloedema are as follows.

Papillitis	Papilloedema
Reduced visual acuity	No visual disturbance
± Central scotoma	May have an enlarged blind spot
Diminished pupillary light reflex (Marcus Gunn pupil see p. 290)	Normal pupillary light reflex
May be pain on eye movements	No pain on eye movements

With papillitis there is a rapid loss of central vision over a few hours. There follows a gradual recovery over the following weeks. There are usually signs of optic atrophy months after the event. If all or most of the features described about papillitis are present without signs of a swollen optic disc, this suggests retrobulbar neuritis. In cases of papillitis or retrobulbar neuritis the possibility of multiple sclerosis should always be borne in mind.

Holmes–Adie pupil

This is a slowly reacting or myotonic pupil. If the pupil is exposed to light the pupil may remain dilated for a long period before finally constricting. Conversely in poor light the pupil may remain constricted for a long time before dilating. There are no other neurological complications associated with this condition. There is no ptosis nor any abnormal eye movements, which distinguishes it from cranial nerve abnormalities. There is an association with absent tendon reflexes.

Ramsay-Hunt syndrome

This is the combination of a lower motor neurone facial nerve palsy with herpes zoster infection (shingles). Initially there may be pain in the ear with nothing to find on examination. A few days later the characteristic vesicular eruption of shingles can be seen on the pinna and external auditory canal. The vesicles can contain pus (pustules) or become haemorrhagic, before crusting over to leave a scab and eventually a scar. There may also be VIIIth cranial nerve involvement leading to sensorineural deafness and vertigo.

Acute labyrinthitis

Often acute labyrinthitis or sometimes the term acute vestibular neuronitis is used to describe a condition where a previously healthy patient develops a sudden onset of severe vertigo. There is no hearing loss or tinnitus and the acute attack can last several days. The patient may be bed bound for fear of falling and there is associated nausea and vomiting. The symptoms usually ebb away over a few weeks. Treatment is symptomatic relief with anti-emetics.

Bell's palsy

This is the cause of a lower motor neurone facial nerve palsy of unknown cause. The paralysis occurs suddenly and is complete within 24 h. Symptoms are the result of swelling of the facial nerve within the restrictive facial canal of the skull. If the involvement is extensive the chorda tympani branch may be affected leading to the loss of taste on the anterior two-thirds of the tongue. There may also be hyperacusis due to paralysis of the stapedius muscle (see p. 305). As the eye cannot close it may be vulnerable to damage by foreign body or infection. Therefore a patch may be required temporarily to protect the eye. The condition usually resolves slowly over 2 months.

Subarachnoid haemorrhage

This is a bleed into the subarachnoid space, usually as a result of the rupture of an intracranial aneurysm or arteriovenous malformation (the subarachnoid space is between the pia mater (*pee-a-may-ter*) and the arachnoid mater and allows the circulation of cerebrospinal fluid (CSF)). Clinically this haemorrhage leads to the sudden onset of severe headache 'like being hit with a baseball bat'. If the haemorrhage is severe the patient may collapse and die. Otherwise they may become comatose within hours. They may also develop fits and focal neurological signs (an expanding aneurysm may produce signs prior to a haemorrhage, for example, posterior communicating artery aneurysm leading to a complete IIIrd nerve palsy. Those with milder degrees of haemorrhage may have headache with neck stiffness (neck stiffness may be absent in 30% of cases). The initial investigation is by CT scan to demonstrate blood. If no blood is seen this does not rule out a subarachnoid haemorrhage and a lumbar puncture should be performed to look for xanthochromia (*zan-throw-chrome-ia*) (a breakdown product of blood) in the CSF. This is usually seen 5–12 h following a haemorrhage and can be present in the CSF for up to 40 days. Patients with a proven subarachnoid haemorrhage need cerebral angiography and any aneurysm demonstrated needs clipping to prevent a further bleed.

Meningitis

A variety of infective (and non-infective) agents can inflame the meninges, three protective layers surrounding the brain (the pia-mater, the arachnoid mater, and the dura mater (*dure-a-may-ter*)). Infective causes include viral, bacterial, protozoal, or fungal agents and non-infective causes include drugs and malignant cell infiltrates.

Viral meningitis

Any virus can cause meningitis. It is difficult to get an accurate picture of which organisms are the most common because many people with viral meningitis may not present themselves for medical help. The majority of those that present to hospital will not have viruses isolated (if they are looked for at all). With these reservations, the most common viruses are the enteroviruses such as echovirus and cocksackie (*cock-sacky*) virus. Clinically the patient may have a prodrome of an influenza-type illness, for example, lassitude, muscle and joint pains, and fever. In addition they may develop severe headache and neck stiffness (a sign of meningeal irritation, called meningism). This form of presentation should lead to further investigation including lumbar puncture.

Bacterial meningitis

Bacteria may infect the meninges through blood-borne (haematogenous (*he-mat-todger-nuss*)) spread or there may be more direct spread following complications of head trauma, otitis media, or sinusitis. The most common organisms are neisseria meningitidis (*nice-eerier-men-in-jitty-dis*) (also called meningococcus) (*men-in-go-cock-us*), streptococcus pneumoniae (*strep-toe-cock-us-new-moan-i-ee*) (also called pneumococcus) (*new-mow-cock-us*), and haemophilus influenzae (*heem-off-ee-lus-in-flu-en-zee*). Clinically the patient will present with headache, neck stiffness, photophobia, vomiting, and drowsiness. Later complications such as fits, cranial nerve palsies, or hemiplegias may supervene. There may also be obstruction to the flow of CSF called hydrocephalus leading to a rise in intracranial pressure. Meningococcal meningitis is the form that everybody fears as rapid deterioration can occur with septicaemia and the patient can become comatose within hours. There is a high mortality rate associated with it. One of the signs of septicaemia is the development of a purpuric rash that does not blanch. Lay sources of medical information tell the public to put a glass tumbler over the rash and apply gentle downward pressure. If the rash remains visible then the likelihood is high that this represents a serious development of meningitis. If in doubt the patient should get an immediate injection of penicillin without waiting for confirmatory tests. The investigation of choice is a lumbar puncture. However if focal neurological signs, fits, or depressed conscious level are evident, then a CT scan should be performed first.

Other causes of meningitis

It is worth considering other infective and non-infective causes of meningitis in patients who are immunocompromised, for example, patients with AIDS or leukaemia or transplant patients on immunosuppressive drugs. In these cases unusual organisms such as fungi, amoebae, or tubercle bacilli may be responsible. Suspect these if your patient does not respond to first-line antibiotics (as recommended by your local hospital formulary). Occasionally malignant cells can invade the meninges, for example, leukaemic cells and produce an inflammatory reaction. There should however be clues to the malignant process elsewhere in the body or blood film, as well as clues in the CSF.

Encephalitis

There are a variety of viral agents that can infect the brain. In the UK, herpes simplex is the most common cause of encephalitis, although with the increasing number of HIV infections this will assume greater notoriety in the future. Some organisms seem to have a predilection for certain areas of the brain, for example, herpes simplex—the temporal lobes and the virus in encephalitis lethargica—the basal ganglia. In other countries more 'exotic' viruses may cause spectacular disease and may be transmitted by a range of vectors including mosquitoes and ticks.

Clinically there is an acute onset of headache usually associated with a fever. There is usually a fluctuating conscious level and there may be evidence of focal signs such as cranial nerve palsies or hemiparesis. There may be meningism and seizures may occur. Investigations usually include a CT scan to rule out other pathology such as brain tumour, a lumbar puncture, and sometimes electroencephalolography, because the diagnosis may still not be clear following these procedures. The treatment includes supportive measures such as intravenous fluids, anti-convulsive therapy, and intravenous acyclovir (*ay-sigh-clo-veer*) if herpes simplex encephalitis is suspected.

Lumbar puncture

This is the introduction of a special lumbar puncture needle into the spine to withdraw CSF. This is usually performed between the L3–L4 or L4–L5 vertebrae because the spinal cord terminates at L2 and this minimizes the risk of injury to it. The CSF circulates in and around the brain and spinal cord and therefore analysing the fluid withdrawn from the lumbar spine approximates to the fluid around the brain. This feature is used in the diagnosis (or differential diagnosis) of a central neurological disease. The CSF is examined for glucose, protein, white and red cells, and micro-organisms (CSF pressure should be measured also but is not often done). Any abnormalities in any of these parameters can suggest a diagnosis. Diseases that can be diagnosed include meningitis (the most notorious), encephalitis, spinal cord tumours, Guillain-Barré Syndrome, subarachnoid haemorrhage, and BIH. Care must be taken when doing a lumbar puncture. Physicians should always be aware of the possibility of raised intracranial pressure because if the procedure is done in this situation, the pressure difference generated by the removal of CSF will force the brainstem down through the foramen magnum of the skull (a phenomenon known as 'coning') and lead to a rapid death. If at all possible a CT scan should be performed before doing a lumbar puncture. In areas where CT is not readily available, the decision is a clinical one. The physician should always examine the eyes for papilloedema (see p. 293) as a potential marker for raised intracranial pressure.

Benign intracranial hypertension

This is also called pseudotumour cerebri (*serry-bry*) and idiopathic intracranial hypertension. This is a condition where intracranial pressure rises for reasons that are unclear. It affects females more than males, particularly those who are overweight. It has a peak onset between the ages of 20 and 40 years. It can occur suddenly or have a gradual onset. Symptoms are those associated with raised intracranial pressure, including headache, nausea, and vomiting. Fundoscopy will usually demonstrate papilloedema (unless the onset is sudden and the eyes have not had time to develop changes). A CT scan is required to rule out a space-occupying lesion. Following a normal scan a lumbar puncture should be performed and the CSF pressure measured. If the pressure is raised this confirms diagnosis of BIH. Some cases resolve spontaneously. Others respond to diuretics or steroids. Treatment may also require repeated lumbar punctures to remove CSF in a bid to relieve the pressure. In refractory cases shunts may be used to divert CSF from the cerebral ventricles but these procedures have risks and complications of their own.

Benign paroxysmal positional vertigo

This is the hallucination of movement that is triggered by certain positions of the body. Our understanding of the condition is advancing. Knowledge of the vestibular apparatus will aid your understanding. Each inner ear has three SCCs that are orientated in perpendicular planes. Within each canal is fluid and the direction of flow can be detected by the cupula (*cup-you-la*), which is deflected by the fluid and generates an electrical signal that is transmitted to the brain. A recent theory, the canalithiasis (*canal-lith-i-ay-sis*) theory (meaning canal stones) proposes that calcium carbonate debris collects in the SCC. When the patient changes position, these particles, after a lag period, tumble down the canal and stimulate the cupula. These signals are not congruous with the motion of the patient's head and produce nystagmus, vertigo, and nausea. If the patient then reverses their position, these stones will roll back in the direction they started in but this time the direction of the nystagmus will reverse (think about pebbles in a tyre and visualize how they tumble around the inner tube as they roll in one direction and then in reverse). Once the motion has ceased, the stones settle and the nystagmus and vertigo abate. It is postulated that this debris can be created in young adults through head injury and develop in old age through degenerative changes in the labyrinths. A subclassification of BPPV can be made on the basis of the SCC affected, that is, posterior superior SCC, posterior inferior SCC, and lateral SCC. Clinically a patient may develop sudden vertigo when changing positions. The vertigo is intermittent and may last 30 s before wearing off. Examination is usually unremarkable and nystagmus may not be elicited while the patient is still. The Hallpike-Dix manoeuvre will confirm the diagnosis (see p. 316). Recently a treatment has been developed for the condition, the Epley (*ep-lay*) manoeuvre.

Ménière's syndrome

This is a syndrome comprising attacks of vertigo, hearing impairment, and tinnitus. The cause is unknown but the end result is the accumulation of excessive endolymphatic fluid in the endolymphatic sac. It affects females more than males and usually occurs between the ages of 35 and 55 years. Hearing loss may precede an attack; it is sensorineural in origin and affects the lower frequencies preferentially. It is the vertigo that is debilitating and brings the patient to medical attention. There may be the sensation of pressure in the affected ear before the onset of vertigo. The vertigo may last several hours and may be accompanied by tinnitus. There may be several attacks of vertigo over several weeks but the natural history of the condition is one of gradual recovery. The treatment is symptomatic with antiemetics with or without sedatives. β-Histidine (*beater-hiss-ti-dean*) (serc) is often given although its efficacy is limited. Occasionally in severe cases surgical decompression of the endolylmphatic sac or surgical division of the vestibular nerve is undertaken.

Acoustic neuromas

These are benign tumours arising from the vestibular part of the VIIIth cranial nerve. Ninety-five per cent are unilateral and 5% are bilateral. There is an association with neurofibromatosis especially with bilateral tumours. Sensorineural hearing loss is the initial symptom and it may be gradual enough to be dismissed by the patient as part of the ageing process. Occasionally hearing loss can be sudden (any sudden hearing loss warrants investigation by an ENT surgeon). Other symptoms include tinnitus and vertigo. The tumour is slow growing and may enlarge over many years. As it enlarges it may compress surrounding cranial nerves and neural structures. There may be a lower motor neurone, facial nerve palsy. The trigeminal nerve may be affected, leading to a depressed corneal reflex and facial numbness. Very large tumours can occasionally cause dysphagia by affecting the lower cranial nerves IX and X. They may also compress the brainstem and cerebellum causing raised intracranial pressure and ataxia. The investigation of choice is an MRI scan, although high-resolution CT scanners can detect tumours as small as 1 cm. The treatment is surgical excision.

Meningiomas

These are benign slow-growing tumours that arise from the dura mater. They account for 20% of intracranial tumours. They cause symptoms depending on where they are situated.

Migraine

Migraine is an episodic headache that usually lasts between 4–72 h. It affects females more than males. Migraine tends to be unilateral and may cause headaches of such severity that it disrupts the patient's life (many taking to their beds in a darkened room). The pain is usually described as throbbing or pounding and is usually associated with nausea, photophobia, phonophobia, or osmophobia. Many sufferers endure one to five attacks per month but exceptions at both extremes of frequency exist. Some patients recognize triggers to their migraines including stress, diet, fatigue, loss of sleep, oversleeping, bright lights, and hormonal changes in women.

Migraine used to be described as classical if an aura was experienced and common if not. Now this is simply called migraine with or without an aura. Visual disturbances include photophobia and blurring of vision. A variety of visual aura can be experienced including flashing lights or colours (photopsia) and zig-zag shapes (fortification spectra or teichopsia). Later scotomas or visual field defects may develop. Auras usually last about 30 min and rarely last more than 2 h. More unusual manifestations of migraine include paraesthaesiae, numbness, paralysis (hemiplegic migraine), speech disturbances, vertigo, and ataxia. Many of these symptoms may precede the onset of headache by several hours and in some circumstances it can be difficult to determine whether the patient has suffered a transient ischaemic attack rather than a migraine attack.

The diagnosis of migraine is made through the history. Examination and investigations such as CT head scans are to rule out the possibility of other disease. Always be suspicious of anyone who develops migraines for the first time over the age of 40 years old. The treatment of migraine includes the use of analgesia and anti-emetics in the acute attacks. In those prone to more severe headaches there is ergotamine or 5-hydroxytryptamine (serotin) agonists, for example, sumatriptan, which are particularly useful during an acute attack. If a migraineur (*me-grain-err*) suffers frequent attacks every attempt should be made to unearth any triggers and failing this drugs such as pizotifen (*pies-hot-i-fen*), β-blockers, and methysergide (*meth-ee-surge-hide*) (resistant cases) can be used as preventatives.

Tension headache

This is the most common form of headache. It is usually bilateral and tends to get worse in the evening. It is usually associated with stress. It can be a generalized dull ache in the frontal or occipital regions and sometimes it can be experienced as a tight band or a feeling of pressure of the top of the head. It is unusual for it to be associated with photophobia or phonophobia. The underlying cause of tension headaches is not known although there may be abnormal muscular contraction (hence the old term contraction headache). It does not respond readily to analgesics but some may respond to amitryptylline (an anti-depressant with analgesic properties). Occasionally patients who have chronic headache that has been assumed to be tension headache may respond to migraine treatment suggesting some overlap in symptoms between these two conditions.

Cluster headaches

Cluster headaches produce severe, excruciating pain and affect males more than females. They tend to affect people between the ages of 20 and 50 years. The pain is usually unilateral and experienced around and behind the eye. The pain has been described as sharp, stabbing, or burning in nature and is so severe that the patient can literally bang their heads against walls out of despair. The affected eye may become red and watery and there may be rhinorrhea (a runny nostril) on the ipsilateral side. There may also be an associated Horner's syndrome. In some cases the headache can be triggered by alcohol. Some may experience one to two attacks in the day but this can be as many as seven in a day for others. As the name suggests the headaches occur in clusters and there can be attacks spanning up to 2 months before symptoms abate. Treatments that are used for migraine are often used for cluster headaches with good effect. There is a tendency for cluster headaches to burn out in the fourth or fifth decade.

Finals section

For revision read the examination summary (p. 282) and the keypoints throughout the chapter and do the questions on p. 328. See Tables 11.9 and 11.10 for day-to-day and Finals cases, respectively. It will be extremely unusual for you to get a case where you will have to do a full cranial nerve examination as this is very time consuming. You are more likely to be asked to perform an aspect of the examination, for example, assess the facial nerve, perform fundoscopy, or assess eye movements. Whether the Finals is of the old-fashioned clinical type or an Objective Stuctured Clinical Examination (OSCE) your technique remains the same. Even if your medical school uses OSCEs for assessment, it is still likely that your clinical teaching on the wards will follow the old-fashioned format of oral instruction and verbal interaction.

The following routine represents a quick checklist for your examination of the cranial nerves. Be *au fait* with it and be prepared to perform any aspect of it at a moment's notice.

TABLE 11.9 Day-to-day cases

Fundoscopy
Diabetic retinopathy
Hypertensive retinopathy
Facial nerve palsy
Homonymous hemianopia

TABLE 11.10 Final cases

Day to day cases plus
Ocular palsies
Fundoscopy
Optic atrophy
Papillodema
Horner's syndrome
Bitemporal hemianopia
Bulbar palsy/nystagmus

1. **Introduction.** 'Hello, I'm Vladimir Kernig, a final-year medical student. Do you mind if I examine your face and eyes?'
2. **Olfactory nerve.** (Sense of smell.) 'Do you have any problems with your sense of smell? Is this a new thing? Have you got a cold or blocked nose? How long has it been like this? Are there any smells in particular that you are having difficulty with?'
3. **Optic nerve.** (Eye inspection.) 'Do you wear glasses or contact lenses? Are you short or long sighted? Could you take off your glasses for me please?'
4. **Visual acuity.** 'Can you cover your right eye with your right hand and read the top line for me?. Now can you cover your left eye with your left hand and read the second line?'
5. **Visual fields.** 'I want you to look directly into my eyes and if you can, don't look to the sides. Tell me when you can see my fingers moving. Are my fingers moving? Uncover your left eye, sir and now cover your right eye with your right hand.'
6. **Pupillary light refex.** 'I am going to shine a light into your eyes ... it is a little bright ... and now the other side.'
7. **Pupillary accommodation reflex.** 'Look at the clock on the far wall and now ... look at my finger!'
8. **Fundoscopy.** 'Look straight ahead please, where the ceiling joins the wall, even if I get in the way. Can you look directly into the light for me ... I know it is difficult.'
9. **Oculomotor, trochlear, and abducens nerves.** (Eye movements.) 'I want you to follow my finger by moving your eyes only. I'll hold your chin to help you. Please tell me if you see double at any time.'
10. **Trigeminal nerve.** (Facial sensation). 'Close your eyes please and say "yes" if you can feel me touching you and it feels like you would expect cotton wool to, or say "no" if it feels different.'
11. **Muscles of mastication.** 'Clench your teeth for me. Relax now, open your mouth and let it hang loose.'
12. **Jaw jerk reflex.** 'I am going to tap very gently with this tendon hammer onto my finger ... it won't hurt!'
13. **Corneal reflex.** 'I am going to dab this piece of cotton wool onto your eye, it is a little uncomfortable and it may make you blink. Look straight ahead for me and keep your eyes wide open.'
14. **Facial nerve.** (Facial muscles.) 'Wrinkle your forehead. Close your eyes tight and stop me opening them. Blow your cheeks out and stop me pressing them together. Show me your teeth. Thank you.'
15. **Vestibulocochlear nerve.** (Hearing acuity.) 'I am going to rub your earlobe and I want you to repeat the numbers I whisper to you.'
16. **Rinnés test.** 'Do you hear this buzzing? Is it the same loudness in both ears?'
17. **Weber's test.** 'Tell me when you stop hearing this vibrate. Do you hear it vibrating now?'
18. **Glossopharyngeal, vagus, and hypoglossal nerves.** (Soft palate movement combined with tongue movements.) 'Can you open your mouth please, sir. Can you put your tongue out for me and move it from side to side. Put your tongue down to the bottom of your mouth. I'm just going to hold your tongue down for a moment.'
19. **Gag reflex.** Do not perform this.
20. **Accessory nerve.** (Trapezius and sternomastoid muscles.) 'Turn your head to the right. Keep your head in that position and stop me pushing it back to the middle ... and if you could turn your head to the left side now. Thank you for your help.'

Key diagnostic clues and some advice relating to examination problems

As the cranial nerves require a disparate set of techniques for individual cranial nerves, there is no critical set of clues that stand out in importance. Unfortunately there is no substitute for having a good working knowledge of the function of all the cranial nerves and their anatomical relationships with each other.

Problem. You are asked to examine a fundus but find that you cannot get an adequate view.

Solution. Step back and quickly check the size of the pupil. If it is constricted this will impede your examination. Rather than struggling vainly trying to view the fundus piecemeal, be bold and say to your examiners, 'I am afraid the pupil is too constricted to allow a proper visualization of the fundus.' This will alert your examiners to a problem that is out of your control. They should be fair minded and if there is any doubt they may even try to examine the fundus themselves to appreciate your problem. Remember preparations for examinations do not always run smoothly and eye drops may well wear off during the course of the day.

Problem. You are asked to assess the visual fields of a patient and you are unsure whether to use your fingers or a neurological pin as the target.

Solution. Either would be acceptable although clearly your finger is a cruder target. I would argue that in an examination situation, the likelihood of an abnormality is so great that I would use the neurological pin straight away. You will be able to map out areas of visual loss more accurately and the whole examination looks more polished.

Good luck!

Questions

The more stars, the more important it is to know the answer.

1. How is the sense of smell assessed? **
2. How do you tell the difference between an upper motor neurone facial nerve palsy and a lower motor neurone facial nerve palsy? *****
3. Give six causes of a lower motor VIIth nerve palsy. ****
4. What is Rinné's test? **
5. What is Weber's test? **
6. How is Rinné's test performed? ***
7. How is Weber's test performed? ***
8. What is a homonymous hemianopia? Name a cause. ****
9. What is a bitemporal hemianopia? Name a cause. ****
10. What are the signs of a IIIrd nerve palsy? ****
11. Name three causes of a IIIrd nerve palsy. ***
12. What are the signs of IVth nerve palsy? ****
13. Name three causes of a IVth nerve palsy. ***
14. What are the signs of a VIth nerve palsy? ****
15. Name three causes of a VIth nerve palsy? ***
16. What is the difference between pendular and jerky nystagmus? **
17. What is an acoustic neuroma? ***
18. What are the signs of the jugular foramen syndrome? ****
19. What are the characteristics of a migraine headache? *****
20. What are the characteristics of a tension headache? ****
21. In what conditions might you find nasal regurgitation of fluids? ****
22. What is benign paroxysmal vertigo? ***
23. What is Ménière's syndrome? ***
24. What is vertigo? **
25. What is Kernig's sign? ****
26. What is the most common cause of encephalitis in the UK? *
27. What is a complex partial seizure? ***
28. What is the macula? **
29. What is anosmia? *
30. What is an aura in migraine and epilepsy? ***
31. What is the difference between a primary and secondary generalized fit? **
32. What is a Holmes–Adie pupil? **
33. What is papilloedema? ****
34. What are the causes of papilloedema? ****
35. What is the difference between papilloedema and papillitis? ****
36. What is syncope and pre-syncope? ***
37. What is a Snellen chart? *
38. What is a bulbar palsy? ****
39. What is a pseudobulbar palsy? ****
40. Describe three features of the headache associated with raised intracranial pressure. ****
41. What is ptosis? **
42. What is retinitis pigmentosa? **
43. What is the function of the chorda tympani nerve? ***

Score. Give 4 marks for 4 stars, 1 for 1 star, and so on. At the end of the third year, you should be scoring 70-plus and by Finals, 90-plus; 110-plus is very good.

Further reading

Bull TR. *Colour atlas of ENT diagnosis*. 3rd edn. London: Wolfe; 1995.

Dhillon RS, East CA. *Ear, nose and throat, and head and neck surgery*. 2nd edn. Edinburgh: Churchill Livingstone; 1999.

Hawkes C. *Smell and taste complaints*. Amsterdam: Butterworth Heinmann; 2002.

Khaw PT, Elkington AR. *ABC of eyes*. 3rd edn. London: BMJ Publishing Group;1999.

Ludman H. *ABC of otolaryngology*. 4th edn. London: BMJ Publishing Group; 1997.

CHAPTER 12

Neck

Chapter contents

Introduction

The neck provides support for the head and can be regarded as a large biological tunnel with important structures passing through it from the head to the rest of the body and vice versa. As a result there are few symptoms that are specific to the neck alone. Some structures may be affected within the neck and cause symptoms that have already been discussed in the relevant chapter, for example, dysphagia in the abdominal system. The most clinically important organ in the neck is the thyroid gland and this will be discussed in detail. Another organ, the parathyroid gland, is also described. The neck normally comes under the spotlight because of a lump that has been noticed by the patient, a relative, or a friend. Therefore the emphasis of this chapter is mainly on the clinical examination of the neck.

Symptoms

A neck swelling can produce both local and generalized symptoms. If you suspect a swelling to be of thyroid origin, there are more detailed questions you should ask (which you will learn later). It is exceedingly rare for the parathyroid glands to present as a neck swelling. However they have an important role in calcium balance and can cause distinct signs and symptoms if their function becomes disordered.

Local symptoms

Pain is an important local symptom. The majority of swellings are symptomless (unless they grow large enough to press on surrounding structures—see p. 346). Occasionally an organ may become painful due to infection, for example, acute lymphadenopathy secondary to tonsillitis. Other local symptoms you may encounter are discussed in the relevant chapters and include

- hoarseness (see Chapter 5)
- stridor (*stride-or*) (see Chapter 5)
- dysphagia (see Chapter 6)
- neck pain (see Chapter 13).

Generalized symptoms

If faced with a neck swelling it is worth asking about constitutional symptoms, which could be relevant in a number of conditions. The most important symptoms to ask about are weight loss, fever, and night sweats. The presence of involuntary weight loss is always a worrying sign (see Chapter 6). In the context of a neck swelling, weight loss could indicate a malignancy with lymphatic spread to nearby lymph nodes. Examples of these include thyroid cancer, bronchial cancer (see p. 116), and gastric cancer (Troisier's (*twa-ziers*) sign, see p. 154). However it could represent a solitary toxic nodule in the thyroid gland and the resultant hyperthyroidism could lead to weight loss (see p. 350). The combination of weight loss, fever, and night sweats should make you think of two key conditions (both of which are treatable). These are tuberculosis and lymphoma (*lim-foe-ma*). Lymphoma is a malignant process of the haemopoietic (*he-mow-poe-i-et-ic*) system (that is, the blood-producing cells of the body including the bone marrow, liver, and spleen). There are different types of lymphoma but the most common you will hear about are Hodgkin's lymphoma and non-Hodgkin's lymphoma. They can manifest as a localized swelling of lymphoid tissue, for example, lymph node group or tonsils or be more widespread affecting many lymph node groups, liver, spleen, and so on. In the context of lymphoma, the presence of weight loss, fever, and night sweats are classified as B symptoms and this modifies the stage of the disease (staging is a process where a disease is coded according to its severity and distribution—the stage of a disease will influence the treatment that can be offered and the ultimate prognosis). Weight loss should be more than 10% of the patient's original weight (it is sensible to use a weight from at least 6 months prior to presentation although this may be difficult to achieve practically). You will find the majority of patients cannot quantify their weight loss. Night sweats should be sufficient to drench the nightclothes and there should be an unexplained fever of >38°C. The classical fever termed Pel–Ebstein fever (*Pieter Klaases Pel (1852–1919), Dutch physician, Wilhelm Ebstein (1836–1912), German physician*) with high swinging intermittent temperatures that recur after a few weeks is not often seen (and therefore should not be regarded as classical).

Thyroid

The thyroid is a gland situated at the level of the second and third tracheal rings. It consists of two lobes connected together by a thin bridge of tissue called the isthmus (*iss-th-muss*) (see Fig. 12.1). Normally it is impalpable in most men and about 50% of women. Its function is to produce the hormones thyroxine (*thigh-rocks-in*) (T4) and tri-iodothyronine (*try-eye-owe-dough-thigh-roe-nin*) (T3). These hormones are responsible for regulating the metabolic processes of the body. In simple terms if insufficient hormone is secreted the

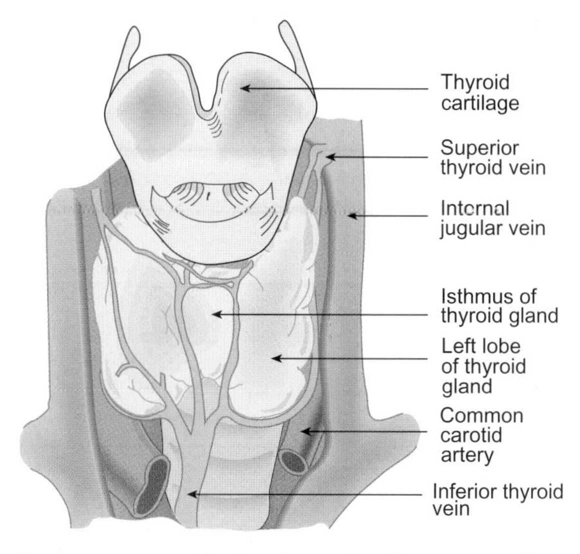

Fig. 12.1 Anatomy of the thyroid. Reproduced by permission of Oxford University Press from **Fig. 12.12** (p. 227), *Human physiology: the basis of medicine*, by G. Pocock and C. Richards (1999).

metabolic processes slow down (in hypothyroidism) and if excessive hormone is produced these processes become over-active (in hyperthyroidism—see later). Thyroid disorder may present clinically in one of five main ways:

(1) over-activity of the thyroid gland (called hyperthyroidism or thyrotoxicosis (*thigh-roe-toxic-owe-sis*));

(2) under-activity of the thyroid gland (called hypothyroidism or myxoedema (*mix-ee-deem-a*));

(3) goitre (*goy-ter*) (an enlarged thyroid gland);

(4) a discrete swelling or nodule in the thyroid;

(5) eye signs in Graves' disease of the thyroid.

Note that each category is not mutually exclusive and you can have a combination of more than one presentation, for example, a patient may have a goitre, eye signs, and hyperthyroidism in Graves' disease of the thyroid. The symptoms due to an over-active and under-active thyroid (presentations 1 and 2) will be discussed below. Presentations 3–5 will be dealt with in later sections of the chapter.

Hyperthyroidism

The patient with hyperthyroidism is likely to be agitated and fidgity (which you may notice during your consultation). This behaviour could be mistakenly rationalized as understandable anxiety in the consultation or just the person's personality. The exception to this presentation is the apathetic hyperthyroid patient. This patient is elderly and appears lifeless and lethargic and the condition can often be mistaken for hypothyroidism.

Questions to ask about hyperthyroidism

1. **'Has there been any change in your weight?'** The patient with hyperthyroidism will lose weight despite a normal or increased appetite.

2. **'Has there been a change in bowel habit?'** With hyperthyroidism the patient usually develops diarrhoea.

3. **'Do you feel uncomfortable in warm rooms when other people are comfortable?'** This question is an exploratory question to look for heat intolerance. If a person responds 'no', then clearly they do not have heat intolerance. If the answer is 'yes', they may still not have heat intolerance due to thyroid disorder because many 'normal people' dislike warm environments. Supplement this question with the following one.

4. **'Do you have to open windows or switch off heating as a result of the heat?'** If the answer is 'yes' to this, then it increases the likelihood that this could be due to hyperthyroidism.

5. **'Do you have chest pain?'** Some patients with hyperthyroidism (particularly elderly patients) may develop angina. If they have chest pain then you need to ask the relevant questions to see if their description of pain is consistent with angina. Patients with pre-existing angina may find the frequency or severity of angina may increase.

6. **'Do you have palpitations?'** There is an increased risk of arrhythmias with hyperthyroidism, particularly supraventricular tachycardia (SVTs) and atrial fibrillation (AF) (if the answer is 'yes' ask the relevant questions in the Chapter 4).

7. **'Do you suffer with shortness of breath?'** Patients with hyperthyroidism can develop high output cardiac failure (if the answer is 'yes' prepare to ask further questions as per Chapter 4).

8. **'What are your periods like?'** Women with hyperthyroidism may have scanty periods (oligomenor-hoea) (*olly-go-men-no-rear*) or absent periods (amenorrhoea).

In addition to the above questions do not forget to take a thorough history and ask about medications (some drugs can precipitate hyperthyroidism—see later) and a family history (some autoimmune diseases, for example, Graves' disease can be familial.

Tip

Always consider hyperthyroidism in any patient presenting with weight loss despite an increased appetite.

Hypothyroidism

The patient with hypothyroidism is likely to be lethargic and apathetic. In addition there is a slowing of mental function and poor concentration. These features can be mistaken for general apathy or diseases such as depression or dementia. They may even be dismissed simply as a function of ageing.

Questions to ask about hypothyroidism

1. **'Has there been any change in your weight?'** The patient with hypothyroidism will gain weight despite a poor appetite (occasionally this weight gain can be due to the retention of fluid because of cardiac failure).
2. **'Has there been any change in your bowel habit?'** With hypothyroidism the patient usually develops constipation.
3. **'Do you feel uncomfortable in cold rooms when other people are comfortable?'** This is an exploratory question to look for cold intolerance. If the answer is 'no', then cold intolerance is not a problem. As with hyperthyroidism, if the answer is 'yes', this does not mean that the patient has cold intolerance due to thyroid involvement, as many 'normal people' are intolerant of the cold. Supplement this question by asking the following one.
4. **'Do you have to put on a heater or dress in several layers of clothing just to keep warm in a room (that others find comfortable)?'**
5. **'Do you have chest pain?'** Angina is common in hypothyroidism as well.
6. **'Do you get short of breath?'** Congestive heart failure is a complication of hypothyroidism.
7. **'What are your periods like?'** Women may experience very heavy menstrual bleeding (menorrhagia) (*men-owe-rage-ia*).

For a comparison of symptoms in hyperthyroidism and hypothyroidism, see Table 12.1.

TABLE 12.1 Comparison of symptoms in hyperthyroidism and hypothyroidism

System	Hyperthyroidism	Hypothyroidism
General	Agitated/listless, sweating, heat intolerance*	Fatigue/lethargy, cold intolerance*
Cardiovascular	Angina, breathlessness, palpitations	Angina, breathlessness, palpitations
Gastrointestinal	Weight loss*, diarrhoea*	Weight gain*, constipation*
Reproductive	Oligomenorrheoa, amenorrheoa	Menorrhagia

* The most discriminating symptoms for each condition.

Tip

Always consider the possibility of hypothyroidism in cases of depression or dementia (particularly in the elderly).

Tip

Always consider hypothyroidism in any patient with weight gain despite a poor appetite (in the absence of oedema).

Keypoints

- Always consider tuberculosis and lymphoma if faced with a neck swelling associated with weight loss, fever, and night sweats.
- The combination of weight loss (despite an increased appetite), diarrhoea, and heat intolerance is highly suggestive of hyperthyroidism.
- The combination of weight gain, constipation, and cold intolerance is highly suggestive of hypothyroidism.

Parathyroids

The parathyroid glands are four small glands imbedded in the substance of the thyroid gland. They are involved in the regulation of calcium balance. They are rarely palpable even when they function abnormally and they usually create problems through disturbance of calcium metabolism. Like the thyroid, the parathyroids can be under-active or over-active. When over-active they produce excess parathormone (*para-thor-moan*) (PTH) and this process is called hyperparathyroidism (*high-per-para-thy-roid-ism*). Hyperparathyroidism is usually classified as primary, secondary, and tertiary. Parathormone causes an elevation of calcium in the blood (amongst other effects). With primary and tertiary hyperparathyroidism this elevation is above the upper limit of normal for calcium and therefore causes hypercalcaemia (*high-per-cal-seem-ya*). Secondary hyperparathyroidism is the response to low plasma calcium (*hypocalcaemia*) and represents the body's attempt to correct this. Therefore there is no hypercalcaemia in this situation. When the glands are underactive the result is hypocalcaemia and the disease process is called hypoparathyroidism (for more details on these conditions see p. 352). The symptoms and signs of symptomatic hypoparathyroidism and hyperparathyroidism are summarized in Table 12.2.

Tetany is one important sign (and should not be confused with tetanus caused by infection with clostridium tetani. With tetany there is spasm of the upper and lower limb termed carpopedal spasm (the spasm of the lower limb occurs less frequently) due to hypocalcaemia or a decrease in the ionized fraction of calcium in the blood, for example, due to hyperventilation. In the upper limb there is flexion of the wrist and metacarpophalangeal joints and hyperextension of the proximal and distal interphalangeal joints. In the lower limbs there is internal rotation of the legs and plantarflexion of the feet. Latent tetany can be demonstrated by performing two clinical tests—Trousseau's (*true-sews*) test (*Armand Trousseau (1801–1867), French physician*) and Chvostek's (*sh-vost-ex*) test (*Frantiesek Chvostek (1835–1884), Austrian surgeon*).

Trousseau's test

Trousseau's test is a test for hypocalcaemia (or a decrease in the ionized concentration of calcium, for example, following hyperventilation). It may also be positive in hypomagnesaemia and occasionally in normal people. A sphygmomanometer cuff is placed around an arm and inflated to a pressure above the systolic blood pressure of the patient. This can be maintained for a number of minutes (it is wise not to go beyond 3 min) and you are looking for a spasm of the hand. If this occurs, there is flexion of the metacarpophalangeal (MCP) joints and extension of the interphalangeal joints together with opposition of the thumb. This hand posture is called main d'accoucheur (*man-da-coo-sher*) (see Fig. 12.2).

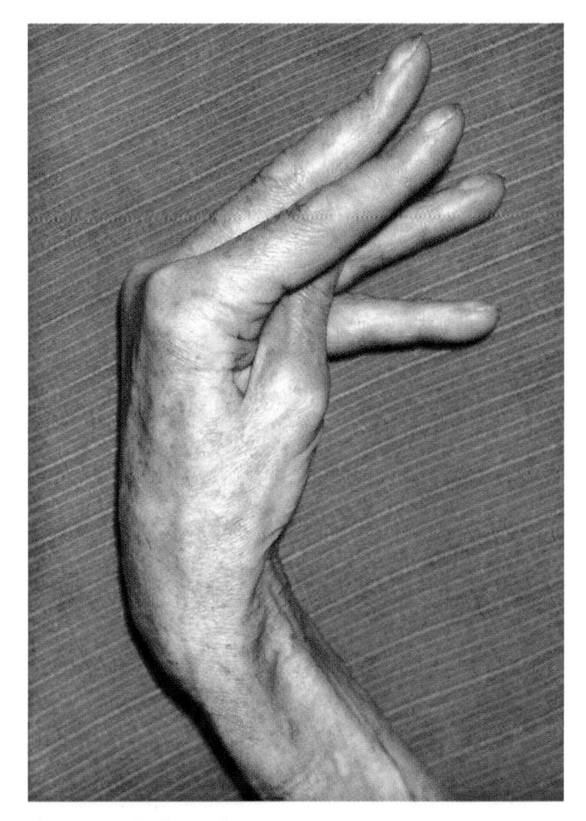

Fig. 12.2 Main d'accoucheur.

TABLE 12.2 Comparison of symptoms in hyperparathyroidism and hypoparathyroidism

System	Hyperparathyroidism (hypercalcaemia)	Hypoparathyroidism (hypocalcaemia)
Gastrointestinal	Anorexia, nausea, vomiting, constipation	
Renal	Polyuria, polydipsia*, nephrocalcinosis (*nef-roe-cal-sin-owe-sis*), renal stones	
Neurological	Lethargy, confusion	Paraesthesia in hands, feet, and around mouth, tetany†, seizures, calcification in basal ganglia—rare cause of parkinsonism
Eyes	Metastatic calcification in conjunctiva and outer margin of the cornea (limbus)	Cataract

* Polydipsia = thirst.

Chvostek's test

Chvostek's test involves tapping the facial nerve as it exits the stylomastoid foramen to supply the muscles of the face. Practically, this is just a few centimetres in front of the lower lobe of the ear. Feel for the ridge of bone, which runs horizontally at the level of auditory meatus of the ear (this is the zygomatic (*zy-go-mat-ick*) arch). Let your fingers drop below this ridge and about 2 cm anterior to the lobe of the ear. Now tap this area gently. A positive test is where that side of the face twitches in response. This test is felt to be less specific than Trousseau's test (in one study up to 25% of normal patients responded positively). See Fig. 12.3

The importance of examining the neck

There are a variety of lumps that can appear in the neck. The purpose of your examination is to identify them where possible and to determine if they are benign (so you can reassure your patient) or if they herald serious disease (and therefore require further investigation and treatment).

Examination of the neck summary

1. Introduce yourself to the patient.
2. Get the patient into position.
3. Inspect the neck for swellings.
4. Ask the patient to stick out their tongue.*
5. Ask the patient to swallow (have a glass of water handy).*
6. Palpate the neck.
7. Auscultate the swelling.
8. Check for lymphadenopathy.
9. If you suspect a thyroid swelling, palpate the thyroid.*
10. Percuss for retrosternal extension of a goitre.*
11. Auscultate the thyroid swelling or goitre for a bruit.*
12. Check for lymphadenopathy.*
13. Assess the thyroid status.*
14. Perform any further relevant examination.
15. Wash your hands.
16. Presentation.

Examination of the neck in detail

1. Introduce yourself to the patient.

Extend your hand to shake their hand and say something like, 'Hello I'm Marie Curie, a fourth-year medical student. Do you mind if I examine your neck?'

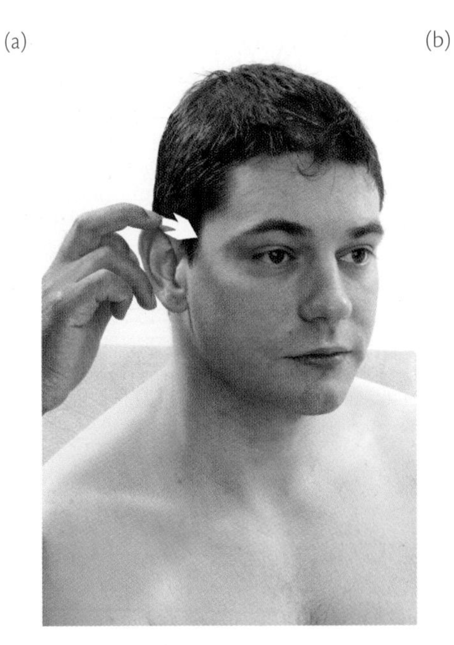

Fig. 12.3 Chvostek's test: (b) percussion over the facial nerve as it exits the stylomastoid foramen.

*Instructions for swellings of thyroid origin.

CASE 12.1

Problem. A 39-year-old woman has been admitted for a partial thryoidectomy and is on her second day after the operation. The procedure took longer than anticipated but she has made a good recovery. Early on the morning of the second day she noticed pins and needles in her finger ends and around her lips, lasting about 10 min. She initially dismissed these symptoms but after midday they returned together with spasms of her hands and wrists. She was able to attract the attention of a nurse but shortly after this she suffered a seizure. What is happening?

Solution. An event so close to an operation should immediately make you suspicious of a surgical complication. The operation took longer than expected and this suggests that it may have been a difficult procedure with the possibility of damage to surrounding structures. The paraesthaesia of the hands and lips, together with the spasm of the hands and wrists, points to hypocalcaemia (and possibly hypomagnesaemia). Profound hypocalcaemia can also lead to seizures. During the operation it is possible to interfere with the blood supply to the parathyroid glands. This may be temporary or permanent. The glands can also be inadvertently removed, but great care is usually taken to identify and preserve them during a thyroidectomy. As the patient is symptomatic she needs treatment with calcium.

Keypoints

- Parathyroid glands secrete PTH, which has an important role in calcium regulation in the body.
- Hyperparathyroidism causes hypercalcaemia in primary and tertiary hyperparathyroidism.
- Hypoparathyroidism causes hypocalcaemia.

2. Get the patient into position.

Unlike most examinations, the best position to examine the neck is with the patient sitting upright in a chair. The best chair to use is one with a low back so that you can palpate the neck from directly behind the patient.

3. Inspect the neck for swellings.

Get your patient to elevate their chin slightly. This exposes more of the chin including the submandibular area and can accentuate any swellings in the mid-line. Be systematic in your inspection so that you observe all aspects of the neck. Note the position of any abnormality because you will need to examine it in more detail later.

4. Ask the patient to stick out their tongue.

This request is conditional and should only be used for a discrete swelling at or near the mid-line of the neck. At first glance this seems a strange request but it uses a very simple principle that can identify certain types of swellings usually of thyroid origin, that is, thyroglossal (*thigh-roe-gloss-al*) cysts.

It is useful to know a little about the development of the thyroid to understand what a thyroglossal cyst is and how it behaves. The thyroid develops in the foetus as an out-pouching at the base of the tongue. This descends in the neck as the thyroglossal tract ('thyro'—thyroid, 'glossal'—tongue). The thyroid matures as it descends until the isthmus comes to rest at the level of the second to fourth tracheal rings. The thyroglossal tract usually disappears when the thyroid reaches its destination, however parts of the tract may persist and may fill with fluid, producing a thyroglossal cyst. Sometimes, thyroid tissue is found in these cysts and rarely this may be the only site that functioning thyroid tissue can be found. As the thyroglossal tract is attached to the hyoid bone (and hence the base of the tongue), when the tongue is protruded the thyroglossal cyst is pulled up.

To examine, first fix your eyes on the swelling, then without shifting your gaze, say to your patient, 'Can you stick your tongue out please!' If the lump elevates a couple of centimetres as the tongue is protruded it is likely that the swelling is a thyroglossal cyst (there are even rarer swellings that may elevate with tongue protrusion but you do not need to know these). The swelling should then return to its original position when the patient retracts their tongue.

5. Ask the patient to swallow (have a glass of water handy).

This request is designed to detect swellings of thyroid origin. The mature thyroid lies at the front of the neck in the mid-line and is covered by connective tissue (the pre-tracheal fascia (*fasher*)), which is attached to the trachea. Therefore when your patient swallows and the larynx elevates, the thyroid (normal or abnormal) will also elevate.

To examine, it is best to first fetch a glass or cup of water. It is remarkable how dry a person's mouth can get when they are being examined (this includes patients and students!). Say to them politely, 'Take a sip of water and don't swallow until I say.' As they take a sip of water make sure the swelling is visible and keep your eyes focused on it. Then say, 'Swallow now!', see

Fig. 12.4. As your patient swallows, watch the swelling and see if it rises a few centimetres in the neck before returning to its original position. If it does the swelling is of thyroid origin. An important point to note is that thyroglossal cysts will also elevate with swallowing as well as tongue protrusion.

6. Palpate the neck.

When you palpate the neck, any swelling you identify on inspection needs to be assessed for a number of features: site, size, consistency, mobility, tenderness, margin, pulsatility, and transillumination.

- **Site.** The neck is divided anatomically into two triangles by the sternomastoid muscle (see Fig. 12.5). These are the anterior and posterior triangles. It is convention to locate any swelling found into one of these triangles. It is also important to have a working map of where the major organs are situated in the neck as this may give a valuable clue as to the identity of any lump found, for example, a mid-line swelling below the 'Adam's apple' could represent a thyroid nodule.
- **Size.** It is important to determine the size of any swelling. This can be done crudely with a tape measure. Baseline dimensions allow any changes in size to be monitored over time. A persistent increase in size raises the spectre of malignancy.
- **Consistency.** Determine how soft or hard a swelling is and whether this is uniform throughout its substance. A soft swelling may represent fat- or a fluid-filled structure (cyst). A firm or rubbery swelling may indicate an enlarged organ or tissue, for example, salivary glands or lymph nodes. Hard swellings may represent malignant infiltration or calcification within its substance.
- **Mobility.** Some swellings exhibit a degree of mobility under the skin and this characteristic should be examined. Thyroid swellings will move upwards with swallowing (see previously). If this feature is absent from a known thyroid swelling this could indicate that there is malignant infiltration of the thyroid with fixing to the surrounding structures. Lymph nodes are also mobile glands but may also become fixed if affected by malignancy or tuberculosis. When assessing mobility, hold the swelling between your thumb and index finger then try and move it back and forth in a horizontal and then a vertical plane. If it moves freely it is more likely to be benign.
- **Tenderness.** As a rule you should always check if a swelling is tender before beginning palpation. If tenderness is present this suggests an inflammatory mass such as an abscess or an organ that is inflamed secondary to infection.
- **Margin.** Assess the border of any swelling and see if it is well demarcated, for example, representing the capsule of an organ or if it is ill defined, which could suggest infiltration by a neoplastic or inflammatory process.

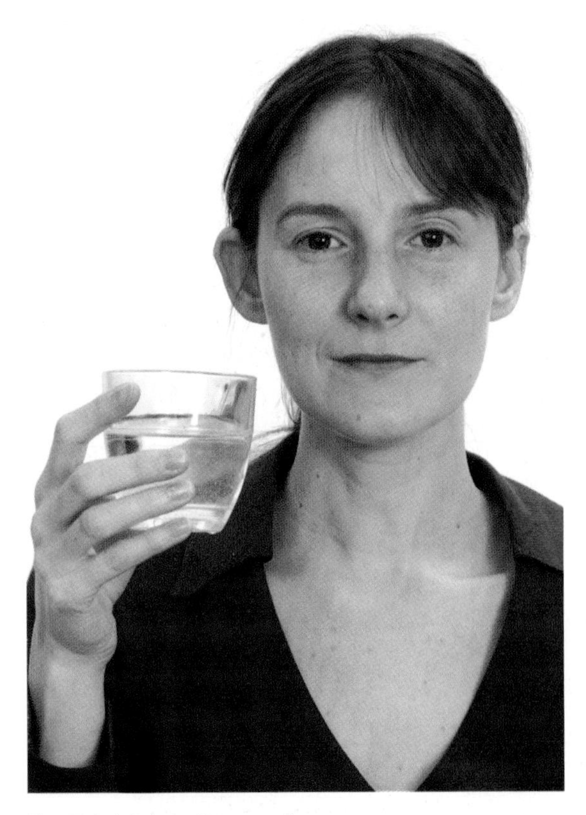

Fig. 12.4 Ask the patient to swallow.

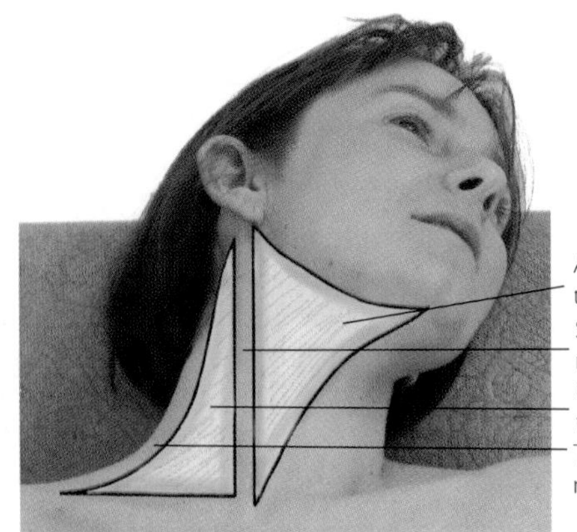

Fig. 12.5 The anatomical triangles of the neck.

- **Pulsatility.** Very few neck swellings will exhibit this property because the only major arteries in the neck are the carotid arteries. One rare swelling that exhibits this feature is a carotid body tumour (also called a chemodectoma (*key-mow-deck-toe-ma*)).
- **Transillumination.** This is a feature that can be demonstrated in fluid-filled lesions. Light from a pen torch can be directed on to one end of a swelling. If it is solid the light will be blocked. If it is a fluid-filled swelling, light will shine through it. This manifests itself as an orange glow within the swelling that diverges from the tip of the pen torch. This is best viewed in dimmed light or a blacked-out room (although this is not essential).

7. Auscultate the swelling.

This aspect of the examination of a swelling is frequently forgotten. Place the diaphragm of your stethoscope over the swelling and if a bruit is present this indicates that it is either vascular in origin or it has an increased blood supply (see later).

8. Check for lymphadenopathy.

This must always be done for any neck swelling, including the thyroid. Enlarged, hard, and irregular lymph nodes may represent spread from a malignant primary. See Table 12.3 for causes of a neck swelling.

TABLE 12.3 Causes of a neck swelling

Causes of a neck swelling
Lipoma (*lie-poe-ma*)
Epidermal cyst
Cervical lymphadenopathy
Thyroid nodule or goitre (see text)
Thyroglossal cyst (see text)
Pharyngeal pouch (see p. 176)
Branchial (*brank-i-al*) cyst
Cystic hygroma (*high-grow-ma*)
Cervical rib
Carotid body tumour
Salivary gland disease

See 'Diseases and investigations of the neck' section for a description of those neck swellings without a reference.

9. If you suspect a thyroid swelling, palpate the thyroid.

If you suspect a thyroid swelling, because of its site (at or near the mid-line) and its elevation with swallowing,

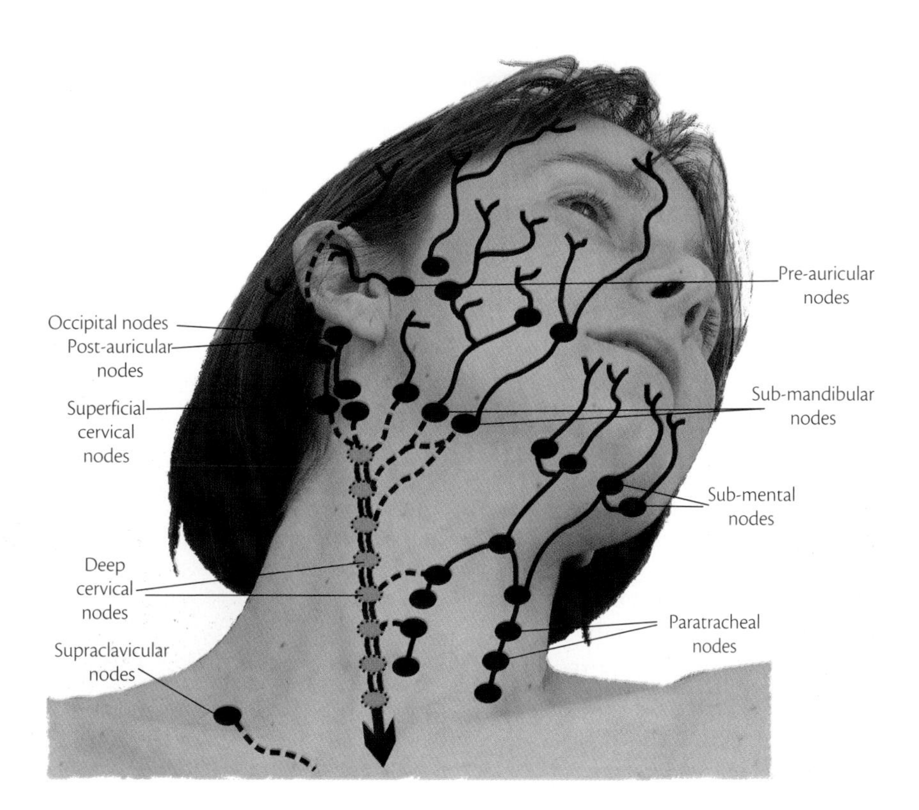

Fig.12.6 Lymph node chains.

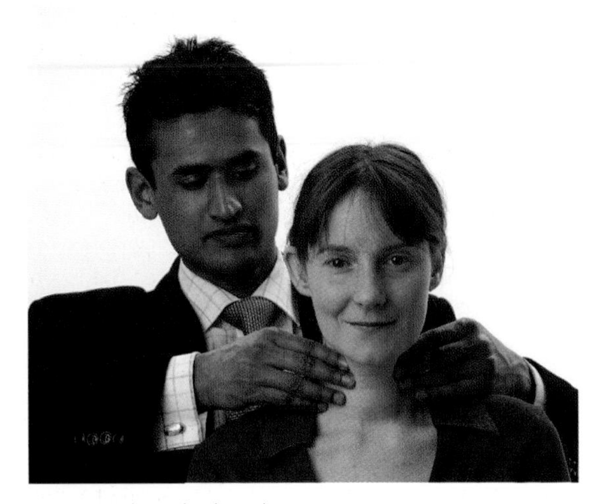

Fig. 12.7 Palpate the thyroid.

then begin palpation of the thyroid (see Fig. 12.7). Stand behind your patient and get them to depress their chin marginally to relax the strap muscles. Place your fingers on either side of the neck and map out the lobes of the thyroid. The tip of your index and middle fingers will do the work. Run your fingers around the margins of any swelling you observed earlier. Are they well demarcated or ill defined? Your analysis of a thyroid swelling or goitre should be no different to that of any other swelling. You will have already noted the site and measured the dimensions of the swelling. Now feel the consistency of the thyroid—is it soft or firm (this suggests normal thyroid tissue) or is it 'rock hard' (this suggests thyroid cancer)? Nodules tend to be firm or hard but this does not necessarily mean malignancy (a thyroid isotope scan may be needed to determine this—see later). Check for tenderness of the thyroid as inflammation of the thyroid (thyroiditis) can occasionally cause this.

10. Percuss for retrosternal extension of a goitre.

Percussion has a limited application in the neck. Occasionally a goitre may extend behind the sternum and rarely this may be its sole position (when it is called a retrosternal goitre). Percuss using the technique described on p. 100) (see Fig. 12.8). Begin just below the suprasternal notch and descend towards the sternal angle. Normally this area is resonant. If it is dull this suggests retrosternal extension of a goitre or a retrosternal goitre (in this context).

11. Auscultate the thyroid swelling or goitre for a bruit.

See Fig. 12.9. Place the diaphragm of your stethoscope over the thyroid swelling or goitre. If a bruit is heard, this suggests overactivity of the gland (because of the requirement for an increased blood supply). If a bruit is not heard this does not rule out the possibility of hyperthyroidism.

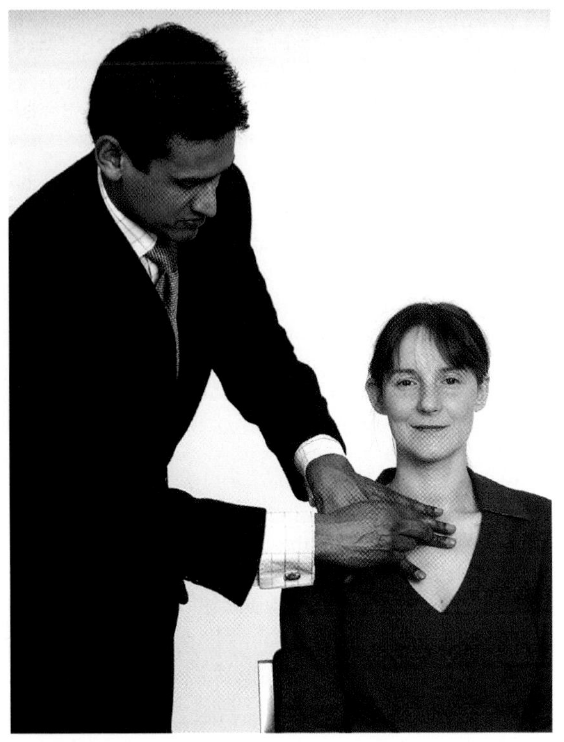

Fig. 12.8 Percussion for a retrosternal extension of a goitre.

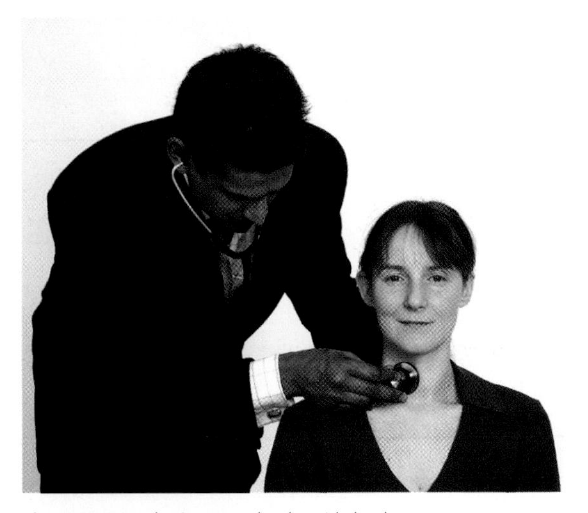

Fig. 12.9 Auscultation over the thyroid gland.

CASE 12.2

Problem. You listen over a goitre but you are not sure if the bruit originates from the goitre or from the carotid artery.

Discussion. Sometimes this distinction can prove difficult particularly if the dimensions of the goitre are such that the diaphragm of your stethoscope overlaps the carotid artery at auscultation. It is always worth checking the aortic area to make sure that you are not hearing the radiation from the murmur of aortic stenosis. If you are still unsure remember that you should not consider this sign in isolation. If the patient has weight loss, heat intolerance, a tremor, lid-lag, and a tachycardia, the chances are that they are thyrotoxic and a bruit is consistent with their disease status. If your patient has weight gain, constipation, bradycardia, and so on, a thyroid bruit is not consistent with the clinical circumstances.

12. Check for lymphadenopathy.

Hard irregular lymph nodes in relation to a thyroid swelling could represent spread from a thyroid cancer.

13. Assess the thyroid status.

When you find a thyroid nodule or goitre you must assess the activity of the thyroid clinically. It can only be one of three possible states:

- normal activity—euthryoid;
- over-active—hyperthyroid.
- under-active—hypothyroid;

You may already have clues from your history as to what the thyroid status might be, for example,

- heat intolerance, diarrhoea, weight loss—hyperthyroid;
- cold intolerance, constipation, appetite, weight gain—hypothryoid.

Now is the time to confirm your suspicions!

- **Observe the patient.** Are they restless and fidgety?—hyperthyroid? Are they relatively relaxed?—euthyroid? Are they lethargic and disinterested?— hypothyroid?
- **Shake the patient's hand.** Are the palms sweaty?—hyperthyroid?
- **Get your patient to hold out their hands (place a piece of paper over their hand).** Is there a tremor present?—hyperthyroid?
- **Feel the pulse**. Tachycardia—hyperthyroid? Bradycardia—hypothyroid? Pulse rate 60–80 beats/min—euthyroid? Atrial fibrillation—associated with both hypo- and hyperthryoidism.
- **Check the eyes for lid-lag and lid retraction.** The phenomenon of lid-lag is associated with Graves' disease and is not strictly a test of thyroid status. Nevertheless it should be performed as part of your thyroid routine. Normally when the eyes follow an object that descends from above, both the globe of the eye and the eyelids move downwards in unison. With hyperthyroidism, the movement of the eyelids is delayed and lags behind that of the globe. To test, provide a target by holding your index finger or the tip of a pen above the head of your patient about 0.5 m in front of their face. Your patient should be able to see the target comfortably without straining their eyes or tilting their head upwards. Say to your patient, 'Keep your head still and follow my finger/this pen with your eyes only!' Now slowly move the target vertically downwards until the patient is staring down at it without straining or tilting their head. While doing this, focus on their eyes and eyelids and note if they move downwards in unison or if there is a brief delay before the eyelids follow the globe of the eye.

Lid retraction is where the upper eyelid retracts backward exposing an arc of white sclera above the cornea. In normal people the sclera is not visible except with fear, anxiety, or anger (the wide-eyed stare). The muscle controlling elevation of the eyelid (levator palpabrae superioris) is under sympathetic control. Any condition that increases circulating adrenaline or noradrenaline will cause this muscle to contract. In the context of thyroid disease these hormones are increased in hyperthyroidism. Note that this is a non-specific sign that can be seen in other conditions including fear, anxiety, or anger for the reasons just discussed. To examine, simply look for a crescent of white sclera above the apex of the cornea.

Tip

If you notice a crescent of white sclera below the bottom of the cornea (with the eye looking forwards naturally), this is not lid retraction. This is exophthalmos (*ex-op-thal-moss*). The cause of exophthalmos is not related to thyroid status but is autoimmune mediated (see later).

6. **Examine the reflexes.** The sign to demonstrate here is the slow-relaxing reflex. This should only be attempted if you suspect hypothyroidism. Classically it is taught that the ankle jerk should be elicited, but those of you who are sharp eyed may notice (given the opportunity) that this can be observed at other sites, for example, biceps and triceps. The reflex is elicited in exactly the same way as you would in a neurological examination. You may notice a brief, brisk contraction followed by a more prolonged relaxation phase. In absolute terms, the whole reflex action is over in just over a second so concentration is crucial.

Tip

You must examine many normal reflexes before you can appreciate the duration of the contraction and relaxation phases and hence when the latter is delayed.

Tip

In working life, no one diagnoses hypothyroidism from slow-relaxing reflexes alone. It is a supplementary sign: one to elicit to delight your friends and colleagues when you already know the diagnosis.

During your evaluation of thyroid status if you suspect a particular state, for example, hypothyroidism, then only examine relevant features from the list above, for example, hypothyroidism—bradycardia, AF, slow-relaxing reflexes, and so on. Once your examination is complete you should confirm the thyroid status of the patient by taking blood for thyroid function tests (see later).

14. Perform any further relevant examination.

Other signs associated with hyper- and hypothyroidism are contrasted in Table 12.4. Although many of these signs are associated with hyper- and hypothyroidism, they are not reliable indicators of thyroid status and therefore do not feature in the routine above. These signs do not have to be present for the respective diagnoses to be tenable.

Wash your hands

15. Wash your hands.

De rigueur!

TABLE 12.4 A contrast of signs associated with hyperthyroidism, hypothyroidism, and Graves' disease

Hyperthyroidism	Hypothyroidism	Graves' disease
Palmar erythema	Dry skin	Pre-tibial myxoedema
Spider naevi	Alopecia	Thyroid acropachy (*a-crow-patchy*)
Gynaecomastia	Erythema ab igne (*erry-theme-a-ab-ig-ney*)	
Proximal myopathy	Xanthelasma	
Hyperreflexia	Hypercarotenaemia* (*high-per-carrot-en-ee-mia*)	
Osteoporosis	Carpal tunnel syndrome, cerebellar ataxia, myopathy, pleural effusion, pericardial effusion, ascites	

* Hypercarotenaemia is the finding of large amounts of β-carotene in the blood. In the context of hypothyroidism, there is the decreased conversion of β-carotene to retinol (vitamin A) in the liver leading to a large concentration in the blood. Deposition in the skin can lead to a yellow/orange pigmentation.

Presentation of findings

16. Presentation.

If the diagnosis is straightforward, mention this up front and support it with findings from your examination. If you are unsure of the diagnosis, describe your findings and give a reasonable differential diagnosis. For example, 'This young woman has Graves' disease of the thyroid. She has exophthalmos and a small, diffusely enlarged goitre. The goitre moves freely on swallowing and there is no retrosternal extension and no lymphadenopathy or bruits audible over the gland. On further examination she also has pre-tibial myxoedema. She is clinically euthyroid with a pulse rate that is 82 beats per minute and regular and there is no evidence of a tremor, sweating, or lid-lag.'

Tip

Never forget to mention the patient's clinical thyroid status when presenting a thyroid case.

Or another example, 'This man has bilateral cervical lymphadenopathy. The nodes are rubbery, firm, and mobile, with some mild tenderness on palpation. In the absence of a history, the differential diagnosis is wide, including viral infections such as infectious mononucleosis (glandular fever), bacterial infections such as brucellosis, multi-system disorder such as systemic lupus erythmatosus (SLE), and neoplastic disease such as lymphoma.'

Diseases and investigations of the neck

Earlier in this chapter, I have mentioned various medical conditions. In this section I will now describe them. In general these descriptions are brief though certain aspects not well described in other textbooks are discussed in some detail

Lipoma

This is a benign fatty tumour due to the growth of adipose tissue. It is a mobile subcutaneous mass. It exhibits fluctuance although it is not cystic in nature. It does not transilluminate.

Epidermal cyst

This used to be called a sebaceous cyst. These cysts occur anywhere where there are hair follicles. They can be small or grow to several centimetres. Keratin rather than sebum is produced within them hence the term sebaceous cyst is a misnomer. They are soft/firm, mobile, painless, and entirely benign.

Cervical lymphadenopathy

This is the most common cause of a neck swelling. There are over 300 lymph nodes in the neck. These drain areas such as the face, scalp, nose, mouth, larynx, and pharynx and can be enlarged by a variety of disease including infections, skin disease, multi-system disorders, and malignancy.

Branchial cyst

This cyst develops from the remnants of the second branchial clefts. The branchial clefts are four grooves seen on either side of the neck during the development of the foetus. The second, third, and fourth clefts usually disappear while the first cleft persists as the external auditory meatus. This cyst may present in late adolescence or adulthood and can be found in the upper neck over the sternomastoid muscle. The cyst is fluctuant and may transilluminate. It can be tender if it becomes infected.

CASE 12.3

Problem. A 78-year-old woman is sent to the hospital's assessment unit by her general practitioner (GP). She has complained of abdominal pain and poor appetite over the last 3 days and has not opened her bowels for 5 days. The GP suspects constipation but would like to exclude an acute abdomen. The GP has also referred her to the psychiatrist because over the last 2 months she has become more withdrawn. She has lost interest in her hobbies and her usually immaculate house is in a state. The GP feels she is depressed and requires urgent treatment. The senior house officer (SHO) takes one look at the letter, has a quick glance at the patient, and diagnoses hypothyroidism. Are they right?

Discussion. On this occasion yes! The GP's assessment has been good and their response has been appropriate. Profound constipation can mimic bowel obstruction with vomiting, decreased appetite, and colicky abdominal pain and therefore a surgical opinion may be necessary to exclude obstruction. However clearly there is more going on than just an abdominal problem. The loss of interest in everyday activities could be due to depression or even a dementia (although the time course is rapid and so this would have to be an atypical variant). The SHO's powers of deduction could become the stuff of legend after this end-of-the-bed diagnosis. However it is based on sound medical thinking and a little bit of luck. The SHO has remembered that hypothyroidism has neuropsychiatric features that can mimic depression. Patients slow down and lose interest in life. In addition they reasoned that constipation is also a manifestation of hypothyroidism. A quick glance at the patient may have revealed coarse, thinning hair, an apathetic appearance, and perhaps erythema ab igne (a brown reticular pattern on the skin of the inner thigh or abdomen where the patient has huddled close to a heat supply to keep warm). Despite the suggestive nature of this evidence the SHO still needed a modicum of luck as this could still have been a case of depression and they have yet to take a full history or examine the patient. The message here is that hypothyroidism is an insidious condition that can be easily missed. The key to making the diagnosis is to be constantly aware of its possibility because it is a condition that can be readily treated.

CASE 12.4

Problem. You see a 48-year-old woman who is referred to the gastroenterology clinic with chronic diarrhoea spanning 2 months. She opens her bowels between four and six times on some days and passes loose motions with no blood or mucus. During this time she has lost half a stone in weight. The GP has sent two stool samples for culture but no pathogens have been seen. You examine her and notice she looks anxious, with a tremor and has eyes that seem to stare. She has a sinus tachycardia of 110 beats/min and abdominal examination including a rectal was unremarkable. What is the cause of her diarrhoea and weight loss?

Discussion. This is a classical case of hyperthyroidism. However it is only obvious when all the facts are presented in this fashion. In the real world of busy clinicians it is easy for any doctor to focus on the obvious problem, for example, GP refers because of diarrhoea. The same error can be compounded by the hospital specialist, who may not see beyond their own area of expertise. Pausing to consider other possibilities may sometimes reap dividends. In this case the diarrhoea was chronic and no infective agent had been found. There was nothing in the stools to suggest an active colitic process from the history given. Clues to a cause outside the gastrointestinal tract could be recognized from the outset. The anxiety, tremor, and staring eyes do suggest thyrotoxicosis (and possibly Graves' disease). The sinus tachycardia also adds further weight. Other features to look for include heat intolerance, a goitre, and a fuller assessment of the patient's thyroid status.

Cystic hygroma

This is also called a cavernous lymphangioma. This is a congenital lesion due to the abnormal development of the lymphatic system. The cyst develops from primitive lymph sacs found in the neck between the subclavian and jugular veins in the embryo. The cyst is usually found in the lower third of the neck in the posterior triangle and sometimes enlarges upwards towards the ear (other areas can be affected including the tongue, chest, and axilla). It also transilluminates.

Cervical rib

Occasionally people may have a seventh cervical rib. It may be attached to the first rib or the sternum or may have no distal attachment at all. The swelling is hard, painless, and immobile. Cervical ribs can also be fibrous bands rather than bone. These bands often cause more complications than their bony counterpart. Vascular complications include narrowing of the subclavian artery, aneurysm formation, thrombus formation, embolization, and ischaemia. Neurological complications include compression of the first thoracic nerve or brachial plexus lesions.

CASE 12.5

Problem. You are on a GP attachment and your GP sees a 52-year-old man who has come for a follow-up visit. He presented a week ago with a sore throat and a flu-like illness. The GP suspected tonsillitis and prescribed analgesia and antibiotics. However, his throat still feels sore and he feels 'edgy' and 'lousy'. You examine his mouth and pharynx, which are normal. As you feel his neck for lymph glands you become aware that he is tender over his thyroid gland. You also notice he has a slight tremor and sweaty palms and you check his pulse and blood pressure, which are 92 beats/min and 130/50 respectively.

Discussion. This is a case of subacute viral thyroiditis. It usually begins with a viral illness. The pain in the thyroid can often be mistaken for a 'sore throat'. In some cases thyrotoxicosis can ensue which is self-limiting and this explains his continuing ill-health (he has a tremor, sweaty palms, and a tachycardia). Treatment will be further analgesia for his pain and a β-blocker to counteract the symptoms of thyrotoxicosis. He will need further review to decide when to stop his treatment.

Carotid body tumour

This is also called a chemodectoma. This is a slow-growing tumour arising from the chemoreceptor cells in the carotid body at the carotid bifurcation. It is slowly growing, painless, and exhibits pulsatility. It is mobile in the horizontal plane but not the vertical. As a highly vascular tumour it will also have a bruit on auscultation. Finally this is one swelling that should not be biopsied.

Salivary gland disease

There are three main salivary glands: the parotid, the submandibular, and the sublingual glands. The most relevant gland for the neck is the submandibular gland.

A number of diseases can cause the glands to enlarge. Acute infection with bacteria can lead to a swollen, extremely tender gland. A stone can often be felt within the duct of the gland and pus can sometimes be expressed into the mouth. Viral infection with a paramyxovirus (*para-mix-owe-virus*) causes mumps, which leads to enlarged glands, particularly the parotids. The gland is not as tender as in bacterial infections. Sjogren's syndrome is the combination of dry eyes and dry mouth in conjunction with a connective tissue disorder such as systemic sclerosis. The salivary glands are often painlessly enlarged in this condition. The salivary glands can also be affected by tumours. Tumours are rare and the majority of them are benign. There are many pathological forms but all tend to be firm and mobile. The malignant tumours tend to be hard and can become fixed to surrounding tissues. They spread via the blood and lymphatics and some can infiltrate along their own nerve supply.

Control of thyroid hormone production

The thyroid produces two hormones, T4 and T3. They are produced from the modification of the amino acid tyrosine, a process that includes the incorporation of iodine extracted from the diet. Once T4 and T3 are manufactured they are stored within the thyroid gland for release at a later date. Once released into the bloodstream the hormones are protein bound (and in this form are inactive). Only a small proportion of hormone is free and it is this proportion that is biologically active. The thyroid gland is under the control of the anterior pituitary gland and is stimulated to function by the pituitary peptide thyrotropin (*thigh-row-trow-pin*) (also known as thyroid stimulating hormone (TSH)). In turn the pituitary is under the control of the hypothalamus via thyrotrophin-releasing hormone (TRH). The whole process is finely tuned by a negative feedback mechanism that ensures that just the right quantity of T3 and T4 are produced to maintain biological processes at their optimum rate. Essentially if the T3 and T4 levels are too low this is 'sensed' by the anterior pituitary, which will increase the production of TSH to drive further production of T3 and T4. Conversely if the levels of T3 and T4 are too high, the production of TSH is reduced to allow the level of T3 and T4 to normalize (see Fig. 12.10).

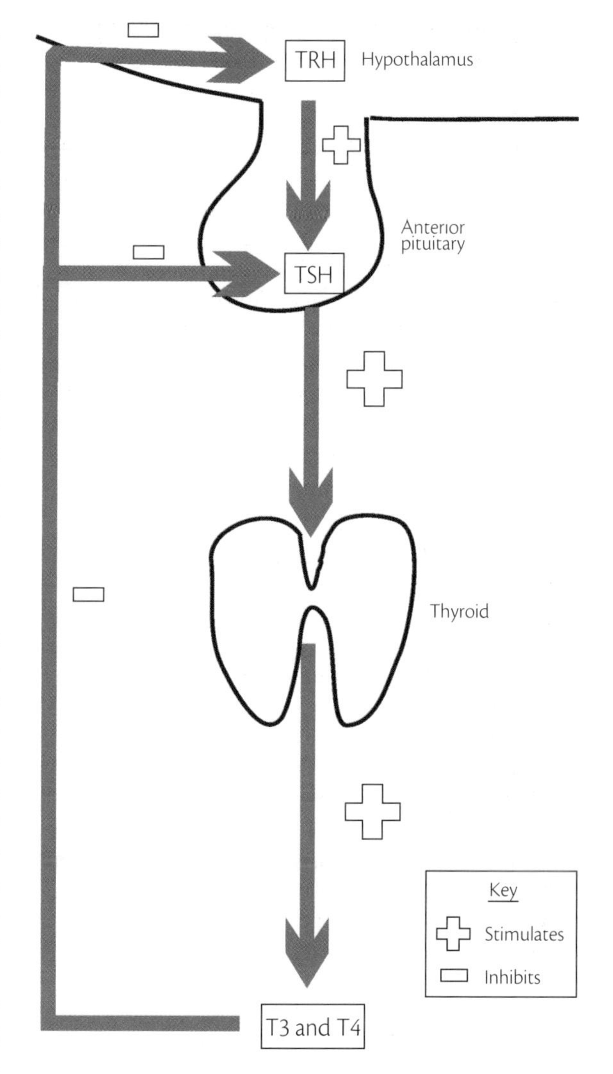

Fig. 12.10 The control of thyroid hormone production.

Goitre

This term means the enlargement of the thyroid gland. Goitres can be classified in the following way:

- diffuse
- simple
- iodine deficiency
- due to Graves' disease
- due to Hashimoto's (*hash-ee-mow-toes*) thyroiditis
- due to subacute viral thyroiditis
- multi-nodular goitre.

Diffuse goitre

Diffuse goitre is a goitre where there is enlargement of both lobes of the thyroid and tends to be symmetrical. A simple goitre is a type of diffuse goitre where there is no disturbance of thyroid function (sometimes called a non-toxic goitre). A small, simple goitre may sometimes be found in some women at puberty or during pregnancy. Iodine deficiency is a common cause of a diffuse goitre worldwide. Iodine is an important co-factor in thyroid hormone synthesis and is normally found in the diet. In regions where iodine is poor in the diet, this form of goitre is common hence the term endemic goitre is also used. In the past Derbyshire in the UK was one such area, where goitres were common enough to lead to the term 'Derbyshire neck'. In the early stages the goitre is small and diffuse but later it can become large and multi-nodular. In some cases the patient may sometimes become hypothyroid. This has led to the introduction of programmes to introduce iodine supplementation in salt or flour which has been successful in treating this problem in some areas of the world.

Subacute viral thryoiditis

This is also called Dequervain's *(de-qwe-veins)* thyroiditis *(Fritz De Quervain (1868–1940), Swiss surgeon)*. This is due to a viral infection and tends to affect females more than males. Usually flu-like symptoms are experienced, for example, headache and muscle aches and pains and sometimes swallowing may be painful because of inflammation of the thyroid gland (this may lead to confusion with pharyngitis or tonsillitis). Patients may exhibit transient thyrotoxicosis, as stored thyroid hormone is released into the blood stream. Note that because there is no glandular over-activity this is not hyperthyroidism. If the disease is mild no treatment is required. The patient may require analgesia for neck discomfort. If thyrotoxicosis is problematical, then treatment with a β-blocker should suffice until symptoms settle. Occasionally the patient may go on to experience hypothyroidism, which usually lasts between 3 and 6 months.

Hashimoto's thyroiditis

Hashimoto's thyroiditis *(Hakaru Hashimoto (1881–1934), Japanese surgeon)* is also called chronic lymphocytic thyroiditis. It affects females more than males. It is an autoimmune disorder due to antibodies that react to the cells of the thyroid gland. Antibodies called thyroid microsomal antibodies are produced by lymphocytes, which infiltrate the thyroid gland and destroy thyroid cells. The condition follows a relapsing and remitting course. Early in the disease patients develop a small goitre. Occasionally some patients develop thyrotoxicosis lasting weeks or months, which may resemble Graves' disease. This is sometimes called hashitoxicosis. This phase is usually short lived as the thyroid gland is progressively destroyed. Later titres of thyroid microsomal antibodies become low or undetectable. Eventually the burden of destruction leads to hypothyroidism. Treatment is essentially symptom control. If the gland is painful analgesia can be used. If the goitre is large or there is a worry about malignancy, surgery may be contemplated. When hypothyroidism supervenes then treatment is with T4.

Graves' disease

Graves' disease *(Robert Graves (1797–1853) Irish physician)*, is an autoimmune condition affecting the thyroid. Antibodies are produced that stimulate the thyroid cells leading to their overactivity and subsequent thyrotoxicosis. It is more common in females than males. It causes a diffuse painless goitre. See Figs 12.11 and 12.12. Other features peculiar to Graves' disease include

- ophthalmopathy
- pre-tibial myxoedema
- thyroid acropachy.

1. **Ophthalmopathy.** See Figs 12.13 and 12.14. This can be found in up to 60% of patients with Graves' disease. In some patients the eye signs may precede

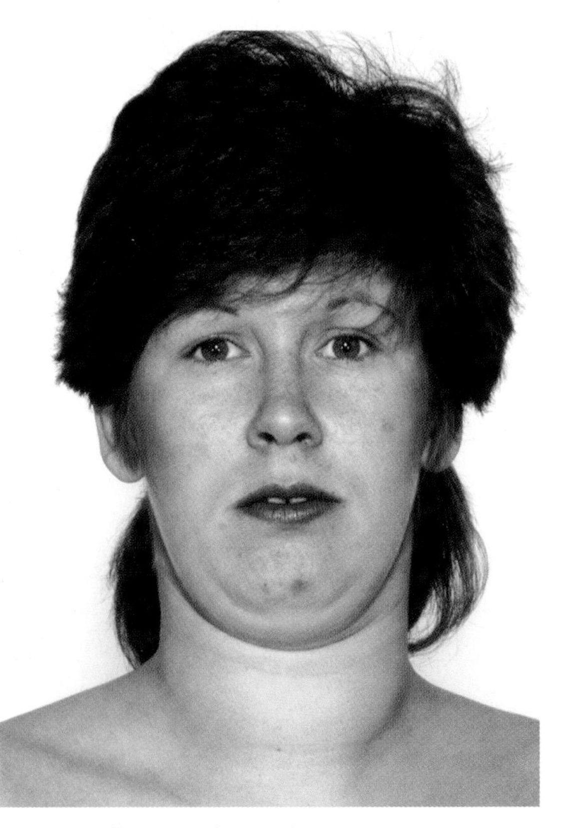

Fig. 12.11 Diffuse goitre of Graves' disease.

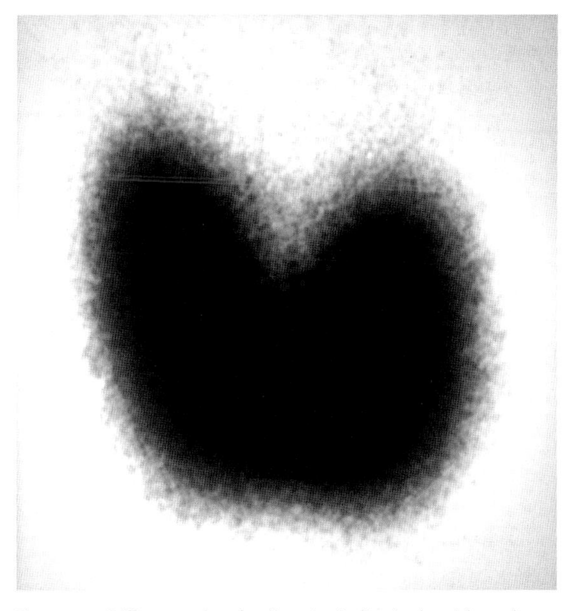

Fig. 12.12 Diffuse uptake of radioactive iodine in thyroid uptake scan in Graves Disease.

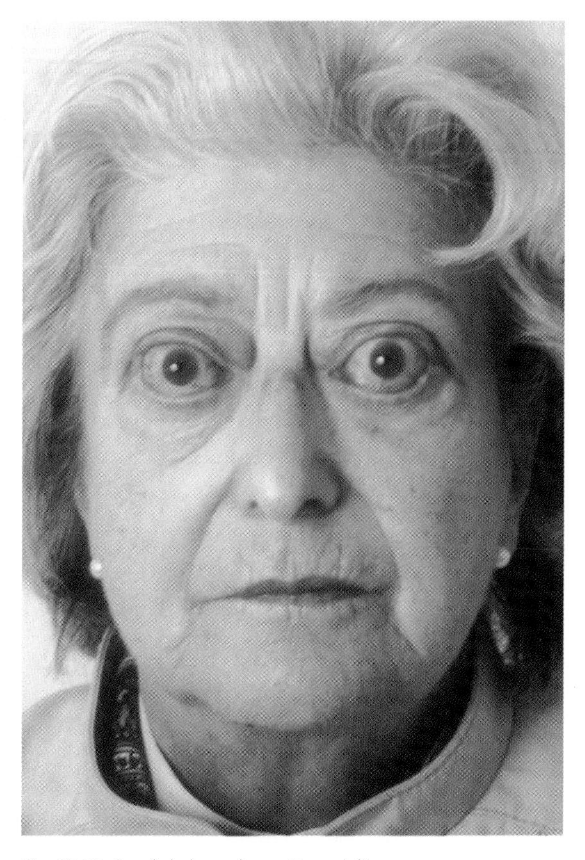

Fig. 12.13 Exophthalmos due to Graves' disease.

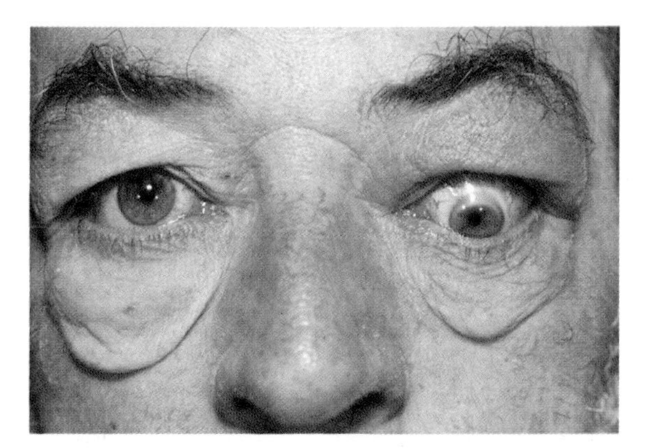

Fig. 12.14 Exophthalmoplegia.

the development of the thyrotoxicosis and goitre. Expoththalmos is the most recognizable sign. This is the protrusion of the eye from its orbit. This process is also called proptosis but exopthalmos is reserved for protrusion of the eye of endocrine origin. Exophthalmos occurs independently of thyroid status. It is an autoimmune phenomenon leading to the deposition of mucopolysaccharide (*mew-co-polly-sack-a-ride*), lymphocyte infiltration, and subsequent oedema behind the eye. There is also lymphocyte infiltration and eventual thickening of the retro-orbital muscles. This combination of changes leads to protrusion of the eye. This process may impair conjugate eye movement leading to diplopia (this is called ophthalmoplegia) (*op-thal-mow-plea-jah*). Chronically there is thickening and fibrosis of the retro-orbital muscles further compounding ophthalmoplegia. Further features may develop including peri-orbital oedema, conjunctival oedema, and oedema of the cornea (chemosis) (*key-mow-seize*). In severe cases the eye is at risk of blindness because of raised intra-ocular pressure on the optic nerve. This is called malignant exophthalmos and is an emergency. Treatment is with high-dose steroids and occasionally surgery to decompress the orbit.

2. **Pre-tibial myxoedema.** See Fig. 12.15. This is an uncommon condition that occurs in 1–5% of patients with Graves' disease. It is a coarse, plaque-like thickening of the skin usually over the shin (hence pre-tibial) but can occur elsewhere. It can be purple/blue, orange, or brown and is due to the deposition of mucopolysaccharides in the subcutaneous layer of the skin. Why a small proportion of people with Graves' disease develop this problem is unknown.

(a)

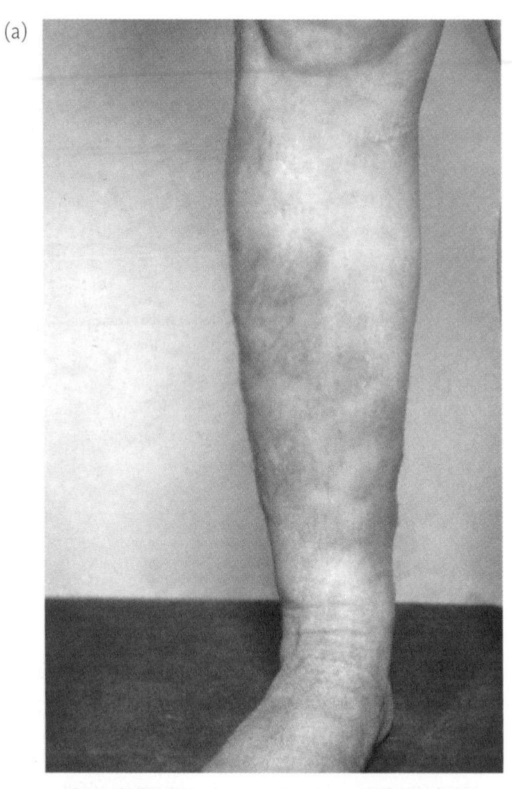

(b)

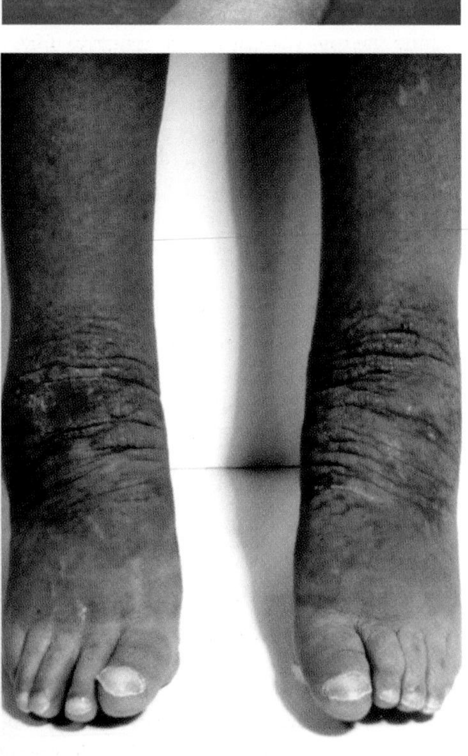

Fig. 12.15 Pre-tibial myxoedema.

3. **Thyroid acropachy.** This is an even rarer manifestation of Graves' disease, which affects the fingers (and toes) and resembles clubbing.

Thyroid nodule

A nodule is simply a lump in the thyroid. It may be a solitary nodule or be one of a number of nodules in a multi-nodular goitre. A nodule is palpable if it exceeds 1 cm in diameter.

Multinodular goitre

See Figs 12.16 and 12.17. This is a goitre where one or more nodules can be felt. With the advent of high-resolution ultrasound, impalpable nodules only a few millimetres in diameter can be detected. Therefore patients who were initially felt to have a solitary nodule can be reclassified as having a multi-nodular goitre. Multi-nodular goitres are more common in areas of iodine deficiency and affect women more than men. Nodules tend to develop in long-standing goitres and can evolve from a simple, non-toxic goitre. If nodules contain functioning thyroid tissue they can eventually

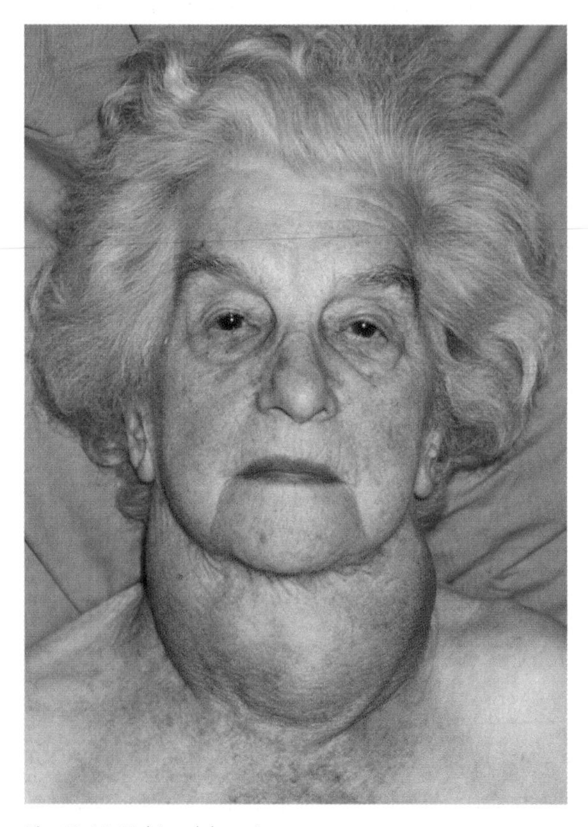

Fig. 12.16 Multi-nodular goitre.

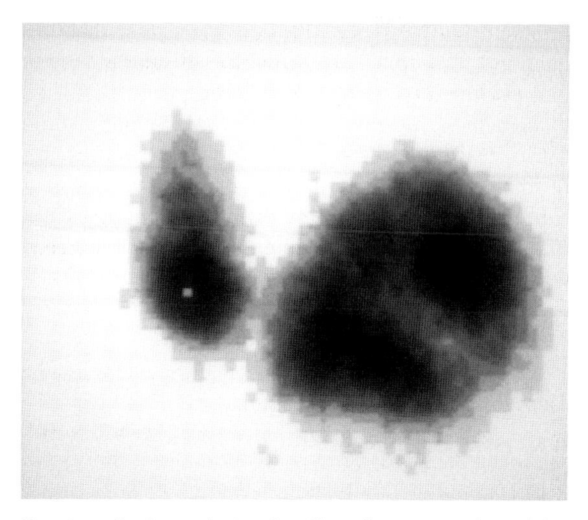

Fig. 12.17 Patchy uptake in a thyroid uptake scan in multi-nodular goitre.

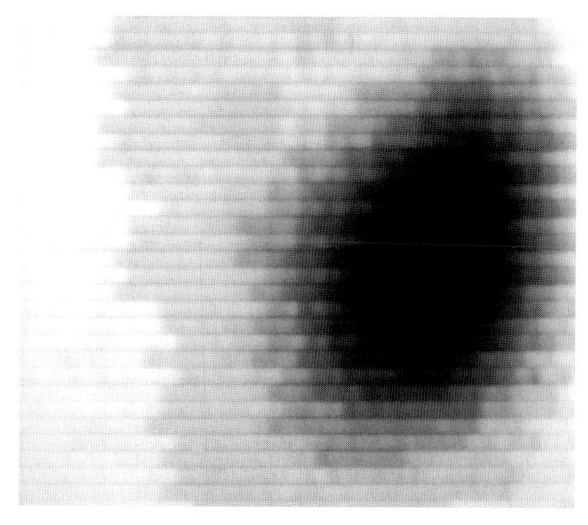

Fig. 12.18 Uptake in a solitary thyroid nodule.

secrete excess thyroid hormones leading to thyrotoxicosis. Patients are described as having a toxic, multi-nodular goitre. This tends to happen in the older patient and the classical signs of thyrotoxicosis (described earlier in the chapter) may not be apparent. They usually present with complications such as heart failure or atrial fibrillation. Complications of a large goitre (of any cause) include

(1) dysphagia (due to compression of the oesophagus);

(2) recurrent pneumonia (due to the compression of a bronchus and infection distal to the narrowing);

(3) stridor (due to compression of the trachea);

(4) hoarseness (due to compression of the left recurrent laryngeal nerve);

(5) venous engorgement (due to the compression of the great veins in the mediastinum).

Treatment includes anti-thyroid drugs to control symptoms if the patient has thyrotoxicosis. Definitive treatment is radioiodine therapy or surgery (particularly with complications due to a large goitre).

Solitary nodule

See Fig. 12.18. The underlying nature of a solitary nodule must always be determined. A nodule can be a cyst, adenoma—a benign collection of glandular cells (of thyroid origin), and cancer. Note that an adenoma can be non-toxic, that is, it does not produce excess thyroid hormones. Or it may become progressively more active and secrete excess T3 or T4, leading to thyrotoxicosis. It is then called a toxic adenoma. This overactivity can be sufficient to suppress activity of the rest of the thyroid gland through negative feedback. There are four ways of determining the nature of a nodule:

- ultrasound scanning
- radionuclide scanning
- fine-needle aspiration
- excision biopsy.

1. **Ultrasound scanning**. This has limited value. It can determine whether the nodule is solid or cystic (if it is cystic it is more likely to be benign). Also it may detect small nodules that are impalpable, which would suggest a multi-nodular goitre, a feature that would make malignancy less likely.
2. **Radionuclide scanning.** A radioactive isotope (either radioiodine or technetium) is injected into the bloodstream. The isotope is taken up and concentrated preferentially by the thyroid gland. Areas of high concentration of isotope reflect increased thyroid activity and are usually described as 'hot'. Areas of low activity are conversely described as cold. A useful guide is that a functioning 'hot' nodule is unlikely to be cancerous. The majority of cancers are cold nodules. Note that although the

majority of cancers are cold nodules, the majority of cold nodules are **not** cancers. Only about 10% of cold nodules are due to cancer.

3. **Fine-needle aspiration.** This is the best technique for identifying a thyroid nodule. A fine needle is inserted into the thyroid and a sliver of tissue is removed for histological examination. In expert hands a diagnosis can be made on most occasions. Sometimes not enough tissue is obtained or the cell morphology cannot lead to a precise diagnosis. In cases of doubt either the aspiration can be repeated or the patient can be referred for surgery.
4. **Excision biopsy.** Very occasionally, in cases of doubt, surgery is warranted. The nodule is removed along with surrounding thyroid tissue (usually a hemithyroidectomy), to provide both a diagnosis and sometimes a cure (as the nodule is removed).

Thyrotoxicosis

Thyrotoxicosis is the clinical syndrome that occurs due to an excess of free-circulating thyroid hormones T3 or T4. Hyperthyroidism should strictly be reserved for those cases where there is over-activity of the thyroid gland although hyperthyroidism and thyrotoxicosis are often used interchangeably. Cases of thyrotoxicosis that are not due to hyperthyroidism are listed under 'Other' in Table 12.5. Hyperthyroidism is termed primary when the main source driving the glandular over-activity is the thyroid gland itself. Secondary hyperthyroidism is where the source driving the over-activity is remote from the thyroid, for example, excess TSH production by the pituitary gland. In old textbooks you may see the term tertiary hyperthyroidism. This used to describe hyperthyroidism due to a hypothalamic cause. However currently hypothalamic causes are regarded as a secondary cause too.

See Table 12.5 for causes of thyrotoxicosis. Graves' disease, toxic multi-nodular goitre, toxic adenoma, hashitoxicosis, and subacute viral thryoiditis have already been described.

TABLE 12.5 Causes of thyrotoxicosis

Primary hyperthyroidism
Graves' disease
Toxic multi-nodular goitre
Toxic adenoma
Hashitoxicosis
Drug induced
Secondary hyperthyroidism
Thyrotropin-secreting tumour of the pituitary
Other tumours
Other
Subacute thyroiditis
Thyroxine ingestion (thyrotoxicosis factitia)

All causes in italics are very rare.

Drug-induced thryotoxicoxis

This may occur because of

- excessive ingestion of T4
- iodine-containing drugs.

1. **Excessive ingestion of T4.** Some people may take excess T4 for a number of reasons. Over-prescription by doctors rarely occurs because thyroid function tests are routinely checked and doses amended accordingly. Some patients may take excess T4 because it gives them a high. Others may take them as part of an abnormal illness behaviour while pretending that they have not taken any (this is called thyrotoxicosis factitia (*fack-tisha*)). This usually occurs in a person with a clinical background, for example, a nurse. This can be detected by the pattern of thyroid function tests, with a raised T4, a normal T3, and a low or undetectable TSH.
2. **Iodine-containing drugs.** These drugs include amiodarone, some cough preparations, and intravenous contrast media and they can induce thyrotoxicosis in susceptible individuals (this is called the Jod–Basedow (*jod-bas-eh-dough*) phenomenon) (*Karl Adolph Von Basedow (1799–1854), German physician; Jod = iodine in German*).

TSH-secreting tumour

A tumour of the pituitary may rarely secrete TSH and drive the production of excess thyroid hormone. The key to the diagnosis of this condition is the finding of elevated T3 and T4 levels with a high or normal level of TSH (normally TSH would be undetectable because of negative feedback). The tumour can be demonstrated on magnetic resonance imaging or a computed tomography scan and surgery is usually required.

Other tumours causing thyrotoxicosis

Rarely a tumour of the ovary may contain thyroid-like tissue that secretes excess T4 or T3. In old-fashioned textbooks this is called struma ovarii (*strew-ma-oh-vary-eye*). Thyroid isotope scans will show no uptake in the thyroid but increased uptake in the ovary. Also tumours of the testis, ovary, or bronchus can rarely secrete a peptide that behaves like TSH and stimulates the thyroid to produce excess thyroid hormone.

Hypothyroidism

See Fig. 12.19. Hypothyroidism comprises the clinical signs and symptoms caused by the decreased production of thyroid hormones due to an under-active thyroid gland (the symptoms and signs of hypothyroidism have already been described). See Table 12.6 for causes of hypothyroidism. Hashimoto's thyroiditis has already been described.

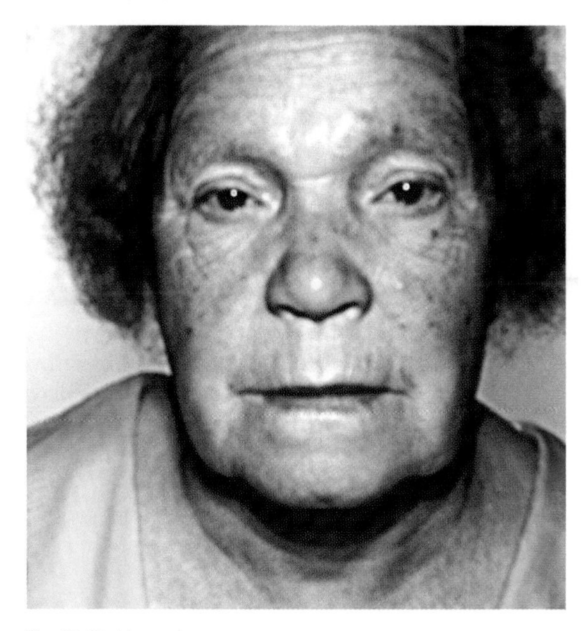

Fig. 12.19 Myxoedema.

TABLE 12.6 Causes of hypothyroidism

Hashimoto's thyroiditis
Idiopathic/spontaneous atrophy
Previous treatment with radioiodine or thyroidectomy
Anti-thyroid drugs
Drugs
Iodine deficiency

Idiopathic atrophic hypothyroidism

This is due to lymphocytic infiltration of the thyroid gland because of an unknown autoimmune trigger. Hashimoto's thyroiditis and idiopathic atrophic hypothyroidism are sometimes grouped together under the umbrella term lymphocytic thyroiditis to emphasize their common autoimmune pathogenesis. Unlike Hashimoto's thyroiditis there is no goitre in this condition. It is more common in women than in men.

Previous treatment for thyrotoxicosis

If the treatment is excessive or too long in duration, then hypothyroidism may occur. It is difficult to prescribe a precise dose for radioactive iodine and hypothyroidism is a recognized complication of this treatment. Ten per cent of patients in their first year will become permanently hypothyroid. After 20 years approximately 80% of patients will develop hypothyroidism. Therefore patients undergoing this treatment require regular follow-up. If hypothyroidism does develop, treatment is with T4 replacement. Surgical treatment with thyroidectomy can lead to hypothyroidism in 20% of cases.

Thyroid function tests

Thyroid function tests are assays for the thyroid hormones T4 and T3 as well as TSH levels. Different laboratories vary in what they test for and their reference ranges but the majority now detect levels of free T3 and T4 (and TSH) that are independent of protein binding. Older assays used to detect total levels of T4 and T3 that are dependent on plasma protein concentrations. This led to problems of interpretation if the patient's plasma protein concentration varied for any clinical reason, for example, the normal increased protein concentration during pregnancy would lead to an increased total T4 level suggesting hyperthyroidism or the decrease in plasma protein concentration in nephrotic syndrome would lead to a decrease total T4 level suggesting hypothyroidism. In both cases, there is no true derangement of thyroid function. Some laboratories only provide T4 and TSH levels to keep costs down and only offer T3 in situations where it is felt the patient is clinically thyrotoxic but with a normal T4 level (possible T3 toxicosis). Interpreting thyroid function tests is easy if you understand the negative feedback mechanism described earlier in the control of the thyroid.

Key
$\uparrow$ = above laboratory reference level
$\downarrow$ = below laboratory reference level
$\rightarrow$ = normal range

Hyperthyroidism
T3↑, T4↑, TSH↓
Hypothyroidism
T3↓, T4↓, TSH↑
Rarer causes
T3 toxicosis
T3↑, T4→, TSH↓
Thyrotropin-secreting pituitary tumour
T3↑, T4↑, TSH↑ (or →)
Thyrotoxicosis factitia
T3→, T4↑, TSH↓

Control of calcium metabolism

The majority of the body's calcium is contained in the bony skeleton. Less than 1% is found in extracellular fluid. About 50% of this is bound to albumen and the rest circulates in plasma in the ionized form. The calcium in bone and in the extracellular fluid are in dynamic equilibrium and small concentrations can be mobilized from the skeleton or replaced (a process that is under hormonal control). The principle hormones involved include PTH and vitamin D. Parathormone is a peptide hormone secreted from the parathyroid glands and elevates plasma calcium by increasing bone resorption, increasing the intestinal absorption of calcium with the aid of vitamin D and increasing the renal tubular reabsorption of calcium. Vitamin D is produced in the skin from sunlight. It is metabolized in the liver and kidney to its active metabolite 1,25 hydroxycholecalciferol (*hide-rocks-i-coal-ee-cal-siffer-ol*) (sometimes called calcitriol (*cal-si-try-ol*)). It increases intestinal uptake of calcium. A third hormone, calcitonin (*cal-si-toe-nin*), is produced in the parafollicular C cells of the thyroid. It decreases bone resorption and decreases renal reabsorption of calcium but it is thought to play little role in the physiological control of calcium.

Primary hyperparathyroidism

This is usually due to a parathyroid adenoma secreting excess PTH. Rarely it may be due to hyperplasia of the glands (overactivity of the glands), multiple adenomas, or a functioning carcinoma. Most commonly the patient is asymptomatic with a mild rise in plasma calcium. If the glandular activity is great enough the calcium rise can be sufficient to cause symptoms. The calcium level at which symptoms occur will vary among individuals. This is because many of the symptoms of hypercalcaemia are insidious, for example, constipation, confusion, polyuria, and polydipsia and they may go unrecognized by the patient early in the disease. Primary hyperparathyroidism can be diagnosed by finding normal or elevated levels of PTH in the presence of hypercalcaemia (normally PTH is low in the presence of hypercalcaemia because of negative feedback).

Secondary hyperparathyroidism

This is the response of the parathyroid glands to chronic hypocalcaemia. The most common cause is chronic renal failure (other causes include malabsorption and osteomalacia (*os-tea-owe-mal-ay-sha*)). The parathyroid glands increase their activity producing more PTH in an attempt to try and normalize the plasma calcium.

Tertiary hyperparathyroidism

This describes those cases of primary hyperparathyroidism where the parathyroid glands become autonomous and no longer respond to the normal feedback mechanisms. In these situations the plasma calcium levels can be very high.

Other causes of hypercalcaemia

See Table 12.7.

Hypoparathyroidism

This is an uncommon condition leading to decreased secretion of PTH and hypocalcaemia. The most common cause is after thyroidectomy and can be due to disturbance of the blood supply to the parathyroid glands or accidental removal of the glands. Hypocalcaemia can be transient or permanent. Idiopathic hypoparathyroidism is associated with other autoimmune disorders. Antibodies against the parathyroid gland have been demonstrated but their role in the causation of the disease is not clear. Clinical features include hypocalcaemia, cataracts, calcification of the basal ganglia,

TABLE 12.7 Other causes of hypercalcaemia

Multiple myeloma
Malignancy
Secondary to bony metastasis
Secondary to parathormone-like hormone secreted from tumour
Sarcoidosis
Vitamin D toxicity (usually drug related)
Hyperthryoidism
Immobilization in Paget's disease of bone*

* Sir James Paget (1814–1899), UK surgeon.

cutaneous thrush, short stature, and short fourth and fifth metacarpals.

Pseudohypoparathyroidism

This condition is rare and is due to the resistance of the target tissues to PTH. It shares many of the features of hypoparathyroidism including hypocalcaemia.

Pseudopseudohypoparathyroidism

This describes the condition where the patient has the external features of pseudohypoparathyroidism such as short stature, ectopic calcification, and short fourth and fifth metacarpals but does not have any biochemical abnormality such as hypocalcaemia. (Thankfully there is no condition called pseudopseudopseudohypoparathyroidism.)

Other causes of hypocalcaemia

See Table 12.8.

Finals section

The emphasis of this section is on the short cases as this format usually causes the most uncertainty. The Objective Structured Clinical Examinations (OSCEs) usually have more straightforward and standardized instructions. Despite the different formats the clinical approach remains the same. For revision read the examination summary (p. 336) and the keypoints throughout the chapter and do the questions on pp. 354–5. See Tables 12.9 and 12.10 for day-to-day and Finals cases, respectively.

TABLE 12.8 Other causes of hypocalcaemia
Malabsorption
Chronic renal failure
Osteomalacia or rickets
Acute pancreatitis

TABLE 12.9 Day-to-day cases
Hyperthyroidism
Hypothyroidism
Multinodular goitre
Cervical lymphadenopathy

TABLE 12.10 Finals cases
Day to day cases
Thyroid nodule
Metastatic lymphadenopathy

Some advice relating to examination problems

The instruction

The examiner may say, 'Look at the patient, what is the diagnosis?' This will usually be a spot diagnosis, for example, exopthalmos and goitre = Graves' disease of the thyroid. A variant of this instruction could be, 'Look at the patient's neck, what do you notice?' This could still be a spot diagnosis but it may also be a request to find a sign that could be the prelude to an examination in a different system, for example, Corrigan's sign (see p. 67), requiring a cardiovascular examination looking particularly for aortic incompetence. If the instruction is 'examine the neck' only, this suggests a thorough examination of the neck and in this circumstance a thyroid diagnosis will be high on the list of probabilities, so be prepared to execute your full thyroid routine.

Problem. You are asked to examine the neck and you do not know where to start.

Solution. Keep calm and have a strategy worked out. The most common diagnosis will be thyroid related, so it is worth glancing in three key areas:

(1) the eyes, looking for exophthalmos and lid retraction;

(2) the neck in the mid-line, looking for a goitre or nodule;

(3) the surrounding environment, looking for a glass of water.

If none of these features are present, then think laterally and look for abnormal pulsations in the neck, that is, raised jugular venous pressure or Corrigan's sign or look for swellings in other areas such as the supraclavicular fossa.

General look

Continue your overall observations and look at the general demeanour of the patient.

1. **Are they listless and fidgety?**—hyperthyroidism?
2. **Are they apathetic and lethargic?**—hypothyroidism?
3. **Do they look cachexic?** —malignancy?

Inspection

You should have performed this already especially if you adopt the solution in the problem above. Get your patient to lift their chin slightly as this may make a swelling more pronounced.

Protrusion of tongue

If the swelling is at or near the mid-line, get the patient to protrude their tongue and observe if the swelling elevates.

Swallowing

If you suspect a thyroid swelling, get the patient to swallow and observe if it elevates.

Palpate the neck

Get the patient to flex their neck slightly to relax the sternomastoid muscles. Any swelling should be assessed for site, size, consistency, tenderness, temperature, mobility, pulsatility, and transillumination and auscultated.

Thyroid swelling

Palpate from behind the patient using the pulps of your fingers:

(1) do not forget to percuss for retrosternal extension of a goitre;

(2) do not forget to auscultate;

(3) do not forget to check for lymphadenopathy.

Check thyroid status

This can be

(1) hyperthyroid—irritability, tremor, sweaty, tachycardia, lid retraction, and lid-lag;

(2) hypothyroid—apathetic, bradycardia, and slow-relaxing reflexes (check ankle jerks);

(3) euthyroid—relatively relaxed and normal pulse rate (on average between 70–90 beats/min).

Look for other signs

Other signs include the following:

(1) hyperthyroid—palmar erythema, spider naevi, gynaecomastia, proximal myopathy, and hyper-reflexia;

(2) hypothyroid—dry skin, alopecia, erythema ab igne, xanthelasma, hypercarotenaemia, carpal tunnel syndrome, cerebellar ataxia, myopathy, pleural effusion, pericardial effusion, and ascites.

(3) Graves' disease—pre-tibial myxoedema, thyroid acropachy, and exophthalmos.

You should be able to observe the majority of these signs with the minimum of fuss. In the short cases section do not get bogged down trying to find every single sign that might be present. Some signs require a thorough routine all of their own, for example, proximal myopathy or ascites and so should not be looked for unless requested or unless you have picked up on a further clue, for example, distended abdomen.

Problem. In a case of thyroid disease your examiners follow up by instructing you to ask some relevant questions.

Solution. This one is simple. The examiners are just testing your depth of knowledge of thyroid disease.

1. If your case is a goitre, do not forget to ask about dysphagia, stridor, breathlessness, and hoarse voice. You could also ask about the possibility of previous investigations requiring contrast media, whether the patient is on medications such as amiodarone, or whether there has been any recent flu-like illness, which could cause a goitre.
2. If your case is hyperthyroidism ask about heat intolerance, increased appetite, weight loss, and diarrhoea.
3. If your case is hypothyroidism ask about cold intolerance, decreased appetite, weight gain, and constipation.

Good luck!

Questions

The more stars, the more important it is to know the answer.

1. What is a goitre? *
2. Name three possible complications of a large goitre. ****
3. In what condition would you find tetany? **
4. Why does a thryoid swelling elevate on swallowing? ***
5. Why does a thyroglossal cyst elevate on protrusion of the tongue? ***
6. What is exophthalmos? **
7. What is lid retraction? **
8. What is the differential diagnosis of a thyroid nodule? ****
9. Which neck swelling exhibits pulsatility? *
10. How do you demonstrate lid-lag? ***
11. What 10 features should you examine for in any neck swelling? *****
12. How do you examine thyroid status? ****

13. Why do you percuss when examining a goitre? ***
14. Which electrolyte is elevated in primary hyperparathyroidism? **
15. If primary hyperparathyroidism is symptomatic, what symptoms may a patient complain of? ****
16. What is the significance of a bruit over the thyroid gland? **
17. If a thyroid swelling does not elevate with swallowing give one important reason for this. ***
18. What is the best investigation to determine the nature of a thyroid nodule? ***
19. What cardiovascular features can you find with hypothyroidism? ****
20. In what clinical circumstance might you find a slow-relaxing reflex? **
21. What are the two triangles the neck is divided into anatomically? **
22. Name four symptoms of hyperthyroidism. ****
23. Name four symptoms of hypothyroidism. ****
24. What is thyroiditis? **
25. Name two types of thyroiditis. **
26. What is Trousseau's sign? **
27. In what condition might you find calcification of the basal ganglia? *
28. A tumour of which organ can cause a lower motor neurone VII palsy? ***
29. Which tumour exhibits lateral mobility but no vertical mobility? *
30. Which swellings may transilluminate in the neck? **
31. If faced with fever, night sweats, and weight loss, together with a neck swelling, name three possible causes. ****
32. What is the most commone cause of hyperparathyroidism? **
33. Name three causes of hypercalcaemia. ****
34. Name three causes of hypocalcaemia. ****
35. What is Chvostek's sign? **
36. What is struma ovarii? **
37. What happens to the TSH in hypothyroidism? ***
38. In what condition would you find pre-tibial myxoedema? ***
39. What is Derbyshire neck?*
40. Name the three main salivary glands. **
41. What is a branchial cyst? **
42. What is transillumination? ***
43. What is hypercarotenaemia? **

Score. Give 4 marks for 4 stars, 1 for 1 star, and so on. At the end of the third year, you should be scoring 60-plus and by Finals, 90-plus; 100-plus is very good.

Further reading

Bayliss RIS, Tunbridge WM. *Thyroid disease, the facts*. 3rd edn. Oxford: Oxford University Press; 1998.

Brook CGD, Marshall NJ. *Essential endocrinology*. 4th edn. Oxford: Blackwell Science; 2001. pp. 78 and 119.

Hall R, Evered DC. *A colour atlas of endocrinology*. 3rd edn. London: Wolfe; 1989.

CHAPTER 13

Joints

Chapter contents

Introduction

Joints (and connective tissue) come under the field of rheumatology. The most common rheumatological conditions are osteoarthritis and rheumatoid arthritis. Osteoarthritis is usually ascribed to wear and tear or ageing (but this is incomplete and an over-simplification). Rheumatoid arthritis is a multi-system disorder that may affect many organs as well as joints. In 60–70% of cases an autoantibody called the rheumatoid factor can be isolated and such cases are termed seropositive (for rheumatoid factor). How this factor is generated is still not fully understood. In contrast there is a family of conditions called the seronegative spondyloarthritides (*spon-dee-low-arth-ritty-deez*). These are a range of diseases with similar or overlapping presentations and are unified by the absence of the rheumatoid factor. These include ankylosing spondylitis (*ank-ee-low-zing-spon-dee-light-iss*), Reiter's (*writers*) syndrome, and psoriatic (*sore-ee-attic*) arthropathy.

In the following section the bulk of the history taking will focus on symptoms from the groups above but less common groups of diseases such as the crystal arthropathies, for example, gout and pseudogout and the vasculitides (*vas-cue-litty-deez*), for example, systemic lupus erythmatosus (*systemic-loo-pus-erith-mat-owe-suss*) (SLE) and temporal arteritis will be touched upon. You will also learn not to restrict your thoughts to joints alone but to the possible systemic complications that a disease may produce or to medical disease, which may have an impact on the joints.

Symptoms

The most common presentation of joint disease is pain. As with pain elsewhere there are a number of key questions you need to ask.

Joint pain

1. **'Where do you feel the pain?' (Site.)** This is a crucial question. People can be vague about where they experience pain. Do not be satisfied with a vague waft of the hand. Get them to be specific and make them demonstrate exactly where it is. If the pain is localized to a joint it is likely that you are dealing with an arthropathy (an all-embracing term meaning an abnormality of a joint; arthralgia (*arth-ral-jah*) is a term you may also see which means pain in a joint and arthritis means inflammation in a joint). If the pain is more diffuse then it could be due to a chronic pain syndrome, for example, fibromyalgia (*fie-bro-my-al-jah*) (see p. 387). Another possibility is polymyalgia rheumatica (*polly-my-al-jah-room-attic-a*) (p. 389).
2. **'Are there other joints affected?'** Always ask if there are other joints affected. Patients may be so consumed by the pain of the offending joint that they neglect to tell you about the less troublesome joints. If one joint is affected this is called a monoarthritis, if two to four joints are affected it is called an oligoarthritis (sometimes pauci-arthritis (*paw-si-arth-right-iss*)), and if more than four joints are affected it is called a polyarthritis. The causes of joint pain are usually different for a monoarthritis compared with a polyarthritis with some overlap in an oligoarthritis (*olly-go-arth-right-iss*)(see Table 13.1). When faced with a single hot joint, the most important diagnosis you must consider is a septic arthritis. This is an acute infection within the joint (usually due to staphylococcus aureus (*staff-ee-low-cock-us-aw-ree-us*)). If it is not recognized quickly, the joint can be destroyed irreparably. It is important that a single hot joint is aspirated and any fluid analysed for possible infection.
3. **'How long have you had the pain?' (Duration.)** Acute joint pain (arthralgia) may be fleeting, for example, following a viral infection where joints may ache transiently for several hours. During such an episode there is usually no inflammation of the joints. Some systemic infections may cause arthralgias that last longer and some may cause a reactive arthritis, for example, brucellosis (*brew-sell-owe-sis*). Crystal arthropathies can cause exquisite pain in a joint for several weeks although they can be as short lived as a couple of days. Diseases such as rheumatoid arthritis or osteoarthritis may cause chronic pain. Sufferers may be plagued with pain

TABLE 13.1 Causes of a monoarthritis and polyarthritis

Monoarthritis
Septic arthritis
Crystal arthritis, for example, gout
Seronegative spondylarthritides
Polyarthritis
Rheumatoid arthritis
Osteoarthritis
Seronegative spondlyoarthritides, for example, ankylosing spondylitis

This table reflects the likelihood of a diagnosis related to the number of joints affected. It does remain possible that an unusual presentation of a disease may occur, for example, rheumatoid arthritis presenting initially with a monoarthritis or gout as a polyarthritis.

for years. The natural history of chronic pain may include episodes of more severe pain, which may represent a 'flare up' of disease. Other processes such as trauma, infection, or other rheumatological disease, for example, gout can also lead to an exacerbation of pain. Therefore you must be prepared to consider other conditions and fully evaluate your patient before finally accepting that you face a disease flare.

4. **'Does the pain go anywhere?' (Radiation.)** This question is of limited diagnostic value with the exception of radicular pain (*rad-ick-you-lar*) (see p. 199) due to root or nerve entrapment, for example, sciatica. This question may also reveal that the pain is not truly joint pain but pain that just happens to span a joint. So pay special attention to how the pain is described particularly if it seems ill defined and seems to radiate to the whole of a limb (which would favour a chronic pain syndrome). Another trap for the unwary is referred pain. In this circumstance, pain is experienced remote from its site of origin, for example, the pain caused by arthritis in a lumbar vertebra may be experienced over the hip. Diagnosing referred pain is not easy and requires the doctor to have an index of suspicion. Consider this possibility if after examination and an X-ray a joint appears normal. You may get more joy examining a joint that is more proximal.
5. **'How severe is the pain?' (Severity.)** This question will establish how much of a problem the pain is and how it affects the patient's life. Ask the patient to score their pain out of 10, with 10 being the worst pain they have ever experienced. You will, however, have to make a judgement about the patient's personality as the same pain can be experienced differently by different individuals. A stoical individual may play down excruciating pain and conversely those with low pain tolerance may complain bitterly of the most exquisite agony. This judgement will come with experience.
6. **'Is there anything that makes the pain better or worse?' (Relieving or aggravating factors.)** In most cases inflamed arthritic joints will be more painful with usage or stress on the joint, for example, weight bearing. There may be a history of trauma, which may aggravate pre-existing arthritis or even cause a haemarthrosis (*he-mar-throw-sis*) (blood within a joint). Ankylosing spondylitis is unusual in that back pain is worse when resting. It tends to be worse at night and eases when the patient moves during the day (unlike mechanical back pain). Most sufferers will have tried painkillers to ease their pain, usually with varying degrees of success. As a rule, a good response to non-steroidal anti-inflammatory drugs (NSAIDs) suggests an underlying inflammatory arthritis (but remember osteoarthritis may also respond to these medications).

Stiffness

Stiffness is a subjective symptom. Many people will have experienced some joint stiffness after unaccustomed exercise or trauma to a joint or muscle. In rheu-

CASE 13.1

Problem. A 28-year-old man presents with a painful big toe. The day before he played football and missed his evening meal. He remembered stubbing his toe during the match, but could not remember which one. Afterwards he retired to the bar where he celebrated his team's victory with copious amounts of beer. He is on no medication and has never been in hospital before. On examination, his right big toe is swollen, red, and very tender. The rest of the examination is unremarkable. What is the diagnosis?

Discussion. This patient has an inflammatory monoarthritis affecting the first metatarsophalangeal (MTP) joint. It is possible that he suffered trauma to his big toe. However, he has performed heavy exercise on an empty stomach, which he filled preferentially with alcohol! All these factors can predispose to acute gout. Furthermore acute gout is extremely painful and classically affects the first MTP joint. The diagnosis can be confirmed by joint aspiration although it is technically difficult (and painful) with a small joint.

Keypoints

- Joint pain is the most common presentation of joint disease.
- Ask especially about the site of pain and the number of joints affected.
- Determine whether the patient has a monoarthritis, an oligoarthritis, or a polyarthritis.
- Try to ascertain whether the arthritis is inflammatory or non-inflammatory in nature.
- Always ask if painkillers have been taken (including over-the-counter remedies).

matological conditions stiffness is not transient but a persistent feature. In an inflammatory arthritis, for example, rheumatoid arthritis, stiffness is usually more pronounced when a joint is first used, for example, in the morning (morning stiffness). This stiffness is prolonged and can last more than hour (note that morning stiffness for longer than 30 min is more suggestive of an underlying (inflammatory) arthritis). Ask, 'Is your/are your joints stiff?' If the answer is yes probe further.

1. 'How long are they stiff for?'
2. 'At what time of the day is your joint stiffness worse?'
3. 'Is the stiffness related to activity or rest?'

With degenerative or mechanical arthritis, stiffness and pain tend to be worse following prolonged activity. This tends to be experienced towards the end of the day. In one particular condition, polymyalgia rheumatica (see p. 389), pain and stiffness are prominent symptoms. This condition affects the proximal muscles preferentially, that is, shoulder and pelvic girdle and can be so disabling that a patient has difficulty rising from a chair or combing their hair. If you suspect this condition ask the following.

1. 'Do you have difficulty combing you hair?'
2. 'Do you have difficulty reaching for objects on high shelves?'
3. 'Do you have difficulty rising from a chair?'
4. 'Do you have difficulty climbing stairs?'

Also consider asking questions about temporal arteritis (see pp. 386, 390 as polymyalgia rheumatica and temporal arteritis may co-exist).

Keypoints

- Prolonged joint stiffness of greater than 1 h suggests an inflammatory arthropathy.
- Stiffness when a joint is first used (that is, morning stiffness) suggests an inflammatory arthropathy, for example, rheumatoid arthritis.
- Stiffness following prolonged activity suggests a 'degenerative'/mechanical arthropathy, for example, osteoarthritis.
- The stiffness associated with ankylosing spondylitis improves with exercise and worsens with rest.
- Stiffness and pain in the distribution of the proximal muscles should make you think of polymyalgia rheumatica.

Swelling

Ask if there has been swelling of the affected joint. Swelling may be due to soft tissue swelling, for example, synovitis (*sign-owe-vie-tiss*) (inflammation of the joint lining), new bone formation due to osteophytes (*os-tea-owe-fights*), or the accumulation of fluid within a joint (effusion). Swelling may also occur around tendons (tenosynovitis) (*tea-no-sign-owe-vie-tiss*) and tendon sheaths may develop nodules. It is important to verify that swelling exists during your examination because some people will claim their joints are massively swollen even when no swelling is apparent. As joint swelling is a dynamic process it is possible that the swelling has subsided before presenting to you. This could represent a spontaneous remission or could be as a result of therapy, for example, NSAIDs or steroids. If this is the case it is worth keeping an open mind and reviewing at a later date. The concept of 'subclinical synovitis' is increasingly popular, that is, inflammation that is present and sufficient to cause symptoms, but not apparent on examination. This is important because it may still result in joint damage. The increasing use of imaging techniques, for example, ultrasound and magnetic resonance imaging, have demonstrated this and show that clinical examination can be misleading.

Keypoints

- Swelling must be objectively verified.
- Joint swelling may be due to soft tissue growth, for example, synovial thickening, bony overgrowth, for example, osteophytes, or fluid, for example, effusion.
- Arthritis may occur in the absence of clinical signs, that is, subclinical synovitis, but may still result in joint damage.

Extra-articular features

Some rheumatological conditions, for example, rheumatoid arthritis, can affect other organs as well as joints. Multi-system disorders, for example, SLE, may affect joints as well as other organs. When you perform your review of systems you will detect many of these symptoms (if they exist). Generalized symptoms such as anorexia, weight loss, night sweats, and fever are common. Fatigue is an extra-articular feature that patients complain about commonly. Table 13.2 shows the more 'organ-specific' features that should be looked for.

TABLE 13.2 Extra-articular features of other medical disease

Feature	Associated condition
Diarrhoea	
Inflammatory bowel disease	
Reactive arthritis	
Rash	
Psoriasis	
SLE	
	Malar flush
	Photosensitivity rash
	Livido reticularis (*live-ee-dough-re-tick-you-lar-iss*)
Behçets syndrome (see p. 389)	
Vasculitis	
Raynaud's phenomenon (see p. 362)	
Systemic sclerosis/scleroderma (limited/diffuse)	
SLE	
Primary Raynaud's	
Mouth	
Ulcers	
	SLE
	Reiter's syndrome
	Behçets syndrome
Dry mouth	
	Sjögren's syndrome (see p. 391)*
	Rheumatoid arthritis
	SLE
	Systemic sclerosis
Eyes	
Scleritis/episcleritis (see p. 272)	
	Rheumatoid arthritis
Scleromalacia perforans (*s-clear-owe-mal-ay-sha-per-fur-anz*)	
	Rheumatoid arthritis
Iritis (eye-right-iss) and uveitis (*you-vee-eye-tiss*)	
	Ankylosing spondylitis
Other seronegative spondyloarthropathies, for example, reactive arthritis	
Loss of vision	
	temporal arteritis
Respiratory	
Pleural effusion	
	Rheumatoid arthritis
	SLE
	Other vasculitides
Fibrosing alveolitis	
	Rheumatoid arthritis
	Vasculitis and other connective tissue disease
Cardiovascular	
Pericarditis	
	Rheumatoid arthritis
	SLE
	Other vasculitides
Pericardial effusion	
	Rheumatoid arthritis
	SLE
	Vasculitis
Thromboembolic disease	
	Anti-phospholipid (*anti-foss-foe-lip-id*) syndrome
Neuropsychiatric	
Psychosis	
	SLE
Stroke	
	SLE
	Temporal arteritis
	Other vasculitides
Epilepsy	
	SLE
Depression	
	Most causes
Carpal Tunnel syndrome	
	Rheumatoid arthritis
	Severe osteoarthritis
Genitourinary	
Urethritis (*you-reeth-right-iss*)	
	Reiter's syndrome
Cervicitis (*serve-i-site-iss*)	
	Reiter's syndrome
Obstetric	
Recurrent miscarriages	
	SLE and anti-phospholipid syndrome

SLE, systemic lupus erythmatosus.
*Henrik Samuel Conrad Sjögren (1899–1986), Swedish ophthalmologist.

Raynaud's phenomenon

What is it?

Raynaud's (*ray-nose*) phenomenon (*Maurice Raynaud (1834–1881), French physician*) is a common condition in which there is abnormal spasm of the arteries of the hands or feet in response to the cold. It is common with the highest incidence occurring in young females. It affects the hands more than the feet and is usually bilateral. It is important to consider a cervical rib as a possible cause of unilateral Raynaud's phenomenon. Classically the hands change colour three times, from white to blue and finally red. The white colour occurs due to spasm of the arteries, resulting in decreased blood in the peripheral vessels of the hands. The poor blood flow causes cyanosis and the bluish discolouration. The hands ultimately turn red as vasoactive metabolites build up in the vessels causing dilatation of the arteries. During the three stages the hands become increasingly painful and numb. In severe cases of Raynaud's phenomenon ulceration of the hands can occur. For causes of Raynaud's phenomenon, see Table 13.3.

Questions to ask about Raynaud's phenomenon

1. 'Do your hands become painful in cold weather?'
2. 'Do your hands change colour in the cold and what colour do they change to?' Try to elicit whether there is a triphasic colour change, that is, from white to blue and then red. The white represents the pallor of the hand as the vessels go into spasm restricting its blood supply. The blue represents peripheral cyanosis as the sluggish blood flow returns. The red phase represents a circulatory over-compensation (reactive hyperaemia (*high-per-ee-mia*) as blood surges back into the hand). This phase is also painful.
3. 'How long have you had this problem?'
4. 'What precautions do you take to prevent this happening?' In severe Raynaud's, people may wear gloves indoors. This question may enable you to gauge the severity of the patient's condition.
5. 'Are you taking any medication?'
6. 'What is your occupation?' Are they a builder or someone who works with vibrating tools? (This can cause Raynaud's phenomenon.)

If you think the patient has CREST (an acronym for major symptoms, that is, **c**alcinosis (*cal-sin-owe-sis*), **R**aynaud's phenomenon, **oe**sophageal dysmotility, **s**clerodactyly, and **t**elangiectasia) or systemic sclerosis, ask the following.

1. Do you have any chest or breathing problems? (Associated pulmonary fibrosis.)
2. Do you have any swallowing difficulties? (Oesophageal dysmotility problems.)

TABLE 13.3 Causes of Raynaud's phenomenon

Idiopathic	Known as Raynaud's disease
Connective tissue disorders	Systemic sclerosis/CREST syndrome, systemic lupus erythmatosus, polymyositis, rheumatoid arthritis, and Sjögren's (*show-grens*) syndrome (see p. 391)
Cervical rib, cervical spondylosis	
Increased plasma viscosity	Waldenstrom's macroglobulinaemia (*wal-den-stroms-macro-glob-you-lin-eem-ia*)* and cryoglobulinaemia (*cry-owe-glob-you-lin-eemia*)
Drugs	β-Blockers and ergot
Vibrating tools	Pneumatic drills
Endocrine	Hypothyroidism and diabetes mellitus

* Jan Gösta Waldenstrom (1906–1996), Swedish physician.

Drug history

A drug history is always important. Take the opportunity to check if analgesia or anti-inflammatory drugs have been used and how effective they have been (do not forget to ask about over-the-counter medications at the chemist and alternative or herbal remedies). Also anticipate possible side-effects from medication, for example, NSAIDs—indigestion, oedema, gastrointestinal haemorrhage, renal dysfunction, and so on. Some medications can contribute to an arthropathy, for example, diuretics can precipitate an attack of gout by decreasing the renal excretion of uric acid. An arthropathy may also be the result of a severe allergic response to any drug. This will be in the context of a severe illness affecting multiple organs including the skin. Do not forget to ask about illicit drugs, for example, intravenous heroin.With the prevalence of intravenous drug abuse increasing in this country, there has been a corresponding rise in unusual infections such as tuberculosis, hepatitis B and C, and HIV, all of which can cause arthritis.

Genitourinary history

Where appropriate take a sexual history. This is important because reactive arthritis caused by chlamydia infection is becoming increasingly common. Also a urethritis or cervicitis are potential symptoms of Reiter's syndrome.

Family history

Some rheumatological conditions are familial including:

- osteoarthritis
- rheumatoid arthritis
- ankylosing spondylitis (and other seronegative arthritides).

A family history of skin psoriasis is important because its presence may be indicative of psoriatic arthropathy.

Impact of illness

During your enquiries it is useful to find out what the impact of illness is on the patient's life (handicap) and their ability to function (disability). This can be done while taking a 'social history'. As you explore the patient's occupation and domestic situation find out how the disease is affecting their life. This will also guide your treatment of the patient. If you are unable to cure their disease then appropriate aids may transform their lives, for example, a 'bathing chair' may enable a patient to have a bath safely. Also enquire about the patient's occupation, their ability to work, and the time they have taken off work—this is being increasingly used as an outcome measure in rheumatology.

The importance of examining the joints

Rheumatological problems directly affect the joints, muscles, and bones, but perhaps more importantly they affect function. Many have manifestations in other systems, for example, rheumatoid arthritis can affect the cardiorespiratory system. Similarly many general medical conditions like diabetes mellitus and acromegaly can affect the joints. For this reason it is important to look closely at a patient's joints when performing a general examination.

Keypoints

- Any organ in the body can be affected by a range of rheumatological conditions.
- Never forget a drug history.
- Also ask about illicit drug use as intravenous drug abusers are at particular risk of infections including hepatitis, tuberculosis, and HIV.
- Always assess the impact of arthritis on the patient's life.

CASE 13.2

Problem. A 40-year-old Afro-Caribbean woman who has been hypertensive for several years presents with aching muscles and a rash over her arms, legs, and face. She takes bendrofluazide (*bend roe-flu-a-zide*) 2.5 mg once daily to control her blood pressure. Her mother, who she has recently visited in the Caribbean, suffers from osteoarthritis. She has had one child who is fit and well, but four pregnancies in total. Five years ago she was treated with warfarin (*war-fa-rin*) for a deep-vein thrombosis (DVT). On examination, she is obese, but well. There is no evidence of arthritis affecting the large joints, but her left wrist joint is swollen and tender. The rash is erythematous and there are plaques affecting her cheeks, but not her nose. Elsewhere it is urticarial (*err-tick-ariel*) in nature. She has patchy hair loss. What is going on?

Discussion. This case highlights the need to be on your guard. Any one symptom could easily be explained away in isolation, for example, aching muscles and a rash could simply be a viral infection. However if you stand back and draw the disparate threads together you will find a unifying diagnosis. In this case the diagnosis is SLE. As you become more familiar with conditions such as SLE you will have more of a chance of spotting them so long as you remain alert. Typically SLE affects women, particularly of Afro-Caribbean origin and it is characterized by a 'butterfly' rash on the face. However, any type of rash is possible. Alopecia (*allo-pea-sha*) (the loss of hair) is also a feature. Myalgia (*my-al-jah*) (muscle pain) is common and most small joints can be affected. Patients with SLE can suffer abnormalities of coagulation and there is often a history of DVT. Miscarriages are also more frequent than in the general population. The patient may have longstanding essential hypertension with a degree of renal impairment, but another possibility is lupus nephritis causing hypertension. Further blood tests may add weight to the diagnosis. In this case the anti-nuclear antibodies were positive (see p. 391).

Examination of the joints summary

1. Introduce yourself to the patient and ask for permission to examine.
2. Ask the patient to get on to bed (if not already on the bed). You may need to help!
3. Expose the relevant joint adequately.
4. Whilst doing 1–3, have a 'general look' Discomfort? Any aids or adaptations visible?
5. Before examining any joint ask if it is painful.
6. With all joints, think 'Look! Feel! Move!'
7. Examine the hands and feet.
8. Examine the shoulder joint.
9. Examine the hip joint.
10. Examine the knee joint.
11. Examine the spine.
12. The GALS assessment.
13. Wash your hands
14. Presentation.

Examination of the joints in detail

Getting started

1. Introduce yourself to the patient and ask for permission to examine.

Put out your hand to shake the patient's hand (do not squeeze too hard!). Say something like, 'Hello I'm Abraham Colles, a third-year student. Do you mind if I examine your xxxx?' (where xxxx is any joint under consideration).

2. Ask the patient to get on to bed (if not already on the bed). You may need to help!

Usually this will be no problem, but if the patient is unable to get on to the bed on their own, offer your assistance. If their stability seems extremely dodgy get professional help to lift them on to the bed properly.

3. Expose the relevant joint adequately.

Make sure you can see not only the joint, but the major muscle groups around the joint and the joint proximal and distal to the one you are examining. It is probably best that you demonstrate the whole limb if examining a joint affecting an arm or leg and the patient should strip to their underclothes if you are going to examine the spine. In this way you may appreciate any muscle wasting as a result of disuse or perhaps some subtle neurological lesion that may be contributing to a joint disorder, deformity, or swelling. Remember keyhole surgery may be desirable but keyhole examinations are not!

4. Whilst doing 1–3, have a 'general look' Discomfort? Any aids or adaptations visible?

As soon as you meet your patient you should be assessing their general demeanour. Do they look in discomfort? Are they unwell? Note the patient's posture and ability to move. Also glance around the immediate environment and see if you can see any walking aids, for example, walking stick, zimmer frame, or adaptations such as foam-handled cutlery to aid grip in an arthritic hand.

5. Before examining any joint ask if it is painful.

Before examining any joint, ask if it is painful. It is essential that you do not inflict any unnecessary pain with a thoughtless grab of a painful joint. This is not only undesirable and unprofessional, but you may also lose the co-operation of your patient (and fail an exam!)

Keypoints

- Always check if a joint is painful before examining it!

6. With all joints, think 'Look! Feel! Move!'

Look! Feel! Move! Remember this mantra before you examine any joint and in the majority of cases you will perform an adequate examination (particularly if you have a mental blank).

1. **Look.** When looking at the joint(s) in question, identify any evidence of inflammation, such as redness and swelling and any obvious deformity. An old Latin summary of the signs of inflammation is
   rubor—redness
   tumor—swelling
   calor—heat
   dolor—pain
   functio laxio—lack of function.
2. **Feel.** When feeling the joint(s) use your fingertips to identify any evidence of inflammation, such as heat. Similarly, you will be able to locate any source of pain or swelling. Bimanual palpation of a joint is the most sensitive method of palpation. Can you feel the joint line clearly? If so, inflammation is unlikely. Synovitis is usually felt as a boggy swelling (like feeling a grape) and is usually tender. Bony swelling is usually hard and non-tender. Feel along

the tendons while moving the joint—you should be able to palpate any tendon sheath swelling or tenosynovitis, which may cause crepitus (*crep-it-us*) (a crackling feeling beneath your fingers on movement of the joint—see later) or a tendon nodule.

3. **Move.** Ask the patient to move the relevant limb in all plains (active movement) and compare that with passive movement (you move the limb for the patient). A restricted range of movement may be due to pain, muscle weakness, mechanical problems, effusion, or inflammation.

Some joint examinations do not follow the pattern of look, feel, move very readily, for example, hand and knee. However, if you analyse the steps closely, looking, feeling, and moving are still vital components of the assessment.

Keypoints

- The classical features of inflammation are redness, pain, heat, swelling and loss of function
- Remember **'Look! Feel! Move!'**

Hands and feet

7. Examine the hands and feet.

As the hands are the most important functionally these will be concentrated on exclusively (although many aspects of hand examination are relevant to the foot). You should first be aware of the anatomy of the hand (see Fig. 13.1). The hand examination is straightforward (see Fig. 13.2).

Expose the forearms and elbows. Ask the patient if they can do this for you. Gently help them if they cannot. This will give you an idea of the degree of function they have. Now crouch down next to the patient. You should have a systematic order in which you examine hands. The author tends to use the following routine:

- nails
- skin
- bones and joints
- muscles
- elbows
- function
- neurological examination
- vascular examination.

Nails

Examine the nails very carefully. Look for signs shown in Table 13.4. See Fig. 13.3.

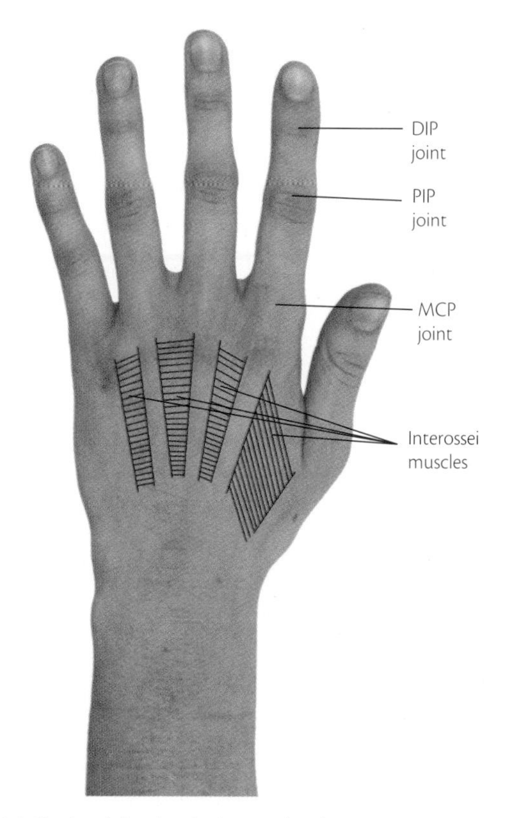

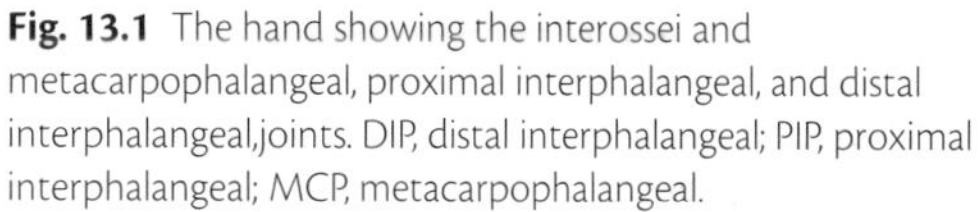

Fig. 13.1 The hand showing the interossei and metacarpophalangeal, proximal interphalangeal, and distal interphalangeal,joints. DIP, distal interphalangeal; PIP, proximal interphalangeal; MCP, metacarpophalangeal.

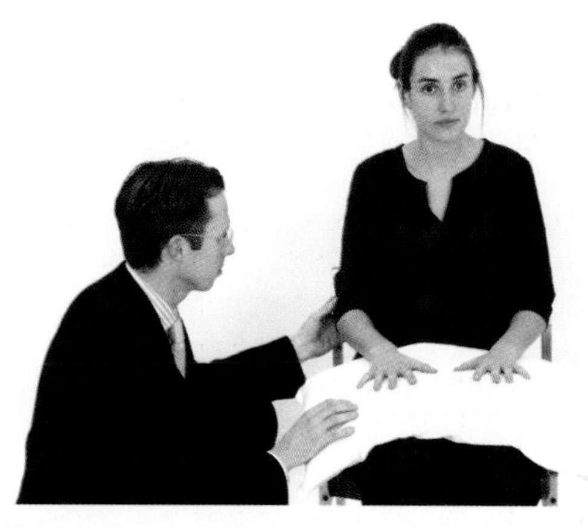

Fig. 13.2 Correct position for examining the hands.

Tip

It may be helpful to rest the hands on a pillow placed across the patient's lap for comfort. If not **be gentle** when holding their hands.

TABLE 13.4 Comparing nail signs with their associated diseases

Sign	Description	Disease suggestive of
Pitting and splitting	Multiple tiny nail depressions	Psoriatic arthropathy
Onycholysis (*on-ee-coal-lie-sis*)	Separation of the nail plate	Psoriatic arthropathy
Hyperkeratosis (*high-per-kerra-toe-sis*)	Exuberant nail growth	Psoriatic arthropathy
Longitudinal ridging	Small ridges along the nail length	Rheumatoid arthritis
Nail fold infarcts	Tiny black streaks	Vasculitis
Nail fold capillaries	Tiny nail blood vessels	Scleroderma/SLE
Periungal (*perry-un-gwal*) erythema	Redness of the nails	Connective tissue disease
Gottran's papules	Scaling pink/purple papules over knuckles	Dermatomyositis
Sclerodactyly (*s-clear-owe-dack-tilly*)	Skin tightening	Scleroderma
Raynaud's phenomenon	White fingers in the cold, changing to blue and then red on warming	Systemic sclerosis, scleroderma/SLE, and primary Raynaud's

SLE, systemic lupus erythmatosus.

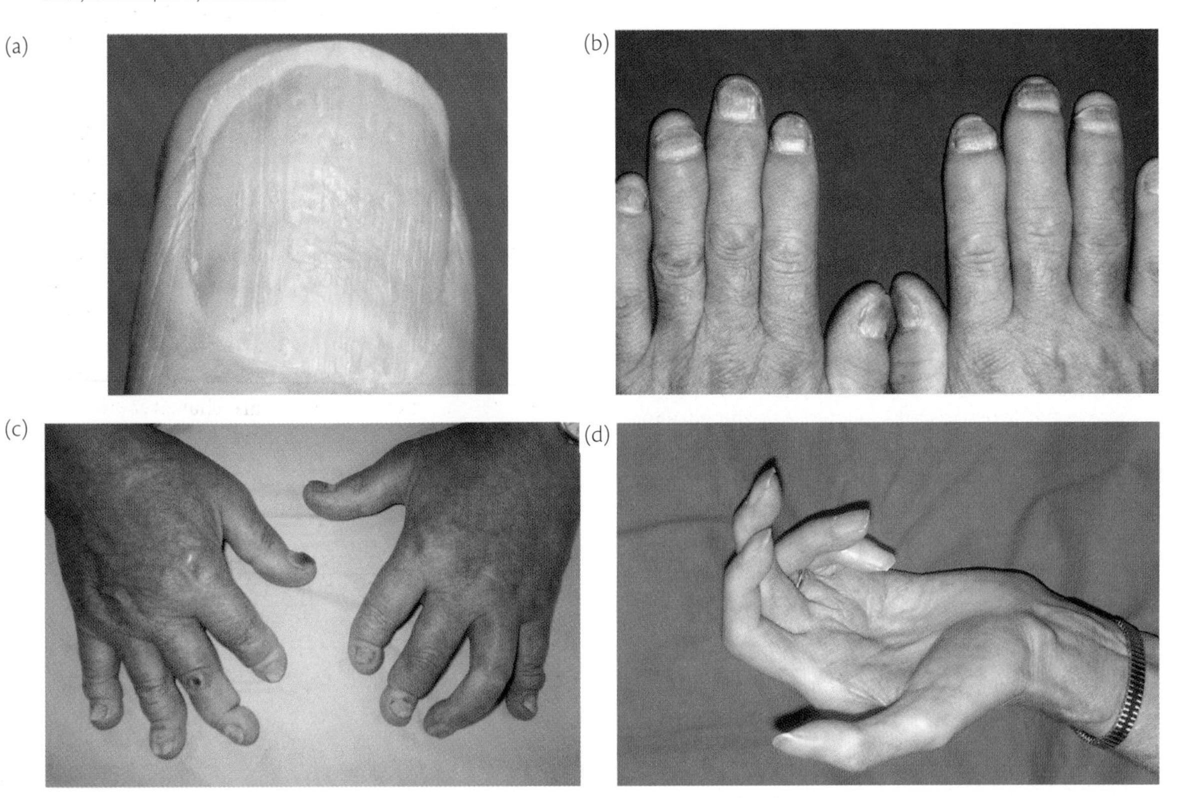

Fig. 13.3 Nail and hand signs. (a) Nail pitting, (b) onycholysis and joint swelling due to psoriatric arthropathy, (c) onycholysis and arthritis mutilans, (d) sclerodactyly.

Skin

Look at the skin carefully. Do not restrict your gaze to the hands but also look at the arms and face. Look for steroid-induced purpura associated with the treatment of rheumatoid arthritis; the skin will also be papery thin (also check for a 'moon face' and 'buffalo hump' suggesting steroid-induced Cushing's syndrome, see p. 405). Also look for the signs shown in Table 13.5. See

TABLE 13.5 Comparing skin signs with their associated diseases

Signs	Disease suggestive of
Psoriatic plaques on extensor surfaces	Psoriatic arthropathy
Telangiectasia	Systemic sclerosis
Tophi (*toe-fie*)	Chronic tophaceous gout
Rheumatoid nodules (elbows)	Rheumatoid arthritis
Palmar erythema	Rheumatoid arthritis
Tight, thick, shiny skin	Systemic sclerosis
Papery thin skin with purpura	Steroid treatment—likely to be rheumatoid arthritis
Atrophy of the pulp of the finger	Systemic sclerosis
Calcinosis	Systemic sclerosis
Scleroderma facies (*fay-seize*) (beaked nose, small mouth, and telangiectasia)	Scleroderma

Fig. 13.4. Look for linear scars suggesting previous surgery such as decompression of the carpal tunnel or tendon sheaths or joint replacement.

(a)

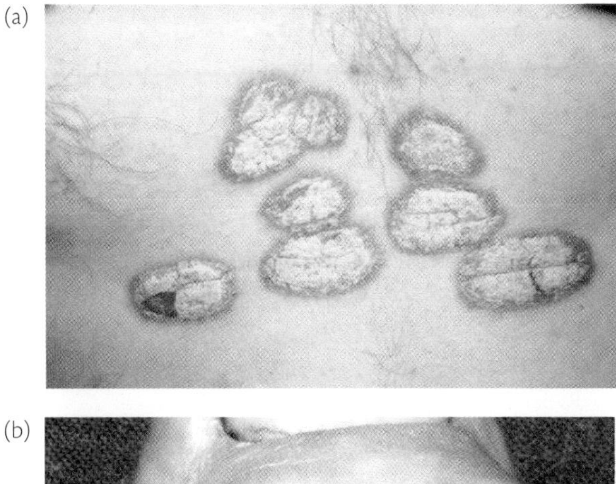

(b)

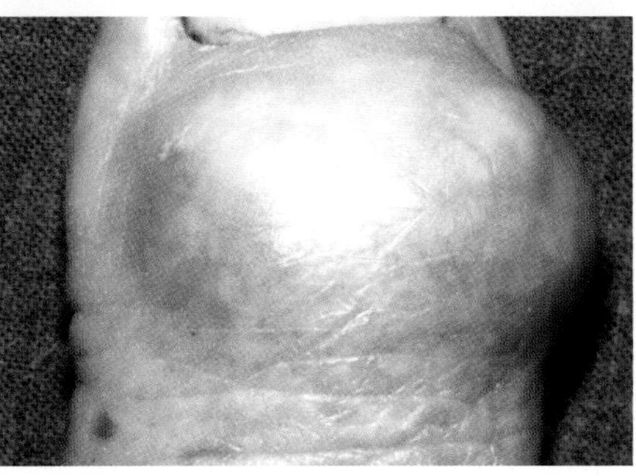

Fig. 13.4 (a) Psoriatic plaques and (b) gouty tophus.

Bones and joints

Inform the patient that you are now going to concentrate on the bones and joints in the hands. Note that DIP = distal interphalangeal, PIP = proximal interphalangeal, MCP = metacarpophalangeal, IC = intercarpal, and CMC = carpometacarpal. Say, 'I am now going to look at the bones and joints in your hands. I am going to gently squeeze over the joints, tell me if they hurt.' You should look, feel, then move the bones and joints. Are there any bony deformities, such as Heberden's (*hebber-dens*) nodes (*William Heberden Sr (1710–1801), English physician*) to suggest osteoarthritis? Osteophytes (small bony outgrowths around the joint margin) develop in osteoarthritis; when found at the DIP joints, they are called Heberden's nodes (those found at the PIP joints are called Bouchard's (*boo-shards*) nodes) (*Charles Joseph Bouchard (1837–1915), French physician*). Look and feel for joint swelling–is there any synovitis (boggy soft tissue swelling around the joint)? Carefully palpate along the digits. If the MCP joints look swollen, ask the patient to clench their fist. Normally, you will see the knuckles clearly defined. If synovitis is present there will be generalized swelling around the knuckles obscuring their definition. Remember that swollen joints may be painful. Joints may become dislocated (displacement of the ends of bones forming a joint so that they do not touch) and subluxed (partial dislocation, so that there is some contact with the ends of bones within the joint). These changes occur typically in rheumatoid arthritis. See Table 13.6 for some signs of joint disease. The hand changes in rheumatoid arthritis are characteristic and should be learned as they are common (see Fig. 13.5 and Table 13.7). Remember to expose and look at the elbows for any rheumatoid nodules. They are also found over many of the extensor tendons and along the ulna border of the forearm. Ask the patient to both flex and extend the wrist joints. Again joint swelling or pain will restrict this movement. It is also worth considering the patterns of symptoms and signs. The existence of a symmetrical MCP synovitis may indicate rheumatoid

TABLE 13.6 Some signs of joint disease

Sign	Disease suggestive of
Heberden's nodes	Osteoarthritis
Bouchard's nodes	Osteoarthritis
Synovitis	Often associated with rheumatoid arthritis
Subluxation	Rheumatoid arthritis

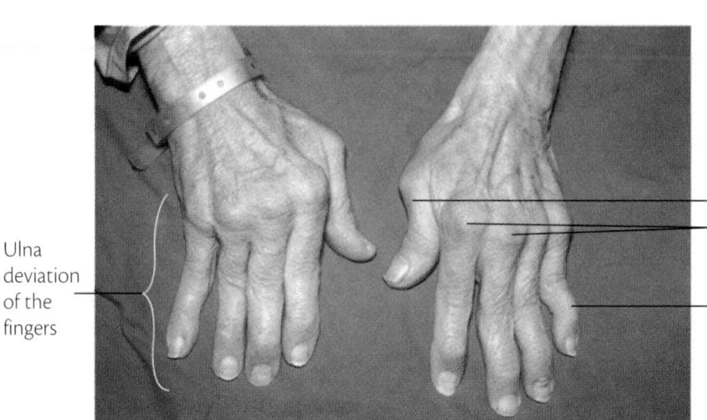

Fig. 13.5 Rheumatoid hands.

TABLE 13.7 The hand changes of rheumatoid arthritis

Changes	Explanation
Swelling of the MCP and PIP joints	Synovial thickening/synovitis
Swan neck deformity	Hyperextension of PIP joints with fixed flexion of MCP and DIP joints
Boutonnière (*boot-on-knee-airs*) deformity	MCP flexion deformity of PIP joint with extension contracture of DIP and PIP joints
Z deformity of the thumb	Subluxation at the base of the thumb
Palmar erythema	
Triggering of the finger	Flexor tendon nodule interrupting smooth movement of tendon in tendon sheath
Ulnar deviation of the fingers	Subluxation at the MCP joints
Rheumatoid nodules	Fibrinoid material surrounded by inflammatory cells

MCP, metacarpophalangeal; PIP, proximal interphalangeal; DIP, distal interphalangeal.

arthritis, whereas DIP and large joint involvement suggest a seronegative spondyloarthritides such as psoriasis.

Muscles

The muscles can be normal or wasted. You should concentrate on the pattern of wasting:

(1) **disuse atrophy**—generalized wasting of the muscles of the hand;

(2) **ulnar nerve lesion**—wasting of the hypothenar eminence and dorsal and palmar interossei (*inter-ross-ee-eye*) (intrinsic muscles of the hands) with sparing of the thenar eminence;

(3) **median nerve lesion**—wasting of the thenar eminence.

Generalized wasting of the small muscles of the hand is common in chronic arthritides affecting the hands. Specific wasting relating to a mononeuropathy is less common. However, carpal tunnel syndrome secondary to rheumatoid arthritis is the cause of a median nerve palsy (see Chapter 9). The affected muscles will demonstrate a reduction in power and there will be sensory loss in the distribution of the nerve.

Elbows

An essential part of the examination of the hands is to look at the elbows. Ask the patient if you can look at their elbows (show them how you want them to be positioned—see Fig. 13.6). Look carefully at the elbow joint and also along the ulnar border of the forearm. Gently run your fingers over these areas. You should be looking and feeling for rheumatoid nodules and gouty tophi. Note that the presence of rheumatoid nodules in a patient with rheumatoid arthritis increases the

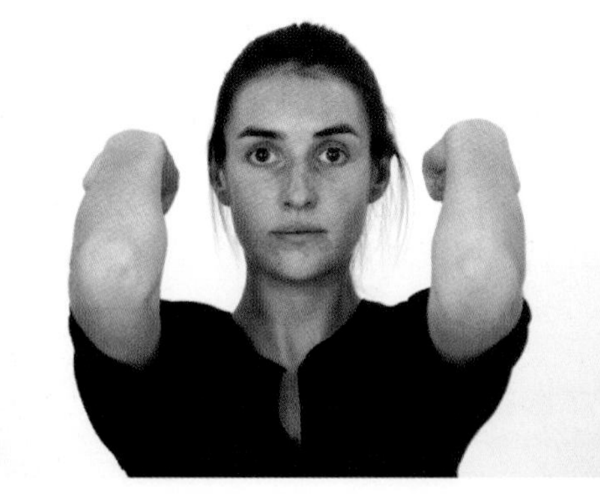

Fig. 13.6 Correct exposure of elbows.

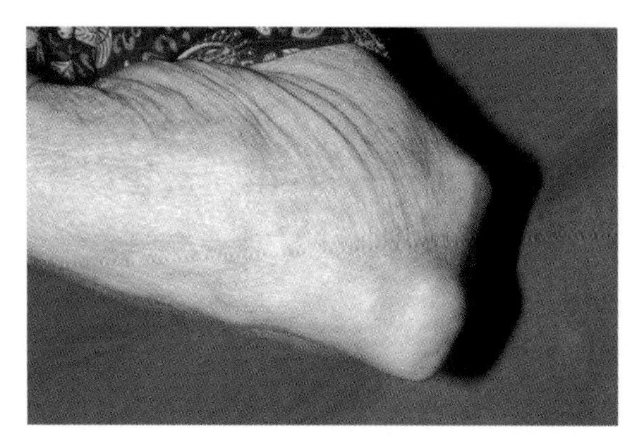

Fig. 13.7 Rheumatoid nodule at the elbow.

chance of them being seropositive for the rheumatoid factor (over 80%) (see Fig. 13.7). Ask the patient to place their hands back on the pillow, but this time with palms facing upwards. You should quickly re-examine the hands from this angle. Look for palmar erythema, Dupuytren's contracture, any muscle wasting in the palms, and any scars of previous surgery.

Function

It is extremely important to assess function. The author assesses gross function by asking the patient to perform five specific tasks.

1. Undo and redo a button.
2. Remove a pen top and demonstrate how they would write a letter.
3. Unscrew the top of a small container or medicine bottle (it is useful to carry one with you into an examination, see Fig. 13.8).
4. Demonstrate how they comb the back of their hair (this also assesses external rotation of the shoulder).
5. Pick different sized coins up from a table, see Fig. 13.8.

Remember that these functions will be limited by pain or deformity secondary to the arthritis so ask, 'Is pain stopping you from doing that task?' as it may not always be obvious.

Neurological examination

Any examination of the hands should include a neurological assessment. This is covered in Chapter 9.

Vascular examination

Also palpate the ulna and radial pulses (see Chapter 4).

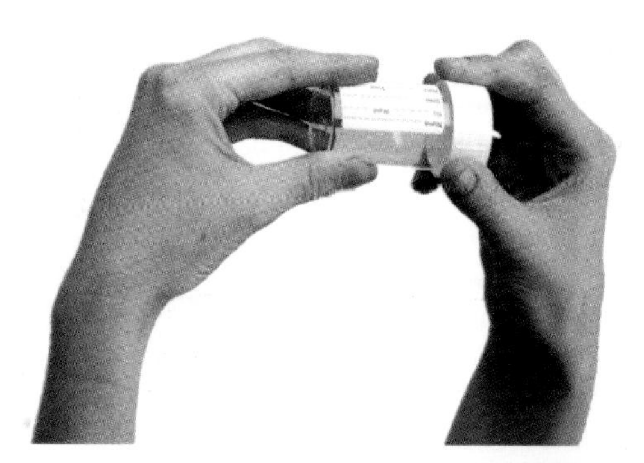

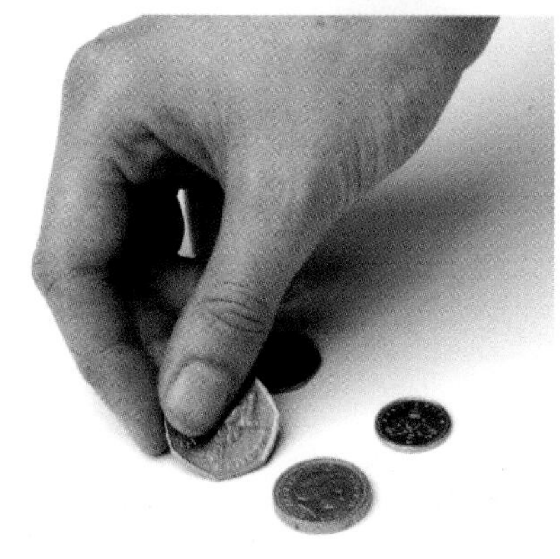

Fig. 13.8 Testing hand function.

Keypoints

- Always inspect for nail changes.
- Observe the skin for thinness, purpura, and rashes.
- Note any deformities of the hand. Are they symmetrical and characteristic of rheumatoid arthritis?
- Look for the pattern of muscle wasting. Disuse? Carpal tunnel syndrome?
- Never forget to inspect the elbows especially for rheumatoid nodules or plaques of psoriasis.
- Never forget to check function.

Shoulders

8. Examine the shoulder joint.

The primary function of the shoulder is the placement of the hand. It is a mobile joint, but as a consequence is less stable. Stability is provided by the rotator cuff, a collection of muscles and tendons that surround the shoulder joint. The muscles involved are supraspinatus (*soup-ra-spin-ay-tus*), infraspinatus (*in-fra-spin-ay-tus*), subscapularis (*subs-cap-you-lar-iss*), and teres (*terrys*) minor. Ask the patient to remove their shirt. This will provide you with an ideal opportunity to observe the shoulders (you may instantly see which shoulder is affected).

1. **Look.** Look at the shoulders from all angles, comparing each side with the other. Look for areas of skin discoloration, swelling, and muscle wasting. Swelling may represent an effusion or if overlying the clavicle a previous fracture. Muscle wasting affecting the deltoids will result in a flattened shoulder. This could be secondary to a neuropathy. Supraspinatus and infraspinatus (the muscles running from the scapula to the shoulder joint) will waste in chronic tendonitis or acute tear. Ask the patient to flex their biceps (ideally against resistance) looking for a ruptured biceps tendon. You will see a tightly contracted mass of biceps muscle either sitting high in the arm or distally near the elbow. See Fig. 13.9. Now ask the patient to push against a wall. This will reveal any winging of the scapula. Any pathology affecting the long thoracic nerve or the muscle it supplies (serratus (*sir-rate-us*) anterior) will cause the scapula to 'wing' or rotate so that it becomes a prominent bulge through the muscles of the back.
2. **Feel.** Gently palpate the shoulder and feel for swelling or crepitus. Crepitus is a grating, crunchy sensation you feel when a joint moves while your fingers are applied to it (it can sometimes be heard). It indicates degenerative changes within the joint. Swelling may be due to effusions, bursitis, dislocation, or old fractures and crepitus may be due to degenerative changes within the glenohumeral (*glean-owe-humour-al*) or acromio-clavicular (*a-crow-me-owe-cla-vick-you-lar*) joints. Palpate over the dorsal spine and the interscapular area. These areas are called trigger points and pain here may be suggestive of fibromyalgia (a benign, functional condition, giving rise to various aches and pains in muscles). There are many definitions for fibromyalgia, which include specific numbers of tender points throughout the skeleton. Remember tenderness in the interscapular area could equally be related to muscle spasm from a problem related to the thoracic spine. Check the supraclavicular fossa for any evidence of lymphadenopathy and sternoclavicular joints for evidence of arthropathy
3. **Move**. See Fig. 13.10. Assess both the active and passive movements of the shoulder joint and try to quantify them in terms of degrees of movement. When testing shoulder movement it is important to make sure you are not simply getting scapula movement contributing to movements of the shoulder. So observe the scapula during your assessment. Assess
   - abduction
   - adduction
   - flexion
   - extension
   - internal rotation (with the elbow flexed at 90°)
   - external rotation (with the elbow flexed at 90°).

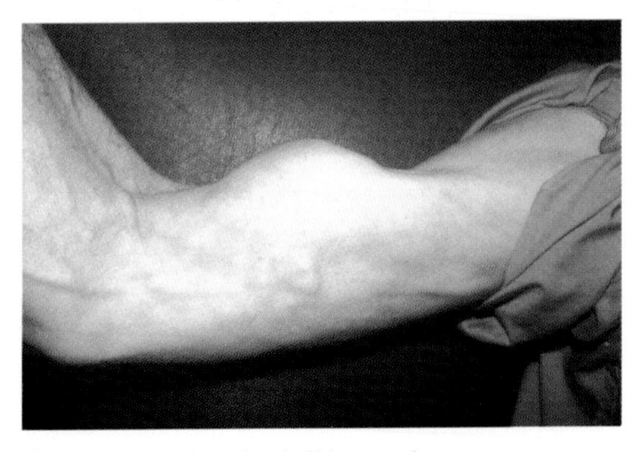

Fig. 13.9 Ruptured long head of biceps tendon.

Any limitation of movement is significant and may reflect underlying pathology affecting the glenohumeral joint. Other causes of impaired movement are capsular or subacromial bursitis, subacromial (*sub-a-crow-me-al*) impingement, rotator cuff tear, and tendonitis. Usually abduction is affected first. There may be signs of inflammation or an effusion. Limitation of active movement **only** suggests pathology of the muscles and tendons around the shoulder joint (the rotator cuff). Active movement is often painful. Limitation of active **and** passive movement suggests pathology of the shoulder (glenohumeral) joint itself. Limitation of movement may be due to pain or be 'mechanical' (bony or joint capsule) or inflammation. There are exceptions to any rule and capsulitis (*cap-sue-light-iss*) is one of these. With capsulitis, there is loss of passive as well as active movement yet the glenohumeral joint is normal. Perform a brief examination of the acromioclavicular joint. Look and feel the joint: undertake the scarf test—ask the patient to touch their opposite shoulder with the tip of their index finger. Observe the movement and note any tenderness. Other signs include mid-arc pain, which suggests rotator cuff tendonitis and subacromial impingement. Loss of external rotation suggests capsulitis.

(a)

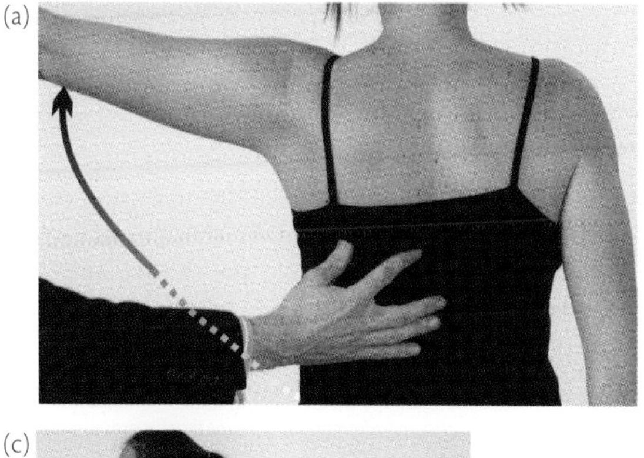

(b)

(c)

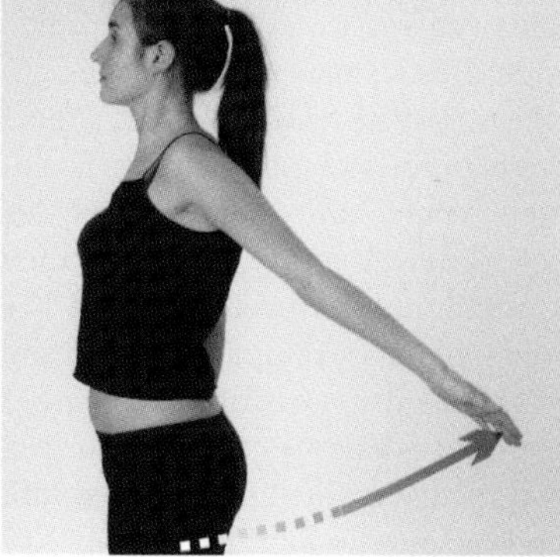

(d)

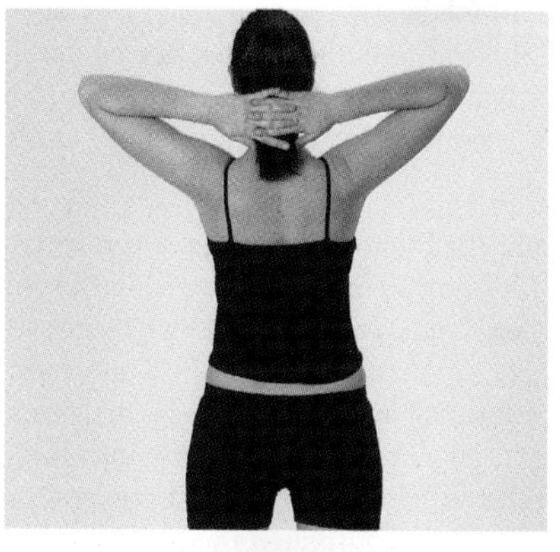

(e)

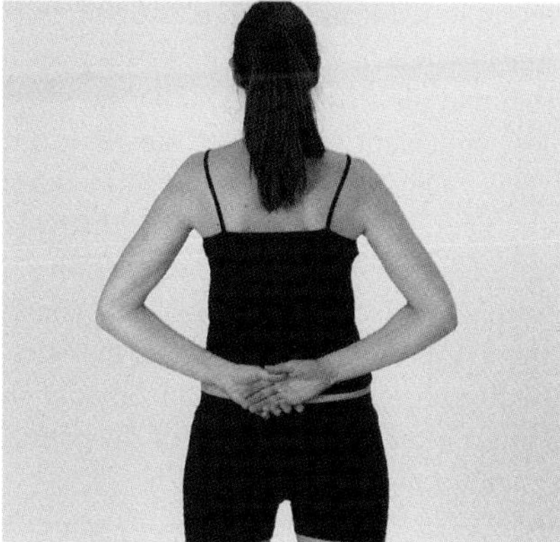

Fig. 13.10 Assessing shoulder movements. (a) Abduction, (b) flexion, (c) extension, (d) external rotation, (e) internal rotation.

Keypoints

- The shoulder is a mobile joint and is relatively unstable hence it is prone to dislocation and subluxation.
- A major contribution to the stability of the shoulder is by the rotator cuff muscles.
- Movements at the shoulder joint include abduction, adduction, flexion, extension, and internal and external rotation.

Hips

9. Examine the hip joint.

The hip is a ball and socket joint and has a major role in weight bearing. Disorders of the hip will present with pain and a limp. Examine the following:

- observe the gait
- measure leg length
- hip flexion
- hip abduction

CASE 13.3

Problem. A 45-year-old woman is referred to clinic with stiff swollen and painful joints. Her symptoms are worse in the morning and have been bad enough to keep her off work for the last 2 weeks. Her hands and feet are mostly affected. She complains of being tired, having a poor appetite, and being feverish. Recently she has had a rash over her front and back that disappeared quickly. She describes tiny non-tender lumps at the back of her ankles. She suffers from migraines and has had a DVT and chronic back pain secondary to a 'disc' in her back. She was found to be anaemic by her general practitioner who also performed X-rays of her hands that were reported to be normal. What is the diagnosis?

Discussion. This woman describes a symmetrical inflammatory polyarthropathy involving the small joints of her hands and feet and the diagnosis is likely to be rheumatoid arthritis. Patients often have constitutional symptoms such as malaise and fever and transient rashes are not uncommon. X-rays can often be normal in the early stages of rheumatoid arthritis. Although the rheumatoid factor was not analysed it has some diagnostic utility. However the absence of rheumatoid factor does not rule out rheumatoid arthritis. To make the diagnosis, the most important criteria are the clinical features. Patients must satisfy four out of seven criteria to receive a diagnosis of rheumatoid arthritis (see 'Diseases and investigations of the joints'): five are clinical, rheumatoid factor and radiological changes are the others. Laboratory tests such as markers of acute phase response and rheumatoid factor should always be interpreted in the context of the patient's clinical presentation.

- hip adduction
- internal rotation
- external rotation.

1. **Look.** Look as your patient walks into a clinic or on the ward. Do they have an antalgic gait. This is a limp secondary to pain in any part of the leg. With hip disease the patient will lean towards the affected side to minimize movement of the hip on walking. A Trendelenberg (*trend-ellen-burg*) gait (*Friedrich Trendelenberg (1844–1924), German surgeon*) is usually due to chronic hip disease. Here the patient will lean away from the affected hip. The pelvis on the unaffected side drops when they stand on the affected leg (in fact, you should ask the patient to stand on one leg then the other to emphasize this—this is called Trendelenberg's sign).

Tip

Do not forget to look for neurological causes for an abnormal gait.

Now measure the leg length from the anterior iliac spines (the bony protuberance over the upper pelvis) to the medial malleolus (*mal-lee-owe-lus*) (over the ankle joint) of the same side. This is called the true leg length because it simply measures the femur plus tibia/fibula (a difference of 1 cm between right and left legs is normal). But the patient could have identical true leg lengths and still look as though one leg is shorter than the other! This is usually due to problems with the pelvis or hip joint (or spine, for example, scoliosis) and for this reason you should also measure the apparent leg length. The apparent leg length is from the umbilicus to the ipsilateral medial malleolus and takes into consideration the pelvis and hip joint (a difference of greater than 2 cm is significant). Any tilting of the pelvis, for example, from curvature of the spine, will produce unequal apparent leg length despite the true leg length being equal.

2. **Feel.** Feel around the hip joint for any area of local tenderness. Feel over the greater trochanter (*trow-canter*) (this can easily be seen and felt when the patient is on their side, it is the bony protuberance on the lateral aspect of the upper thigh and is an important site of muscle insertions). The most common problem here is trochanteric bursitis (painful inflammation of the bursa overlying the greater trochanter).
3. **Move.** You can test all the movements of the hip (except hip extension) whilst the patient is supine. Start with passive movements and follow this order.
   1. **Hip flexion.** See Fig. 13.11. Flex the hip with knee bent. It should reach 120°.
   2. **Hip abduction.** See Fig. 13.12. Keep the legs straight and stabilize the pelvis with your left hand by placing it over the anterior iliac spine. Draw the right leg towards you (or left leg away from you) using your right hand to support the calf muscles. Once the pelvis starts to deviate (you will feel it start to abduct in line with the leg), this is the point of maximum hip abduction. It is usually about 45°.

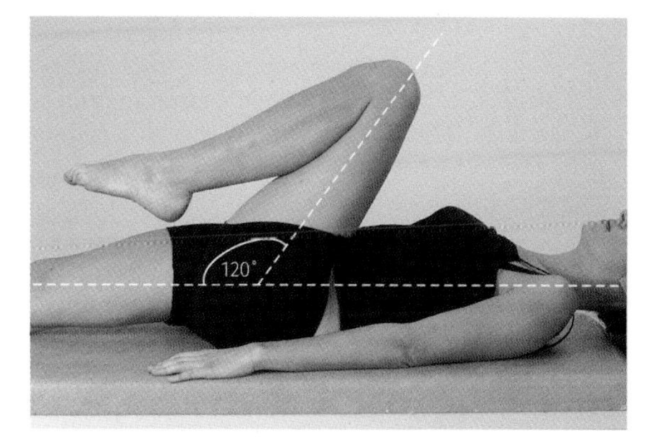

Fig. 13.11 Hip flexion.

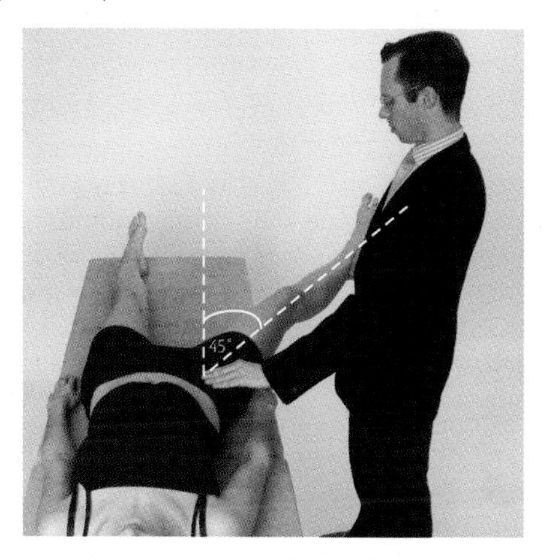

Fig. 13.12 Hip abduction (ensure the pelvis is stabilized).

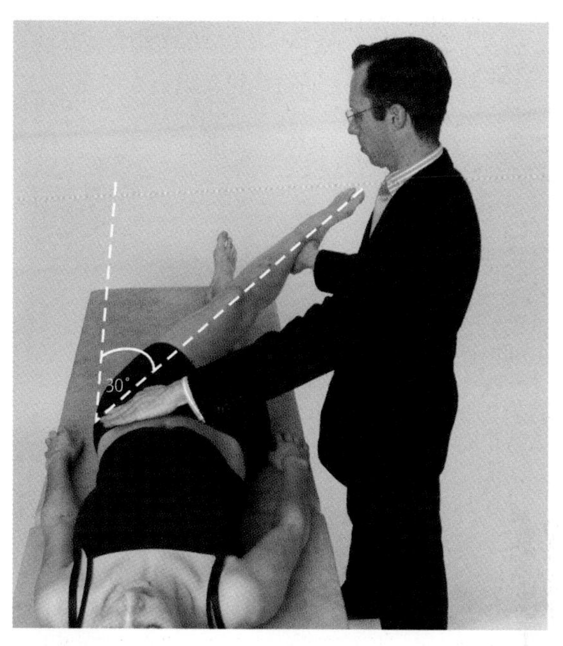

Fig. 13.13 Hip adduction.

3. **Hip adduction.** See Fig. 13.3. You can keep you hands in the same position as for abduction, but this time move the right leg away from you across the mid-line (or left leg towards you). Again, keep the leg straight and pelvis still. The normal angle of adduction is about 30°.
4. **Internal and external rotation of the hip.** See Figs 13.14 and 13.15. This is one of the earliest and most reliable signs of hip disease. Flex the knee to 90° and rotate the foot laterally, thereby turning the hip inwards. Similarly with external rotation, rotate the foot medially. You should be able to achieve 45° of both internal and external rotation.
5. **Extension of the hip.** Ask the patient to turn over so that they are prone; keeping the leg straight extend the hip. After performing the passive movement for each action get the patient to repeat the movement actively and note any pain or limitations of movement.

(a)

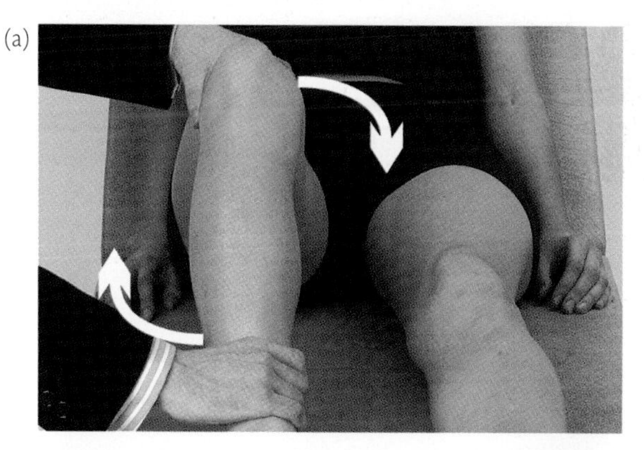

(b)

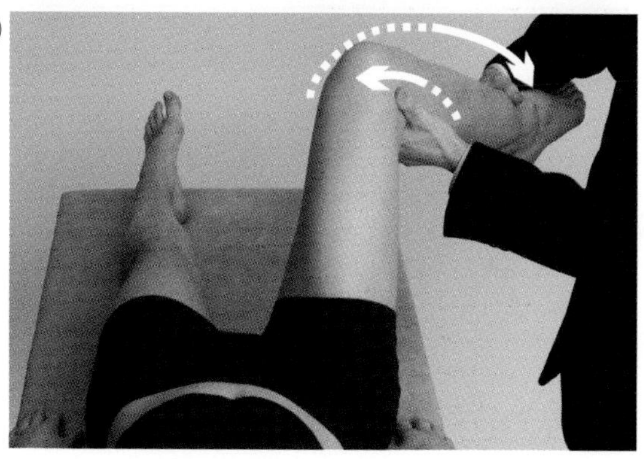

Fig. 13.14 Internal rotation of the hip.

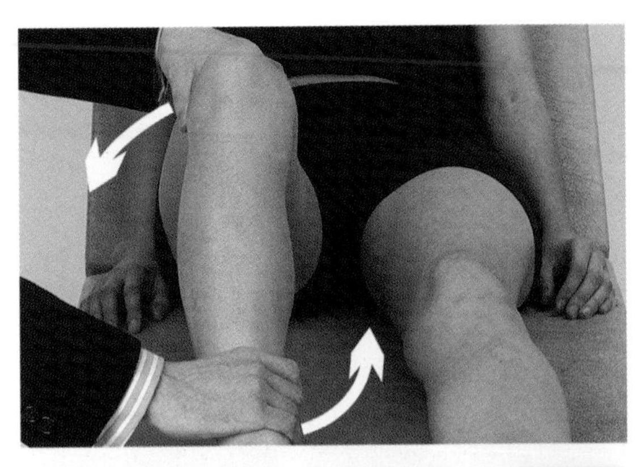

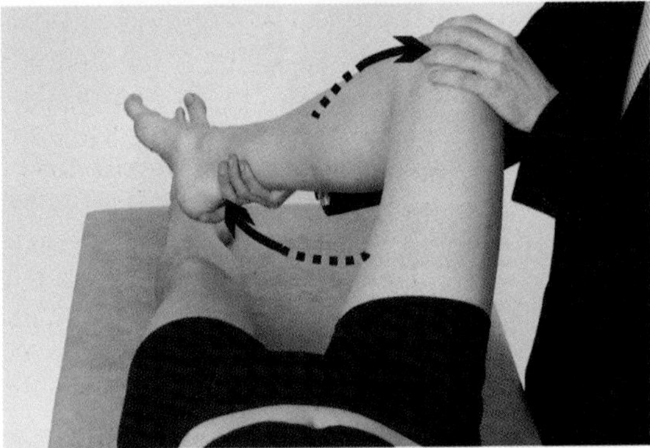

Fig. 13.15 External rotation of the hip.

Keypoints

- Always examine the gait of a patient with hip problems.
- Movements at the hip joint include abduction, adduction, flexion, extension, and internal and external rotation.
- Difficulty with internal rotation of the hip is one of the earliest signs of hip disease.

Knees

10. Examine the knee joint.

The knee joint is a modified hinge joint. Its stability depends on internal structures (cruciate (*crew-she-ate*) ligaments and menisci (*many-sky*)) and external structures (collateral ligaments and surrounding muscles). The menisci are crescent-shaped pieces of cartilage found in the medial and lateral aspect of the knee joint. They are relatively unstable and susceptible to injury. Both the seronegative spondyloarthritides (such as psoriatic arthropathy and ankylosing spondylitis) and rheumatoid arthritis commonly affect the knee.

Observation of the knee

Remove clothing covering the patient's lower limbs, but remember to cover the patient's groin to protect their modesty. Now look at the legs. There are certain features to look out for:

- genu varum (*jen-oo vair-um*)
- genu valgum (*jen-oo val-gum*)
- genu recurvatum (*jen-oo re-curve-ate-tum*)
- muscle wasting.

Genu varum

See Fig. 13.16. This is medial displacement of the tibia on the femur causing an outward bowing of the leg. Such 'bowing' of the legs can be due to rickets, injury, or infection. Sometimes an abnormality of the epiphyseal (*epi-fizzy-al*) growth plate or of the medial aspect of the knee may also cause genu varum.

Genu valgum

See Fig. 13.17. This is lateral displacement of the tibia on the femur. Again this may be due to injury, infection, or abnormalities of either the epiphyseal growth or of the lateral compartment of the knee. It is seen more commonly in inflammatory joint disease such as rheumatoid arthritis.

Genu recurvatum

See Fig. 13.18. This is hyperextension of the knee beyond 10°. This may be associated with hypermobility syndromes. For example, Ehlers–Danlos (*err-luz-dan-loss*) syndrome or pseudoxanthoma elasticum (*sue-dough-zan-though-ma-elastic-um*). Benign hypermobility syndrome is the most common cause where lax ligaments due to

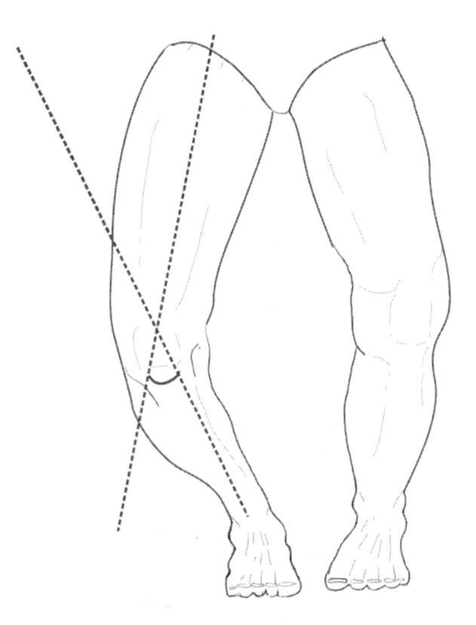

Fig. 13.16 Genu varum.

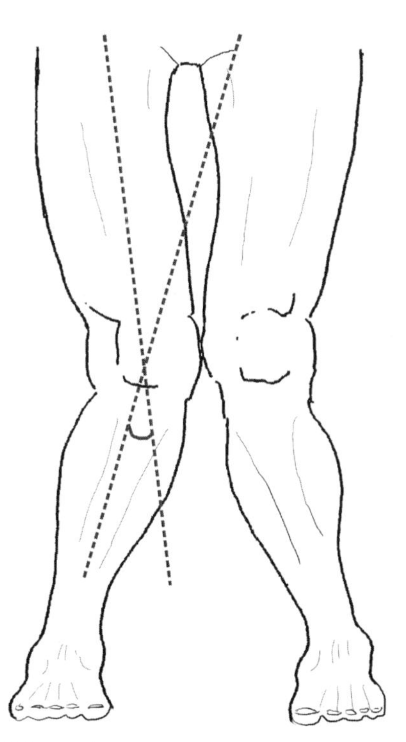

Fig. 13.17 Genu valgum.

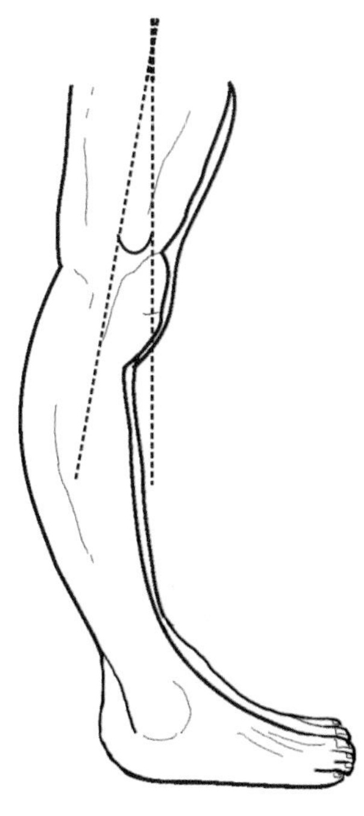

Fig. 13.18 Genu recurvatum.

abnormal collagen synthesis permit excessive movements at joints (in lay terms 'the double-jointed').

Muscle wasting

Look at the quadriceps muscle bulk. Any chronic painful knee condition will cause it to waste. You will need to examine many quadriceps muscles before you can appreciate subtle loss of muscle bulk. To monitor the rate of muscle wasting or recovery, it may be necessary to measure the circumference of the quadriceps. Do this at 10 cm above the superior pole of the patella.

Examination of swelling

There are many causes of a swollen knee. Often in a young fit person it is secondary to trauma causing a haemarthrosis. However, there are several inflammatory conditions that may cause it (see Table 13.8). The swelling can be due to fluid, bony growth, or synovial thickening. Swellings secondary to fluid are either generalized (an effusion) or localized (a bursa). There are a few clinical tests for effusions. For each test, start with the patient sitting on a couch or bed with their knees extended and exposed. First, inspect the knee for either an obvious suprapatellar pouch effusion or loss of the normal contours of the parapatellar gutters (see Fig. 13.20). Then perform the following more specific tests.

TABLE 13.8 Causes of a swollen knee

Septic arthritis
Rheumatoid arthritis
Osteoarthritis
Pseudogout
Gout

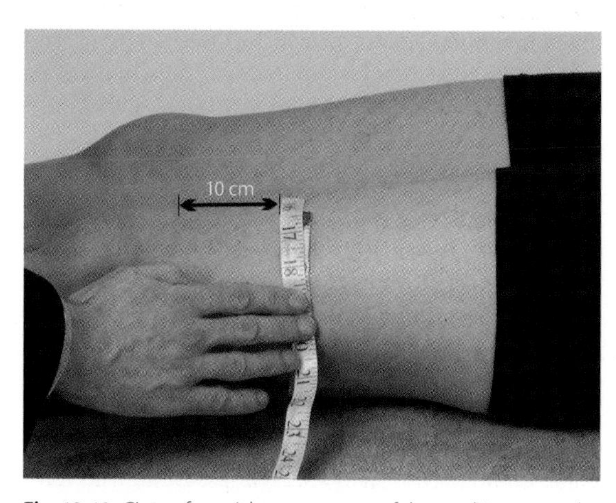

Fig. 13.19 Circumferential measurement of the quadriceps muscle.

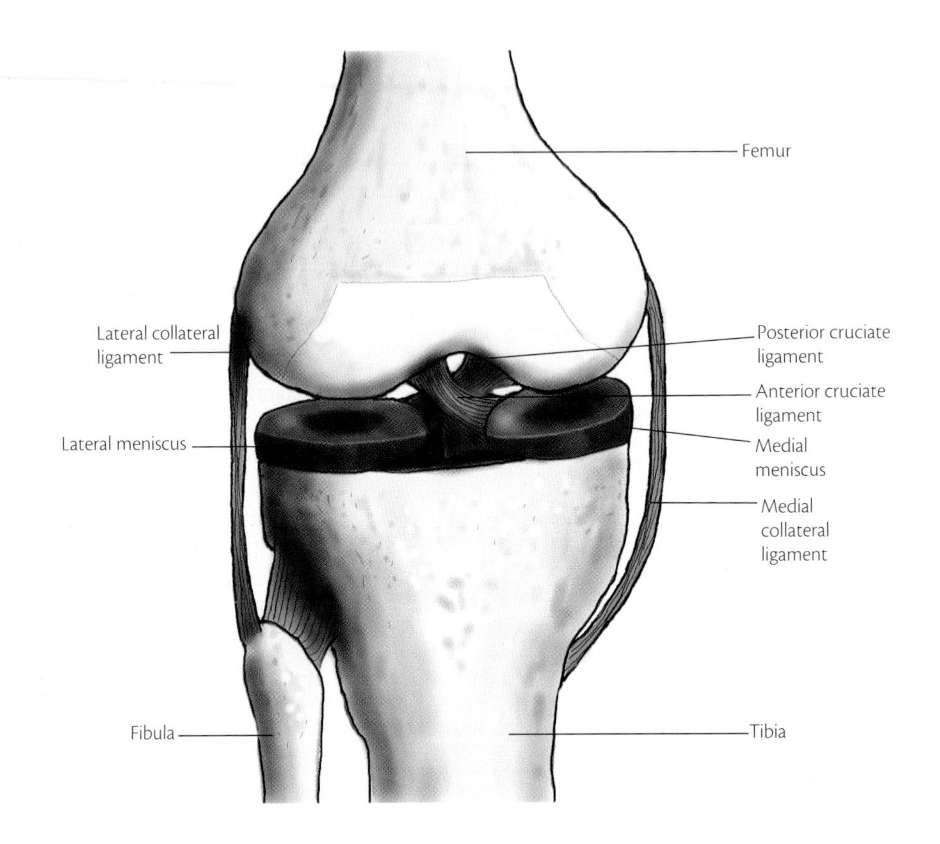

Fig. 13.20 Anatomy of the right knee joint.

Bulge test

See Fig. 13.21. This is a test for small effusions. Stroke the fluid around the knee with the palm of your right hand from the medial joint line proximally into the suprapatellar pouch. Now place your left hand across the medial aspect of the joint margin with the thumb resting on the patella. This will prevent any fluid passing back down the medial side of the knee. You can now stroke the fluid from the suprapatellar pouch back down the other (lateral) side of the knee using the dorsum of the right hand running down the lateral joint line. A bulge of fluid at the medial patella gutter confirms a small effusion.

Patella tap

See Fig. 13.22. This is a test for larger effusions. With the knees extended, place your left hand on the suprapatellar pouch (to contain the effusion within the pouch) and gently milk any fluid towards the patella, making sure you maintain downward pressure on the thigh (see Fig. 13.22). Now place your right hand on the patella and tap it. If fluid is present you will feel the patella descend before tapping against the underlying bone. Compare this with yourself (assuming you have no effusion). There should be no downward displacement of the patella or 'tapping' sensation. Note that if the effusion is very tense these tests will be less accurate. If the swelling looks localized, then consider a bursitis. Check its position and see if it correlates anatomically with a bursa. With any localized swelling define the consistency, dimensions, tenderness, presence of pulsation, reducibility, and transillumination (if a swelling transilluminates, it will glow when you shine the light from a pen torch through it—indicating the presence of fluid).

Ruptured Baker's cyst

A Baker's cyst (*William Morrant Baker (1839–1896), English surgeon*) is a swelling of clinical importance. It lies in the popliteal fossa (at the back of the knee) and if it ruptures precipitates sudden calf pain. The knee swelling may reduce and the calf may become swollen with pitting oedema. The most important differential diagnosis is that of a DVT as both produce similar signs (calf swelling, oedema, pain, and often redness). Patients presenting in this way should be investigated with an ultrasound scan of the veins of the leg (to check their patency) or a venogram (contrast is injected into the veins of the foot to see if there is good flow back up the leg. If the flow is blocked this suggests a clot in the vein). Ultrasound is particularly useful because it can also be used to confirm any

(a)

(b)

(c)

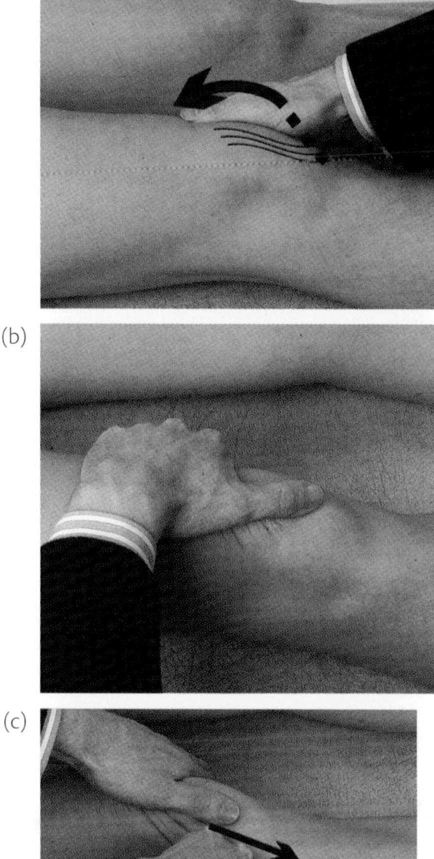

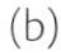

Fig. 13.21 The bulge test. (a) Stroking fluid proximally into the suprapatellar pouch, (b) holding the fluid in the suprapatellar pouch, (c) stroking fluid distally from the suprapatellar pouch.

fluid in the knee joint, any remnants of the baker's cyst, or any evidence of soft tissue oedema.

Examination for stability

The knee depends on a number of structures for its stability. This includes the cruciate ligaments, the collateral ligaments, the capsule of the knee, and the menisci. You should test for the stability of the collateral ligaments and the cruciate ligaments.

There are two collateral ligaments, the medial and lateral collateral ligaments.These ligaments run vertically on either side of the knee and prevent any medial

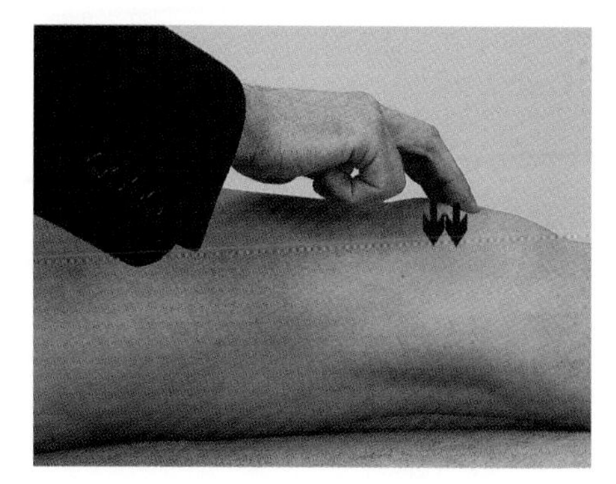

Fig. 13.22 The patella tap.

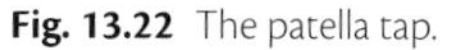

(varus) or lateral (valgus) movement. To test the collateral ligaments, the knee should be flexed at about 20°. Hold the ankle with one hand and support the thigh with the other. To stress the lateral collateral ligament, apply a valgus (lateral) force to the joint. If you are examining the right leg, you do this by pushing the ankle

(a)

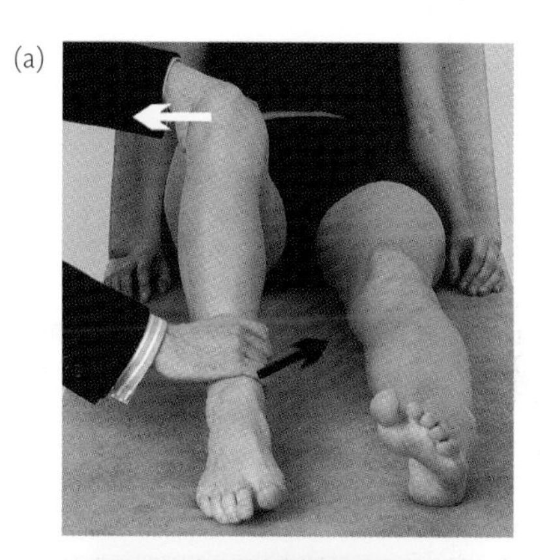

(b)

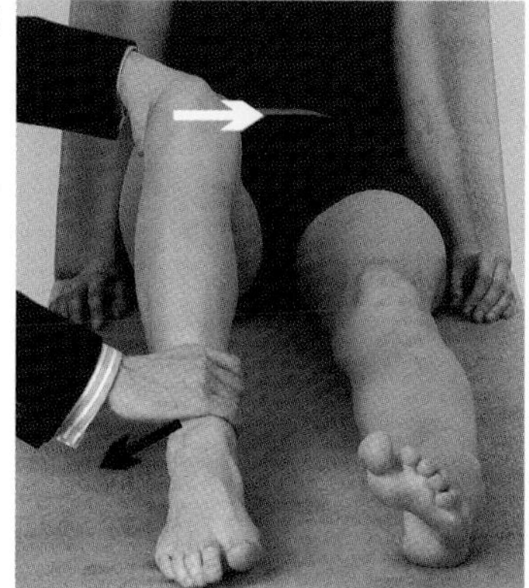

Fig. 13.23 Assessment of the collateral ligaments. (a) Stressing the medial collateral ligament: the white arrow represents the force generated by the left hand to stabilise the knee (to prevent its movement). The right hand attempts to move the ankle medially. (b) Stressing the lateral collateral ligament.

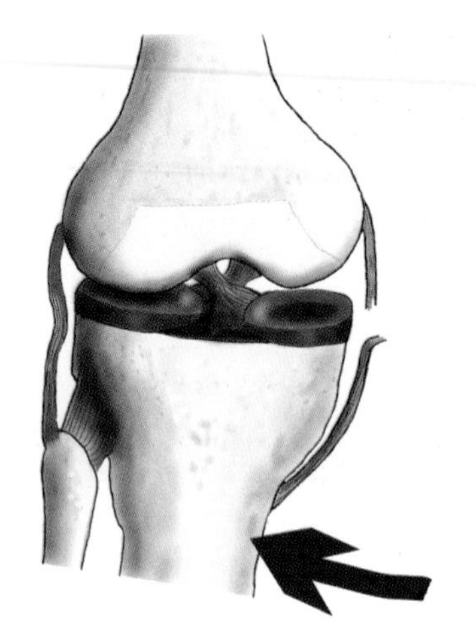

Fig. 13.24 Collateral tear showing angulation and separation. Any lateral movement of the tibia will cause undue displacement and angulation.

medially (away from your body) with your right hand and simultaneously pulling the inner aspect of the knee laterally with your right hand. To stress the medial collateral ligament, apply a varus (medial) stress to the knee, pull the ankle laterally (towards **your body**) with your right hand while simultaneously pushing the outer aspect of the knee medially with your left hand. Check the joint line between the tibia and femur for any separation. Any weakness or tear of the collateral ligaments will become apparent as a lateral (or medial) movement associated with a widening of the joint line on the opposite side of the knee. See Figs 13.23 and 13.24.

There are two cruciate ligaments, the anterior and posterior cruciate ligaments. The anterior cruciate ligament runs from the anterior aspect of the femur to the posterior aspect of the tibia. Similarly, the posterior cruciate ligament runs from the posterior aspect of the femur to the anterior aspect of the tibia. They prevent any anterior or posterior movement of the femur on the tibia. The anterior cruciate prevents the tibia slipping forward in a horizontal plane from the femur (and is essential for climbing down a flight of stairs). The posterior cruciate prevents the tibia slipping backwards on the femur.

Anterior cruciate assessment

Lachman's (*lack-mans*) test is used. The knee should be flexed at about 30°. Hold the femur securely by placing your left hand at the back of the thigh. Now hold the tibia with your right hand over the back of the calf muscles. Try to pull the tibia forwards on the femur. An intact anterior cruciate ligament will prevent any anterior movement. Any movement greater than 5 mm anteriorly is suspicious.

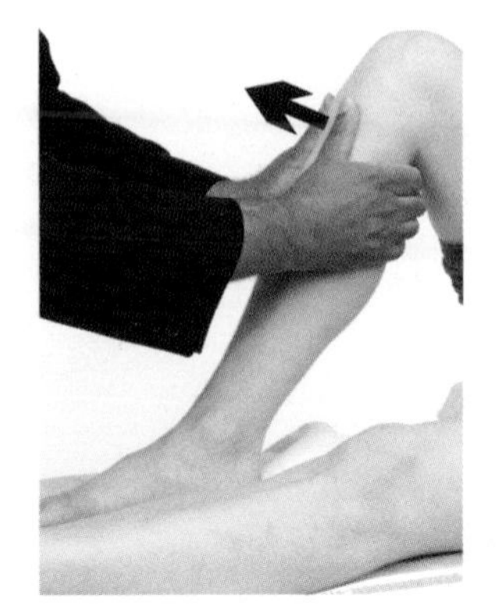

Fig. 13.25 The anterior drawer test: stressing the anterior cruciate ligament..

Anterior cruciate assessment

The anterior drawer test is used; it is similar to the Lachman's test, but the knee is flexed at 90°, see Fig. 13.25. The hip should not be in internal or external rotation as this prevents the anterior cruciate being assessed. For this reason it is inferior to the Lachman's test. If the tibia is internally rotated inadvertently it tightens the posterior cruciate. If there is now any anterior movement this will be due to a posterior cruciate tear.

Posterior cruciate assessment

The posterior drawer test is used. The knee should be flexed at 90°. If there is a posterior cruciate tear, there will be posterior subluxation of the tibia on the femur leading to the loss of convexity of the upper tibia compared with the normal one. See Fig. 13.26. Performing an anterior drawer test will correct this (the posterior drawer sign). As mentioned above you can also perform an anterior drawer test whilet the tibia is in internal rotation to assess the posterior cruciate.

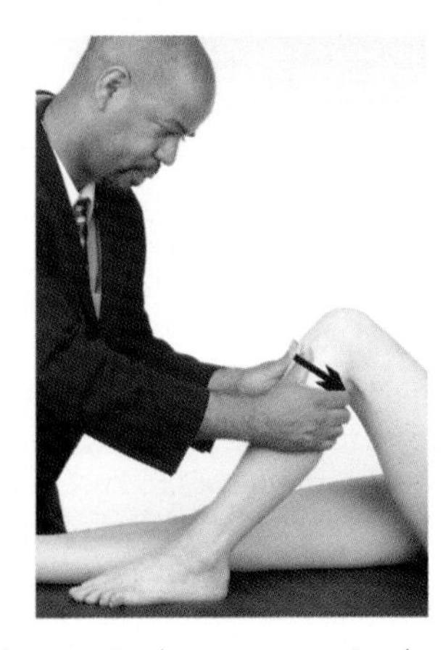

Fig. 13.26 The posterior drawer test: stressing the posterior cruciate ligament..

Range of movement

In testing the range of movement of the knees, there are several steps that you should consider:

- prone-lying test
- active hyperextension of the knee
- quadriceps lag
- passive extension of the knee
- active flexion of the knee
- passive flexion of the knee.

Prone-lying test

A flexion deformity of the knee could be missed on simple observation. The prone-lying test is a good way of demonstrating a flexion deformity. Ask your patient to lie prone on the bed or couch with their feet over the edge. The knees should extend naturally as the anterior aspect of the leg comes to rest on the examination surface. If there is a flexion deformity, the affected leg will remain elevated above the couch from the knee down. Chronic hamstring tightness, occurring in sportsmen and sportswomen, will produce a flexion deformity. The resistance to extension will be gradual on passive examination. A locked knee will produce a sudden painful resistance to extension and it represents the presence of intra-articular debris, for example, from meniscal tears. This requires orthopaedic attention.

Active hyperextension of the knee

When the patient is in the supine position, ask them to lift their heels off the couch whilst keeping their knees touching it. This is active hyperextension of the knee. Normal individuals should be able to hyperextend the knee joint to no more than 10° above the horizontal (see Fig. 13.27). Hyperextension beyond this is called genu recurvatum. See Fig. 13.18.

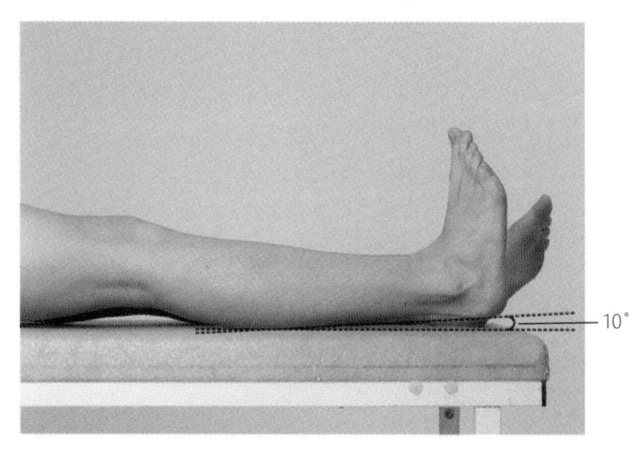

Fig. 13.27 Normal hyperextension of the knee.

Quadriceps lag

Now ask the patient to lift the lower limb off the couch with the knee extended. This will reveal any quadriceps lag, due to weakness. Essentially it takes a little longer for the leg to be raised because it is weaker than the other leg.

Passive extension, active flexion, and passive flexion of the knee

Ask the patient to (actively) flex the knee. Compare both sides. Now passively extend the knee and com-

> **Keypoints**
>
> - Note any deformity of the knee joint (the prone-lying test may unmask a subtle fixed-flexion deformity).
> - Always check the integrity of the knee ligaments with a painful knee.
> - If the knee is swollen perform the bulge test or the patella tap.
> - During active extension of the knee look out for quadriceps lag, which suggests weakness of that muscle group.
> - A ruptured Baker's cyst can mimic a DVT.

> **CASE 13.4**
>
> **Problem.** A thirty-two-year-old man injured his knee while playing football. It had swollen up to the size of a balloon but he did not seek medical help. After a 'few days in bed' the swelling had gone down and he went back to work as an accountant. He has presented to the casualty department because he has found on occasions his knee has 'seized up' and that he is unable to extend his knee. One episode was so painful he had fallen to the floor. What is the problem and what should be done?
>
> **Discussion.** Ideally you should get a clearer account of the mechanism of injury, for example, a direct blow to the knee or a twisting injury, to enable you to predict the possible consequences. However an important complication has ensued. He has developed a locked knee. This is an orthopaedic emergency because if he is not treated promptly he could damage his joint further. He will need arthroscopy to inspect the joint as it is likely that he has damaged a meniscus and a fragment or flap may be impeding the extension of the knee. As part of his examination you should also check the integrity of his ligaments to see if there is any joint instability.

pare it with the other side. Repeat the knee flexion as a passive movement. The range of movements should be full, equal, and painless.

Spine

11. Examine the spine.

Back pain is one of the most common causes of absence from work in the UK. Because the spine has many important functions (scaffold for the limbs, protection for the spinal cord, and a vibration damper), the slightest disorder will affect function dramatically. Patients with back problems usually present to the general practitioner, however, those with acute severe back pain often attend the accident and emergency department. There are several important causes of back pain. Most commonly it results from injury (trauma) through actions such as lifting heavy objects incorrectly or twisting suddenly, but occasionally a patient with back pain will be found to have a more sinister cause. Warning signs for possible serious spinal pathology include

- fever and unexplained weight loss
- bladder or bowel dysfunction
- history of carcinoma
- ill health or presence of other medical illness
- progressive neurological deficit
- disturbed gait or saddle anaesthesia
- age of onset <20 years or >55 years
- steroid use
- HIV infection.

Causes of back pain are shown in Table 13.9. For the purposes of examination, the spine can be divided into three segments: the neck (cervical spine), the upper back (thoracic spine), and the lower spine (lumbar spine). You should ask the patient to remain standing if you are going to examine the whole of the spine. If you are examining the neck, the patient may sit down.

TABLE 13.9 Causes of back pain

Causes of back pain
Trauma
Tumour
Inflammation
Infection
Mechanical/degenerative

Cervical spine

1. **Look.** Watch the patient as they walk into the room and study how they are holding their neck. Ask the patient to sit down if you are examining only the neck. Look at the neck from the front (anteriorly) and from the sides (laterally). When looking at the neck anteriorly, observe whether the neck is held straight

(a)

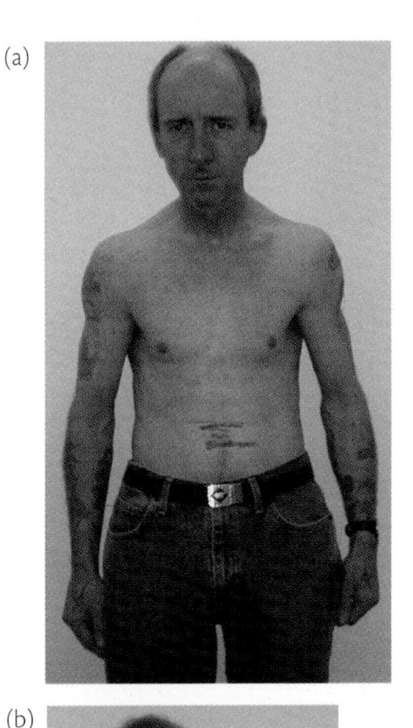

(b)

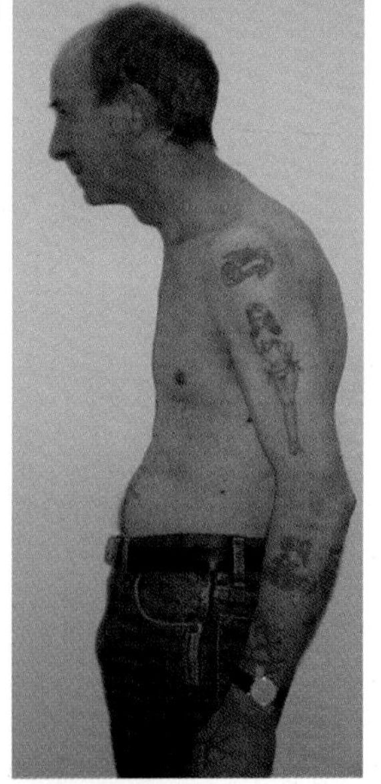

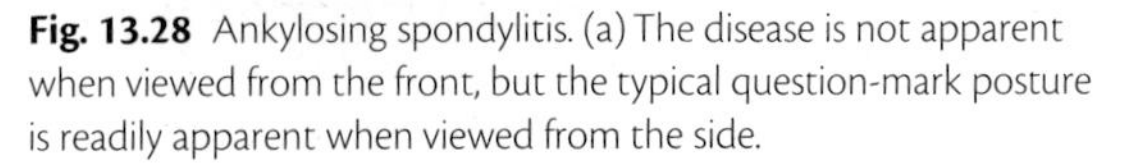

Fig. 13.28 Ankylosing spondylitis. (a) The disease is not apparent when viewed from the front, but the typical question-mark posture is readily apparent when viewed from the side.

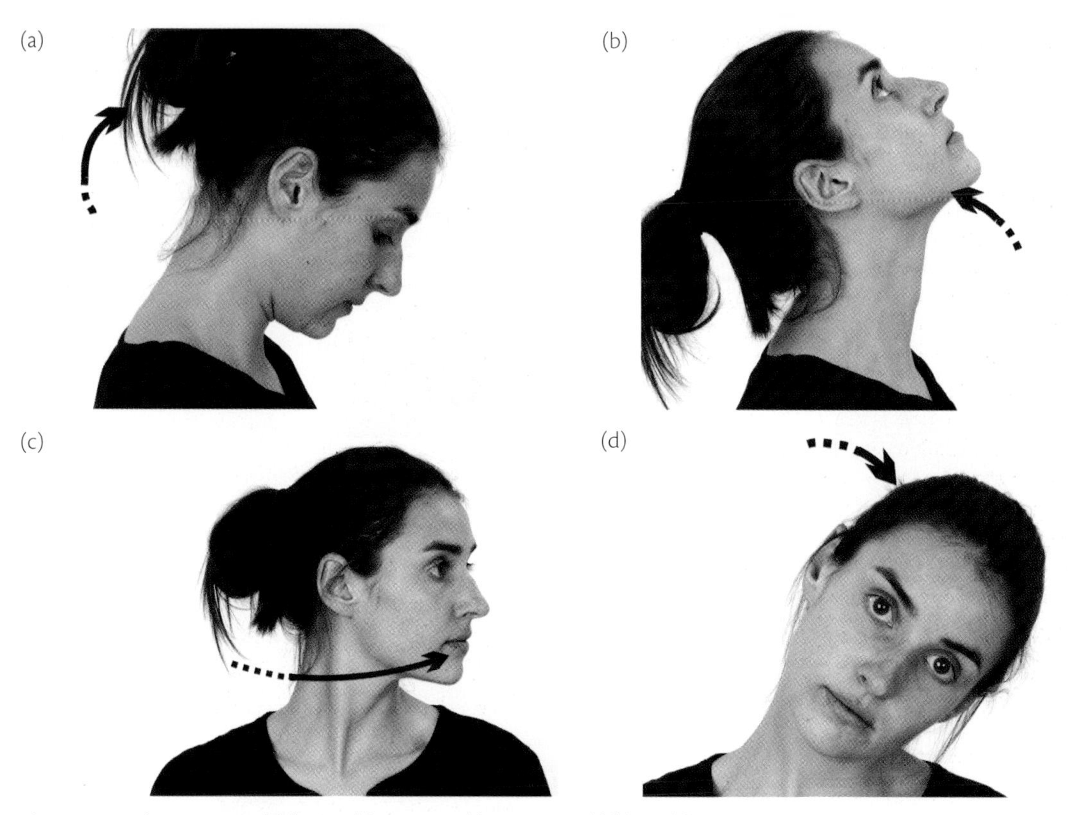

Fig. 13.29 Neck movements: (a) flexion, (b) extension, (c) rotation, and (d) lateral flexion.

or if it is twisted (torticollis) (*taut-ee-coll-iss*). Torticollis in an adult is often due to trauma (injury), chronic scarring of the cervical spine, or disorders of the cervical discs. In infants it can be caused by tumour of the sternocleidomastoid muscle. When observing the neck laterally, look for the normal curvature of the neck (convex forward—lordosis (*lord-owe-sis*)). It becomes exaggerated in ankylosing spondylitis to compensate for the abnormal backward curvature (kyphosis (*kye-foe-sis*)) of the thoracic spine that occurs in this disorder. See Fig. 13.28.

2. **Feel.** Palpate the neck to identify areas of local tenderness, which could represent inflammation or injury. Feel for enlarged lymph nodes. It is easiest to palpate from behind the patient, but remember to tell them exactly what you are about to do, as it is alarming to be grasped by the neck from behind!
3. **Move.** The neck has several basic movements (flexion, extension, lateral flexion, and rotation) that should be assessed (see Fig. 13.29). You should give clear explanations of the exact movement that you would like. It is preferable to show the patient the desired movement yourself. For example, if you ask your patient to place their left ear on their shoulder, they may do so by simply lifting up their left shoulder to touch their ear! This demonstrates good shoulder movement but defeats the purpose of the examination, that is, lateral flexion of the neck.

There are a couple of supplementary tests that should be considered when examining the neck.

1. **Lhermitte's (*ler-meets*) sign (the barber's chair sign).** (*Jacques Jean Lhermitte (1877–1959), French neurologist/psychiatrist.*) Flexion of the neck produces paraesthesia in the arms and sometimes legs due to nerve irritation. This occurs in multiple sclerosis.
2. **Reverse Lhermitte's sign.** This occurs when parasthaesia occurs in the arms on neck extension. It is due to cervical myelopathy (see p. 220).

Thoracic spine

1. **Look.** Observe the spine from the back (posteriorly) and the sides (laterally). The normal thoracic spine curves backwards slightly (kyphosis) (see Fig. 13.30) and the vertebrae should be aligned vertically on top of one another. Any curvature in the lateral plane is abnormal and is called a scoliosis (*scoe-lee-owe-sis*) (see

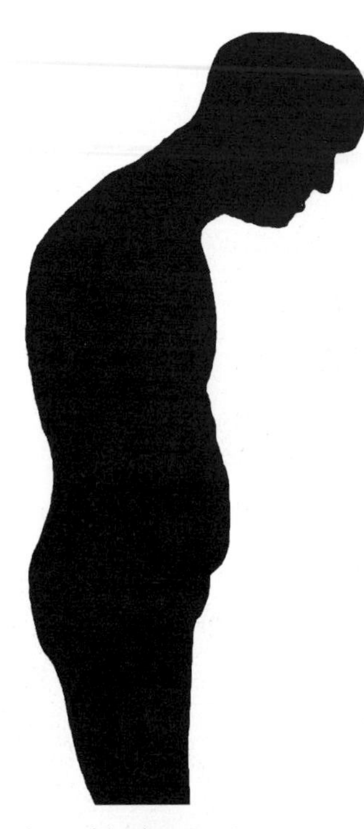

Fig. 13.30 Kyphosis of the thoracic spine.

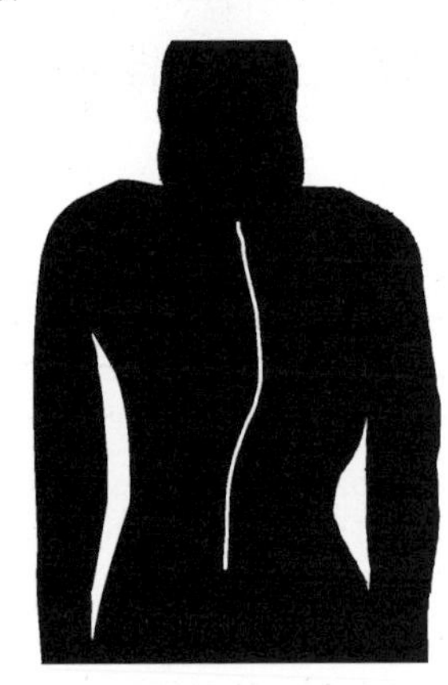

Fig. 13.31 Scoliosis of the thoracic spine.

Fig. 13.31). The normal thoracic kyphosis can increase gradually in chronic disorders such as ankylosing spondylitis, osteoporosis, or degenerative disc disease. It can occur acutely due to infection or fracture of the vertebrae. An angular kyphosis called a gibbus (*gib-bus*) may result. A small degree of lateral curvature is acceptable but more pronounced scoliosis can be due to

- leg length inequality
- postural (only occurs when the patient is sitting down)
- neurological disease (syringomyelia or neurofibromatosis)

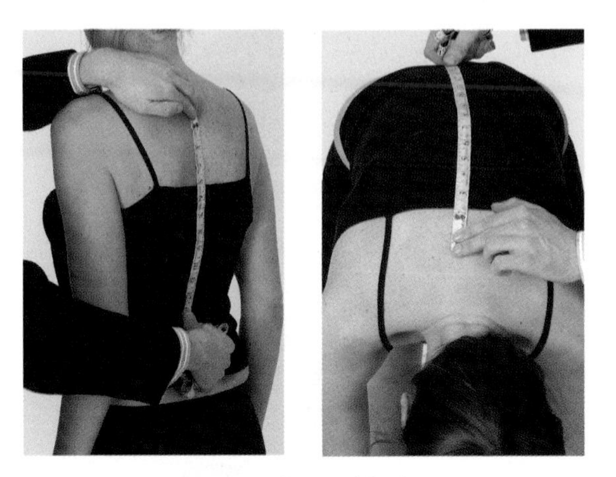

Fig. 13.32 Measuring anterior flexion of the thoracic spine.

- congenital (absent or fused vertebral discs)
- infected vertebral discs
- tumour (primary or metastatic) affecting the vertebrae.

However, commonly no cause is found and the cause is said to be idiopathic.

2. **Feel.** Gently feel along the spine and percuss individual vertebrae to locate areas of tenderness. A painful vertebra is significant and should alert you to the possibility of a collapsed vertebra, infection of the intervertebral disc, or a tumour affecting the spine.

3. **Move.** Measure the distance from the first thoracic disc (D1) to the last (D12) (see Fig. 13.32) (D = dorsal, synonymous with thoracic) and ask the patient to bend over (anterior flexion); the distance between these two points should increase by at least 3 cm. Ask the patient to run one hand down the side of their leg, this is lateral flexion and should achieve about 15° from the mid-line on either side. Next assess rotation by holding the patient's pelvis (or asking them to sit down) and ask them to twist to look over one then the other shoulder. Remember that flexion, extension, and lateral flexion of the thoracic spine are closely linked with that of the lumber spine and can be difficult to separate.

Lumbar spine

1. **Look.** Observe the lumbar spine both laterally and posteriorly. The lumbar spine has a lordosis. Determine whether the lordosis is exaggerated or lost. Is there a co-existent scoliosis? See Table 13.10 and Fig. 13.33.

TABLE 13.10 Causes of a loss of lordosis and exaggerated lordosis

Loss of lordosis
Degenerative disc disease
Exaggerated lordosis
Spondylolisthesis*
Fixed flexion deformity of the hips
Pregnancy
Obesity

* Spondylolisthesis (*spon-dee-loll-iss-thesis*) is the forward movement of a vertebra on the one below it (and tends to occur in the lumbar spine).

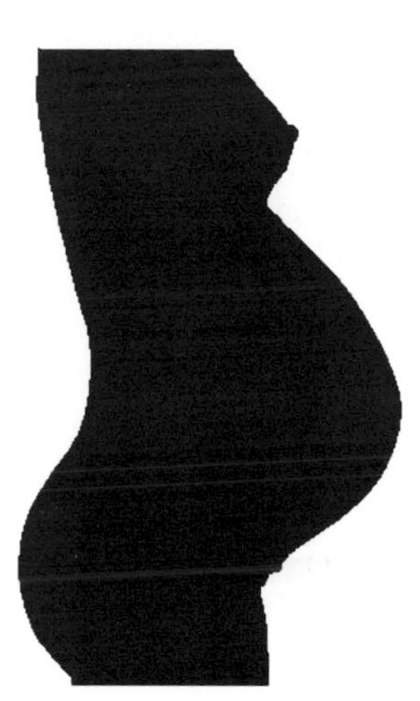

Fig. 13.33 Exaggerated lordosis due to pregnancy.

2. **Feel.** Gently feel along the vertebrae for areas of focal tenderness and percuss each one in turn.
3. **Move.** Movement of the lumbar spine is closely linked with that of the thoracic spine and it is difficult to isolate movements to one particular segment of the spine. In fact, there are specific tests for measuring flexion of the lumbar spine as there are for measuring flexion of the thoracic spine. Schober's (*show-burrs*) test is the best of these. When the patient is standing, identify the posterior superior iliac spines or the dimples of venus, that is, L5 (see Fig. 13.34) and mentally draw a line from one to the other. From the mid-point of this line measure 10 cm upwards and mark this point with a pen. Ask the patient to bend forwards to touch their toes and re-measure the distance from the pen mark back to the mid-point between the posterior superior iliac spines. The distance should be at least 15 cm. A reduction in flexion is often seen in ankylosing spondylitis. Normally the length of the lumbar spine should increase when bending forward. Also assess lateral flexion and rotation to see if they are full and equal.

(a)

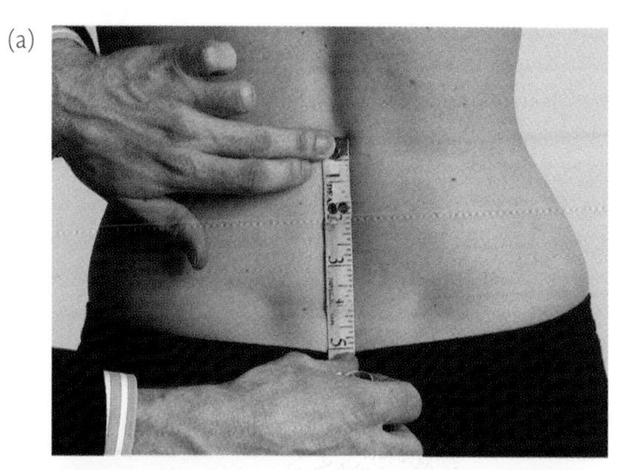

(b)

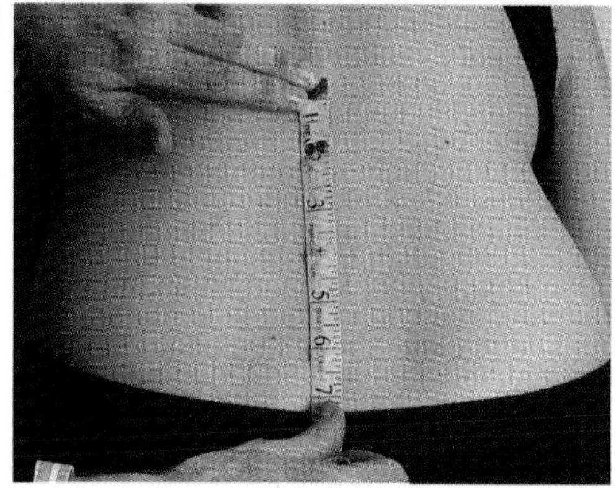

Fig. 13.34 Schober's test: (a) standing, (b) touching toes.

Keypoints

- The spine provides a scaffold for the limbs and organs, is a shock absorber, and protects the spine.
- The spine is conveniently divided into the cervical, thoracic, and lumbar regions.
- Normally the cervical spine has a lordosis, the thoracic spine a kyphosis, and the lumbar spine a lordosis. Look out for loss or exaggeration of these curvatures,
- Palpate and percuss each vertebra (and paraspinal area) and look for tenderness.
- Perform Schober's test to quantify flexion of the lumbar spine.

CASE 13.5

Problem. A seventy two-year-old male smoker is admitted with severe back pain. This occurred after he tried lifting a heavy bag of compost while leaning forward in an awkward position. He took solpadol, which gave some temporary relief but the pain is as strong as ever. On examination, he has a kyphosis and is tender around D10–D12. The pain is severe enough to restrict any movement of the spine. An X-ray reveals generalized osteopenia of the spine and wedge fractures of D9–D12. How should he be managed?

Discussion. Clearly he has sustained fractures of several vertebrae resulting from when he attempted to lift a heavy weight with a poor technique. Osteoporosis is prevalent in old age and leads to fragile bone architecture, which can predispose to fractures (even with trivial forces). It is a disease that affects women predominantly (one in three women over 50 years) but what is not widely appreciated is that it can affect men too (one in 12 men over 50 years). Despite this, your patient is a 'young fit' older person (assumed, as he is still gardening) and therefore you need to consider other pathological causes of osteoporosis. Check that he is not on steroids and he needs screening for thyrotoxicosis, malabsorption, liver disease, myeloma, and other malignancies including prostate cancer with prostate specific antigen. He will need regular analgesia until his pain settles and treating in the acute setting with the intravenous bisphosphonate (*buy-foss-phone-ate*) pamidronate (*pam-id-roe-nate*) (which also has a good analgesic effect). If no secondary causes of osteoporosis are found he should continue with oral biphosphonate treatment to protect his spine, have a dual energy X-ray absorphometry (DEXA) bone scan to monitor the density of bone and be advised to stop smoking as this is a risk factor for osteoporosis.

The GALS assessment

12. The GALS assessment.

The overall integrity of the musculoskeletal system can be screened very quickly. Indeed, most of the examination can be done without touching the patient, by simply asking the patient to follow your movements (it is easier to show someone what you mean than to describe it to them). The main signs of rheumatic disease are swelling and deformity, plus pain and difficulty with movements. Consequently, the minimum screening examination involves

(1) looking for any swelling or deformity and for any abnormal position or posture of the limbs or individual joints.

(2) Observing the patient move and looking for any difficulty or restriction of movement.

The order in which the system is examined is not important and depends on the situation (outpatients, ward, and so on) and the patient. Essentially four components must be assessed and can easily be remembered using the acronym GALS (**g**ait, **a**rms, **l**egs, **s**pine). This is a rapid and efficient way of assessing the integrity of the musculoskeletal system. It is **not** a diagnostic examination. It is a screening procedure to indicate which aspects of your examination require more detailed assessment. As the patient performs a movement, enquire if it is painful. If abnormalities are noted, examine these in more detail as described earlier. Once you become familiar with all aspects of the rheumatological examination you will be able to perform the GALS screen quickly and efficiently.

Gait

This can be done as the patient walks towards you in any clinical setting. Look for a normal symmetrical gait. Disorders of the musculoskeletal system can lead to a variety of gait abnormalities including loss of symmetry, stiffness, and pain on walking. Some patients need walking aids, others need help with transfers. You should observe how easily they manage to sit and get up from a chair. Look at their knees (varus, valgus, flexion deformity?), look at their feet (pronation, valgus deformity, toe posture?), and look for unsteadiness—especially when turning. Make a note of their posture—look for normal spinal curvatures (cervical lordosis, thoracic kyphosis, and lumbar lordosis).

Arms

Hand

Ask the patient to perform the prayer sign (see Fig. 13.35). It tests wrist extension (and when reversed, flexion), MCP and PIP joint extension, and flexor tendon and soft tissue stretch. Ask the patient to make a fist—are they able to cover their nails? Assess the 'pinch' and 'power' grips (see Fig. 13.36). With the patient's hand extended, look for 'squaring' of the hand, for CMC osteoarthritis, and osteophytes at DIP joints (Heberden's nodes) or PIP joints (Bouchard's nodes). Perform a lateral squeeze by gently and progressively squeezing across MCP joints, noting any tenderness that may be found in an inflammatory

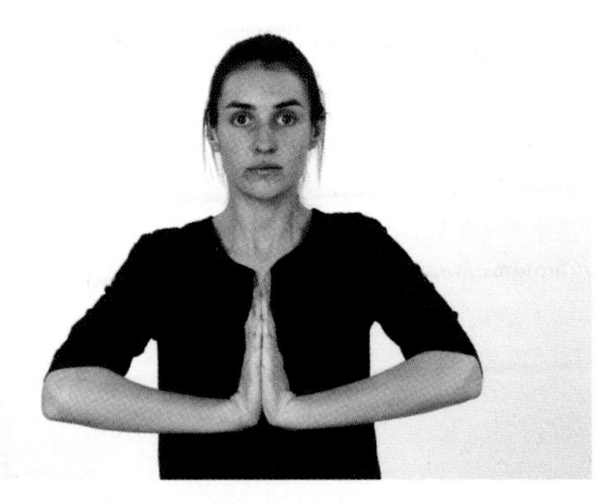

Fig. 13.35 The prayer sign.

(a)

(b)

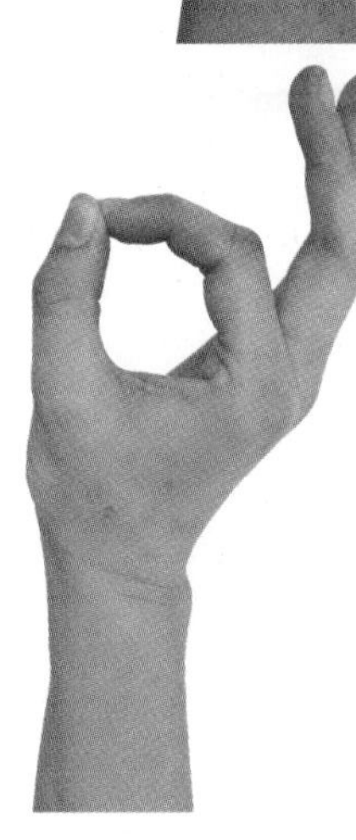

Fig. 13.36 (a) Fist and (b) pinch.

arthritis. Examine for synovial swelling (synovitis) and look for loss of joint contours. Feel for soft tissue swelling obscuring the normal joint outline and for synovitis at the PIP joints. Remember synovial thickening has a similar consistency to a grape! Tendon sheaths are lined with synovium; feel for thickening and crepitus in rheumatoid arthritis and 'triggering' due to a nodule (rheumatoid arthritis or SLE).

Elbow

The elbow extends to at least 180°, but not usually beyond 190°. It flexes to allow the fingers to touch the shoulder easily. Test the proximal radio-ulnar joint with the elbow tucked in. Ask the patient to turn their hand palm down (pronation), then palm up (supination).

Shoulder

Check shoulder abduction and elevation, noting the transition from glenohumeral movement to scapulothoracic movement. Internal rotation is a functionally important movement for dressing. Also assess external rotation; it is especially restricted in lesions of the shoulder capsule

Spine

You cannot examine the spine with the patient fully dressed because you will need to see and feel the anatomy.

Cervical region

The patient may sit or stand for this. The levator scapulae (*le-vay-tor-scap-you-lee*) is often tender to gentle squeeze in cervical spine problems and also in fibromyalgia. The neck becomes stiffer with age so loss of movement does not always indicate disease (lateral flexion is more sensitive for detecting symptomatic lesions).

Dorsal region

Ask the patient to sit (to eliminate rotation at the pelvis and legs) and then rotate their torso.

Lumbar region

With the patient standing ask them to touch their toes noting separation of the lumbar spinal processes. If the patient complains of back pain or if movement is restricted, further assessment is warranted and more so if there is leg pain or paraesthesiae.

Legs

Hip

With the patient supine, check hip flexion.

Knee

Abnormal swelling may be due to fluid, bony, or soft tissue swelling— look for loss of the normal contours and test for effusions.

Foot and ankle

Inspect the sole for calluses, look for abnormal separation of the toes, then gently squeeze the metatarsal heads. Examine for asymmetry or abnormal posture. Pain or observed abnormalities require further assessment.

Wash your hands

13. Wash your hands

Don't bug your patients.

Presentation of findings

14. Presentation.

Now start your presentation. If your findings point to a diagnosis, then be confident and mention this up front, for example, 'The diagnosis is rheumatoid arthritis because there is a symmetrical deforming inflammatory arthropathy with evidence of swan neck and boutonnière deformity of the fingers. There is a Z deformity of the thumb and palmar erythema. There is wasting of the small muscles of the hands and ulnar deviation of the fingers. The distal interphalangeal joints are spared and there are nodules at the elbows. This is consistent with rheumatoid arthritis and the presence of nodules increases the likelihood of the patient being seropositive for rheumatoid factor. I would now like to go on and examine the chest for any signs of pleural effusion, the skin for steroid induced changes, and the eyes for for scleritis.'

CASE 13.6

Problem. a 54-year-old woman is referred to clinic with neck pain. She also has pain in her shoulders, wrists, and hands, which she has had for 2 years and 'nobody has done a thing about it.' She is unable to sleep at night and her appetite is poor. She says she has swelling of all her joints and she is stiff all over every day. She suffers with headaches and has irritable bowel syndrome, which has flared up recently. She works as a secretary and is having a stressful time at the moment. On examination the pain is not limited to any specific joint and there are several points over her neck, trapezius muscle, shoulders, and back that are tender to the touch. Although she says her joints are swollen, they are normal with no signs of inflammation. She has a full range of movement of all her joints. What is the diagnosis?

Discussion. This case seems difficult at first sight and it is easy to be overwhelmed by the amount of pain and the patient's multiple symptoms. Some clues are apparent however. The pain is diffuse and not confined to a joint and despite the patient complaining bitterly of joint swelling there is no objective evidence for this. The pattern of symptoms is not consistent with inflammation, that is, inflamed joints are not stiff all the time and the patient has a full range of movement. With the diffuse nature of the pain and multiple tender spots the diagnosis is likely to be fibromyalgia. This is an ill-defined condition with no discernible pathology (see p. 387) and tends to be linked with disorders such as tension headache, irritable bowel syndrome, and chronic fatigue syndrome. These conditions tend to get worse at times of stress and it is notable that the patient is under pressure at work. It is said that such people should not be over-investigated because this will reinforce the idea that something serious is wrong. This is a sensible approach, although in practice a beleaguered general practitioner may well refer to a number of specialists over time as symptoms recur and an insistent patient pleads for something to be done.

CASE 13.7

Problem. A 72-year-old woman gives a 3-week history of progressive pain and stiffness in her shoulders and hips. It has gradually worsened so that she cannot get out of a chair easily and is unable to climb stairs, forcing her to sleep downstairs. She also has difficulty combing her hair and her scalp feels sore when she attempts this. Getting food out of the top cupboards in the kitchen has been impossible. She has also had drenching night sweats and has lost a stone in weight. Examination revealed very little. There was no joint inflammation and she had good power in all her limbs although movements were limited by pain. There were no rashes but she was tender over her right temporal artery. What is the diagnosis?

Discussion. The history suggests a proximal muscle problem and possibly a myopathy. However the patient's power is preserved and movements are limited by pain only. Other important clues are the tender temporal artery and the soreness when she combs her hair. The diagnosis is polymyalgia rheumatica and it is likely that she has temporal arteritis. Systemic features such as nights sweats and weight loss can accompany temporal arteritis. Even so, it is worthwhile excluding other possible causes, for example, polymyositis, underlying malignancy, and even an atypical presentation of rheumatoid arthritis. Further investigations should include a temporal artery biopsy, creatine kinase (CK) enzyme, rheumatoid factor, and a possible search for malignancy. Treatment with steroids rapidly improved her symptoms.

Diseases and investigations of the joints

In the earlier parts of this chapter, various medical conditions have been mentioned. In this section they are now described. In general these descriptions are brief

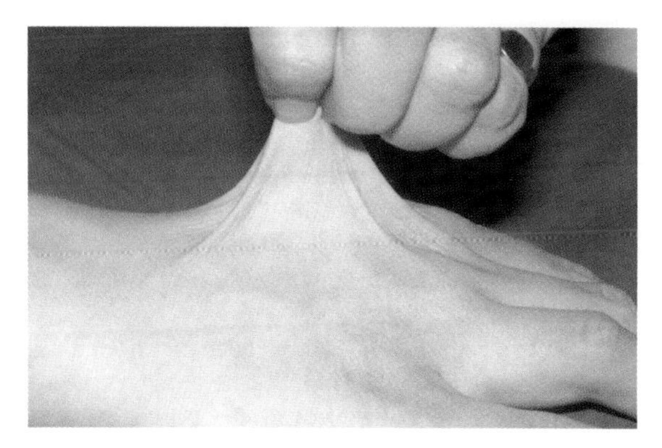

Fig. 13.37 Ehlers–Danlos syndrome. The skin is elastic and distensible.

though certain aspects not well described in other textbooks are discussed in some detail

Ehlers–Danlos syndrome

See Fig. 13.37. Ehlers–Danlos syndrome (*Edvard Lauritz Ehlers (1863–1937), Danish dermatologist, Henri Alexandre Danlos (1844–1912), French dermatologist*) is a disease of connective tissue of which there are different subtypes. The main characteristic of this condition is the hypermobile joints ('double-jointedness'). The skin tends to be thin but elastic. It also exhibits poor healing producing typical 'fish-mouth' scars and pseudotumours (calcified haematomas). The patient may have kyphoscoliosis or genu recurvatum and are prone to spontaneous pneumathorax, gastrointestinal haemorrhage, dissecting aneurysm, ruptured aortic aneurysm, and aortic and mitral incompetence.

Pseudoxanthoma elasticum

See Fig. 13.38. This is an inherited disorder of elastin with different subtypes. The hallmark feature is the appearance of the skin, which resembles a 'plucked chicken'. The skin of the flexures, that is, axillae, neck, antecubital fossa, and groins tends to be loose. The patient has hypermobile joints and may exhibit genu recurvatum. Complications include gastrointestinal haemorrhage, ischaemic heart disease, and aortic and mitral incompetence.

Fibromyalgia

This is one of the chronic pain syndromes. The pain tends to be ill defined and not limited to the joints and the pain is sometimes described as 'all over the body'. There is no identifiable pathology connected with this syndrome yet there may be multiple tender spots all over the body. It tends to occur in patients who exhibit psychiatric symptoms such as poor sleep, lassitude and irritability, and conditions such as tension headaches, irritable bowel syndrome, and chronic fatigue syndrome. This does not mean that this condition is 'all in the mind'. It does however mean that plenty of reassurance is required that there is no life-threatening illness going on and that the treatment (including physiotherapy, graded exercise, improving sleep disturbance, and addressing psychological issues/depression/anxiety) will be different from standard rheumatological regimens.

Gout

Gout is one of the 'crystal arthropathies' and is due to deposits of monosodium urate monohydrate into joints and tendons. It affects men more than women and commonly causes a monoarthritis or oligoarthritis, but polyarthritis resembling rheumatoid arthritis can occur. It produces a hot painful joint (classically the first MTP joint of the big toe). Uric acid is a breakdown product of purines (*pure-eens*) (guanine (*gwar-neen*) and adenosine (*add-den-owe-seen* or *adder-no-seen*) bases in deoxyribonucleic acid (DNA) and ribonucleic acid (RNA)). Increased

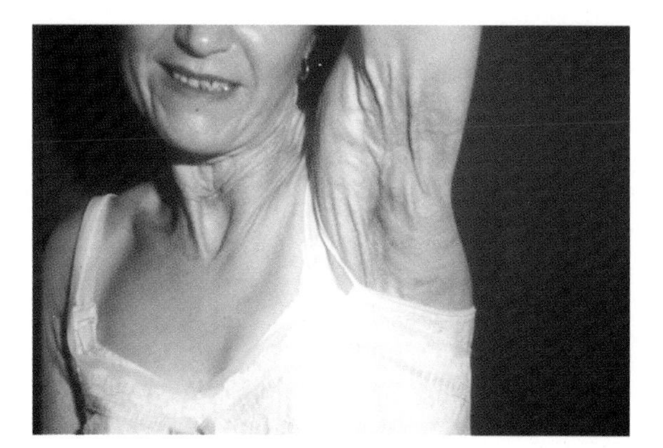

Fig. 13.38 Pseudoxanthoma elasticum.

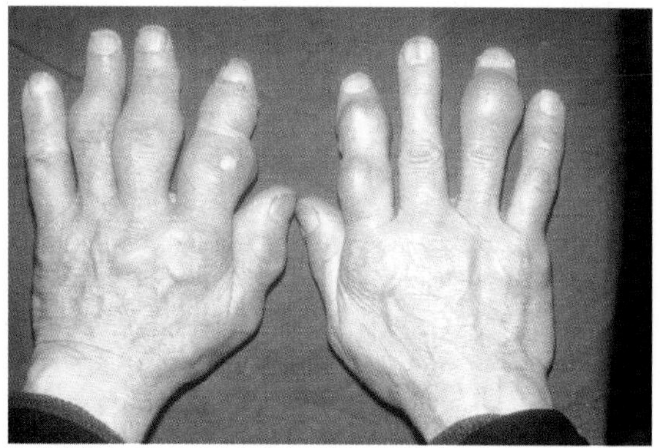

Fig. 13.39 Chronic tophaceous gout.

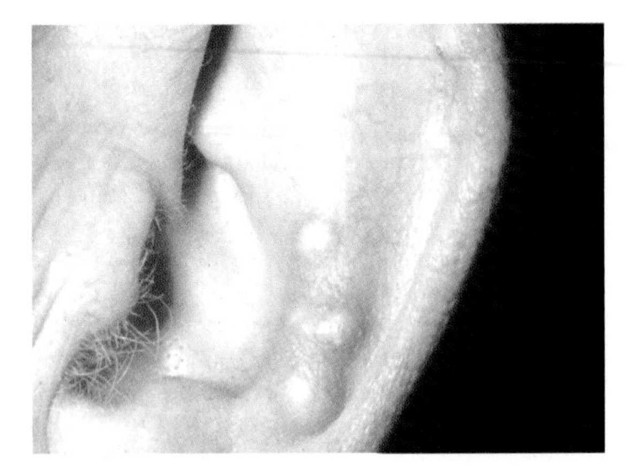

Fig. 13.40 Gouty tophi at the helix of the ear.

serum levels of uric acid (hyperuricaemia) (*high-per-you-reek-ee-mia*) may be due to increased production of uric acid or decreased excretion by the kidney. Although hyperuricaemia is a prerequisite for gout not everybody with high uric acid will develop gout. Gout may be recurrent and can become chronic. In chronic gout a large deposition of uric acid crystals may lead to tophi (a cheesy looking exudate). These tophi can be found in joints, tendon sheaths, and the helix of the ear (see Figs 13.39 and 13.40). The diagnosis of gout is made by joint aspiration and demonstrating the characteristic crystals (needle-shaped, negatively birefringent (*bye-re-fringe-gent*) crystals on polarizing light microscopy).

Pseudogout

This is another cause of a 'crystal arthropathy' due to the deposition of calcium pyrophosphate (*pie-roe-foss-fate*) crystals. As the name suggests pseudogout can mimic gout clinically with the production of one or more hot painful joints. The pain tends to linger longer than in classical gout (may last for weeks). The diagnosis, like that for gout, is made on joint aspiration and finding positively birefringent crystals of calcium pyrophosphate on polarizing light microscopy. Deposition of calcium pyrophosphate in cartilage is called chondrocalcinosis (*con-dro-cal-sin-owe-sis*) and can be seen as fine white lines on the articular surface of the affected cartilage on X-ray. Many metabolic diseases can cause this appearance, for example, myxoedema, hyperparathyroidism, and Wilson's disease. However it is important to note that chondrocalcinosis is often asymptomatic and is therefore distinct from pseudogout.

Septic arthritis

This is due to active infection of a joint by micro-organisms. Usually the infection is bacterial but viral (and in immunocompromised patients fungal) infections can occur. The most common bacterial agent in adults is staphylococcus aureus. This form of arthritis leads to a hot, painful joint, which the patient is reluctant to move. This presentation always warrants a joint aspiration for diagnostic purposes. If this diagnosis is missed irreparable damage may occur. So do not miss it!

Psoriatic arthropathy

Psoriasis is a skin disease with plaques that have a red base with a silvery scaly surface and are found on the extensor surfaces especially over the elbows (see Fig. 13.4), scalp, in the navel and behind the ears. Between 15–20% of patients with psoriasis develop arthritis (in a small number of cases the arthritis may predate the psoriasis). Why joint disease develops in some people and not in others is unclear. Five main patterns of joint disease are seen:

(1) distal joint disease affecting predominantly the DIP joints of the hands and feet;

(2) mono- or oligoarthropathy;

(3) a symmetrical polyarthropathy resembling rheumatoid arthritis;

(4) arthritis mutilans (*mute-till-anz*)—a rare, severe destructive arthritis leading to gross deformity;

(5) sacro-iliitis (*say-crow-eye-lee-eye-tiss*)

There may be overlap between many of the groups above. Psoriatic arthropathy is usually associated with nail changes including

- nail pitting and splitting
- onycholysis (separation of the nail plate)
- hyperkeratosis (exuberant overgrowth of keratin of the nail, see p. 366).

Reiter's syndrome

Classically Reiter's syndrome (*Hans Conrad Julius Reiter (1881–1969), German physician*) has been described as a triad of signs:

- arthritis
- genital tract inflammation
- conjunctivitis.

This syndrome is triggered by a specific infective episode. When first described it was thought to be a sequelae of sexually transmitted disease, for example, chlamydia but now it is also recognized following a diarrhoeal illness. It affects men more than women and predominantly affects young adults. It is classified as one of the seronegative spondyloarthritides and shares many clinical features although the arthritis tends to affect the lower limbs. A characteristic desquamating rash affecting the palms and soles of the hands and feet called keratoderma blenorrhagica (*ke-rat-owe-derma-blen-owe-ra-jicka*) may occasionally be seen. Other features include iritis and painless ulceration of the mouth. Treatment is symptomatic and directed at the underlying cause.

Behçets syndrome

Behçets (*beh-shays*) syndrome (Hulusi Behçets (1889–1948), Turkish dermatologist) is a multi-system disorder that is usually classified with the seronegative spondyloarthritides. It most commonly presents as a monoarthritis or an oligoarthritis. It is associated with mouth and genital ulceration, skin rash, sterile pustules, iridocyclitis of the eyes, and thromboembolic disease.

Seronegative spondyloarthritides

This is a collection of conditions with similar clinical presentations, which share the absence of the rheumatoid factor. Common features include

- inflammation of the sacro-iliac joints (sacro-iliitis)
- an asymmetrical peripheral arthritis
- an enthesopathy (*en-thee-sop-pathy*) (inflammation at the site of tendon insertion)
- an iritis or anterior uveitis.

Ankylosing spondylitis

This is one of the seronegative spondyloarthritides. It is more common in men and is associated with HLA B27. It has a predilection for the spine. Initially it starts as local sacro-iliitis and it can progress to affect the whole spine. Calcification of the interspinous ligaments occurs and in advanced cases there is fusion of the spine (a process called ankylosis). On X-ray this looks like a bamboo cane and is sometimes referred to as a bamboo spine. A compensatory cervical lordosis is required to enable the patient to look forward. When viewed from the side the patient looks like a question mark (hence they are described as having a question mark posture). See Fig. 13.28. Remember to perform Schober's test. They also have poor chest expansion and rely on 'diaphragmatic' respiration. Measure chest expansion using a tape measure and record the circumference of the chest on expiration at the nipple line. This should increase by 4 cm on inspiration but is substantially reduced in ankylosing spondylitis. Other features include iritis, aortitis and aortic incompetence, conduction defects of the heart, and apical fibrosis of the lungs.

Systemic sclerosis

This is a disorder that is recognized by its characteristic skin appearance (tight, hard, and waxy). This may be limited (called CREST) or diffuse (termed scleroderma). Other organs may be affected and the term systemic sclerosis is used (although many people use the term systemic sclerosis and scleroderma synonymously). It affects females more than males and there is a strong association with Raynaud's phenomenon. Other features include reflux oesophagitis and stricture, oesophageal dysmotility, small bowel hypomobility, and bacterial overgrowth leading to malabsorption, lung fibrosis, and renal failure. There is also another variant called limited cutaneous systemic sclerosis (formerly called CREST syndrome; it is worth remembering its earlier name because, as mentioned previously, this is an acronym for its major symptoms).

Polymyalgia rheumatica

This is a condition in which the disease process is poorly understood. There is an overlap with temporal arteritis (see pp. 386, 390) but a vasculitic process cannot explain those cases of polymyalgia rheumatica that occur in isolation. It affects females more than males and tends to affect patients over the age of 50 years and those of Caucasian origin. It causes pain and stiffness (**not weakness**) of the proximal muscle groups (shoulder and pelvic girdle muscles). The stiffness is worse in the morning and lasts for hours. Patients experience difficulty getting out of a chair and climbing stairs and they also experience difficulty combing their hair and reaching for objects over their heads. Other features include non-specific symptoms of anorexia, weight loss, night sweats, and fatigue. There are usually raised inflammatory markers, that is, erythrocyte sedimentation rate (ESR) or plasma viscosity. It is essentially a clinical diagnosis and responds rapidly to steroid treatment. Polymyalgia rheumatica may need prolonged treatment over a number of years as it has a tendency to relapse off steroids.

Rheumatoid arthritis

This is a multi-system inflammatory disorder that affects synovial joints and is characterized in some cases by the presence of the rheumatoid factor. It affects females slightly more than males. Its most common presentation is a symmetrical polyarthritis that develops over weeks or months, although more acute presentations occur. There is morning stiffness for longer than 1 h. The synovial lining of a joint becomes inflamed, which if untreated will lead to erosion of cartilage and bone (typically peri-articular osteoporosis and erosion). Later on in the disease process deformities of the joints may develop. There may be non-specific features such as fever, sweats, anorexia and weight loss, and fatigue. There may be vasculitic features such as nail fold infarcts, digital gangrene, ulcers, scleritis or episcleritis, peripheral neuropathy, and mononeuritis multiplex. Other organs may be involved:

(1) lungs—pleural effusion, lung fibrosis, rheumatoid nodules, bronchiolitis *(bron-key-owe-light-iss)*, and Caplan's *(cap-lanz)* syndrome (rheumatoid nodules and pneumoconiosis) in miners (see Fig. 16.39);

(2) heart—pericarditis and endocarditis—aortic incompetence and myocarditis;

(3) neurological—carpal tunnel syndrome, cervical myopathy, peripheral neuropathy, and mononeuritis multiplex;

(4) keratoconjunctivitis sicca *(ker-rat-owe-con-junk-ti-vie-tiss-sicker)* syndrome or Sjögren's syndrome;

(5) spleen—Felty's syndrome—enlarged spleen and hypersplenism leading to anaemia (occasionally pancytopoenia) *(pan-site-owe-pee-nia)*;

(6) anaemia—of drug-related anaemia—gastrointestinal loss due to NSAIDS, bone marrow suppression due to gold or penicillamine *(penny-sill-am-mean)*, the anaemia of chronic disorders, dietary, for example, folate deficiency, or an association with pernicious anaemia (vitamin B12 deficiency).

Diagnostic criteria have been drawn up by the American Rheumatism Association and the American College of Rheumatology. Seven criteria have been identified:

(1) morning stiffness of greater than 1 h;

(2) arthritis of the hand joints;

(3) arthritis of at least three types of joints (PIP, MCP, wrist, elbow, knee, ankle, and MTP);

(4) symmetrical arthritis;

(5) rheumatoid nodules present;

(6) rheumatoid factor present;

(7) joint erosions on X-rays of wrists and hands.

Four of the seven criteria must be present to establish the diagnosis of rheumatoid arthritis. Criteria 1–4 must be present for at least 6 weeks.

Vasculitis

The systemic vasculitides are a collection of disorders caused by inflammation and fibrinoid necrosis of blood vessels. This inflammatory process can be primary, that is, the underlying cause is not known or secondary to another disease, for example, rheumatoid arthritis. Primary vasculitis can be classified according to the size of blood vessel affected, that is,

(1) large vessel (for example, temporal arterities);

(2) medium vessel (for example, polyarteritis nodosa);

(3) small vessel (for example, Wegener's granulomatosis *(vague-gunners-gran-you-low-mat-toe-sis)* *(Friedrich Wegener (1907–1990), German pathologist)*.

Some conditions are more common at certain ages, for example, Kawasaki *(cower-sack-ee)* disease *(Tomisaku Kawasaki (twentieth century), Japanese paediatrician)*—childhood and temporal arteritis—old age. Other conditions have a predilection for certain organs, for example, temporal arteritis—temporal arteries and Churg-Strauss syndrome *(Jacob Churg born 1910), Polish-born American pathologist, Lotte Strauss (1913–1985), American pathologist)*—lungs. Most diseases can be diagnosed by biopsy of an affected organ and treatment is often steroids with or without steroid sparing agent.

Osteoarthritis

This is a chronic joint disorder resulting in progressive damage to cartilage and subchondral bone. It used to be regarded only as a degenerative disorder because it affected older people. However other factors may play a role including genetic factors (composition of cartilage), mechanical stress, for example, obesity, repetitive high-impact activity, or trauma with disordered repair (increasing evidence is supporting the role of inflammation in the genesis of osteoarthritis). Symptoms include pain that is worse with activity but settles on resting, stiffness after a period of inactivity, and in more advanced cases deformity of the joint. Pathologically there is a gradual thinning of articular cartilage leading to a decrease in the joint space. Later as cartilage destruction is complete (or near complete), underlying bony surfaces may become eroded and sclerose in an attempt at repair. The bone response may be sufficient to produce bony outgrowths at the joint margins called osteophytes. In the hands these osteophytes produce hard swellings at the DIP joints (Heberden's nodes) and at the PIP joints (Bouchard's nodes). If the hands demonstrate these nodes the patient is described as having nodal osteoarthritis (more common in females). Often there is a 'square hand' deformity due to subluxation of the base of the first metacarpal. If more than three joints are affected the condition is known as generalized osteoarthritis

Systemic lupus erythmatosus

Systemic lupus erythmatosus is a multi-system disorder of unknown cause where antibodies are directed against constituents of biological cells including the nucleus and surface antigens. Practically any organ in the body can be affected although certain patterns of disease are seen, for example, skin only (cutaneous lupus). It affects females more than males and it is more common in black people (not Africans). Other features include

(1) **skin**—malar rash in classical 'butterfly distribution', photosensitivity rash, discoid rash called discoid lupus erythmatosus, which can be found in isolation, vasculitic rash, livido reticularis, alopecia (hair loss), and Raynaud's phenomenon;

(2) **mouth**—ulcers;

(3) **cardiovascular**—pericarditis, endocarditis, and myocarditis;

(4) **lungs**—pleurisy, pleural effusion, and pulmonary fibrosis;

(5) **neurological**—psychosis, epilepsy, dementia, strokes, and peripheral neuropathy;

(6) **gut**—chronic active hepatitis and splenomegaly;

(7) **rheumatological**—arthralgia and arthritis;

(8) **gynaecological**—amenorrhoea and recurrent abortions;

(9) **haematological**—anaemia of chronic disease, haemolytic anaemia, hypersplenism, and anti-phospholipid syndrome leading to recurrent thromboses (see p. 363, Case 13.2).

Kerataconjuncitivis sicca syndrome

This affects the eyes and is due to the decrease or lack of production of tears leading to 'dry eyes'. The lack of lubrication results in gritty eyes that can become easily inflamed and infected. It is often found in association with a 'dry mouth' called xerostomia (*zero-stow-mia*), which is another unpleasant condition that can lead to poor dental hygiene and subsequent teeth and gum disease.

Sjögren's syndrome

This can be primary (keratoconjunctivitis sicca and xerostomia on their own) or secondary in association with a connective tissue disease, for example, systemic sclerosis, SLE, or rheumatoid disease.

Inflammatory markers

C-reactive protein, plasma viscosity, and ESR are markers of inflammation. They will be elevated regardless of the cause of inflammation and so are non-specific. They provide a guide to the degree of inflammation and can be used to monitor progress with treatment.

Rheumatoid factor

Rheumatoid factor is an autoantibody and its production may be a way for the immune system to aggregate immune complexes so they can be removed more easily by the spleen and other immune organs. Most assays detect an IgM antibody that is directed against the constant region (Fc) portion of IgG. Enzyme linked immunosorbent assay (ELISA) testing is capable of detecting other classes of rheumatoid factors (IgG, IgA) but these are not widely used clinically. The latex test is reported in a titre with most laboratories considering >1:40 as positive. The nephelometry test is usually reported in international units (IU) and the normal range is dependent on the specific laboratory (usually <20 IU). Rheumatoid factor is not a sensitive or specific test for rheumatoid arthritis. There are a variety of clinical conditions that can be positive for the rheumatoid factor (therefore limiting its specificity). In fact it can be present in up to 10% of the normal population. It is most useful as a prognostic indicator because those who are rheumatoid factor positive typically have a more aggressive disease. It is positive in up to 60% of cases with early disease and 75% with established disease. It is also useful in confirming a clinical impression that a polyarthritis that looks like rheumatoid arthritis is even more likely to be so. It is also used to follow patients with Sjögren's disease to predict the development of lymphoma.

Anti-nuclear antibodies

There are many anti-nuclear antibodies. These are antibodies found in the serum, which are directed against certain components of the nucleus of a cell. Different anti-nuclear antibodies are positive in certain conditions, however they are not entirely specific and so cannot be thought of as a powerful diagnostic tool. They can be divided into anti-nuclear antibodies and extractable nuclear antigens. See Table 13.11. Other important markers include anti-neutrophil cytoplasmic antibody (ANCA). C-ANCA is positive in 90% of patients with active generalized Wegener's granulomatosis, but is frequently seen in polyarteritis nodosa, idiopathic necrotizing, and crescentic glomerulonephritis. P-ANCA is a useful marker for vasculitis-associated crescentic glomerulonephritis, but is present in other systemic necrotizing vasculitic disorders including polyarteritis nodosa and Churg–Strauss syndrome and it is present in <10% of SLE patients. It is commonly seen in ulcerative colitis.

TABLE 13.11 Antinuclear antibodies and their possible associations

Antinuclear antibody	Disease suggestive of
Double-stranded DNA (dsDNA)	SLE
Single-stranded DNA (ssDNA)	Drug-induced SLE
Anti-histone	Drug-induced SLE
Anti-centromere	CREST syndrome
Anti-nucleolus	Systemic sclerosis
Anti-speckled	Systemic sclerosis
Extractable nuclear antigens	**Disease suggestive of**
Smooth muscle (Sm)	SLE
Anti-Ro (SSA)	Sjögren's, SLE, and neonatal lupus
Anti-La (SSB)	Sjögren's, SLE, and neonatal lupus
Anti-Scl 70	Systemic sclerosis
Ribonucleoprotein (RNP)	Mixed connective tissue disease and SLE
Anti-Jo-1	Polymyositis and fibrosing alveolitis

DNA, deoxyribonucleic acid; SLE, systemic lupus erythematosus.

Bone scan

A bone scan, involving the intravenous injection of radioisotopes, is useful for detecting malignant deposits in the bone. Patients may present with bone pain and weight loss. Inflammation can also be detected on bone scans and although a bone scan is not useful for diagnosing one rheumatological disorder from another, it can give information about patterns of inflammation, which may be helpful diagnostically. Note that DEXA bone scans use X-ray beams to measure the density of bone and should not be confused with an isotope bone scan.

Joint aspiration and injection

Most joints can be punctured to either remove fluid (for therapeutic or diagnostic purposes) or to inject drugs. For example, an inflamed knee joint due to rheumatoid arthritis can be punctured to

(1) remove fluid that is causing a painful effusion;

(2) inject steroids and local anaesthetic to suppress inflammation;

(3) exclude another cause, for example, gout, pseudogout, infection, or haemarthrosis.

Alternatively, a patient presenting with a swollen knee, who is not known to suffer from arthritis may have the knee joint aspirated as a diagnostic procedure. The most important differential diagnosis here is septic arthritis. Certain conditions can be diagnosed after examination of the joint fluid. Consequently, fluid removed from a joint should be sent to the microbiology department for microscopy, culture, and sensitivity and to the biochemistry department for examination under polarized light. See Table 13.12. Checking the white blood cell count of the aspirate is not performed routinely nowadays. Gout can be diagnosed and differentiated from pseudogout by the examination of joint fluid under polarized light.

Arthroscopy

Arthroscopy entails the direct examination of the joint. A flexible telescope (arthroscope) is introduced into the joint under local anaesthetic. The arthroscope has a small diameter and many joints can be investigated using this technique. Once in the joint, an examination of the structures can be undertaken and the nature and extent of inflammation assessed. In addition fluid can be removed for diagnostic and therapeutic purposes and drugs can be administered. Occasionally minor surgical procedures can also be performed.

Finals section

The emphasis of this section is on the short cases as this format usually causes the most uncertainty. The Objective Structured Clinical Examinations (OSCE)s usually have more straightforward and standardized instructions. Despite the different formats the clinical

TABLE 13.12 Diagnostic features of joint aspirates

	Normal	Osteoarthritis	Rheumatoid arthritis	Septic	Gout	Pseudogout
Appearance	Clear, thick	Clear, thick	Yellow, thin	Pus, thick	Clear, thin	Clear, thin
White blood cell count	+	+	++	++++	++	++
Crystals	None	None	None	None	Present	Present
Culture	Sterile	Sterile	Sterile	Positive	Sterile	Sterile

TABLE 13.13 Day-to-day cases

Rheumatoid arthritis
Osteoarthritis
Gout

TABLE 13.14 Finals cases

Day-to-day cases
Psoriatic arthropathy
Chronic tophaceous gout
Ankylosing spondylitis
Systemic lupus erythematosus
Raynaud's phenomenon

approach remains the same. For revision read the examination summary (p. 364) and the keypoints throughout the chapter and do the questions on pp. 394–5. See Tables 13.13 and 13.14 for day-to-day and Finals cases, respectively.

Key diagnostic clues

Unlike other systems there is no key diagnostic clue. When dealing with the joints, it is most important to determine if there is a true arthritis or synovitis as the causes are different to joints that are not inflamed. Palpation is the key here. A swollen joint that feels boggy suggests synovitis. If it feels hot to the touch this suggests that the inflammatory process is active.

Some advice relating to examination problems

Rheumatology cases are great for examiners! There is a wide variety of rheumatological conditions to choose from and patients are often well despite their illness. Patients can be used for both long cases and short 'spot' cases. In the spot case cardinal features of rheumatological conditions should prompt a diagnosis, for example, the butterfly rash of SLE. When faced with a spot case be prepared to answer supplementary questions on the disease you have identified (see Chapter 14).

The Instruction

The examiner may ask you 'Look at this patient. What is the diagnosis?' (or some variant). This would suggest a spot diagnosis (see Chapter 14). The more likely instruction would be 'Examine this patient's hands.'

Problem. You are unsure when asked to examine the hands whether to check the joints or to perform a neurological examination.

Solution. Do not panic, your observation is the key. Quickly look at the hands and determine if there are any abnormalities. Thankfully most joint disease will be immediately obvious. Look for swelling or deformities. If these are spotted you are home free (but do not relax too much as there is still work to be done). If there are no obvious abnormalities visible **then** it is sensible to begin a neurological examination.

General look

Before you plunge into your examination of the hand, sneak a peak at the face and the rest of the body. A patient with a plethoric, round face with purpura on the arms may be cushingoid as a result of steroid treatment for rheumatoid arthritis.

Position the hand

If there is obvious deformity, ask the patient if their hands are painful. If a pillow is handy get them to rest their palms on them. If no pillow is present hold the hands very carefully so as not to cause discomfort.

Look

Always start with the nails otherwise the signs could be missed. Look for pitting, onycholysis, and hyperkeratosis (psoriasis) or splinter haemorrhages and nail fold infarcts (vasculitis). Turn the hands over. Is there any palmar erythema? (rheumatoid arthritis?). Also look for any deformity and any obvious pattern, for example, do the fingers deviate to the ulna side? (rheumatoid arthritis). Is there any swan neck or boutonnière's deformity of any fingers? Are the deformities symmetrical, that is, affecting both hands in a similar fashion? (probably rheumatoid arthritis). If asymmetrical this is more likely to be a seronegative spondarthritides or gout (in chronic tophaceous gout look for cheesy looking material exuding from a joint). Now scan the arms quickly for purpura (steroid treatment?), skin plaques of psoriasis, or rheumatoid nodules.

Feel

Now observe all the DIP joints and note any swelling. Do they feel soft and boggy (synovitis?) or hard? (Heberden's nodes). Do the same for the PIP joints (Bouchard's nodes) and the MCP joints. Check the wrist for any deformity and synovitis before running your hand down the ulna border of the forearm to the elbow. You may palpate rheumatoid nodules that were not apparent on inspection. A fluctuant swelling at the elbow suggests olecronon bursitis (gout? rheumatoid arthritis?). Double check and make sure there are no occult plaques of psoriasis on the extensor surface of the elbow.

Move

You need to perform a quick check of function. Get your patient to undo and do up buttons, hold a pen, and so on.

Remember!

You could be shown rheumatoid feet! Do not panic, simply follow the steps for the examination of the hand and the signs are similar.

Supplementary clues

With joint disease of the hands you will usually have an idea what condition you are dealing with early on (you hope). So to add the finishing touches to the examination you can demonstrate extra relevant findings, for example, with rheumatoid arthritis pull down the lower eyelid and inspect for scleritis or episcleritis or with chronic tophaceous gout inspect the pinna of the ear for deposition of gouty tophus. It is important to note that these manoeuvres are not essential but demonstrate that you have a good working knowledge of the disease you are suspecting including their extra-articular manifestations.

Problem. You have finished your examination of rheumatoid hands but you are unsure whether to progress to a neurological examination.

Solution. You realize that a neurological deficit is possible with rheumatoid arthritis but to embark on a 'neuro' examination will be time consuming. Worse still if you hesitate your examiners may (wrongly) assume that you are clueless. The author's approach is to say up front that they have concluded their examination but ordinarily would perform a neurological examination because they are aware that rheumatoid arthritis can cause neurological deficits. Also be alive to any clues such as wasting of the thenar eminence, which could suggest a carpal tunnel syndrome. If this is the case the author would modify their statement and say 'I would normally go on to perform a neurological examination particularly as I have noticed marked wasting of the thenar eminence which raises the possibility of carpal tunnel syndrome.' In this way the examiners will give you due credit for your knowledge and will usually let you know if they expect you to proceed with a neurological examination.

Presentation

Try to be confident—avoid the words 'seems' or 'might'!

Good luck!

Questions

The more stars, the more important it is to know the answer.

1. Name three nail changes in psoriatic arthropathy. ***
2. What are the names of the two forms of nodes found in osteoarthritis? **
3. What is the carpal tunnel syndrome? ****
4. What is genu varum? *
5. What is genu valgus? *
6. What are the causes of a knee effusion? ****
7. How do you perform a patella tap? ****
8. What is the differential diagnosis of a ruptured baker's cyst? ***
9. What is the rheumatoid factor? **
10. Which structures are responsible for the stability of the knee? ****
11. What are passive and active joint movements in joint assessment? ****
12. What is the rotator cuff? ***
13. What is an antalgic gait? **
14. What is a locked knee? ****
15. What is Schober's test?*
16. What is quadriceps lag and its significance? *
17. Describe Trendelenburg's sign **
18. What is Felty's syndrome? **
19. What is Lachman's test? ***
20. What do the terms kyphosis, scoliosis, and lordosis mean? ***
21. What is Lhermitte's phenomenon? *
22. What are boutonnières and swan neck deformities? ***
23. Describe three skin manifestations of systemic lupus erythmatosus. ***
24. What is arthritis mutilans? *
25. What is the difference between apparent and true leg length and how do you measure them? ***
26. Define arthritis, arthralgia, and arthropathy. ***
27. What is keratoconjunctivitis sicca syndrome? *
28. What is Sjögren's syndrome? *

29. Name three possible respiratory complications associated with rheumatoid arthritis. ****
30. What are the five main features of limited systemic sclerosis (CREST syndrome)? ****
31. In which condition would you find a question mark posture? **
32. Give an example of a large vessel vasculitis.*
33. In chronic tophaceous gout, where might you find deposition of tophi? **
34. What is deposited in the joints in pseudogout? *
35. If faced with a single 'hot' joint, what is the most important diagnosis to consider? ****
36. Describe the anterior drawer sign. **
37. How do you perform the bulge test for the knee? ***
38. What is the earliest movement to be affected at the hip? **
39. What is the reverse Lhermitte's phenomenon? *
40. What is an arthroscope and what does it do? ****

Score. Give 4 marks for 4 stars, 1 for 1 star, and so on. At the end of the third year, you should be scoring 60-plus and by Finals, 80-plus; 90-plus is very good.

Further reading

Bellamy N. *Colour atlas of clinical rheumatology*. Lancaster: Kluwer; 1985.

Boyle AC. *Colour atlas of rheumatology*. London: Wolfe; 1986.

Doherty M, Dacre J, Dieppe, Snaith ML. Screening examination of the musculoskeletal system: the GALS system. *Annals of Rheumatological Disease* 1993; **51**:1165–9.

Doherty M, Doherty J. *Clinical examination in rheumatology*. London: Wolfe; 1992.

Snaith ML. *ABC of rheumatology*. 2nd edn. London: BMJ Publishing Group; 1999.

CHAPTER 14

Spot diagnosis

Chapter contents

Introduction

A spot diagnosis is not the diagnosis of acne. Spot cases are an assortment of different diseases with visible signs that can lead to an instant diagnosis. Any system, for example, the endocrine, dermatological, or neurological, can be used and the only factor they have in common is the instruction 'Look at this patient! What is the diagnosis?' (or a similar variation). The spot diagnosis requires a different skill to the ones you have been learning so far. It requires the instant recognition of clinical signs (in contrast to the usual methodical approach). The key to the spot diagnosis is experience. Once you have seen the clinical signs again and again, you will be able to process the information quickly and make that snap diagnosis. It is as simple as that. The only difficulty with some spot cases is that subtle signs can be easily overlooked. However if you can develop a 'trigger' for these conditions, that is, some clue that will prompt your recall, then you will not miss them.

The spot case scenario can be unnerving for any student because rather than plunging into a comfortable, well-rehearsed routine, they are literally put 'on the spot.' The situation is made even more nerve-wracking because **any** system can be affected and where do you start looking? The aim of this chapter is to acquaint you with the more common spot cases that you will encounter as a stude nt and to give you some system of approach to spot diagnosis.

The importance of spot diagnosis

The spot technique is valuable because it can provide a short cut to a diagnosis, for example, while taking a history, you notice the staring eyes of a patient with exophthalmos. You then make the connection with their weight loss and diarrhoea, that is, they have Grave's disease of the thyroid and are thyrotoxic. Everyone is impressed by the clinician who stands at the end of the bed and plucks the diagnosis out of the air without touching the patient. However here is a note of caution about using the spot technique in clinical practice.

1. First impressions can be misleading, for example, the telangiectasia you thought were spider naevi from a distance could be due to other disease on closer inspection, for example, systemic sclerosis (see Case 6.7 and Fig. 14.15).
2. Your diagnosis could be accurate but the disease could have no connection with the patient's symptoms.
3. Your diagnosis could be accurate and relevant but the patient could have other pathology in other systems. This is especially important in the elderly (this is called co-morbidity).

The approach to the spot case

The spot case tests your ability to notice signs and formulate a diagnosis. Sometimes in your finals this is all that is required. More often however, the spot case will be the basis for further examination or questions. This could be an opportunity for you to demonstrate your knowledge of the case. So if you can, seize the initiative. The instruction is all important in the spot case. It may be specific, for example, 'Look at this patient's leg.' The focused case is usually straightforward as you do not have to hunt very far to find the lesion. The only problem you face is not recognizing the sign (if this is the case do not freeze, describe what you see and try and come to a sensible conclusion; if necessary give a differential diagnosis). The more general commands, 'What is the diagnosis?' or 'Look at this patient: what is the diagnosis?' are more difficult. As the range of possible cases is so wide, you have to be more systematic in your inspection. Even then some cases can still be strikingly obvious at first glance.

Start by getting an overall impression of the patient. This first glance may be sufficient for you to reach a diagnosis. If this is the case, spend a few more seconds gathering extra clues that might strengthen the diagnosis before reporting back to the examiners (do not spend too much time or you might appear clueless). If the diagnosis is not immediately obvious, pay attention to the patient's demeanour and mood. Do they seem apathetic and expressionless? (Parkinson's disease? myxoedema?). Are they listless and agitated? (thyrotoxicosis?). Do they have a hunched posture? (which might suggest Parkinson's disease or vertebral fractures due to osteoporosis (Cushing's syndrome?), Paget's (*pah-jets*) disease, or acromegaly). Also check skin colour. Do they appear pigmented (the most common causes are racial or tanning) but in an examination setting this may be more relevant (Addison's disease? haemochromatosis (*he-ma-crow-ma-toe-sis*)?). Does the skin appear yellow (jaundice?). After a brief global assessment if answers are still not forthcoming, it is time to inspect your patient in more systematic detail. The author prefers a 'top-down' approach because they find the majority of information about a person is packed into the head and face. First check the shape of the head. Is the forehead enlarged? (Paget's disease?). Is there unusual balding (myotonia dystrophica) or hair loss (alopecia)? (systemic lupus erythmatosus (SLE)? myxoedema?). Assess the shape of the face. Is it round and 'moon' shaped? (Cushing's syndrome?). Check for symmetry of the face. Is there drooping of one side of the face? (facial nerve palsy?).

Now assess the eyelids and check for symmetry. Is there drooping of one of the lids? Is it a complete ptosis (third nerve palsy?) or a partial ptosis? (Horner's syndrome?). Look at the eyes and again compare both sides. Do they have a staring quality? (exophthalmos?). Or is there evidence of yellow sclerae? (jaundice?). Check the nose. Is it enlarged and bulbous? (acromegaly?). Or is it pinched and 'beak' like? (systemic sclerosis?). Inspect the lips. Are they thin and drawn with radial furrows surrounding them? (systemic sclerosis?). Or are there multiple red 'spots' that could suggest telangiectasia (hereditary haemorrhagic telangiectasia (HHT)?) or speckled pigmentation? (Peutz–Jehger (*perts-yay-ga*) syndrome?). At this point it is worth scanning the rest of the face for other areas of discolouration. There may be telangiectasia on the cheeks (spider naevi?) or a 'butterfly rash' (SLE?).

Now leave the face and study the neck underneath. Is there a diffuse swelling in the mid-line? (goitre?). Or is there a more discrete lump? (multi-nodular goitre or thyroid adenoma?). Trace along the edge of the neck until you reach the clavicles on each side and check for lumps there too (malignant lymph nodes? (on the left side, Virchow's (*ver-coughs*) node?)). Finally study the limbs. If they are exposed, check to see if there are any telangiectasia (spider naevi?) or purpura (Cushing's syndrome?). Is there deformity of the limbs? (Paget's disease?). Are they held in an unusual posture (for example, flexion at the elbow and internal rotation of the arm due to hemiplegia)?

This list may seem daunting but as you see more signs and gain in experience, you will find that you process information rapidly and automatically. Do not try to remember all the conditions that have been mentioned so far. In fact there are many more conditions that could have been added. The aim has been to give you a systematic approach to the spot case, a blueprint for seeking out abnormalities (especially those that are subtle and easily missed). You do not need to stick with the sequence described. You could do it in reverse order or some other personal preference. The important thing is that your adopted routine does not miss anything.

In the next section a number of diseases that are commonly used as spot cases have been chosen. The list is not comprehensive and it is likely that you will face a condition that is not on the list. Here cases that you will have to diagnose from a general look at the patient (rather than a more focused study of part of the body) have been concentrated on. For each case a specific feature (or features) that **triggers** the author's recall of that condition (much as large animal and trunk triggers the image of an elephant) has been picked.

Below the triggers, other features of the disease that can prompt you to search for other confirmatory signs or to ask relevant questions have been summarized. If you can, take charge and be bold in your finals. Tell your examiners what you are suspecting and why and tell them you would like to check (or ask questions) to determine if other features of the condition are present. If they give you permission, go for it. If not, they may have questions about the case they may test you on instead.

Tip

For conditions that are not described try and work out the features that can act as triggers for you.

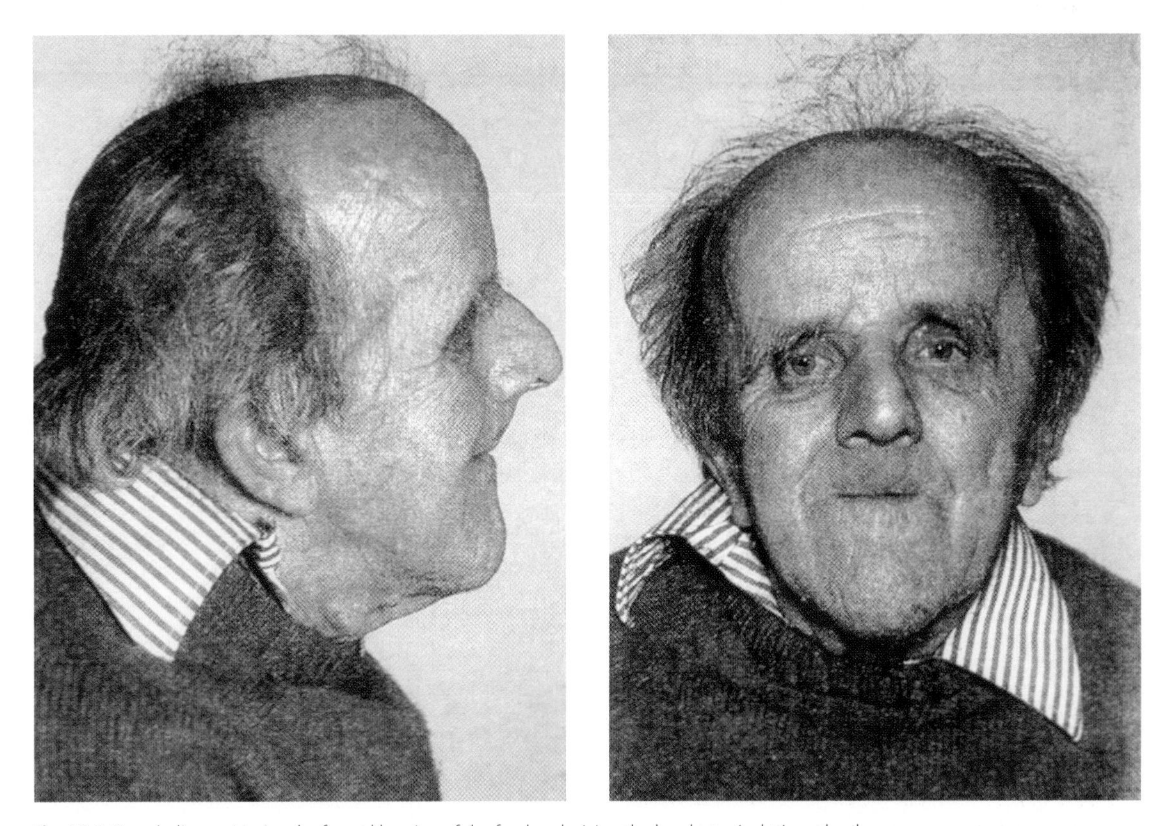

Fig. 14.1 Paget's disease. Notice the frontal bossing of the forehead, giving the head a typical triangular shape.

Tip

Be prepared to ask simple questions on the causes, investigation, treatment, and complications of the disease you have spotted.

Spot cases

Paget's disease

What is it?

It is a disorder of bone of unknown cause, leading to a lack of co-ordination between bone formation and bone lysis (destruction). The result is bone that may be enlarged but soft with poor tensile strength.

Trigger features

- The shape of the head—enlargement of the forehead
- elderly person.

The person is usually elderly and their forehead may be enlarged (called frontal bossing). This can give the face a triangular outline (with the base of the triangle being formed at the top of the head and the point by the chin (see Fig. 14.1). The presence of a hearing aid will reinforce the diagnosis because deafness may be caused by Paget's disease affecting the ossicles (the tiny bones of the middle ear that normally conduct sounds to the inner ear).

Tip

Deafness is prevalent in older people and therefore Paget's disease is not necessarily the cause of hearing impairment.

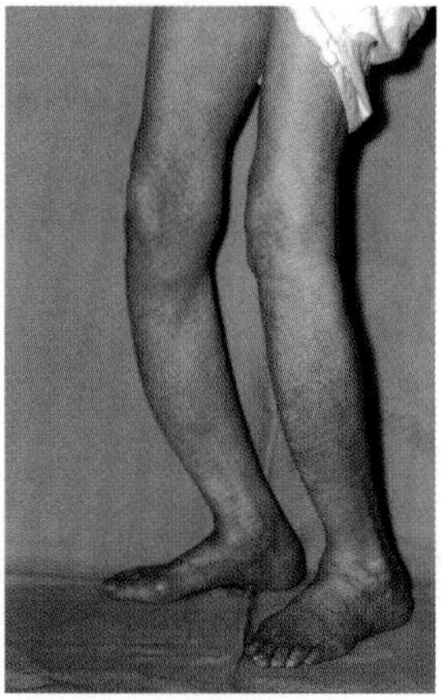

Fig. 14.2 Bowing of the tibia bilaterally.

Other features

- Bowing of the long bones—the humerus, tibia, and femur may bend under the weight of the body (see Fig. 14.2)
- pathological fractures—bones may fracture due to relatively minor stresses
- kyphosis—the spine may curve due to vertebral fractures
- optic atrophy—the second nerve can be trapped by expanding bone leading to atrophy
- high output cardiac failure—the affected bone is very vascular early in the disease and sufficient blood can be shunted into the bone to force the heart to work harder to compensate
- spinal cord compression—this can occur either due to vertebral fracture or more rarely due to brainstem invagination (*in-vaj-in-ay-shun*) (called platybasia (*plat-ee-base-ia*)). Normally, the weight of the skull and its contents are balanced by an upward force, produced by the cervical vertebrae. If Paget's disease affects the base of the skull, this upward force can push the softened base and the brainstem upwards, with disastrous consequences.

Parkinson's disease

What is it?

It is a chronic neurological disorder due to depletion of dopamine in the basal ganglia.

Trigger features

- An apathetic, mask-like face
- usually elderly person
- flexed posture
- pill-rolling tremor.

Examinations are stressful situations for patients as well as students. So if someone appears to be staring blankly without expression you should be suspicious about Parkinson's disease. The patient tends to be elderly, although younger people are afflicted, for example, Michael J. Fox, the actor and they may have a hunched posture. If you see a pill-rolling tremor, breathe a sigh of relief as this helps clinch the diagnosis. This has not been put in as the most important trigger because the tremor is not always produced to order in the examination setting. People have been known to stare for ages in the hope of seeing the tiniest flicker and have been disappointed.

If you are certain you are dealing with Parkinson's disease seize the initiative and tell your examiners,

Tip

If you see a tremor observe the hand closely. Pay particular attention to the thumb and make sure it is pill rolling in nature because there are other forms of tremor that have been mistaken for a Parkinsonian tremor.

'The patient has a mask-like, expressionless face and I suspect they have Parkinson's disease. I would like to assess their tone with your permission.' Most examiners will allow this. Introduce yourself to the patient and ask if you can examine their arms. Then test for cogwheel or lead-pipe rigidity (see p. 206).

Tip

Note the response from the patient when you ask for permission to examine them. If their voice is quiet and lacks volume this is dysphonia, another feature of Parkinson's disease.

Other features

- Slow movements (bradykinesia)
- rigidity (these first two features together with the tremor are the hallmarks of Parkinson's disease)
- greasy skin (seborrhoea)
- excessive drooling (sialorrhoea)
- tiny spidery writing (micrographia)
- shuffling gait
- prone to falling
- postural hypotension.

Exophthalmos

See Figs 14.3 and 14.4.

What is it?

This is the protrusion of the eyes from the orbit due to retro-orbital infiltration and oedema and the most common cause is auto-immune thyroid disease. Sometimes you may hear the term proptosis (*prop-toe-sis*) used. Both terms mean the same thing with the exception that

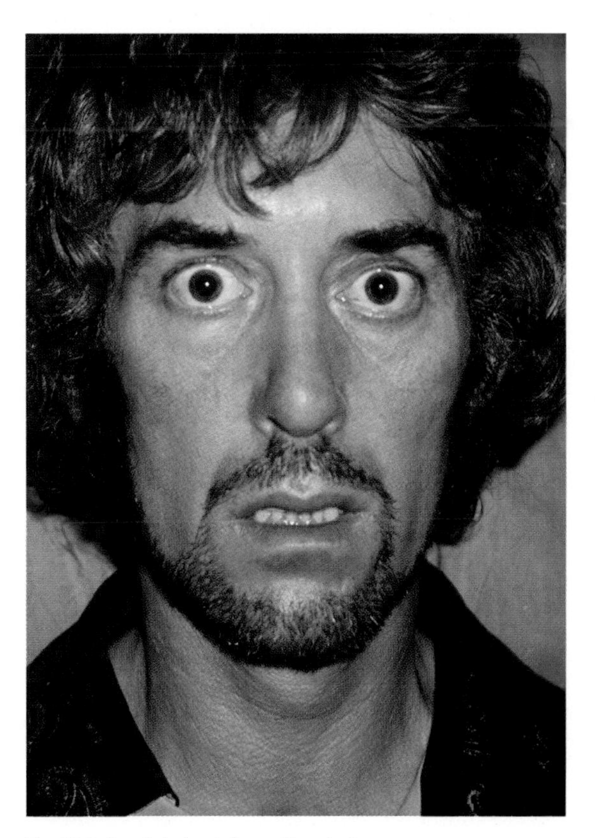

Fig. 14.3 Exophthalmos due to Grave's disease.

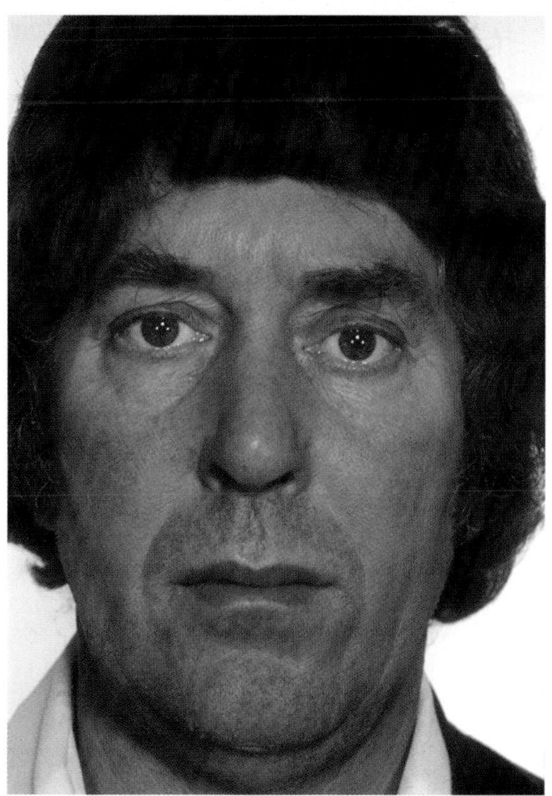

Fig. 14.4 The patient in Fig. 14.3, after treatment .

exophthalmos is usually reserved for proptosis of thyroid origin. Twenty-five per cent of patients with Grave's disease have exophthalmos. Exophthalmos is unrelated to thyroid status (that is, hyperthyroid, euthyroid (*you-thigh-roid*), or hypothyroid see p$) and may precede the development of Grave's disease.

Trigger feature

- Staring eyes.

This spot case is easily missed. The patient (usually a woman) seems to be staring at you (sometimes to the point of rudeness), but then staring can be normal human behaviour. You have to remind yourself that you are in an examination and this may be your only clue. If you make the connection between staring eyes and exophthalmos you are on your way. Look carefully at the eyes, especially around the iris. If you can clearly see white sclera under the bottom margin of the iris (and also possibly the top margin), it is likely that the patient has exophthalmos. Exophthalmos tends to be assymetrical. Some people advocate you look over the top of the patient's head from behind, while they are seated. From this position you can see how far the eye is protruding from the orbit. Although this visually confirms that the eye is protruding, it does not add any further useful information.

Other features

- Corneal ulceration—as the eye protrudes further from the orbit, the cornea becomes exposed and dry (as it loses the lubricating properties of blinking). It then becomes prone to ulceration and infection
- chemosis—as the eye protrudes the venous and lympatic drainage can be obstructed leading to oedema of the conjunctiva and periorbital oedema. In advanced cases the conjunctiva can become very red and swollen
- malignant exophthalmos—the pressure in the orbit becomes so great that it compresses the optic nerve or its blood supply, threatening sight. Note that this is not dependent on the degree of exophthalmos
- ophthalmoplegia—this is where eye movements are affected leading to double vision (diplopia). This occurs because of infiltration and oedema of the ocular muscles. In long-standing cases there may be fibrosis of the muscles leading to further impairment of movement (see Fig. 12.14).
- goitre—this is usually a smooth diffusely enlarged goitre (this may be the subject of a spot case—see later).

Goitre

See Fig. 14.5.

What is it?

This is the enlargement of the thyroid gland.

Trigger features

- Swelling at the front of the neck
- (a glass of water nearby).

This can be easy to miss. However if you stick to your systematic review, which includes the neck, you should pick this up (especially if your patient is a woman). If you see a goitre, quickly check for exophthalmos. Then say to your examiners, 'I have noticed a mid-line swelling in the neck, which is smooth and symmetrical. There is no exophthalmos. The likeliest cause is a goitre. I would like to confirm that it moves with swallowing and check the patient's thyroid status.' If your examiners permit it, get a glass of water (one may be conveniently handy and is a further clue to a thyroid case) and observe if the swelling rises with swallowing. If it does, this confirms that it is of thyroid origin. Also check for lymph nodes around the neck. Then go on to

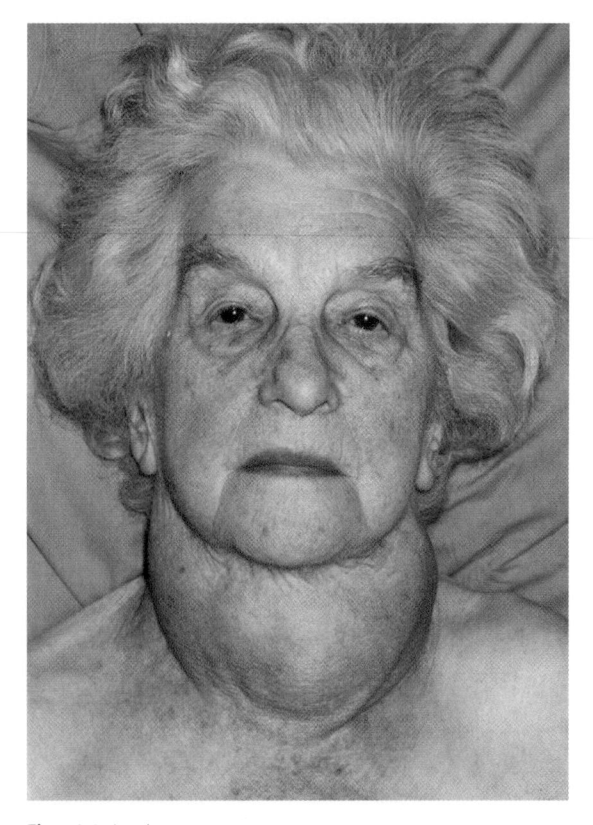

Fig. 14.5 A goitre.

Tip

If you get a case with a discrete nodule or lump in the mid-line, get the patient to stick out their tongue to exclude a thyroglossal cyst (see p. 337) even if you see a glass of water present. Then go on to get the patient to swallow some water to determine if the swelling is a thyroid nodule. You will still need to check for lymph nodes and to assess the thyroid status as before.

check the thyroid status (see p. 341 and 'Thyrotoxicosis' and 'myxoedema' below).

Other features

- Dyspnoea (due to compression or deviation of the trachea)
- cough
- stridor (inspiratory noise due to obstruction of the trachea)
- dysphagia (compression of the oesophagus from large goitre)
- hoarse voice (due to left recurrent laryngeal nerve compression)
- Horner's syndrome (due to compression of the sympathetic nerves in the neck).

Thyrotoxicosis

What is it?

This is a condition due to the excess secretion of thyroid hormones.

Trigger features

- Patient looks anxious, listless, and fidgety
- fine postural tremor.

This is another tricky spot case because there is sometimes very little to go on. Sometimes your examiners may give you some supplementary information to guide you. Your only physical clue may be that your patient (usually a woman) seems listless and agitated. If possible, watch their hands and see if you can glimpse a fine tremor when they move them. In some cases thyrotoxicosis will be combined with Grave's disease and exophthalmos and a goitre may be additional clues. Tell your examiner, 'This young woman looks restless and fidgety and this suggests thyrotoxicosis. There is no obvious exophthalmos or a goitre but I would like to check this patient's thyroid status fully.' If you are on the right lines your wish is likely to be granted. If you are wrong (some people can become anxious when they are on show for an examination), the examiners should give you credit for your thinking and will gently steer you in the right direction. Now check the thyroid status (see p. 341).

1. Observe the outstretched arms for a postural tremor.
2. Check for sweaty palms.
3. Check the pulse for a tachycardia.
4. Check the pulse for atrial fibrillation.
5. Look for lid retraction.
6. Look for lid-lag.

Other features

- Fatigue
- heat intolerance
- increased appetite
- weight loss (despite increased appetite)
- diarrhoea
- angina
- tachycardia
- atrial fibrillation
- heart failure
- spider naevi
- palmar erythema
- osteoporosis
- mild hypercalcaemia
- proximal myopathy
- amenorrhea (absent periods) in women.

Myxoedema

See Figs 14.6 and 14.7.

What is it?

This is a coarse thickening of the skin and subcutaneous tissues due to the deposition of mucopolysaccharides, which occurs in association with an underactive thyroid (sometimes myxoedema is used synonymously with hypothyroidism **but** hypothyroidism can occur without myxoedema).

Trigger features

- Apathetic expression
- coarse thickened facial features
- thinning of the hair.

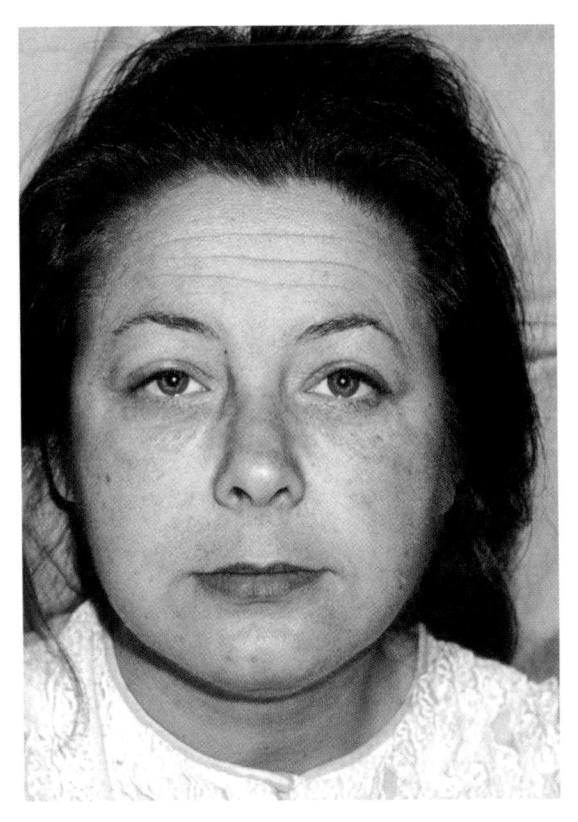

Fig. 14.6 Myxoedema .

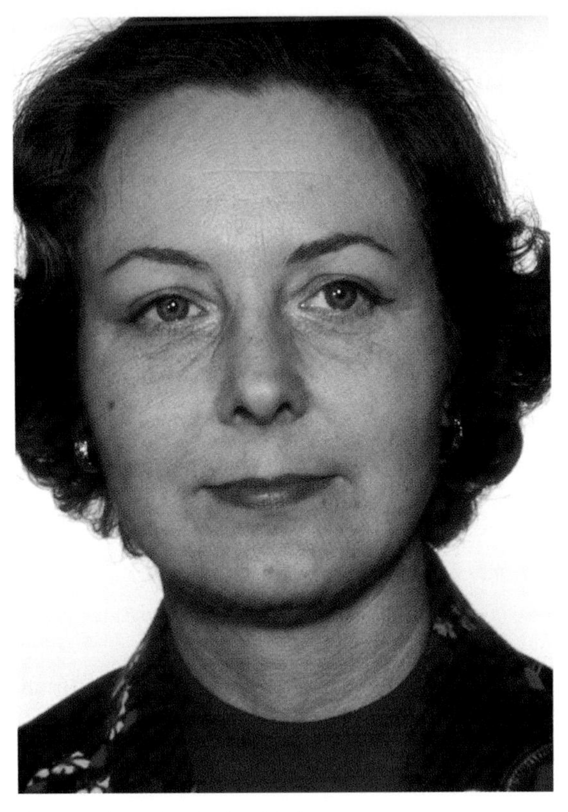

Fig. 14.7 The patient in Fig. 14.6, after treatment.

Myxoedema is a condition that is easily missed. The patient is usually elderly (and female). Sometimes the skin has a yellowish tinge due to hypercarotenaemia (see p. 151, Case 6.8). Also check to see if the patient has exophthalmos or a goitre. Occasionally patients with Grave's disease develop spontaneous hypothyroidism. More commonly it is the result of treatment for thyrotoxicosis with radioactive iodine or thyroidectomy (look carefully for a scar in the collar region of the lower neck— surgeons try to make them as invisible as possible). If you think you are dealing with myxoedema say to your examiners, 'This patient has an apathetic expression and has coarse thickened features and thinning hair. This suggests that the patient has Myxoedema and with your permission I would like to check their pulse and their reflexes.' If permission is granted, introduce yourself to the patient and ask if you can examine them briefly. Listen to their voice when they respond. Is it hoarse and croaky? This is another feature of hypothyroidism. Check to see if the patient has a bradycardia and then assess their ankle reflexes (you are looking for slow-relaxing phase to the reflex).

Tip

If the patient is not in an optimum position for testing the ankle reflexes it is okay to check the biceps or triceps for the same slow-relaxing phenomenon.

Other features

- Fatigue
- cold intolerance
- weight gain
- carpal tunnel syndrome
- angina
- pericardial effusion
- cerebellar ataxia
- depression
- menorrhagia (heavy periods) in women.

Acromegaly

See Fig. 14.8.

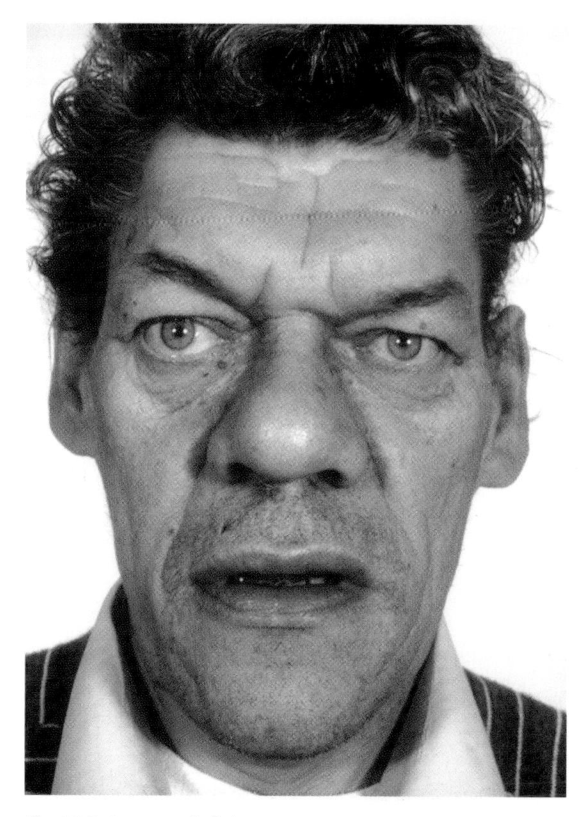

Fig. 14.8 Acromegalic facies.

What is it?

Acromegaly ('acro'—extremities, 'megalos'— big) is a condition that causes enlargement of the bones, soft tissues, and organs of the body. It is due to the excess secretion of growth hormone from a pituitary tumour. The critical feature is that the epiphyses (the growing ends of bones) are fused. If they are not then giantism occurs as the bones can grow without restriction.

Trigger feature

- A large head with large coarse features.

The patient with acromegaly is fairly unmistakable. They have a large head with prominent supra-orbital ridges, a large bulbous nose, and thick lips. They have a prominent lower jaw (prognathism) which can make the lower teeth protrude beyond the upper ones. The teeth may also become widely separated although this will not be obvious until you speak to them.

Other features

- Enlarged hands (see Fig. 14.9) and feet—hands have a 'doughy' feel because of increased thickness of the soft tissues

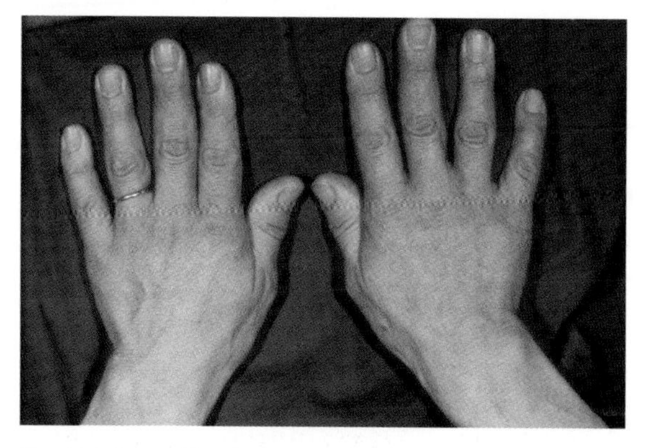

Fig. 14.9 Enlarged hands.

- increased hat size (cap size for the more trendy) and increased glove and shoe size
- greasy skin (seborrhoea)
- kyphosis
- osteoarthritis
- hepatomegaly, splenomegaly, and renal enlargement
- cardiomyopathy
- hypertension
- diabetes
- carpel tunnel syndrome (see p. 239)
- proximal myopathy (see p. 220)
- also features due to pituitary tumour
- headache
- bitemporal hemianopia (see p. 286, Fig. 11.6).

Cushing's syndrome

See Fig. 14.10.

What is it?

Cushing's syndrome (*Harvey Cushing (1869–1939), American neurosurgeon*) is a collection of physical signs and symptoms caused by a chronic excess of cortisol.

Causes

(1) Long-term steroid treatment—the most common cause;

(2) pituitary tumour causing adreno-corticotrophic hormone (ACTH) secretion—this hyperstimulates the adrenals (hyperplasia) to secrete excess cortisol (this is called Cushing's disease);

(3) ectopic ACTH production—this is secreted by tumours, for example, bronchial carcinoma; in some

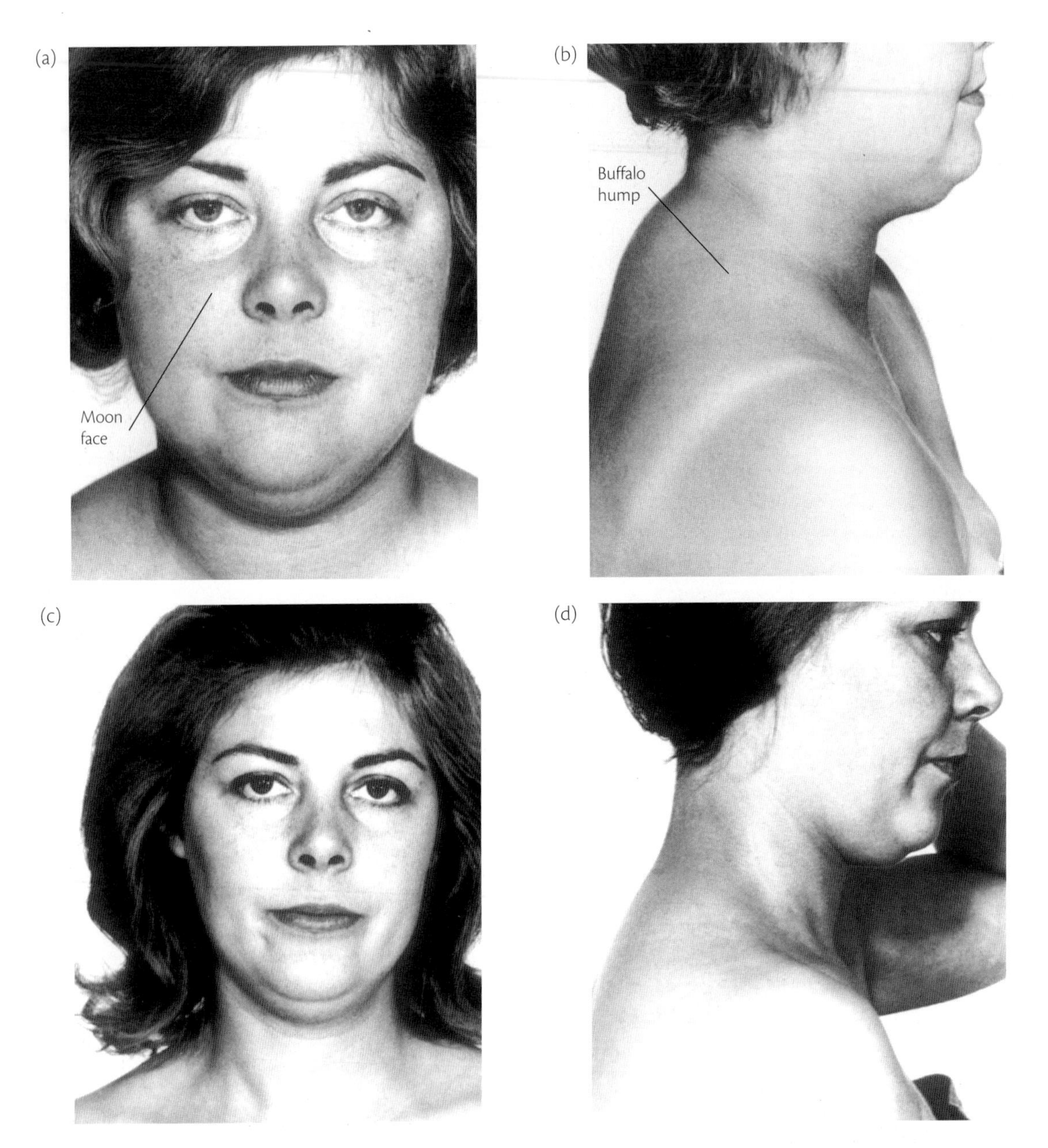

Fig. 14.10 Cushingoid facies. (a) and (b) pre-treatment, (c) and (d) post-treatment.

cases the development of the cancer is so rapid that the full features of Cushing's syndrome are not seen;

(4) adrenal tumours—adenomas and carcinomas.

Trigger features

- Fat, round face (moon face)
- central obesity
- purpura.

If you see a patient with a fat, round face do not dismiss this as simple obesity (especially in an examination setting). The distribution of fat is different in Cushing's syndrome. It tends to accumulate centrally around the neck and trunk (on the neck it causes a 'buffalo hump' and the obese abdomen develops purple stretch marks called striae (see p. 159 and Fig. 14.11). The limbs become thin and wasted, leading to what has

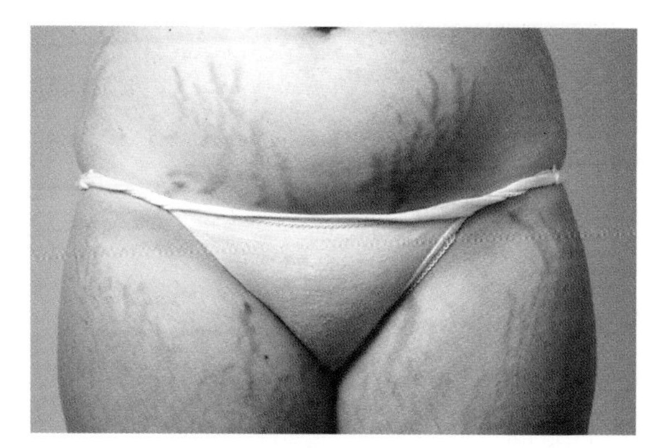

Fig. 14.11 Central obesity and striae associated with Cushing's syndrome.

been called a 'lemon-on-a-stick appearance'). Scan the face and exposed limbs for any sign of bruising. If you see purpura it makes the diagnosis of Cushing's syndrome more likely (it occurs because of fragile dermal blood vessels and thinning of connective tissue that normally supports them).

Other features

- Thin skin
- osteoporosis
- hypertension
- diabetes
- proximal myopathy
- depression
- psychosis
- amenorrhoea (lack of periods) in women.

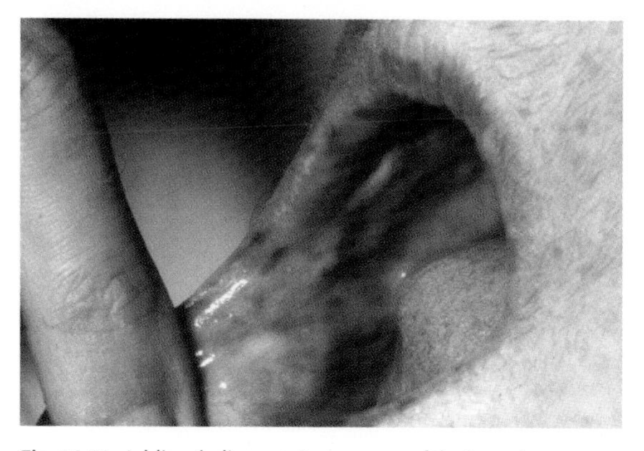

Fig. 14.12 Addison's disease: pigmentaton of the buccal mucosa.

Addison's disease

See Fig. 14.12.

What is it?

Addison's disease (*Thomas Addison (1793–1860), English physician*) is a disorder due to the lack of the hormones cortisol and aldosterone because of damage or destruction of the adrenal cortex.

Causes

(1) Autoimmune;

(2) tuberculosis involving the adrenals;

(3) septicaemia (meningococcal sepsis with adrenal involvement is known as Waterhouse–Friderichson (*waterhouse-frid-er-rick-son*) syndrome) (*Rupert Waterhouse (1873–1958), English physician, Carl Friderichson (1886–1979), Danish paediatrician*);

(4) bilateral adrenalectomy (*a-dren-a-leck-tummy*) (used to be performed for malignant diseases and Cushing's syndrome);

(5) secondary causes of adrenal underactivity occur and include long-term steroid therapy and pituitary or hypothalamic disorders that lead to a decrease in ACTH production.

Trigger feature

- Generalized brown pigmentation of the skin (and recent scars).

This is obviously a non-specific trigger that has other causes. It also highlights what an insidious condition Addison's disease is. Most of its signs and symptoms are non-specific and you need a very high index of suspicion to detect it. If you meet someone who is inappropriately brown and unwell, this disease **must** cross your mind. The pigmentation is due to the lack of adrenocortical hormones, which normally provide feedback to the pituitary. In the absence of these hormones the pituitary secretes even more ACTH and a by-product of this hyper-secretion is the stimulation of melanocytes leading to pigmentation.

Other causes of brown pigmentation

(1) Haemochromatosis (sometimes slate grey);

(2) Nelson's syndrome (this occurs following bilateral adrenalectomy where the lack of adrenocortical hormones produces a hypersecretion of ACTH as before);

(3) ectopic ACTH production (usually from hormone-secreting cancers, for example, small cell tumours of the bronchus).

If you see a pigmented individual, you have to be more flexible in your approach. Tell your examiners, 'I have noticed generalized brown pigmentation of the patient. If they have not been to a hot country for a holiday or been on a sun-bed, then the possible causes include Addison's disease, Nelson's disease, ectopic ACTH production, and haemochromatosis. With your permission I would like to examine the patient further and ask some questions.' If this is allowed, introduce yourself to the patient and ask to examine their hands. Look at the palmar creases and see if they are pigmented. Look at the elbows and for any scars. Note whether these are pigmented too (only recent scars that have formed when Addison's disease has been active will be pigmented). Ask the patient to open their mouths and examine the buccal cavity with a pen-torch. Are there areas of pigmentation here too? Other possible areas of pigmentation include the nipples and areas of friction such as the elbows and knees. If pigmentation is present in these areas then this suggests Addison's disease. If you have time, ask if the patient has had both their adrenals removed (this would suggest Nelson's syndrome). Ask about other symptoms of Addison's disease (see below). See Figs 14.13 and 14.4.

Other features

- Anorexia
- weight loss
- vomiting
- fatigue
- diarrhoea or constipation
- hypotension
- postural hypotension
- hypoglycaemia.

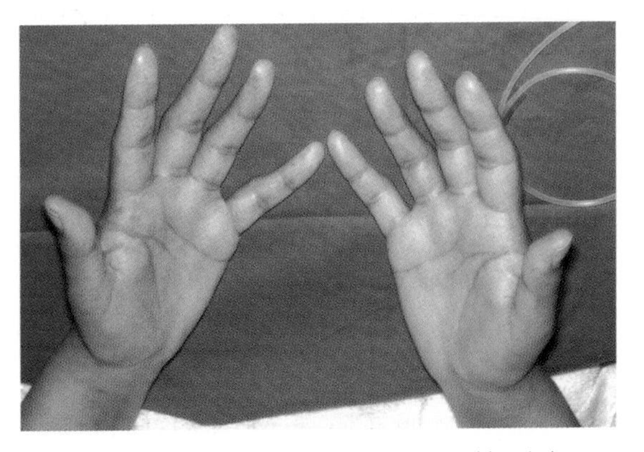

Fig. 14.13 Pigmentation of the palmar creases in Addison's disease.

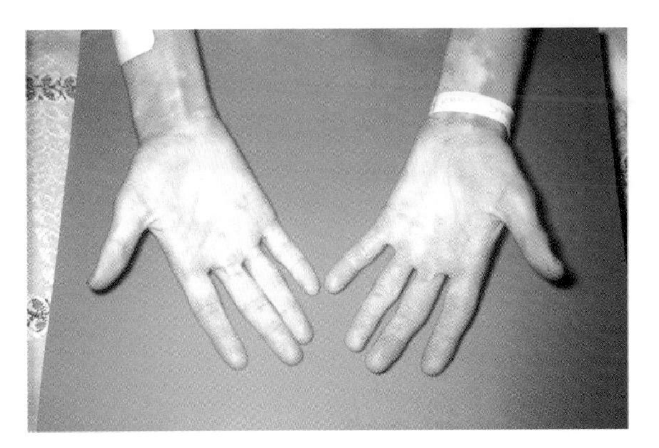

Fig. 14.14 Vitiligo in a patient with Addison's disease.

Systemic sclerosis

See Fig. 14.15.

What is it?

It is a generalized disease of connective tissue that leads to the proliferation of collagen and fibrosis of skin, subcutaneous tissue, small blood vessels, and organs. Its cause is unknown.

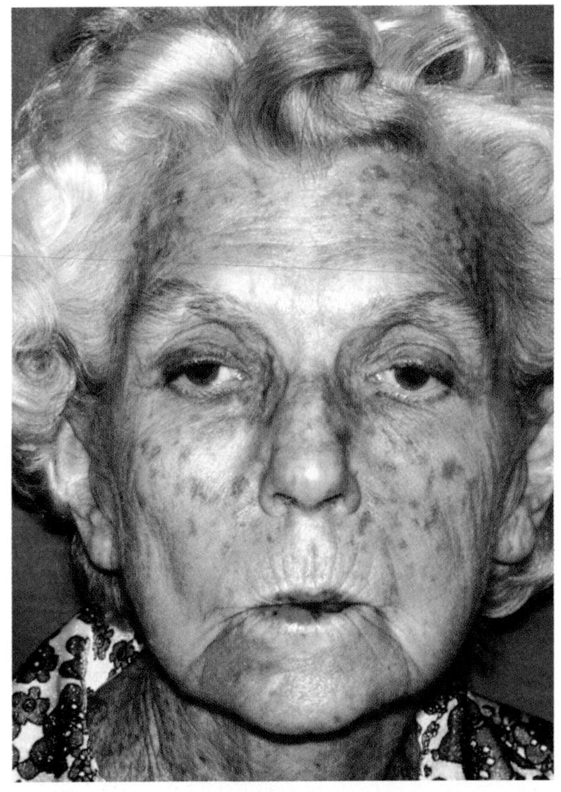

Fig. 14.15 Systemic sclerosis facies. Note the thin drawn mouth with radial furrows (pseudorhagades) and telangiectasia.

Trigger features

- 'Beak'-shaped nose
- thin, drawn mouth
- radial furrows around the mouth (pseudorhagades) (*sue-dough-rag-aids*)
- telangiectasia.

The patient (usually a woman) has an unmistakeable appearance. Despite this each sign on its own can be overlooked unless you are wary. I find the area around the nose and the mouth very helpful in the recognition of this disorder. Once you have twigged the diagnosis, you have an opportunity to demonstrate your knowledge. Tell your examiners that you suspect systemic sclerosis; explain why and say that you would like to examine the hands for evidence of sclerodactyly (*s-clear-owe-dack-tilly*) (atrophy of the fingertips), the changes of Raynaud's phenomenon, and calcinosis.

Other features

- Shiny, waxy-looking skin
- sausage-shaped fingers (early changes of Raynaud's phenomenon)
- dysphagia
- lung fibrosis
- renal failure
- pericardial effusion
- cardiomyopathy.

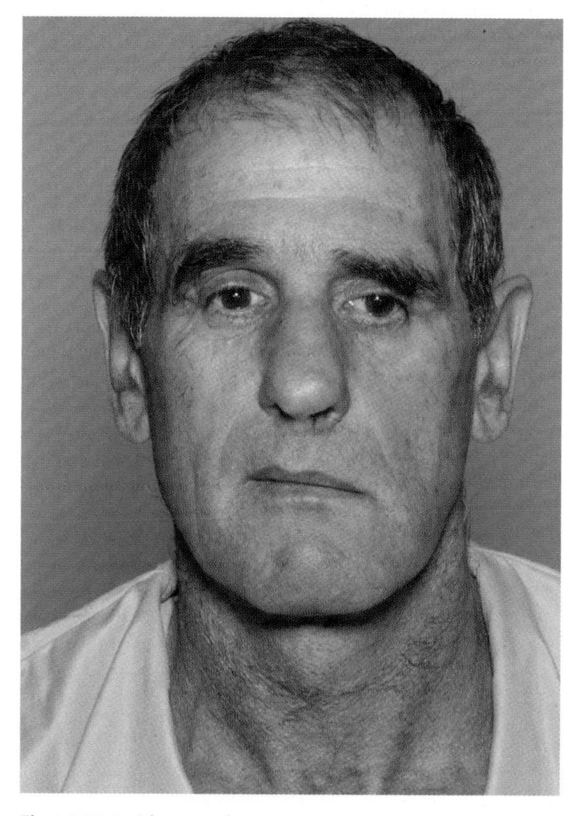

Fig. 14.16 Facial nerve palsy.

Facial nerve palsy

See Fig. 14.16.

What is it?

This is a lesion of the facial nerve, which can be due to an upper or a lower motor neurone cause.

Trigger feature

- Facial asymmetry with drooping of one side of the face (occasionally people can have bilateral facial nerve palsy, which can be difficult to spot but you should not encounter this in an undergraduate examination).

This is one case that should be easy to spot. However there is plenty of work to be done. You need to demonstrate whether the facial nerve palsy is an upper motor neurone or a lower motor neurone lesion. Tell your examiners, 'I can see drooping of the left side of the face, which indicates a facial nerve palsy. I would like to determine whether it is an upper or lower motor lesion and look for clues to its aetiology' (*ee-tea-ollow-jee*) (cause). Introduce yourself to the patient and assess the facial nerve in detail. Get your patient to blow out their cheeks, show their teeth, screw their eyes up tight, and raise their eyebrows. If they are unable to screw their eyes up tight or raise their eyebrows this is a lower motor neurone lesion (see p. 307). Having demonstrated a lower motor neurone lesion, quickly check for any potential causes. Look at the cheeks in the parotid area for signs of a swelling (parotid tumour) or a scar of a previous operation. With a pen-torch, look around the ear and the external auditory meatus for signs of herpetic vesicles (Ramsay–Hunt Syndrome). Very rarely a cerebello-pontine tumour can cause a lower motor neurone lesion. So ask the patient if they have trouble with their hearing (VIIIth nerve, cochlear) or have been falling (VIIIth nerve, vestibular). If you have time, check for nystagmus (see p. 296). If you demonstrate an upper motor neurone lesion, the most common cause is a stroke. Immediately look at the position of the limbs. Is one arm internally rotated with flexion at the elbow and is the corresponding leg internally rotated with the knee in extension and with plantarflexion of the foot? This is the classical position for hemiplegia.

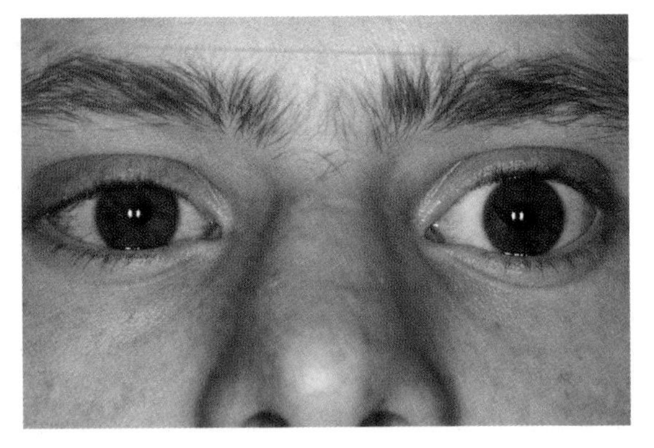

Fig. 14.17 Horner's syndrome. There is a partial ptosis as the right eyelid encroaches on the iris along with miosis of the right pupil.

Horner's syndrome

See Fig. 14.17.

What is it?

This is a collection of four physical signs:

(1) partial ptosis of an eyelid (partial droop of the lid);

(2) small pupil (miosis);

(3) absence of sweating (anhydrosis) (*an-high-drow-sis*);

(4) enophthalmos (the eye sinks back into the socket).

Trigger feature

◆ Slight droop of an eyelid.

A Horner's syndrome is another sign that is very easy to miss. Even its most obvious marker, partial ptosis, can be hard to spot for the unwary. So when inspecting the eyes, spend time checking for symmetry between them. If you do suspect a Horner's syndrome you need to move in closer to confirm your findings. Let your examiners know what you are doing, say, 'I have noticed a partial ptosis of the right eyelid and I am suspecting a Horner's syndrome. With your permission I would like to examine the pupil for miosis.'

Introduce yourself to the patient and see if the relevant pupil is constricted when compared with the other. If it is then it is likely you are dealing with Horner's syndrome.

Tip

Further examination is important because in elderly people a partial ptosis may be a consequence of ageing. This is because the levator muscle can become weak or become detached from the lid.

Tip

In an examination setting there may not be time to do this, but if there is very little difference between the pupils because of bright ambient light take your patient to somewhere gloomy (and explain why, lest they become suspicious of your intentions). In a darker environment, the normal pupil will dilate appropriately and make any differences between the two pupils more obvious.

Tip

To confuse the issue, miosis may be a normal consequence of ageing, plus elderly people may be on eyedrops, for example, for glaucoma, which can constrict (some can dilate) the pupil, so it may be worth asking if they have eye problems and if they are on eye drops.

You can check for anhydrosis crudely by running your index finger down one side of the forehead and then the other. Normal skin sweats slightly and has a soapy feel as you run your finger down it. If there is absence of sweating, the skin is dry, and your finger will glide smoothly without resistance. Demonstrating enophthalmos is not necessary. It is now believed that this is an illusion due to depression of the palpabral fissure.

Hereditary haemorrhagic telangiectasia

See Fig. 14.18.

What is it?

This is an inherited condition (autosomal dominant) whereby patients develop telangiectasia in the skin and mucous membranes. These vessels are weak and may lead to bleeding.

Trigger feature

◆ Red blebs on the face, particularly around the lips.

There are a number of conditions that may cause telangiectasia of the face including systemic sclerosis (see previously) and chronic liver disease (spider naevi). However HHT causes lesions around the lips, buccal mucosa, and tongue. Therefore if you see telangiectasia especially around the lips (and there is no evidence of systemic sclerosis or jaundice), say to the examiners, 'I have noticed lesions reminiscent of telangiectasia on the face and around the lips. I would like to demonstrate that they are telangiectasia and I would like to inspect the buccal mucosa and tongue because I am

(a)

(b)

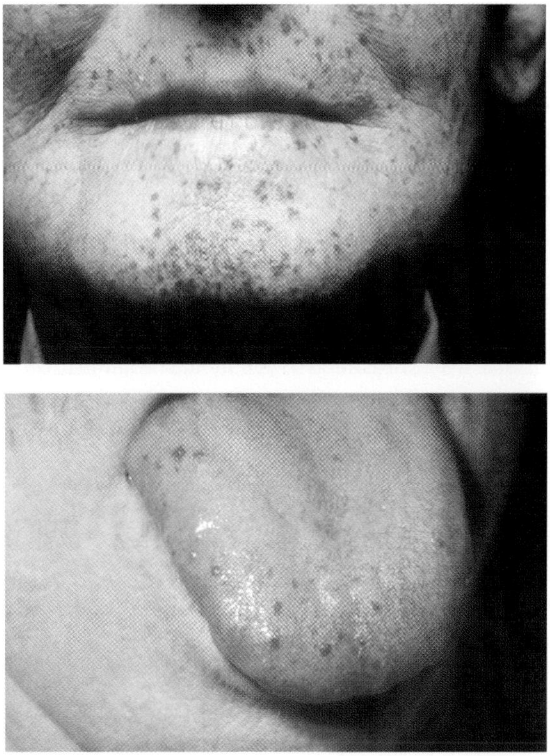

Fig. 14.18 Telangiectasia of hereditary haemorrhagic telangiectasia around the lips and tongue.

suspecting hereditary haemorrhagic telangiectasia.' If allowed, blanch a lesion and see if it refills. Then ask the patient to open their mouth and inspect with a torch. Make sure that you inspect the underside of the tongue. If lesions are present in the mouth the diagnosis is HHT.

Other features

- Iron deficiency anaemia
- gastrointestinal haemorrhage
- haemoptysis
- epistaxis (nose bleed).

Peutz–Jehger's syndrome

See Fig. 14.19.

What is it?

This is an inherited disorder (autosomal dominant), leading to a combination of pigmentation of the skin and mucous membrane and polyposis of the intestines.

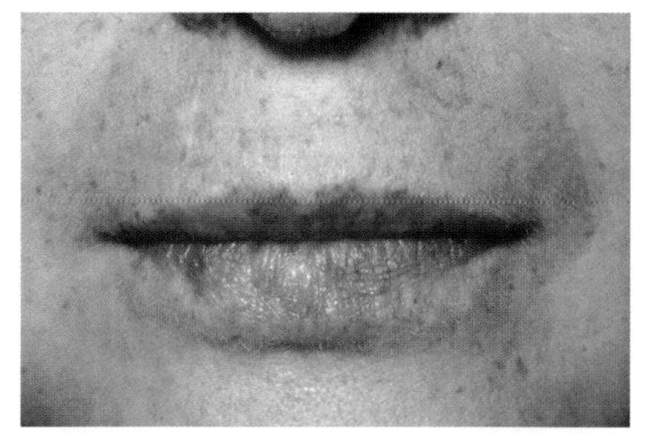

Fig. 14.19 The perioral pigmentation of Peutz–Jehger's syndrome.

Trigger feature

- Brown freckly pigmentation around the lips.

This sign is easy to miss, but if you do home in on this sign then the diagnosis is straightforward. You just need to keep this in mind when you do your systematic scan of the face. Pigmentation can also be found on the hands and feet.

Other features

- Polyps in the bowel (histologically they are hamartomas)
- iron deficiency anaemia
- gastrointestinal haemorrhage
- rarely malignant change.

Jaundice

See Fig. 14.20.

What is it?

Jaundice is the yellow discoloration of the skin and sclerae due to the deposition of the bile pigment bilirubin (see p. 177).

Trigger features

- Yellow sclerae
- yellow skin.

Jaundice can be easy or difficult to spot depending on the underlying cause. A full-blown obstructive jaundice may jump out at you whereas someone with mild Gilbert's syndrome may not be readily noticeable from the end of the bed (it would be unfair for examiners to try to get you to spot the latter without getting you to examine the face closer). If you notice yellow skin, check for scratch marks, which suggest itching (pruri-

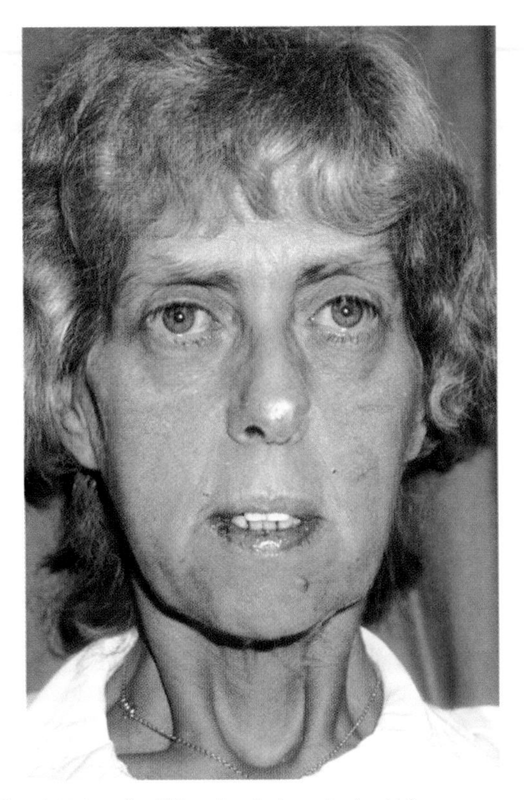

Fig. 14.20 Jaundice. This patient looks cachexic which suggests a malignant cause for her jaundice.

tis) and see if you notice any telangiectasia, which could be spider naevi and might indicate chronic liver disease. Often a spot case of jaundice will be a prelude to a full examination of the gastrointestinal tract. Tell your examiners that you have noticed yellow skin and sclerae and you suspect jaundice. You would like to confirm this and perform a fuller examination of the abdomen to determine a cause and to look in particular for signs of chronic liver disease.

Other features

These depend on the cause of jaundice. Usually this is chronic liver disease and so you should be familiar with the signs (see Chapter 6).

Further reading

Ryder REJ, Mir MA, Freeman EA. *An aid to MRCP short cases*, 2nd edn. Oxford: Blackwell Science; 1986.

CHAPTER 15

The electrocardiogram

Chapter contents

Introduction

Even the slightest mention of the word electrocardiogram (ECG) sends shivers down the spine of many a student! There is often a great fear of being asked to interpret an ECG in an examination. However, it is very unusual to be given an ECG in the examination. The ECG is an essential investigation in many clinical situations. As a newly qualified doctor, you will have to decipher ECGs on a daily basis. They allow us to diagnose myocardial infarctions (MIs), arrhythmias, angina, and structural abnormalities of the heart. In this chapter, a guide to ECG diagnosis will be given. The key to understanding the ECG is knowing what is normal. When you can identify what is normal, you will be able to spot what is abnormal and work out why. With practice you will be able to recognize patterns without working it out from first principles.

What is an electrocardiogram?

Contraction of muscle is secondary to depolarization associated with ionic movement within the sodium, potassium, and calcium channels. This creates electrical activity that can be recorded by electrodes placed on the patient. When the patient is lying still, the only significant muscle electricity produced is from the heart. It is this that is detected by the ECG. The ECG looks at the heart from 12 different directions. Once you understand this concept, the interpretation of the ECG begins to

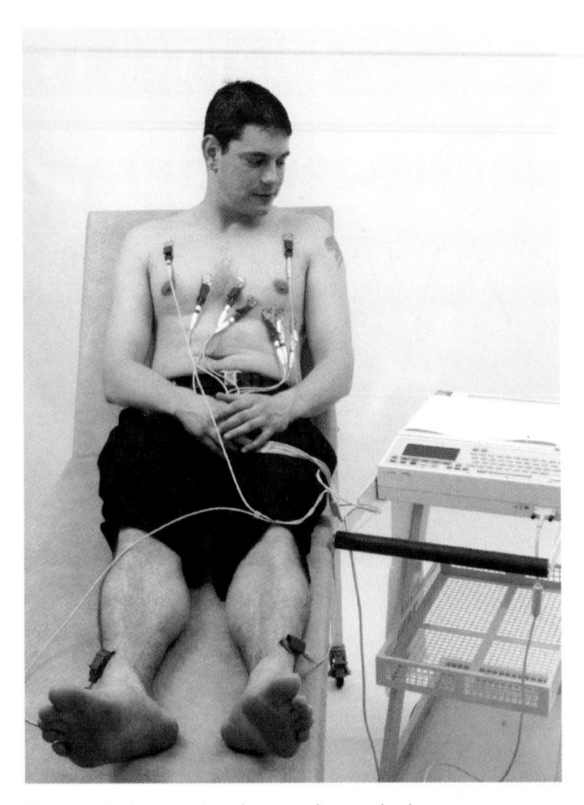

Fig. 15.1 Patient wearing electrocardiogram leads.

make sense. There are six chest leads and four limb leads. The chest leads are placed over the heart on the chest and look at the heart in a horizontal plane. These electrodes enable the anterior, lateral, and occasionally the posterior aspect of the heart to be observed electrically (V_1 - V_6). The four limb leads are placed on the arms and legs and

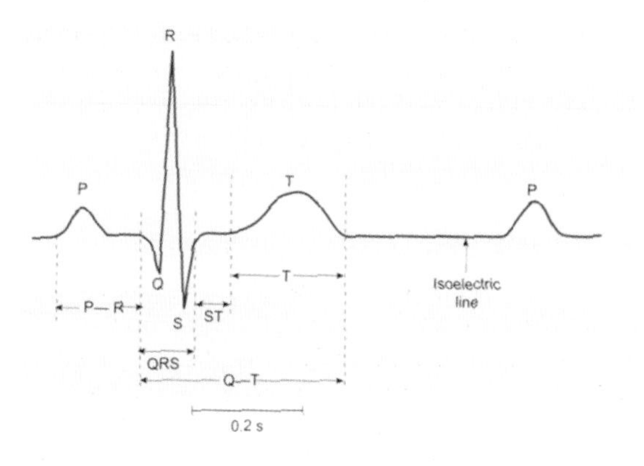

Fig. 15.2 Normal electrocardiogram trace. Reproduced by permission of Oxford University Press from **Fig. 15.9** (p. 304), *Human physiology: the basis of medicine*, by G. Pocock and C. Richards (1999).

the ECG machine interprets the electricity in the four limbs to give us six further directions from which we can analyse the heart (I, II, III, aVR, aVL, and aVF). The limb leads look at the heart in the vertical plane, detecting electrical activity from its inferior and lateral aspect.

Using combinations of these leads, you can focus in detail on specific regions of the heart:

- II, III, and aVF look inferiorly
- V_1 and V_2 look anteriorly (right ventricle)
- V_3 and V_4 look antero-septally (septum of left ventricle)
- V_5 and V_6 look antero-laterally
- I, aVL and V_6 look laterally

A positive charge (a depolarization) flowing towards an electrode will cause an upward deflection. Similarly, a negative charge (repolarization) will cause a downward deflection. Remember though, a positive charge flowing away from an electrode will also cause a downward deflection.

The electrocardiogram trace

See Fig. 15.2. Different parts of the ECG trace are assigned letters:

- P wave (a deflection before the QRS complex)
- Q wave (the first downward deflection)
- R wave (an upward deflection)
- S wave (a deflection below the baseline after the R wave)
- T wave (a deflection after the QRS complex).

P waves represent atrial activity (they are small because the atria are small), QRS waves represent ventricular electrical activity, and T waves represent ventricular repolarization. The size and configuration of each of these waves differs depending on which direction they are being measured from. See Fig. 15.3.

How to analyse the electrocardiogram trace (summary)

1. Patient details.
2. The rate.
3. The P wave.
4. The rhythm.
5. The axis.

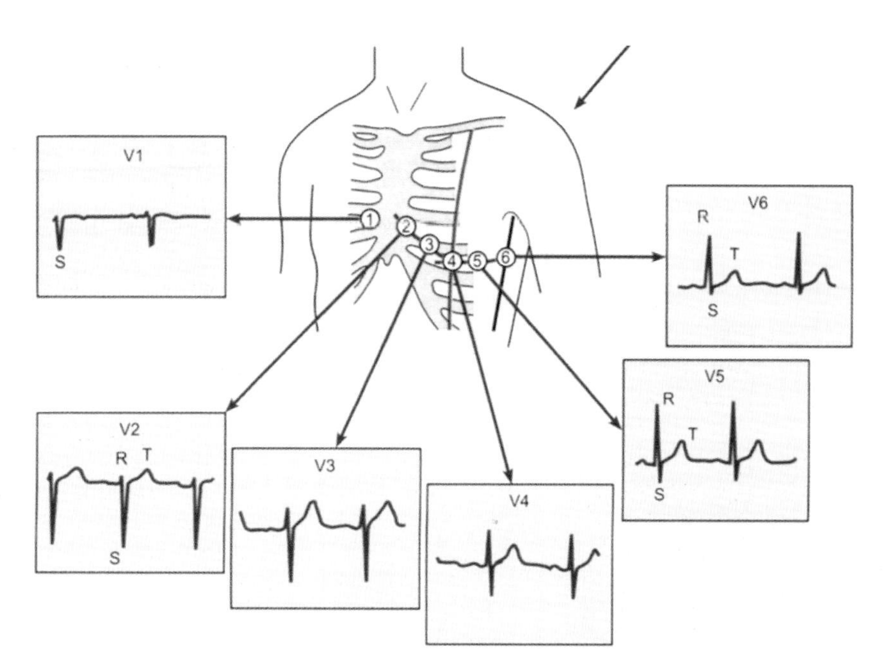

Fig. 15.3 Electrocardiogram trace associated with chest lead position. Note the S wave in VI with the complexes becoming more positive culminating in the R wave in V6. Reproduced by permission of Oxford University Press from **Fig. 15.7** (p. 300), *Human physiology: the basis of medicine*, by G. Pocock and C. Richards (1999).

6. The QRS complex.
7. Specific patterns.

How to analyse the electrocardiogram trace (in detail)

Try to be systematic when you examine the ECG. There follows a suggested order for analysing an ECG.

Getting started

1. Patient details.

Always check the name, date of birth, and when the ECG was taken. This is important because ECGs have been misfiled with the potential for disaster.

Rate

2. The rate.

The ECG usually comprises two sheets of paper. One for the 12-lead analysis and the other with usually three leads showing—the rhythm strip (some portable machines may only use one lead for the rhythm strip). The rhythm strip shows many heartbeats in succession. It allows us to calculate the rate and observe the rhythm. The heartbeat (represented by the ECG) is in sequence: P wave, QRS wave, and then T wave. The trick for calculating the rate is to identify the peaks of two R waves. Each R wave coincides with ventricular contraction and hence with the pulse. Count the number of large squares between R waves. Now divide this number into 300 and this will give you the rate per minute. A rough and ready way of estimating the rate is to remember that an R–R interval of one large square = 300 beats/min, two large squares = 150 beats/min, three large squares = 100 beats/min, and four large squares = 75 beats/min.

The normal heart rate is 60–100 beats/min. Tachycardia (*tacky-card-ia*) (meaning fast heart) is when the rate is greater than 100 beats/min and bradycardia (*braddy-card-ia*) (meaning slow heart) is when it is less than 60 beats/min. A tachycardia of more than 100 beats/min can be normal depending on the status of the patient, that is, if they have just been exercising. A bradycardia of less than 60 beats/min can be normal in fit athletes. See Figs 15.4 and 15.5.

P wave

3. The P wave.

The P wave represents atrial depolarization and subsequent atrial contraction (see 'Rhythm' below). If a P wave is present before each QRS complex the patient is said to be in sinus rhythm (which is the normal state of affairs). This is best appreciated in leads V1 and II. The P wave can sometimes be difficult to see. This occurs especially if there is much artefact (abnormal spikes usually due to patient movement), for example, in patients with Parkinson's disease who have a tremor

Tip

Try and make your first R wave coincide with the beginning of a large square, it makes the counting easier.

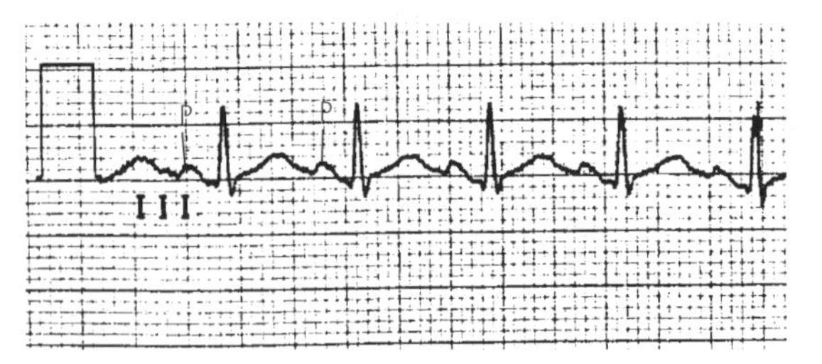

Fig. 15.4 Sinus tachycardia.

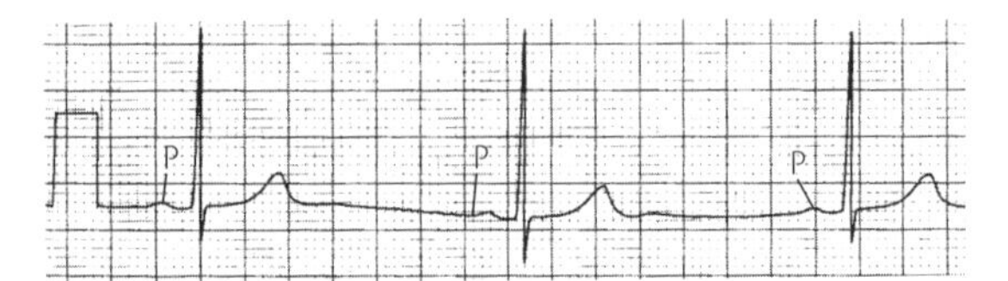

Fig. 15.5 Sinus bradycardia

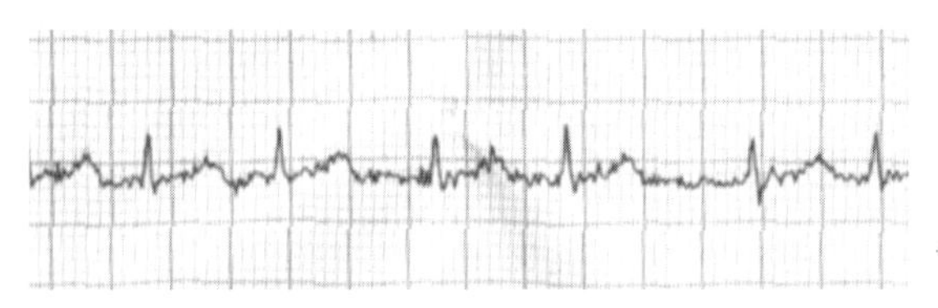

Fig. 15.6 Electrocardiogram in Parkinsonian patient. The tremulous baseline obscures the P waves and to a lesser extent the t waves.

(see Fig. 15.6). It may be difficult to say which deflections are P waves and which is artefact. If the right atrium becomes dilated, the P waves become peaked. This is called P pulmonale (*pee-pull-ma-nail-ee*) and can be caused by pulmonary hypertension or tricuspid stenosis (see Fig. 15.7). If the left atrium becomes dilated, the P waves become bifid (have two peaks). This is called P mitrale (*pee-my-traal-ee*) and can be caused by mitral stenosis (see Fig. 15.8). See Fig. 15.9 for a poor ECG trace.

Rhythm

4. The Rhythm

See Fig. 15.9. Abnormalities of rhythm can be due to abnormalities of the conducting system, ischaemic heart disease, or structural abnormalities of the heart. They can be fast or slow and regular or irregular. Sinus rhythm is the normal rhythm of the heart. The normal heartbeat originates in the sino-atrial node (*sigh-no-ay-tree-al*) of the right atrium. The impulse passes along normal conducting pathways from the atria to the ventricles. This is reflected by the P wave (which represents atrial contraction) preceding the QRS complex (which

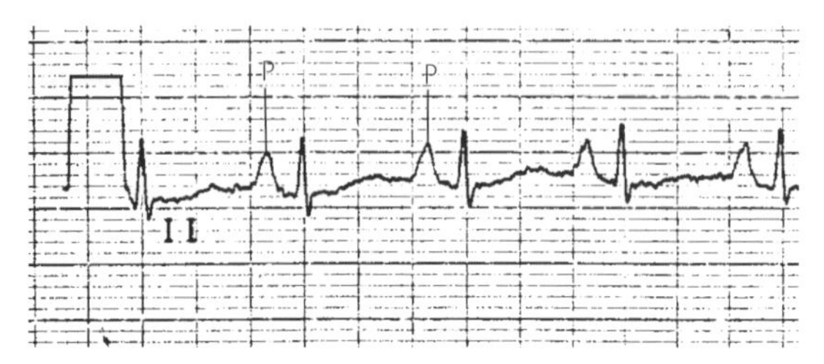

Fig. 15.7 P pulmonale. Note the peaked P waves are almost as tall as the R wave.

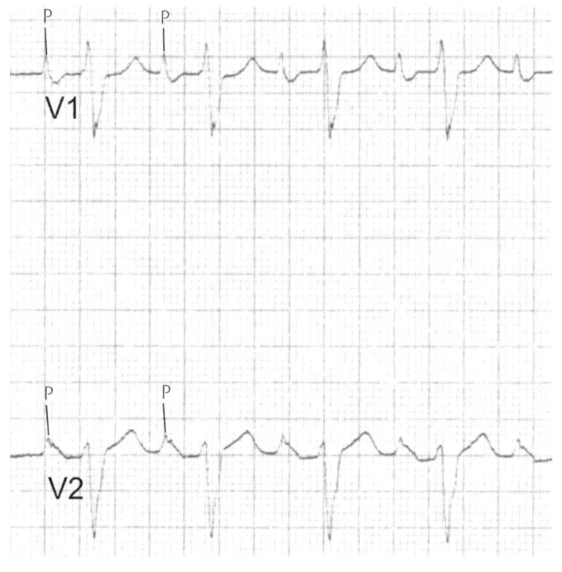

Fig. 15.8 P mitrale.

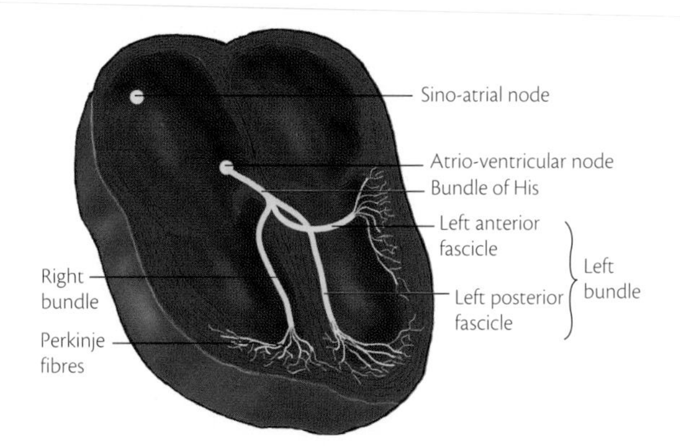

Fig. 15.9 Conducting system of the heart

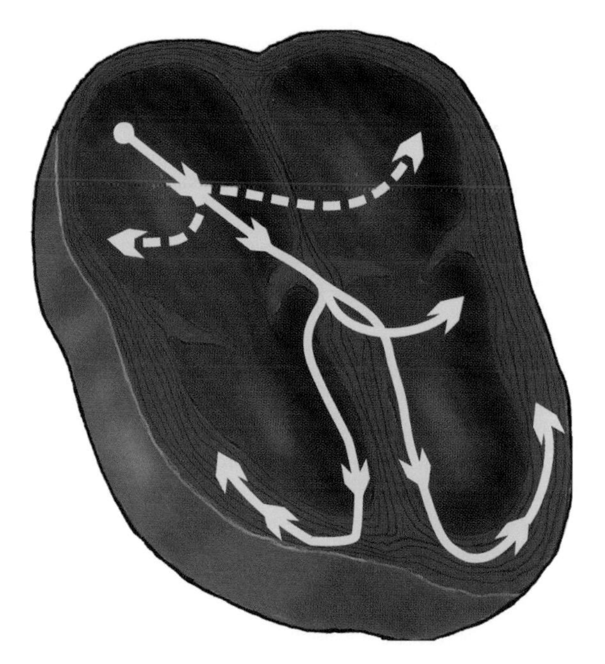

Fig. 15.10 Path of the electrical impulse in sinus rhythm. The impulses originate in the Sino-atrial node which pass to the atria stimulating them to contract. Further impulses travel to the AV node, through the bundle of his to the right and left bundles (left anterior fascicle and left posterior fascicle). Impulses then spread to the ventricles stimulating them to contract in turn.

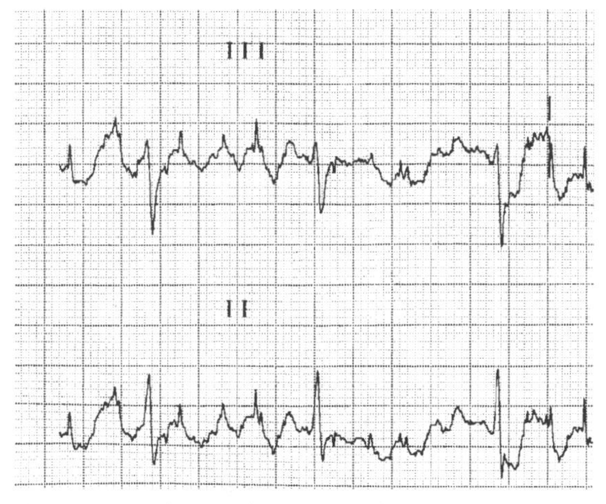

Fig. 15.11 Poor electrocardiogram trace. This restless patient has produced a tracing that simulates atrial flutter (see text). When calm their trace was sinus rhythm.

CASE 15.1

Problem. A patient has become acutely confused and is restless and agitated. What is the diagnosis from this portable ECG tracing (Fig. 15.11)?

Discussion. On the basis of this ECG it is impossible to say. The baseline is all over the place and there is superimposed muscle tremor obscuring any further detail. Although it is possible that an MI or arrhythmia may have caused the confusion you cannot make any inferences from this trace (it was mistakenly identified as atrial flutter with 4:1 block). The person who got this trace deserves credit for getting something out of a difficult situation but the only real alternative is to try and repeat the ECG when the patient is calm.

represents ventricular contraction). This is sinus rhythm. See Fig. 15.10.

It is important to note that sinus rhythm is not always regular. That is, although every QRS complex is preceded by a P wave, the R wave-to-R wave interval varies marginally with respiration. This is a normal variant found in fit adults. It is called sinus arrhythmia (see Fig. 15.12). If you take a deep breath in, your heart rate increases and if you exhale, your heart rate slows. The heart rate speeds up when you inhale due to a reflex inhibition of vagus (*vague-us*) nerve activity (the vagus nerve slows the heart). Another cause of an irregular pulse that occurs in sinus rhythm is extrasystoles (*extra-sis-toe-lees*) (or ectopics). This means extra heart beat. When patients describe their heart 'missing a beat', it is in fact an extra beat followed by a compensatory pause! These extrasystoles can arise from anywhere in the conducting system, so they can be atrial

Tip

One of the key things to do with an ECG is to confirm that the patient is or is not in sinus rhythm by identifying the presence or absence of P waves before each QRS complex.

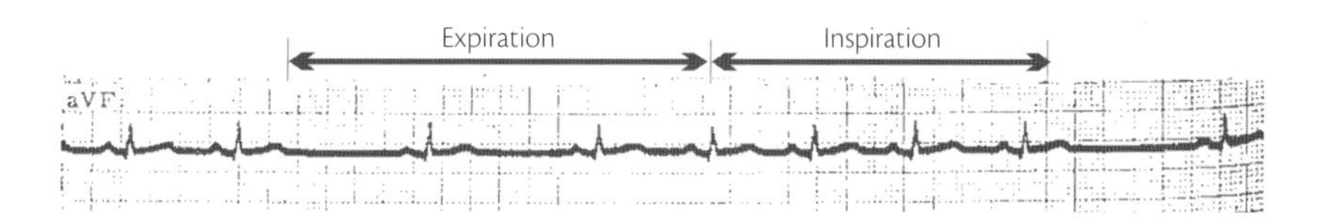

Fig. 15.12 Sinus arrhythmia.

extrasystoles or ventricular extrasystoles, for example (see Figs 15.13 and 15.14). Atrial extrasystoles look exactly like normal sinus beats. This is not surprising because they originate from the sino-atrial node and follow the normal conduction path, so producing normal-looking complexes. The heart then tries to make up for the premature beat by delaying the next one. Ventricular extrasystoles can originate from anywhere in the ventricles. Consequently, they do not follow the normal conduction path. These other routes of conduction are slower (it is like comparing rapid travel on the motorway with that on a slow country lane). Because the conduction is slower, this makes the complexes broader.

There are many types of arrhythmia (meaning lack of rhythm, dysrrhythmia means abnormal rhythm). However, if you remember the sequence of events as an impulse passes down the conducting system and the relationship of each wave of the ECG trace to that cycle, you will be able to work out what the rhythm disturbance is. It just takes time and practice. The arrhythmias to be considered here are

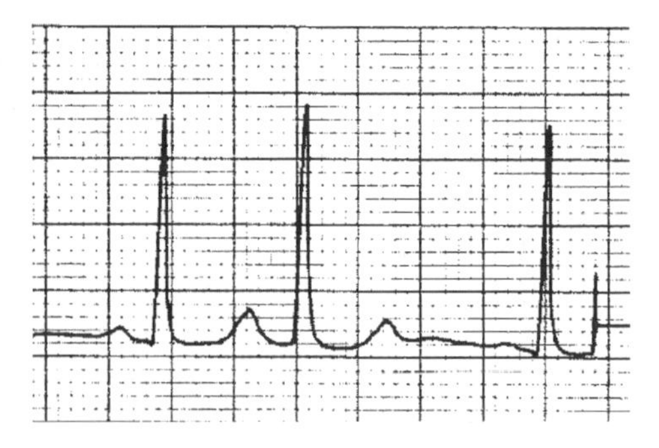

Fig. 15.13 Atrial extrasystole. Note the narrow complex superimposed on the t wave of the preceding complex. It is then followed by a compensatory pause.

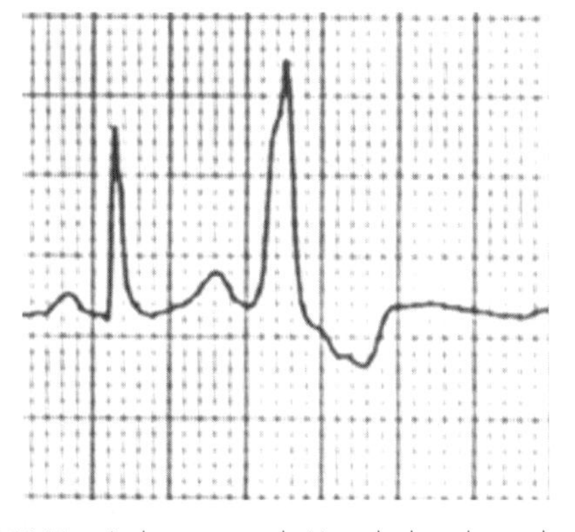

Fig. 15.14 Ventricular extrasystole. Note the broad complex in comparison to Fig. 15.13.

- slow arrhythmias (bradyarrhythmias)
  - the heart blocks
  - asystole
- fast arrhythmias (tachyarrhythmias)
  - supraventricular tachycardia (SVT)
  - atrial fibrillation
  - atrial flutter
  - ventricular tachycardia
  - ventricular fibrillation.

Slow arrhythmias

The heart blocks

There is a block to the conduction of the electrical impulse between the atria and ventricles and this leads to a number of rhythm disturbances (the most common cause is ischaemic heart disease). There are three main types of heart block, with second-degree heart block having two categories:

- first-degree heart block
- second-degree heart block—Mobitz (*mow-bits*) type I (*Woldemar Mobitz (1889–1951), Russian-born German surgeon*) (or Wenkebach (*when-key-back*) phenomenon (*Karel Frederik Wenkeback (1864–1940), German physician*)
- second-degree heart block—Mobitz type II (sustained and non-sustained)
- third-degree heart block (complete heart block).

First-degree heart block (see Fig. 15.15) occurs when each QRS wave is preceded by a P wave, but there is a delay in the conduction between them. This results in the interval between the P and R wave lengthening to greater than one large square (0.2 s). It can cause a normal or slow, regular rhythm and is harmless.

Second-degree heart block occurs when there is intermittent failure of transmission between atria and ventricles. Depending on the pattern, it is either called Mobitz type I or type II. The Mobitz type I (or Wenkebach phenomenon) occurs when the P–R interval gradually length-

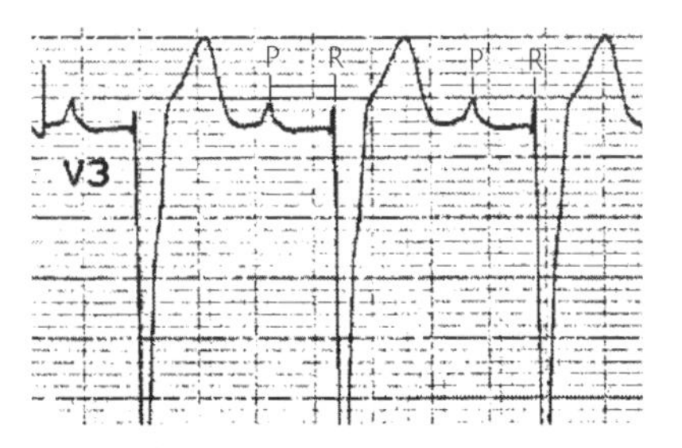

Fig. 15.15 First-degree heart block. There is prolongation of the PR interval of greater than 1 large square.

ens until a QRS complex is missed altogether. This cycle can be repeated producing a regularly irregular rhythm. See Fig. 15.16. The Mobitz type II form of second-degree heart block (see Fig. 15.17) occurs when the conduction between the atria and ventricles is impaired in a specific pattern, occurring just once or on a regular basis. If it occurs regularly, then there may be two, three, or more atrial contractions (P waves) needed before a ventricular contraction is produced. If there are two P waves to one QRS complex this is 2:1 block, if there are three P waves to one QRS complex this is 3:1 block, and if there are four P waves to one QRS complex this is 4:1 block. This needs rectifying with a pacemaker before it enters third-degree heart block. Note that in second-degree heart block the QRS complexes appear at regular intervals albeit delayed. The interval may become irregular if the conduction defect produces a variable block.

In third-degree (or complete) heart block (see Fig. 15.18), the conduction block is more severe. It is so bad that the ventricles are electrically isolated and have to beat at their own intrinsic rate creating a slow regular rhythm (all cardiac muscle has the ability to contract independently and this occurs at different rates depending on the area of the heart: atria—70 beats/ min, nodal (junctional)—50 beats/min, ventricles—30 beats/min). By beating at their own rate (called an escape rhythm), the ventricles ensure that some blood gets round the body. This compensation is inefficient so dizziness, chest pain, or breathlessness on exertion may occur. The ventricles can stop beating altogether leading to collapse and even death. Complete heart block is dangerous and requires the insertion of a pacemaker.

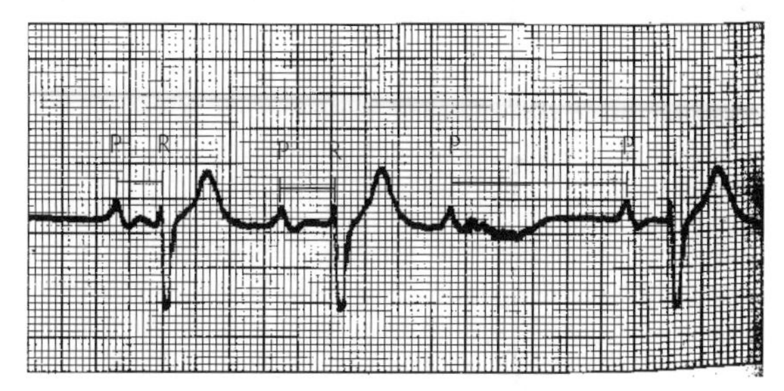

Fig. 15.16 Mobitz type I. Lengthening PR interval before conduction fails altogether through the AV node (i.e. no QRS complex seen.)

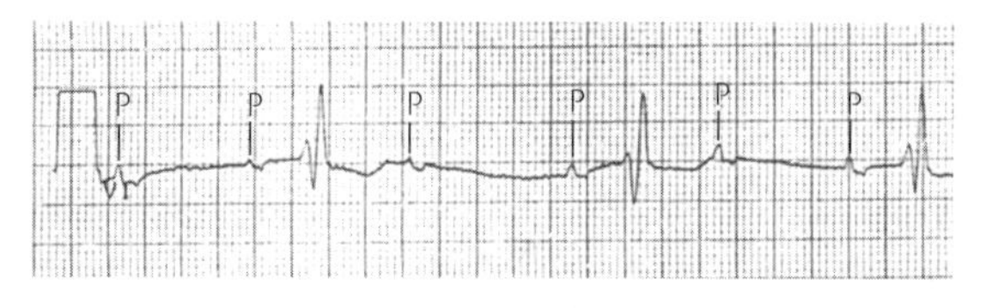

Fig. 15.17 Mobitz type II (2 : 1 block).

Asystole

Asystole (see Fig. 15.19) is where there is no electrical activity in the heart and there is ventricular standstill. It may be the end result of a bradyarrhythmia when cardiopulmonary resuscitation is indicated. It may also be secondary to disease outside the heart (especially respiratory disease) leading to tissue hypoxia. Cardiopulmonary resuscitation is again required but the patient may require ventilation on an intensive care unit. Finally asystole is the final common pathway for many terminal conditions (including severe heart disease). In these circumstances the patient should previously have been identified for palliative care (and should not have a cardiac monitor in any case) and a 'do not attempt resuscitation (DNR/DNAR) order should have been made after consultation with the patient (and with the consent of their relatives).

Fast arrhythmias

Supraventricular tachycardia

Supraventricular tachycardia (see Fig. 15.20) is a common arrhythmia that produces a fast regular rhythm. It can be short lived but if prolonged can cause palpitations, chest pain, or a faint feeling. It occurs because an accessory

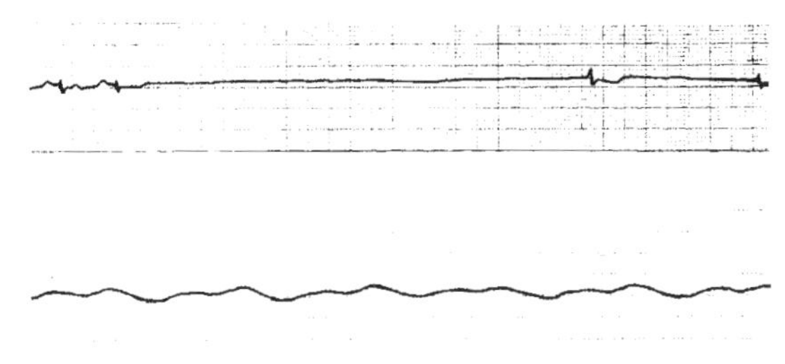

Fig. 15.19 Asystole.

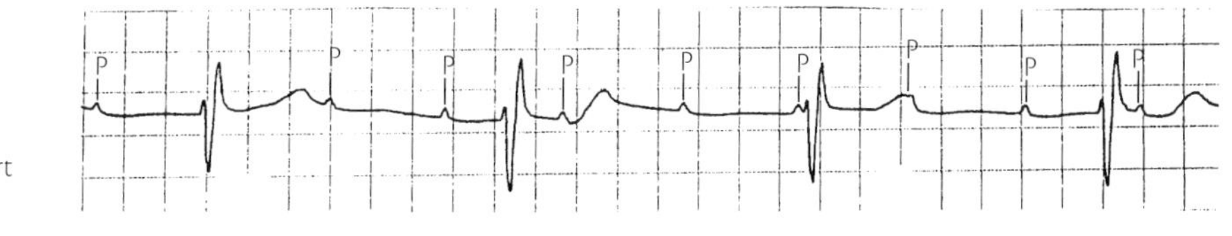

Fig. 15.18 Third-degree heart block.

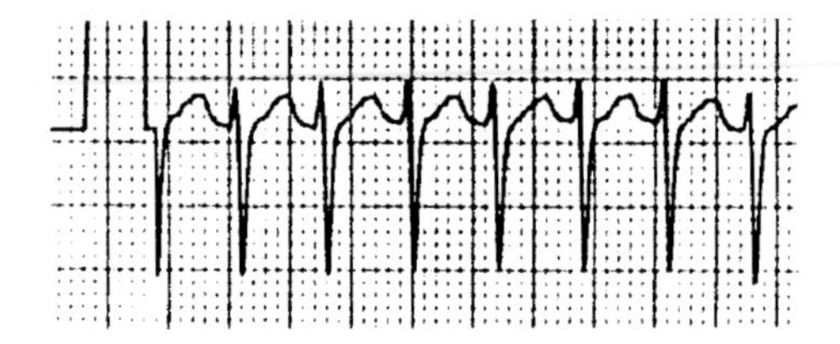

Fig. 15.20 Supraventricular tachycardia.

pathway connecting the atria to the ventricles allows the impulse that has reached the ventricles to travel back up to the atria again (called retrograde conduction). Once the impulse reaches the atria it has the option of returning down the normal conduction pathway again. If the pathway is still capable of conducting (that is, it is not refractory to fresh stimuli) then a vicious cycle can be set up leading to a fast heartbeat, which can be up to 180 beats/min (it is rarely faster).

Atrial fibrillation

Atrial fibrillation (see Fig. 15.21) is a common arrhythmia and when uncontrolled produces a fast irregular rhythm. Fibrillation is the rapid chaotic contraction of muscle. Electrical stimulation of the atria occurs up to 400 beats/min. However, there is no synchrony of muscle contraction. In fact there is very little muscle contraction at all. As a result, there are no P waves, only an irregular baseline due to fibrillation (or F) waves. Rapid, but sporadic, electrical impulses are transmitted to the ventricles. These vary in strength and frequency, so the resulting ventricular contraction will be totally irregular. In this situation we often say the pulse is irregularly irregular.

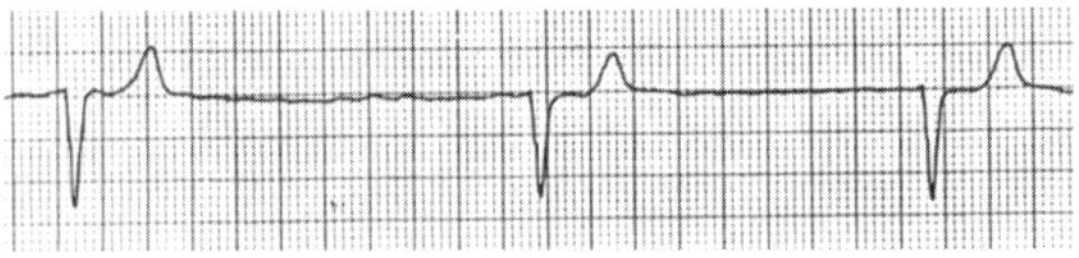

Fig. 15.21 Atrial fibrillation. There are no P waves. The ventricles are beating at 36/minute indicating that this is also complete heart block (this patient also needs a pacemaker)

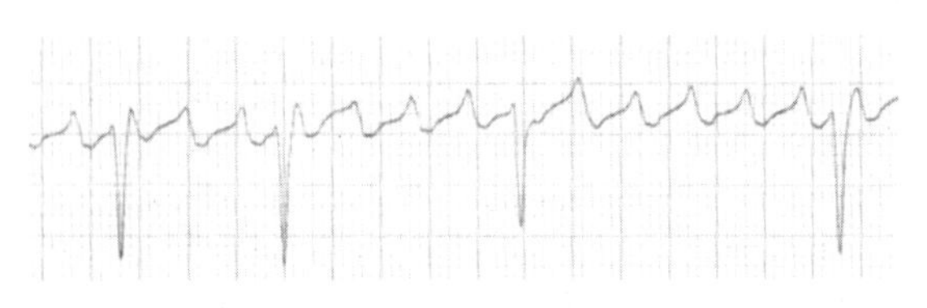

Fig. 15.22 Atrial flutter with variable block. Note the saw-tooth pattern between QRS complexes.

> **Tip**
>
> Place a piece of paper along the top of the R waves and mark on the paper where the R waves occur. Now move the paper along a few centimeters; you will see that it is impossible to match the markings with the new sequence of R waves. This is a quick method of demonstrating an irregularly irregular rhythm, especially if you are not sure of the regularity of the rhythm at first sight.

Atrial flutter

The atrio-ventricular (AV) node cannot conduct any faster than 200 beats/min. If the atria beat any faster than this there will be a natural block to the conduction of some impulses. Atrial flutter occurs when the atria contract at approximately 300 beats/min. The smooth outlines of normal P waves are lost and replaced by a saw-tooth baseline. Atrial flutter can occur with varying lengths of block (see Figs 15.22–15.25). The most notorious is atrial flutter with 2:1 block. Because the atrial rate is 300 beats/min and only every other impulse is transmitted (2:1), the ventricular rate will be exactly 150 beats/min. It is infamous because it is easy to miss. The saw-tooth configuration is not obvious and the flutter wave can be mistaken for a P wave.

Similarly, if the block is 3:1, the rate will be 100 beats/min. Occasionally the block can be variable in which case the pulse will be irregular, but there may still be a saw-tooth baseline pattern. Remember that the only difference between a Mobitz type II variable

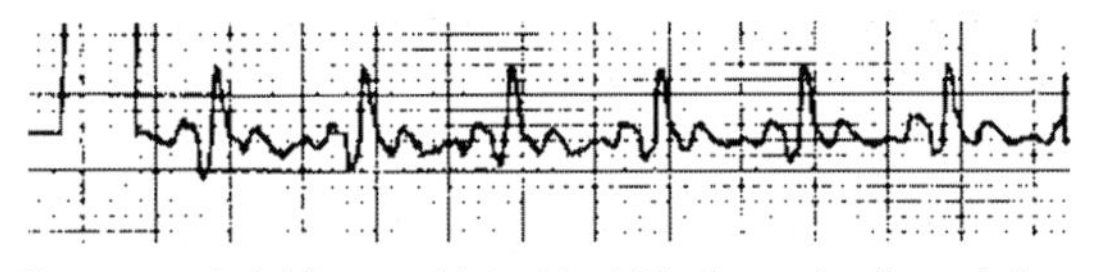

Fig. 15.23 Atrial flutter with 2:1 block. The key to its diagnosis is to consider the possibility when you see an 'SVT' with a rate of 150 beats/min.

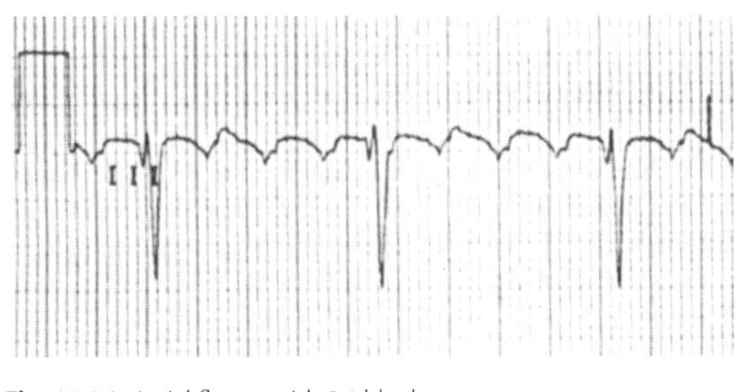

Fig. 15.24 Atrial flutter with 3:1 block.

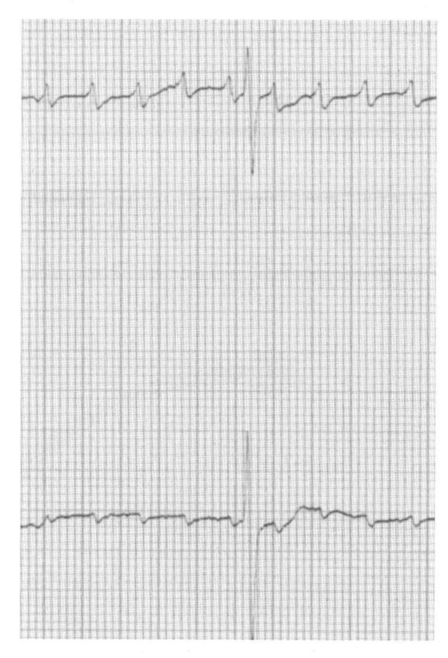

Fig. 15.25 Atrial flutter with 4:1 block.

> **Tip**
>
> Always consider the possibility of atrial flutter with 2:1 block if a patient's pulse rate is 150 beats/min.

block and atrial flutter with variable block is the baseline. Atrial flutter has a saw-tooth pattern, Mobitz type II will show P waves. Similarly, it is easy to distinguish atrial fibrillation from the irregular pulse of atrial flutter with variable block because the baseline in flutter has a saw-tooth pattern.

Ventricular tachycardia

Ventricular tachycardia (see Fig. 15.26) is caused by electrical activity in the ventricles and usually causes a heart rate greater than 120 beats/min. As the electrical activity starts and is transmitted via alternative routes through the ventricles, the complexes are broad. In ventricular tachycardia the rhythm is rapid, regular, and broad. P waves will not be obvious because electrical activity is occurring further down the pathway. It

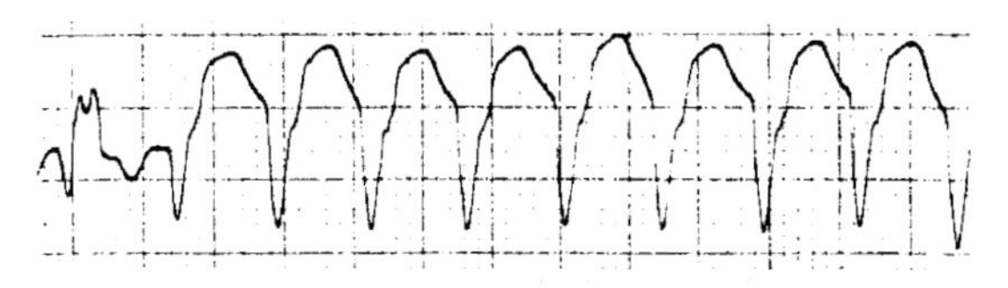

Fig. 15.26 Ventricular tachycardia

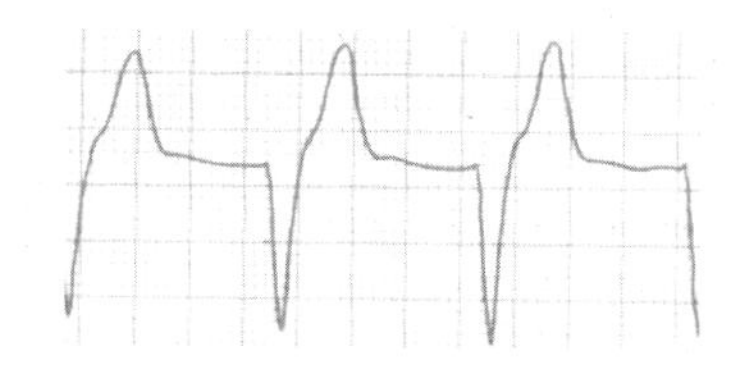

Fig. 15.27 Idioventricular rhythm.

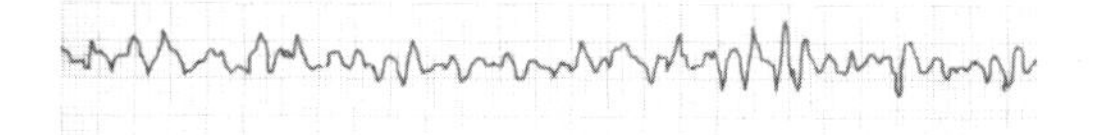

Fig. 15.28 Ventricular fibrillation.

requires prompt treatment with anti-arrhythmic agents. If the rate is less than 120 beats/min, this is called an idioventricular rhythm and requires no treatment (see Fig. 15.27).

Ventricular fibrillation

Ventricular fibrillation (see Fig. 15.28) is probably the easiest arrhythmia to identify. The combination of a typical rhythm strip and an unconscious patient clinches the diagnosis! Rapid chaotic contraction of the ventricular muscle fibres occurs without any synchronized muscle contraction. There is no cardiac output. There is only an irregular wavy baseline on the ECG. This requires urgent electrical defibrillation.

Axis

5. The axis

Electrical activity is dispersed from the heart in all directions. However, on average it tends to flow towards the apex of the heart. This average direction of depolarization is called the cardiac axis (see Fig. 15.30).

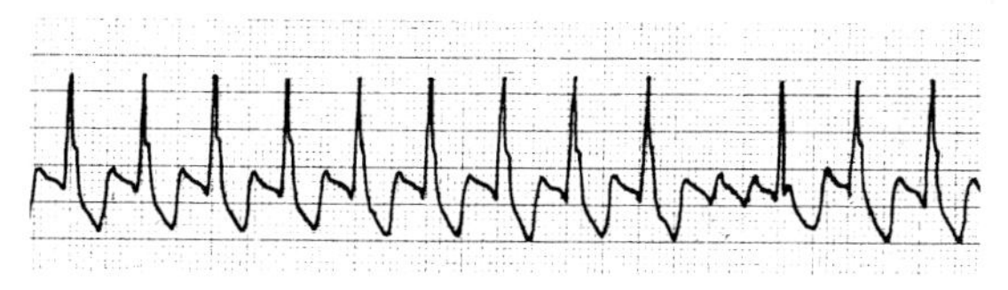

Fig. 15.29 Case 15.2.

> **Tip**
>
> If you see an irregular wavy chaotic trace on an ECG or monitor and the patient is conscious, check to see if the leads are properly applied. You **cannot** have ventricular fibrillation and a conscious patient.

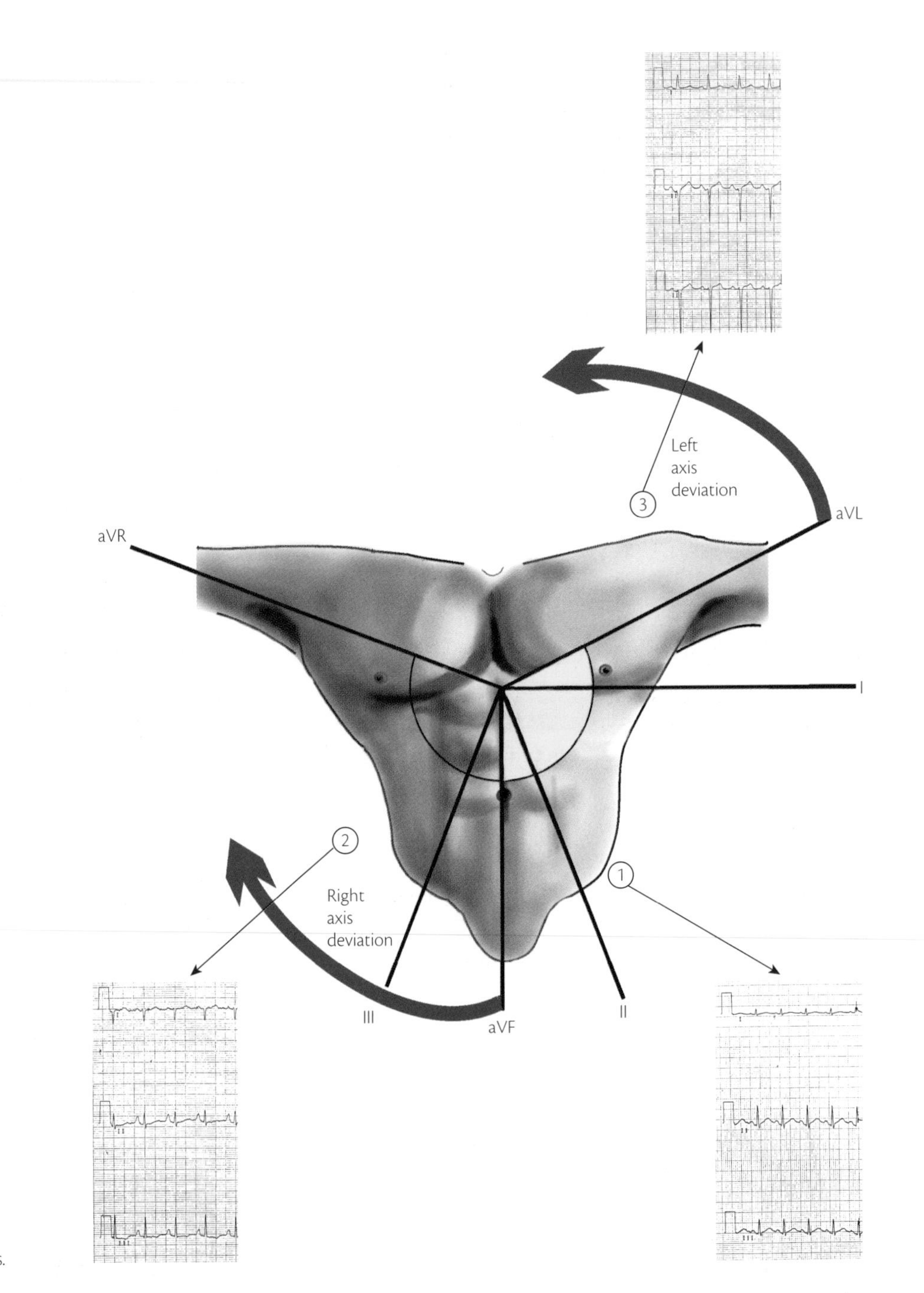

Fig. 15.30 Cardiac axis.

The normal axis ranges from –30 to +90°. Any deviation from this range can indicate pathology particularly if there is a documented change in the axis acutely. There are various mathematical ways of calculating the cardiac axis, but in practice the author finds these unhelpful and relies on the pattern formed in the limb leads I, II, and III to guide interpretation of the axis. In the author's opinion gross deviation requires an explanation, minor deviation (found by calculation) does not. See Figs 15.31–15.33 and Table 15.1.

CASE 15.2

Problem. You have the rhythm strip above in front of you and you have worked out the heart rate at 150 beats/min but you are not sure that you can see P waves. You are wondering if this is an SVT or atrial flutter with 2:1 block (Fig. 15.23).

Solution. Do not worry! Even the experts have difficulty with this one. Thankfully there are tactics you can use to solve the dilemma. Carotid sinus massage, where the carotid artery is rubbed (you should be taught this once you qualify if not before), can increase vagal tone. This can induce a temporary block at the AV node. This may be sufficient to allow you to recognise the underlying rhythm. However in modern times, adenosine (a short acting drug) is used to achieve the same effect. It also has the added advantage that it can terminate a tachyarrhythmia in some cases.

Keypoints

- Always look for P waves preceding each complex to determine if the patient is in sinus rhythm or not.
- Arrhythmias can be fast or slow and regular or irregular.
- There are varying degrees of heart block that must be recognized.
- Complete heart block is a serious complication, which can be fatal.
- Ventricular fibrillation is a medical emergency.

Tip

Determining the axis is not often helpful. It is worth knowing the causes of the shifts in axes but you will always diagnose them using more sensitive methods, for example, echocardiography.

Keypoints

- The cardiac axis represents the average direction of the wave of depolarization.
- Various causes are associated with deviation of the axis to the left or right.
- Determining the cardiac axis has very limited clinical utility.

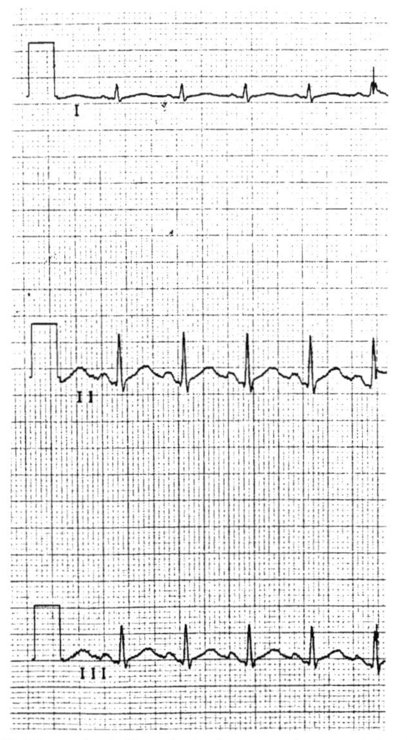

Fig. 15.31 Normal axis. Depolarization spreads towards leads I, II, and III.

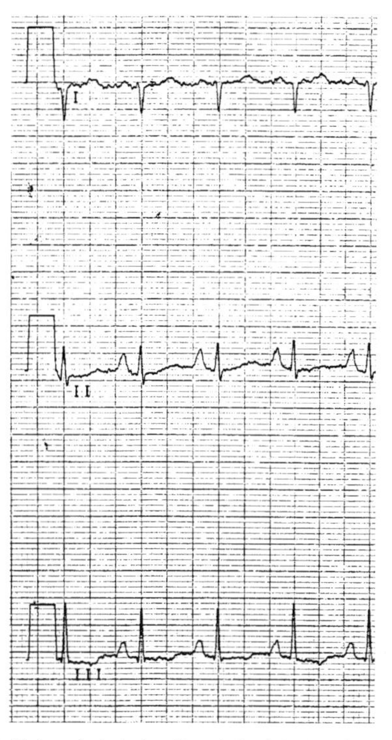

Fig. 15.32 Right axis deviation. Depolarization spreads towards lead III and away from lead I.

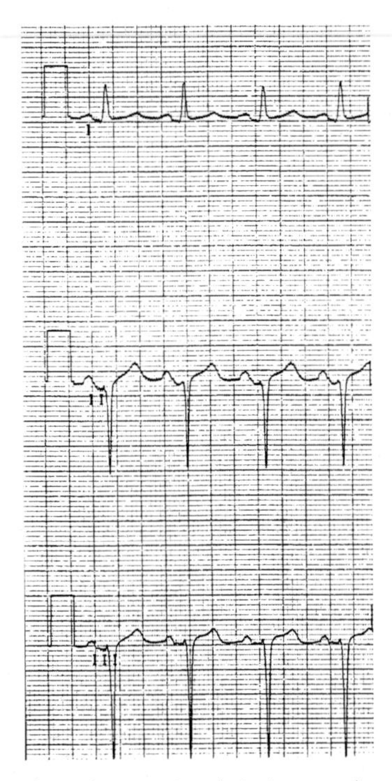

Fig. 15.33 Left axis deviation. Depolarization spreads towards lead I and away from lead III.

TABLE 15.1 Pathology associated with axis deviation

Right axis deviation
Right ventricular hypertrophy
Pulmonary embolism
Cor pulmonale
Pulmonary stenosis
Left axis deviation
Left ventricular hypertrophy
Hypertension
Aortic stenosis
Hypertrophic obstructive cardiomyopathy

QRS complex

6. The QRS complex

There are many disorders that cause abnormalities of the QRS complex. To be able to identify these quickly you should be familiar with the normal ECG (see Fig 15.2). You should concentrate on the chest leads. Essentially, the QRS complex has three features to look out for. It is narrow (less than 3 mm across), it progresses from V_1 to V_6—becoming more positive (the R waves increase in size), and non-pathological Q waves may be seen in V_4—V_6. In normal circumstances, Q waves represent the depolarization of the septum. They are not pathological if they are less than 1 mm across and less than 2 mm deep. Pathological Q waves occur in myocardial infarction (MI). During an MI, an area of heart muscle dies. This area is then unable to conduct electrical current. If you place an electrode over the infarcted area, the initial deflection will be a negative movement, away from the electrode (in healthy muscle it would be conducted towards the electrode). Some people describe the infarcted muscle as 'an electrical window' looking into the heart. The QRS complex can either be too wide or too tall. A bundle branch block makes it too wide and hypertrophy of ventricular muscle makes it too tall.

The bundle branch blocks

Students (and some doctors) find this area difficult. Fortunately there are tricks to identify the two types. Normally, electrical depolarization spread down the correct pathways within the ventricles to give the characteristic ECG pattern. If one of the bundles supplying the ventricles is fibrosed or damaged then transmission of electrical current will be delayed down that bundle. Depolarization will occur in the ventricles, but at slightly different rates depending on which bundle is affected. The shape of the QRS complex is wider (because it takes longer to depolarize) and an abnormal

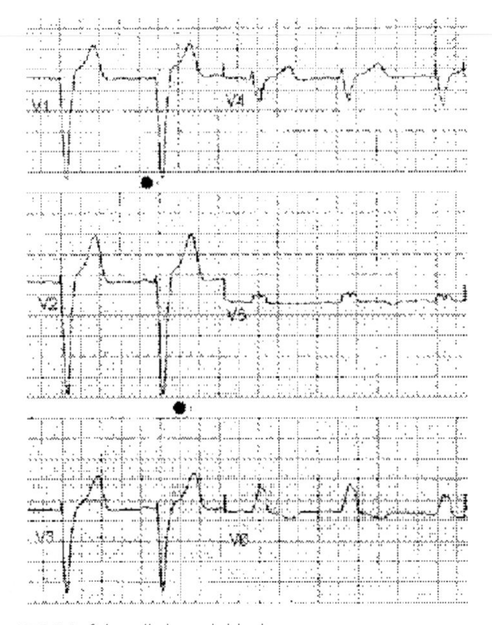

Fig. 15.34 Left bundle branch block.

shape (because the depolarization spreads in a different direction). Each bundle branch block has a characteristic ECG appearance (see Figs 15.34 and 15.35). If the QRS complex looks like an M in V_1 and a W in V_6, this is right bundle branch block (RBBB). Similarly, if the complex looks like a W in V_1 and an M in V_6, this is left bundle branch block (LBBB). It becomes more difficult when the complexes are less typical.

For causes of LBBB and RBBB, see Table 15.2.

TABLE 15.2 Causes of left and right bundle branch block

Causes of left bundle branch block
Aortic stenosis
Hypertension
Left bundle branch fibrosis, for example, after a myocardial infarction

Causes of right bundle branch block
Normal in 1% of young adults
Pulmonary embolism
Cor pulmonale
Congenital heart disease
Right bundle branch fibrosis, for example, after a myocardial infarction

Ventricular hypertrophy

There are complex rules for the calculation of ventricular hypertrophy. Most commonly left ventricular hypertrophy is due to hypertension or aortic stenosis. The recommended best rule of thumb for the assessment of left ventricular hypertrophy is SORF (**S** in V **o**ne plus **R** in V **f**ive is greater than 35 mm indicates left ventricular hypertrophy). Right ventricular hypertrophy is less frequently seen, usually being caused by chronic lung conditions such as chronic obstructive pulmonary disease. Here we will see a positive R wave in V1 (with narrow/normal QRS complexes). See Figs 15.36 and 15.37.

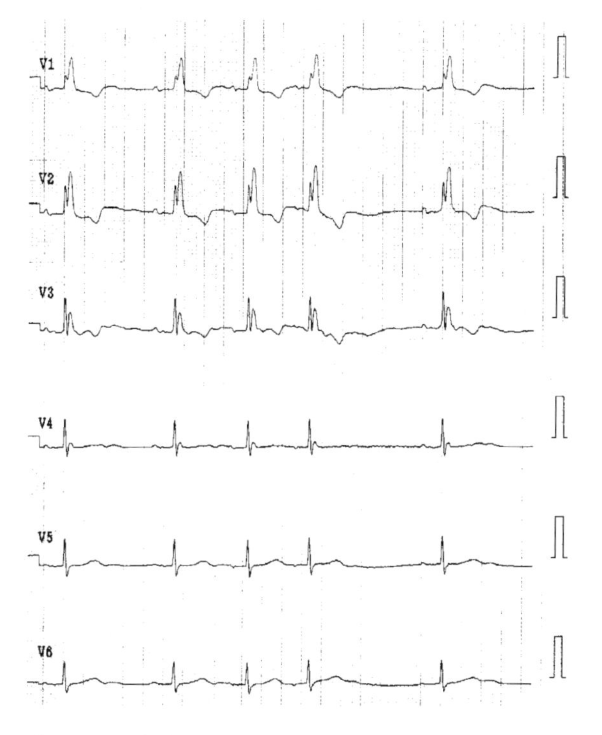

Fig. 15.35 Right bundle branch block.

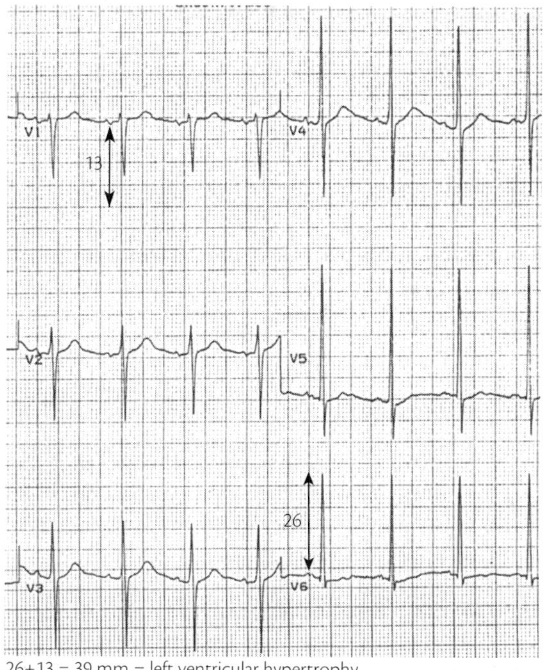

Fig. 15.36 Left ventricular hypertrophy. The sum of s wave in V1 and r wave in V6 is 26 mm satisfying the cirteria for LVH.

Tip

Broad complexes with a WiLLiaM conformation in the chest leads suggests a LBBB. Broad complexes with a MaRRoW conormation in the chest leads suggests a RBBB.

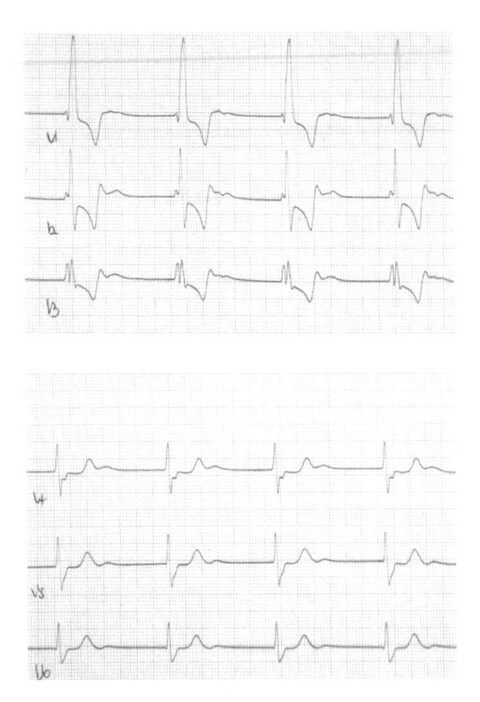

Fig. 15.37 Right ventricular hypertrophy. Note the peaked R wave in V1 and V2. Right ventricular strain is indicated by ST depression in V1–V3 (and there is co-existant partial right bundle branch block).

Keypoints

- The QRS complex is usually no more than three small squares in duration.
- Q waves are pathological if they are >1 mm across and >2 mm deep.
- Bundle branch block cause wide QRS complexes.
- Left ventricular hypertrophy causes QRS complexes that are excessively tall.

Specific patterns

7. Specific patterns

As mentioned earlier, understanding the mechanisms of the ECG trace will help decipher the ECG code. As your confidence and experience grows, you will begin to recognize important patterns. Do not try to decipher all 12 leads *en masse*. Go through the leads one by one. Here are some patterns you will commonly be asked to diagnose especially once you are qualified:

- MI
- left ventricular aneurysm
- acute pericarditis
- high take-off
- myocardial ischaemia
- digoxin effect
- pulmonary embolus (PE)
- hyperkalaemia
- hypokalaemia
- Wolff–Parkinson–White syndrome.

Myocardial infarction

Myocardial infarction is a cardiac emergency. Depending on the age of the MI certain changes can be seen on the ECG (see Table 15.3).

An acute MI will therefore have ST elevation and often, pathological Q waves. An old MI will have pathological Q waves and possibly inverted T waves. Remember that pathological Q waves do not give any indication of the age of the MI; once they develop they are permanent. The area of infarction can be worked out from those leads showing the characteristic changes (see p. 414). To be significant, ST elevation should be greater than 2 mm above the baseline in anterior MIs and at least 1 mm for inferior MIs. Figure 15.38 shows a time sequence of ECG changes in acute MI; Fig. 15.39 shows pathological Q waves in V1–V4 suggesting an old anterior MI; Fig. 15.40 shows typical changes of an acute anterior MI; Fig. 15.41 shows Q waves in III and aVF, suggesting an old inferior MI (note that lead II is not always involved); Fig. 15.42 shows an acute inferior MI.

TABLE 15.3 Electrocardiogram changes with time following myocardial infarction

Within hours	T waves	Abnormally tall
Within hours	ST segments	Rise above the baseline
Less than 24 h	T waves	Inverted
Less than 24 h	ST segments	Return to baseline
Within days	Pathological Q waves	Present
Later	T waves	May or may not remain inverted
Later	Pathological Q waves	Persist

Tip

The order of ECG changes in an evolving MI is ST elevation, then Q wave formation, and then T wave inversion.

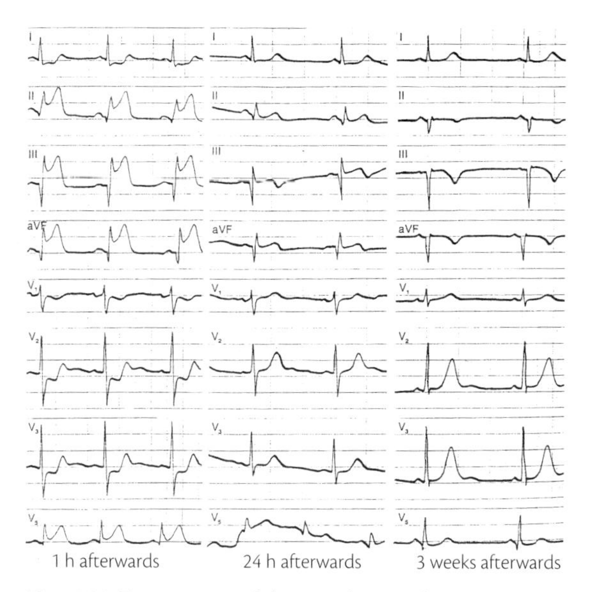

Fig. 15.38 Time sequence of electrocardiogram changes in acute myocardial infarction.

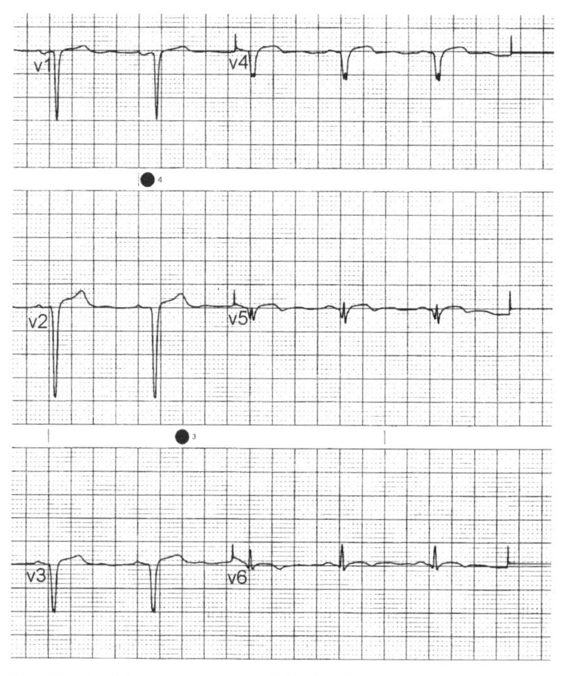

Fig. 15.39 Old anterior myocardial infarction. Note the pathological q waves in V1–V5.

Fig. 15.43 shows an acute posterior MI. These can be easily overlooked. The ST segment is below the baseline in V_1 and there is a positive R wave here too. In fact, this is a mirror image of the normal findings of an acute MI. Lead V_1 can assess the posterior of the heart

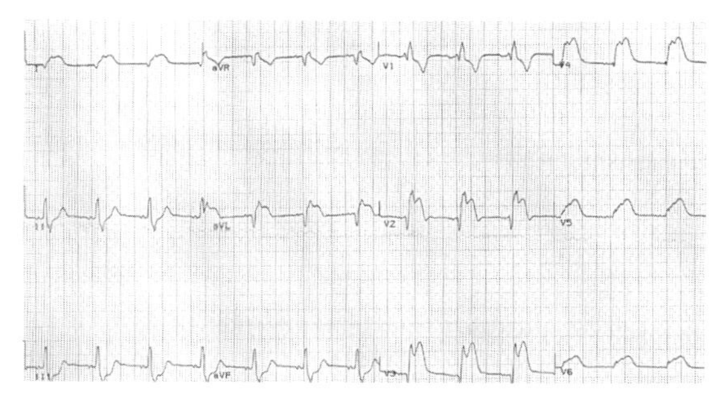

Fig. 15.40 Acute anterior myocardial infarction. Lateral extension is indicated by ST elevation in leads I, AVL, V5 and V6.

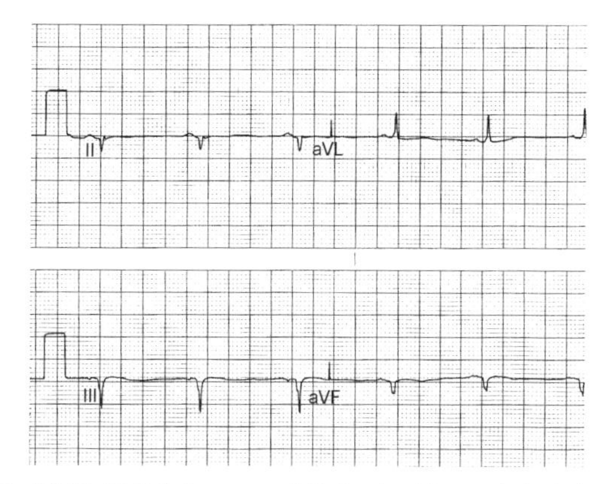

Fig. 15.41 Old inferior myocardial infarction. Note pathological q waves in leads II, III, and AVF.

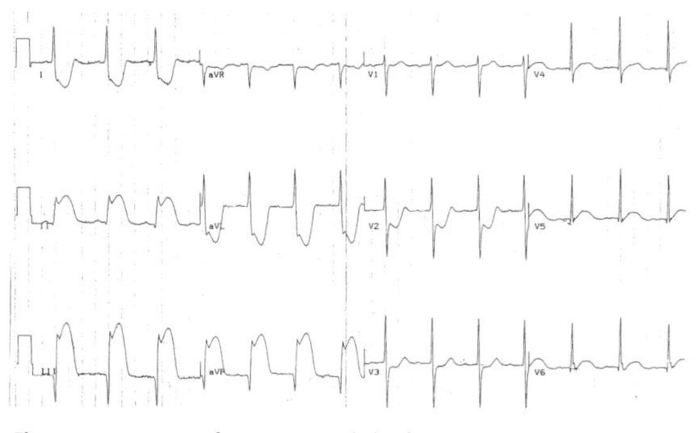

Fig. 15.42 Acute inferior myocardial infarction.

by looking directly through the anterior surface. However any depolarization will be seen in the opposite direction (if you placed a lead on the patient's back to directly assess the posterior of the heart we would see typical changes of an acute MI). Often during an MI, the full thickness of the heart muscle dies, producing the 'electrical window' described earlier. However, occasionally only a partial thickness of heart muscle dies. Consequently, no 'electrical window' is formed

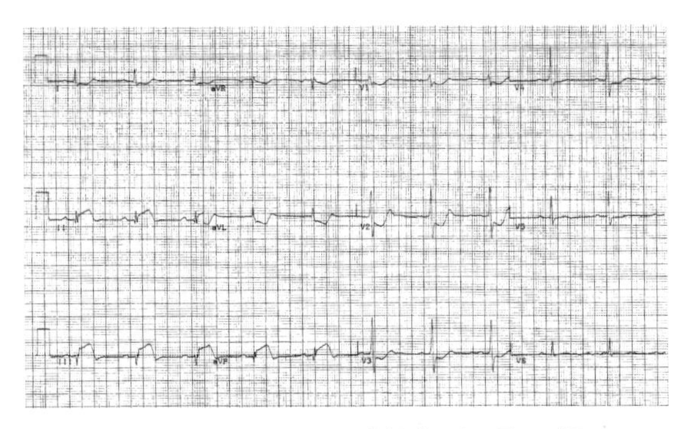

Fig. 15.43 Acute posterior myocardial infarction. The tall R waves in V1 and V2 with significant ST depression in the context of an inferior MI suggests posterior extension.

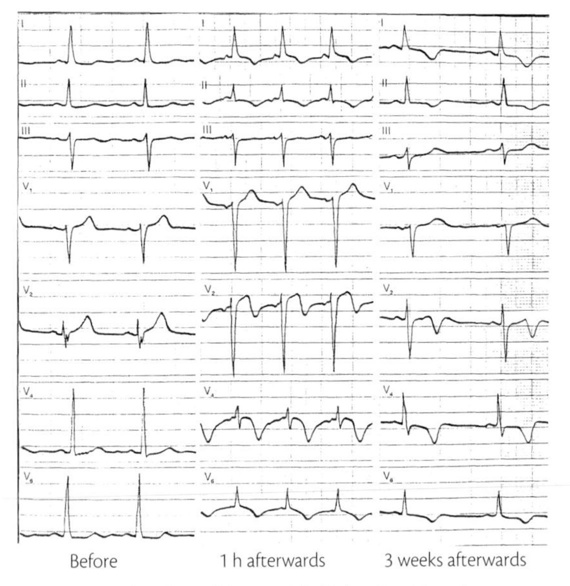

Fig. 15.44 Subendocardial myocardial infarction. Note the developing t wave inversion in leads V4–V6 24 hours after the onset of chest pain.

> **Tip**
>
> Remember, a normal ECG does not exclude a MI.

and there are no Q waves. You might see the initial ST elevation (which later resolves) and T wave inversion. This is called a non-Q wave or subendocardial MI (see Fig. 15.44).

Left ventricular aneurysm

Persistent ST elevation in the anterior leads is characteristic of a left ventricular aneurysm. However, this should be confirmed with an echocardiogram.

Acute pericarditis

See Fig. 15.45. During the first week of illness, the ECG shows ST elevation in all leads facing the surface of the heart (epicardium), that is, the anterior, lateral, and inferior leads. The ST elevation is concave upwards—like a saddle. In MIs, the ST elevation tends to be convex upwards and is usually located in a specific area.

High take-off

This is another cause of ST elevation. It may be difficult to differentiate high take-off from an acute MI, however, it usually occurs in young patients without a history of chest pain. The T wave can also help to discriminate between an MI and high take-off. During an acute MI, the T waves dip below the baseline, whereas in high take-off they are above the baseline.

Myocardial ischaemia

Increased demand or reduced oxygen supply can result in myocardial ischaemia. Electrocardiographically, this is characterized by horizontal or down-sloping ST depression. This is where instead of the S wave coming up to the baseline, it falls below it and blends with the T wave. It may occur at rest or be exercised induced and is often associated with chest pain. See Fig. 15.46.

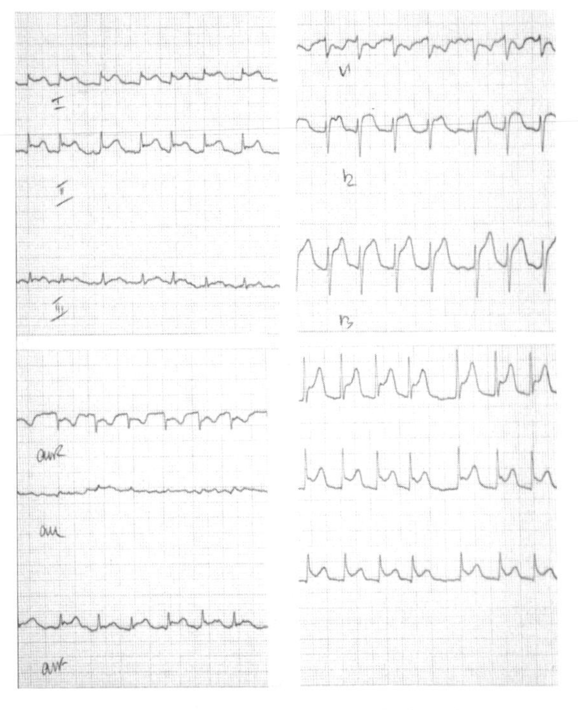

Fig. 15.45 Acute pericarditis. Notice the saddle-shaped ST elevation in the majority of leads.

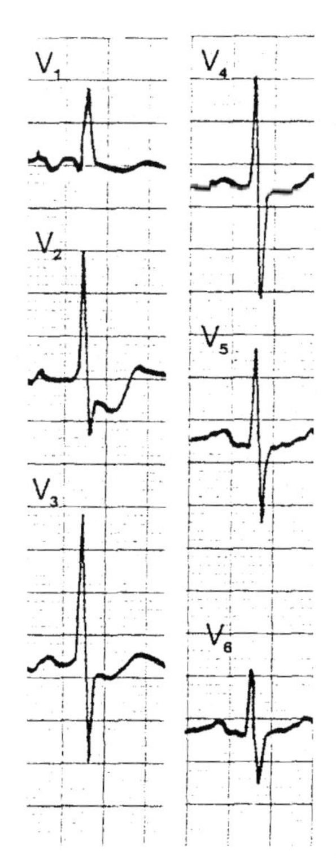

Fig. 15.46 ST depression.

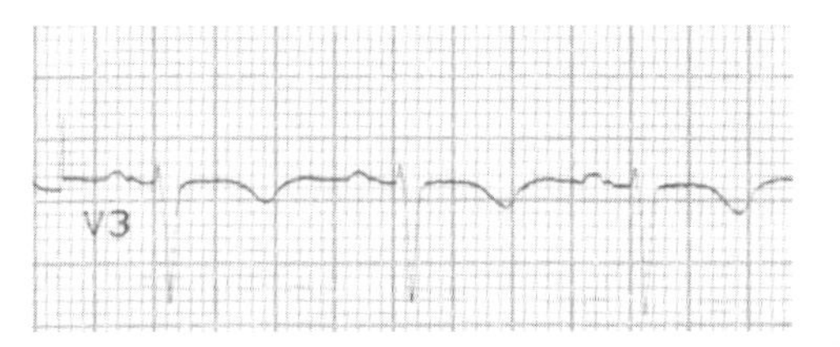

Fig. 15.47 Digoxin-induced ST depression. The 'reverse tick' ST depression of digitoxicity.

Not all ST depression is acute. To decide whether ST depression is new or old, do the following.

1. **Take a history.** If there is no recent chest pain or illness, then it is unlikely to be acute.
2. **Compare with a previous ECG.** When doing so, compare each lead in turn. Comparison of the chest leads may be complicated by the fact that on different dates the leads may be in slightly different positions on the patient's chest. So, instead of comparing V_1 with V_1, V_2 with V_2, and so on, it is probably better to compare chest leads with similar R wave height.

Digoxin effect

See Fig. 15.47. The administration of digoxin can cause T wave inversion. This can be associated with ST depression. Digoxin toxicity can cause many different arrhythmias including bradycardias and tachycardias. Always consider this in patients normally treated with digoxin who then present with an arrhythmia.

Pulmonary embolus

A diagnosis of PE cannot be made on ECG changes alone. However, the ECG is useful when considering the diagnosis. There are some suggestive appearances, plus it can help in excluding other differential diagnoses. The most common abnormality found on the ECG in a patient with a PE is a sinus tachycardia. This is non-specific. Other changes include

- atrial fibrillation
- right axis deviation
- peaked P waves
- RBBB
- tall R waves in V1
- the $S_1Q_{III}T_{III}$ pattern, that is, a deep S wave in lead I, a Q wave in lead III, and an inverted T wave in lead III (see Fig. 15.48) (this is supposed to be classical, but is rarely found in practice).

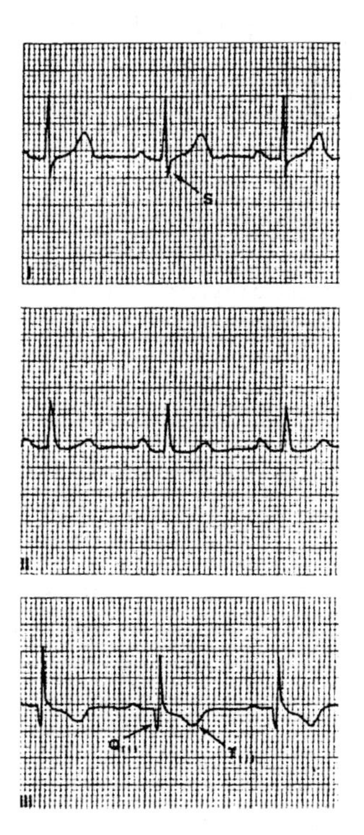

Fig. 15.48 $S_1Q_{III}T_{III}$.

Hyperkalaemia

See Fig. 15.49. Here the classical features are tall, tented T waves. Later there is broadening of the QRS complex and loss of P waves. Check the serum potassium level immediately!

Hypokalaemia

See Fig. 15.50. In this case we will see small T waves and prominent U waves. A U wave is simply a small upward deflection that occurs after a T wave. Both hyper- and hypokalaemia may cause life-threatening arrhythmias.

Wolff–Parkinson–White syndrome

(Louis Wolff (1898–1972), American physician, Sir John Parkinson (1885–1976), English physician, PD White (1886–1973), American cardiologist.) As you will remember from a previous figure, the normal path to the ventricles is through the bundle of His *(hiss)* *(Wilhelm His Jr (1863–1934), German physician)*. In some individuals, there is an alternative route. This extra path (accessory path of Kent) *(AF Kent (1863–1958), English physiologist)* allows rapid conduction

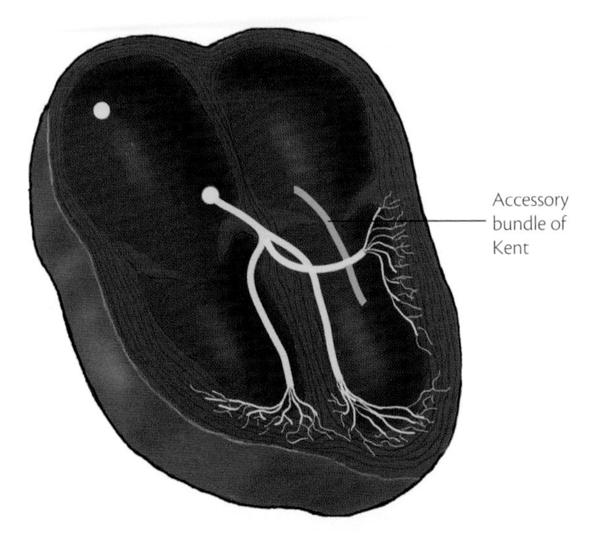

Fig. 15.51 Normal conducting path with Kent's path.

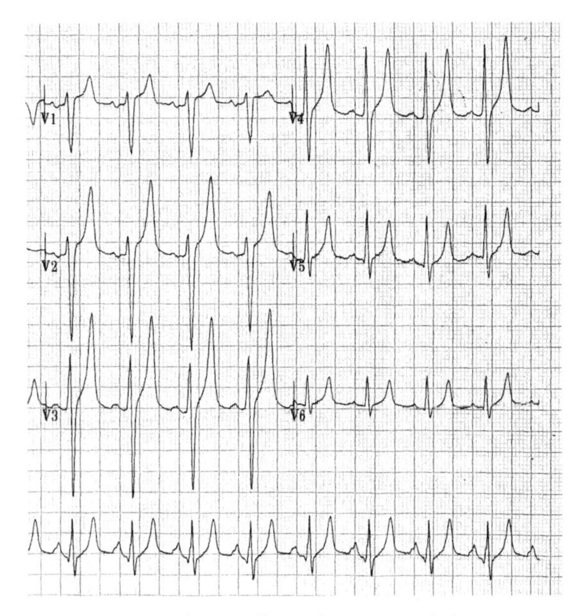

Fig. 15.49 Hyperkalaemia. Tall tented T waves are obvious.

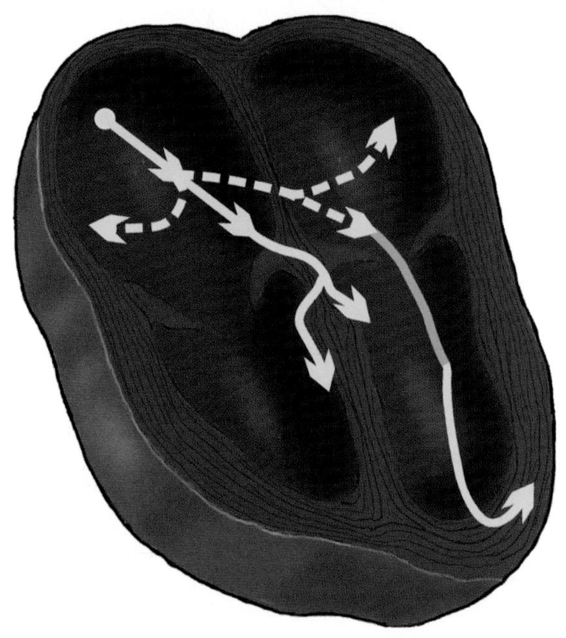

Fig. 15.52 Premature stimulation of the ventricles through Kent's path. In this circumstance impulses in the left atrium bypass the AV node and are fast tracked to the left ventricle leading to premature contraction of the left ventricle (represented by the pre-excitement delta wave in Fig. 15.53). Sometimes impulses can travel up the bundle of His and back down the accessory pathway creating a re-entry circuit leading to dangerous arrhythmias.

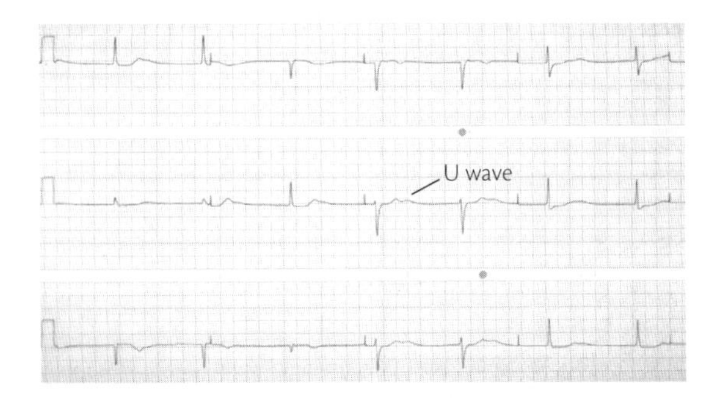

Fig. 15.50 Hypokalaemia.

to the ventricles producing a pre-excitation state. See Figs 15.51 and 15.52. The conduction is faster simply because it bypasses the AV node. The ECG trace will therefore show a shortened P–R interval. The pre-excitation is seen as a slurred upstroke at the beginning of the R wave. This is called the delta wave (see Fig. 15.53). Sometimes the electrical impulse can pass retrogradely up the bundle of His and back down the bundles of Kent creating a circuit that feeds itself. This may lead to a tachyarrhythmia (such as a SVT—see previously). Wolff–Parkinson–White syndrome is congenital. It should be considered when children and young adults present with tachyarrhythmias. Drugs can be used to correct the arrhythmia, but if it is a recurrent problem the accessory pathway can be ablated.

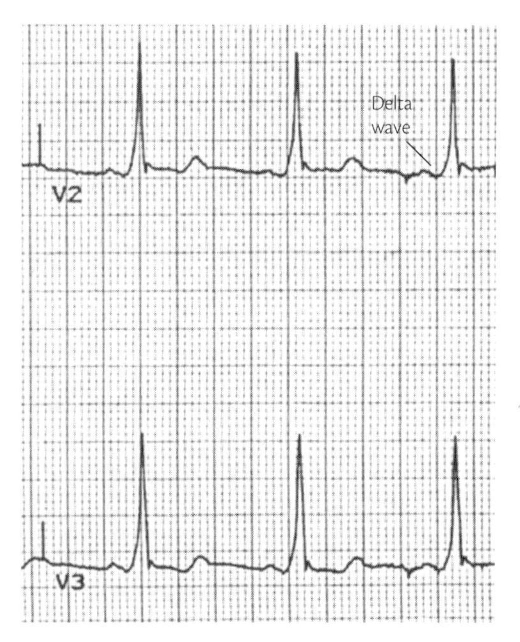

Fig. 15.53 Wolff–Parkinson–White with delta wave.

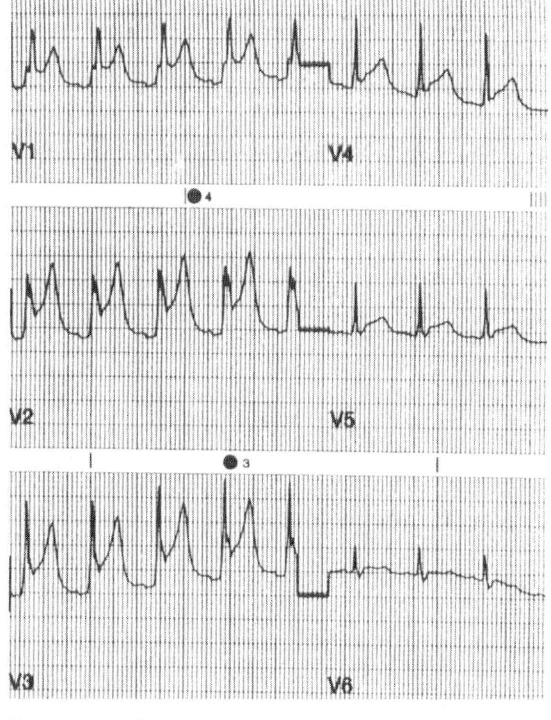

Fig. 15.54 See Case 15.3.

Presentation

If you were asked to comment on the ECG trace in Fig. 15.55, you would say, 'This is an ECG trace of Miss Anne China taken on the 1st January at Leeds General Infirmary at 03.00 hours whilst she was experiencing chest pain. The most obvious abnormality is the appearance of ST elevation in the inferior leads. I will focus on this after I have studied the ECG trace systematically. The rate is 100 beats per minute and the rhythm is sinus. The QRS complexes look normal in size and height. There are however, several ventricular ectopic beats and this is associated with ST elevation greater than 1 mm in leads II, II, and aVF. In the presence of chest pain, the diagnosis is an acute inferior MI complicated by ventricular ectopic beats.'

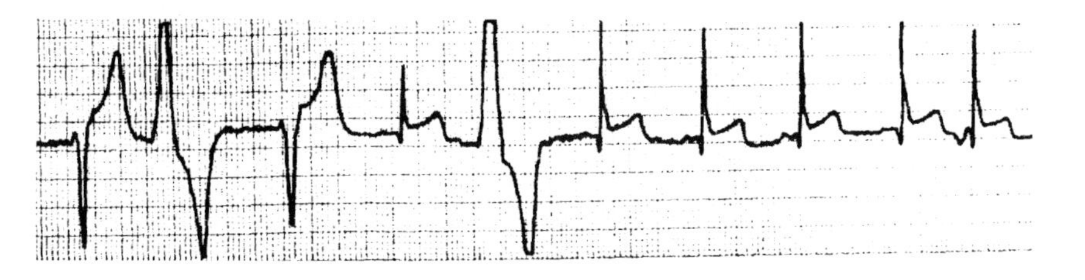

Fig. 15.55 ECG with acute inferior myocardial infarction and ventricular ectopics.

CASE 15.3

Problem. A 42-year-old man is admitted to the coronary care unit with chest pain. He had an influenza-like illness 3 weeks before admission. He is aware of a sharp central pain, which sometimes catches him when he breathes in. He has also noticed that the pain is relieved when he sits forwards in bed. His ECG is demonstrated above; what is the diagnosis?

Discussion. At first sight the obvious abnormality is ST elevation. It is tempting to say that the combination of chest pain and ST elevation is due to an acute MI. However look closely at the shape of the ST segment. It is 'concave upwards'. Further clues are in the history. The pain is sharp and has an occasional pleuritic quality on deep inspiration. More importantly he finds that the pain is relieved sitting forward than when lying down. The shape of the ST segments together with these features point towards an acute pericarditis. The influenza-like illness prior to admission suggests a viral cause for the inflamed pericardial lining. If you listen to the heart you might hear a scratching noise during the cardiac cycle—a pericardial rub. One word of warning though; an MI is a cause of pericarditis, so it is worth doing a series of ECGs and cardiac enzymes just in case.

Keypoints

- There is a range of ECG changes associated with an MI. The order of changes is usually ST elevation, then Q wave formation, and then T wave inversion.
- A normal ECG does not exclude an MI.
- ST depression usually indicates myocardial ischaemia.
- Potassium disturbances can lead to characteristic changes on an ECG.

Further reading

Hampton JR. *The ECG made easy*. 6th edn. Edinburgh: Churchill Livingstone; 2003.

Hampton R. *The ECG in practice*. 4th edn. Edinburgh: Churchill Livingstone; 2003.

CHAPTER 16

The chest X-ray

Chapter contents

Introduction

The chest X-ray (CXR) is one of the most commonly requested investigations. All CXRs will be reported by an experienced radiologist, at a later date. As a junior doctor, after admitting your patient, you will be expected to interpret the CXR straight away. So, it is not surprising that as a student your seniors will test you on the wards or even in examinations!

The CXR is an important investigation. It allows us to diagnose both acute and chronic pathology affecting the cardiorespiratory system. It is a non-invasive, relatively cheap, and easily performed investigation. However, ionizing radiation is potentially harmful. You should be especially aware of exposing pregnant women to X-rays. They can cause radiogenic cancers and hereditary disorders. Radiation protection regulations have been designed to prevent this. The CXR will not occur frequently in the examination setting, but once you have qualified there will be no avoiding it. It is strongly advised that you to master the art of CXR interpretation. It involves recognition of certain patterns. The more you see or indeed look for these patterns, the more easily you will be able to spot them. Of course, you must also think about the clinical features associated with the CXR. Often in the examination, you will be given a short resumé to point you in the right direction. Before the various patterns of CXR pathology are discussed, you must first appreciate how a CXR is produced and be able to identify the normal structures on a CXR.

Keypoints

- Always check for the possibility of pregnancy with a woman patient of reproductive age when making an CXR request.

How X-rays are produced

X-rays are generated in vacuum tubes that produce a beam of radiation. This beam is then directed at the patient's chest. X-rays are absorbed to a variable degree by different body tissue depending on their density. The amount of radiation emerging from the other side of the patient is reflected in different shades of grey on a film that catches the X-rays. Black areas indicate low density tissue (for example, air in the lungs). White areas indicate high density (bone). Strictly speaking, an X-ray is what is produced by the machine and directed at the patient and the radiograph is the picture that we look at. Despite this, most people including doctors refer to the radiograph as an X-ray).

The normal chest X-ray

See Fig. 16.1. CXRs are usually taken on full inspiration. The normal CXR is termed PA, meaning the X-rays pass through the patient from posterior (P) to anterior (A). Sometimes a patient is too unwell to leave their bed and they will have a portable CXR where the radiation beam is directed from the anterior to posterior (this is called an AP CXR).

Chest x-rays (except in a few circumstances) should be taken on full inspiration. The direction from which the film is taken is important. As you can see from Table 16.1, the direction of projection will change the size of structures seen on the CXR. The PA CXR taken on deep inspiration provides most information about the chest

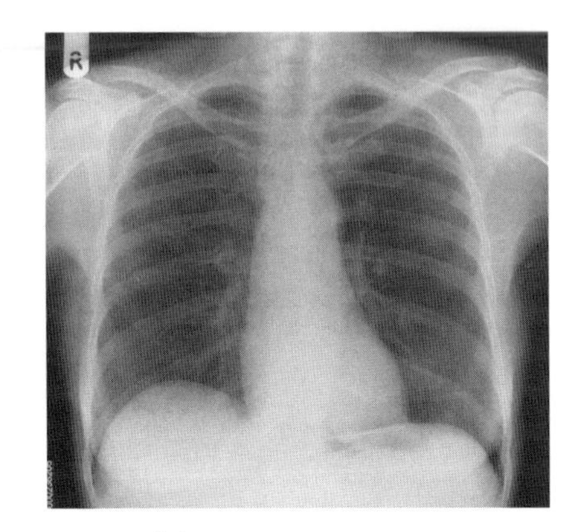

Fig. 16.1 A normal chest x-ray.

Tip

If possible, CXRs should be taken in the radiology department where a good quality PA film can be produced. This maximizes the chance of getting useful diagnostic information.

TABLE 16.1 Differences between PA and AP films

	PA	AP
Heart	Not magnified	Magnified
Scapula	Rotated away from the lungs	Superimposed on the lungs
Clavicles	Cross lungs about 5 cm below apices	Projected above lung apices

TABLE 16.2 Different angles of projections and their indications

Angle	The indication
PA	Gold standard
AP	Unwell, bed-bound, or immobile patient
Lateral	To localize opacities or masses
Expiration	To identify a small pneumothorax, bronchial obstruction, or MacLeod's (*muh-clouds*) syndrome (see p.451)
Lateral decubitus (*de-cube-it-us*)	To identify a subpulmonary effusion (a small amount of fluid may be hidden by the diaphragm in the upright position; getting a patient to lie on their side will allow the fluid to redistribute itself so that it can be seen)

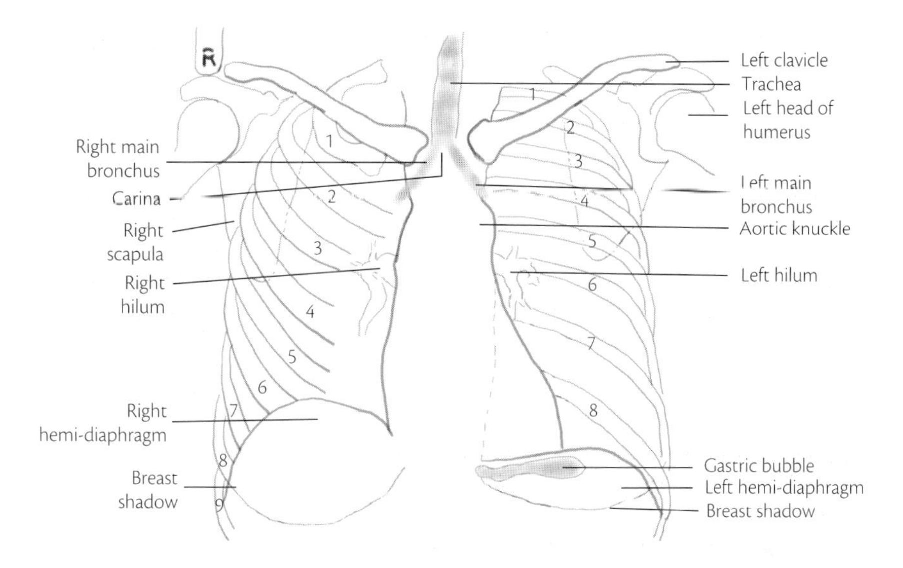

Fig. 16.2 Structures shown on a normal chest X-ray. Numbers on left-hand side of diagram = anterior ribs and numbers on right-hand side of diagram = posterior ribs.

and is the gold standard. Alternative angles of projection may be used for other reasons (see Table 16.2). You must be able to identify the structures and landmarks on a normal CXR before considering any pathology. Figure 16.2 is a schematic diagram of the important features seen on a normal CXR.

How to analyse the chest X-ray (summary)

See Fig. 16.3.

1. Orientation.
2. Patient details.
3. Technical factors (optional).
4. Bones.
5. Trachea.
6. Heart.
7. Mediastinum.
8. Hilar regions.
9. Lungs.
10. Fissures.
11. Diaphragm.
12. Soft tissues.
13. Below the diaphragm.
14. Hidden areas.

How to analyse the chest X-ray (in detail)

There is no single correct method to study a CXR. What matters is how you approach it and whether you follow a routine. An examiner can tell the difference between a candidate, who is familiar with a CXR and one who is not, even if they both get the correct diagnosis! You must therefore have a systematic approach and it is probably best to talk as you go along. The scheme below is the one that the author uses.

Getting started

1. Orientation.

In an examination situation, the film is likely to be correctly orientated on a light box. It is often the examiner's prize CXR. It is essential that you do not touch it! The easiest way to start off on the wrong foot is to mark the CXR with clammy fingerprints or splodges of ink! If they pass you the CXR, then they will expect you to place it on the light box. Do not hold it up to the light (as they often do on television!).

2. Patient details

First look at the label and identify the patient and the date. Say something like, 'This is a plain PA chest x-ray of Hugh Jart taken on the 11 September 1999 at St James's University Hospital.' At this point it is recommended that you tell the examiner that you will be studying the CXR in a systematic order and then stand back and look at the CXR as a whole. This is because if there is a huge lesion in the lung fields that even a mole with cataracts could not miss and you are found

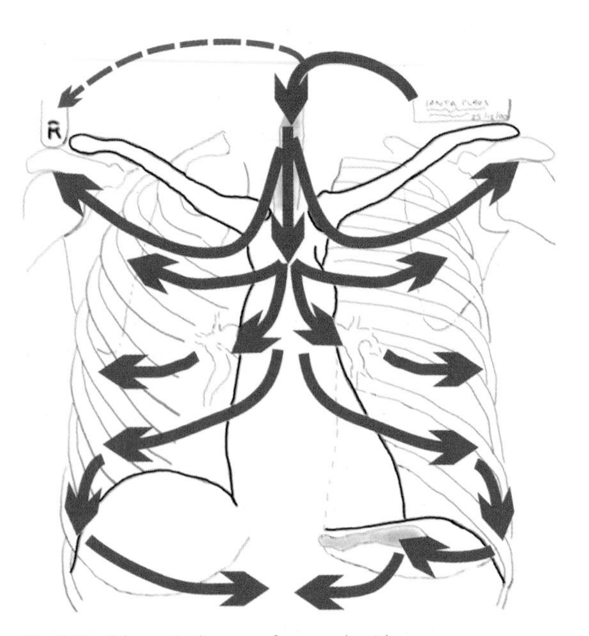

Fig. 16.3 Schematic diagram of approach with arrows.

Tip

Watch out for dextrocardia, it is an examination favourite. In this case the heart will lie on the patient's right side. Examiners may be very crafty and put the CXR on the box **the wrong way round** to mimic a normal CXR. The only clue is that the CXR marker will be on the patient's left (on your right-hand side).

to be studying the intricacies of the bone trabeculations (*tra-beck-you-lay-shuns*), the examiner will become frustrated! It is usually prudent to mention that, 'There is an obvious lesion in the left upper zone, which I will come back to study after I have systematically examined the X-ray.'

Technical factors

3. Technical factors (optional)

If you are feeling brave, you can mention the alignment of the CXR. For a CXR to be central, the medial end of the clavicles will be equidistant from the vertebral spinal processes. If the patient has rotated to the right, then the medial aspect of the right clavicle will be much nearer the vertebral process than the left. See Fig. 16.4.

The CXR should be correctly exposed. If it is over-exposed then the bones will be dark and look transparent (Fig. 16.5). Similarly, if it is under-exposed the bones and lung fields will be white (Fig.16.6). The best way to check is to look at the vertebrae. If you can only just see all the vertebral bodies through the mediastinum (*media-sty-numb*), then it is correctly penetrated (Fig. 16.1).

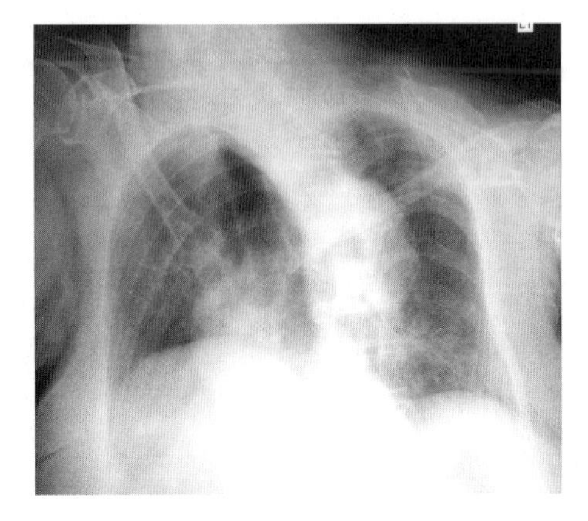

Fig. 16.4 Poorly aligned CXR.

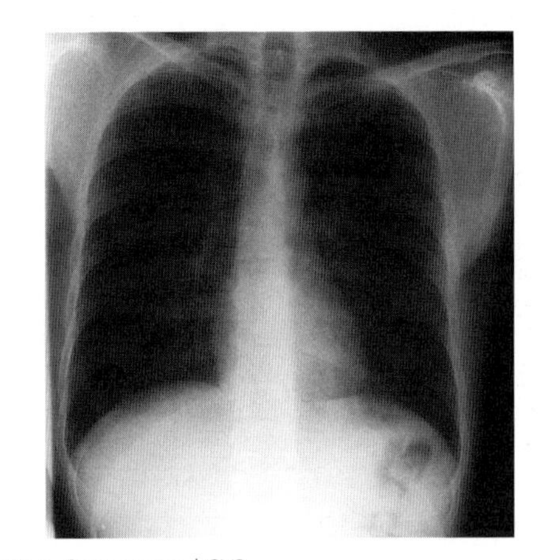

Fig. 16.5 Over-exposed CXR.

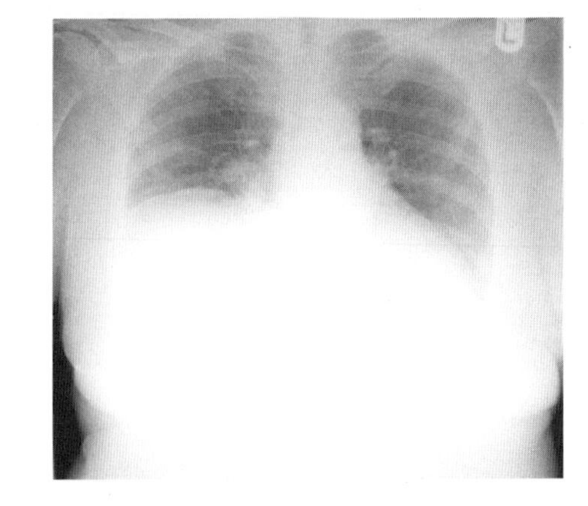

Fig. 16.6 Under-exposed CXR.

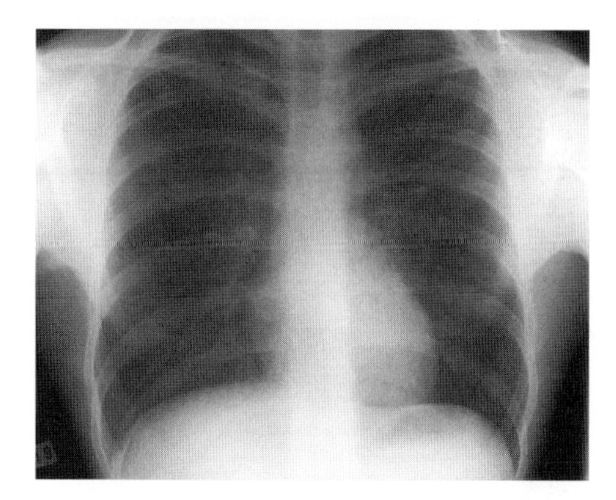

Fig. 16.7 Chest x-ray on inspiration.

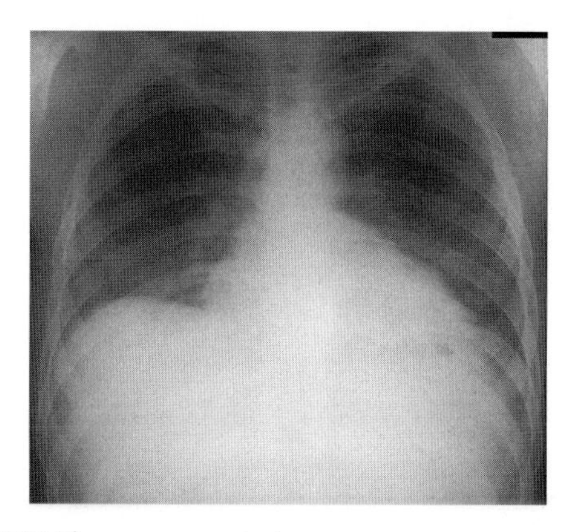

Fig. 16.8 Chest x-ray on expiration.

> **Tip**
>
> Describing the technical features is optional and not advisable unless you know what you are talking about (it is often best left to the radiologists themselves).

CXRs taken during expiration look different from those that are taken on inspiration (as they are normally taken) (see Figs 16.7 and 16.8).

Bones

4. Bones.

You should carefully survey all the bones. Step closer to the CXR. Start in the periphery with the humeri, the clavicles, and then the scapulae. Progress to the vertebrae and eventually the ribs. Look for fractures, bony metastases (*met-ass-ta-seize*), and osteoporosis. Follow the edges of each bone to look for fractures. Look for areas of blackness within each bone (that might suggest bone metastases) and compare the density of the bones, which should be the same on each side. The CXR shows the ribs as they arch around the thorax. For convention, we therefore divide them into anterior and posterior (see Fig 16.2).

Trachea

5. Trachea.

This is central, with a little deviation to the right around the aortic knuckle. If it is not central, there must be some pathology either pulling or pushing it to one side (see Fig. 16.9). It will be pulled to one side by fibrosis or collapse of a lung segment. It will be pushed away by a superior mediastinal mass, such as retrosternal goitre. The angle of the carina (*ka-reen-a*) is 60–70°. It will be widened by dilatation of the left atrium or lymphadenopathy in this area (see Fig. 16.10).

Heart

6. Heart.

Usually only one-third of the heart lies to the right of the mediastinum. The size of the heart should always be determined. We do this by calculating the cardiothoracic

(a)

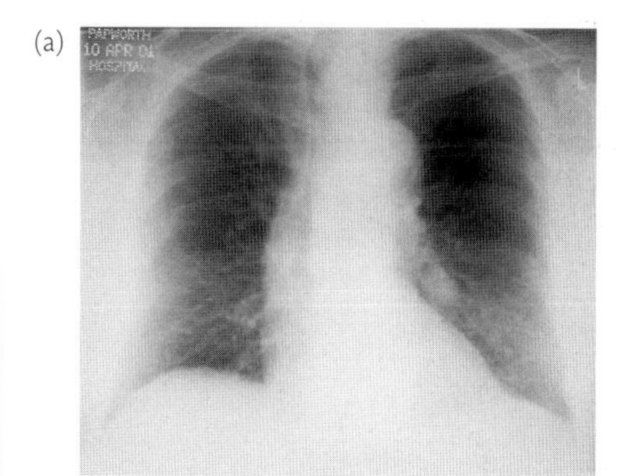

(b)

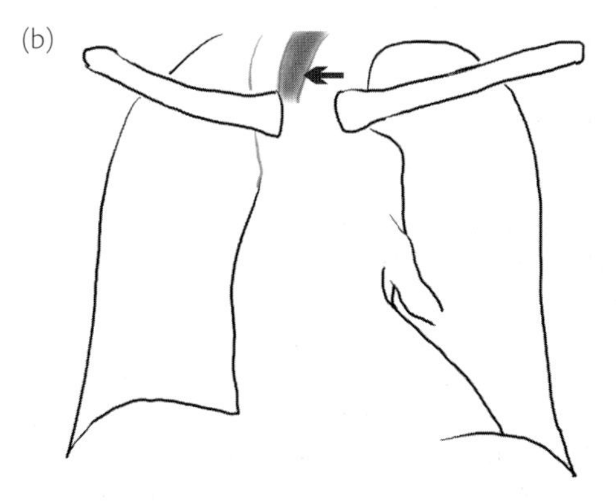

Fig. 16.9 Deviation of the trachea (see arrow) due to thyroid cancer.

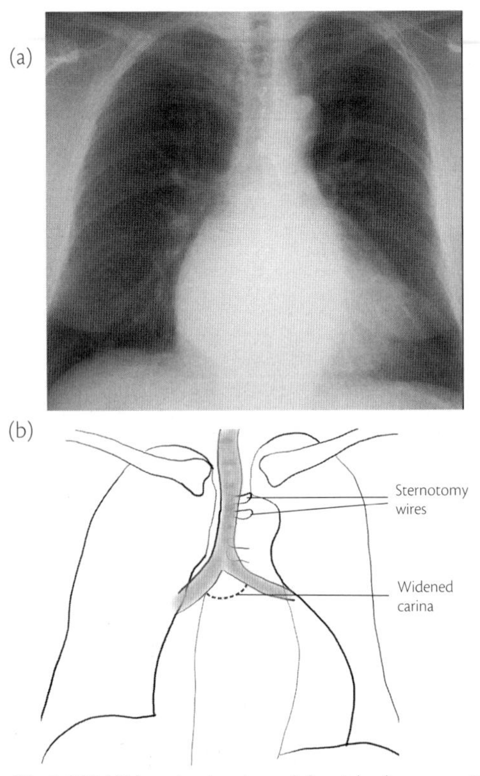

Fig. 16.10 Widened carina due to left atrial enlargement. Note sternotomy wires in (b). In this context this would suggest previous cardiac surgery and with left atrial enlargement the likeliest candidate would be the mitral valve.

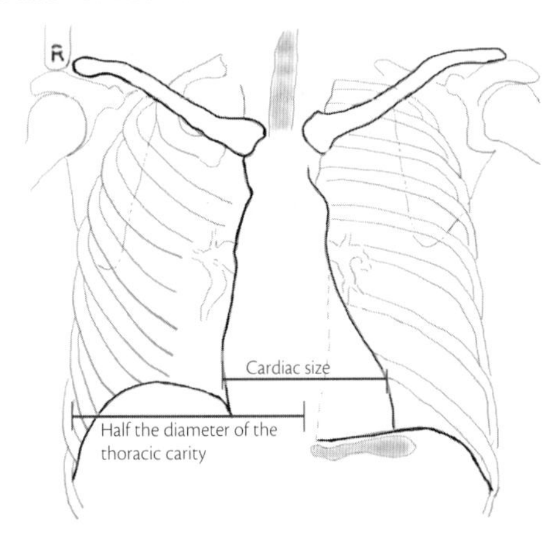

Fig. 16.11 How to calculate the cardiothoracic ratio.

ratio. This is the ratio of the transverse cardiac diameter to the transverse internal thoracic diameter and it should be less than 1:2 (see Fig. 16.11). If it is greater than this, this is called cardiomegaly (see Fig. 16.12). There are at least four important causes that should cross your mind: ischaemic heart disease (IHD), valvular heart disease (VHD), pericardial effusion, and cardiomyopathy. If you are asked to

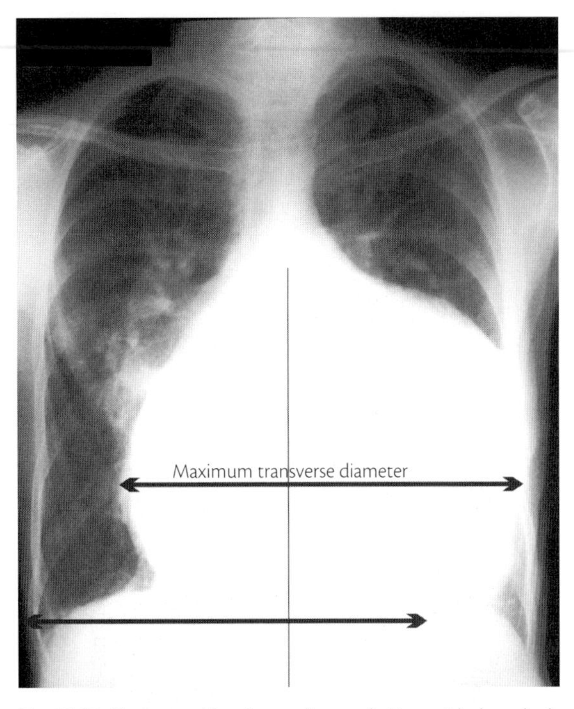

Fig. 16.12 Chest x-ray showing cardiomegaly. Even with the naked eye it can be seen that the heart dominates the whole thoracic cavity.

Keypoints

The heart will always look larger on AP films, supine films, and also on expiration. Therefore you cannot make an accurate judgement on the size of the heart.

compare the heart on successive CXRs, then any increase in transverse cardiac diameter greater than 1.5 cm is significant. Remember that the heart will look larger on AP films, on supine films, and also on expiration.

The composition of the heart shadow is described in Fig. 16.13 and Table 16.3. If we look at the lateral film then the posterior border of the heart is composed of the left ventricle and the anterior border the right ventricle. If we draw a line from the apex to the hilum, then any valvular lesion above the line is aortic and below is mitral. See Fig. 16.14.

Mediastinum

7. Mediastinum.

The edge of the mediastinum should be clear. Some fuzziness is acceptable at the angle between the heart and the diaphragm (the cardiophrenic (*card-ee-owe-fren-ick*) angle), the apices (*ay-pi-seize*), and the right hilum

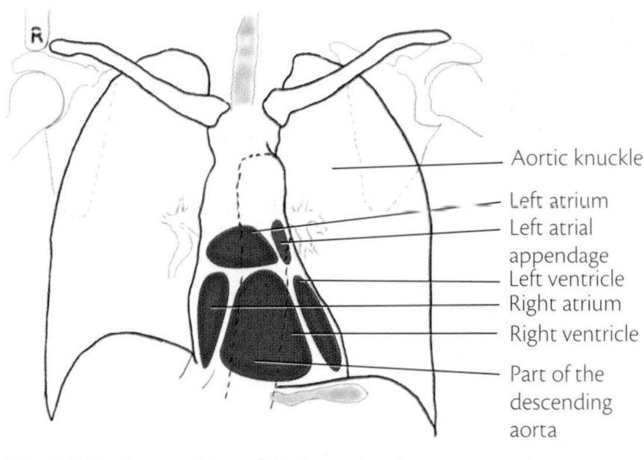

Fig. 16.13 Composition of the heart border.

TABLE 16.3 The composition of the heart border

Heart border	Area	Composition
Right heart border	Right diaphragm to right hilum	Right atrium
	Right hilum and above	Superior vena cava
Left heart border	Left diaphragm to left hilum	Left ventricle
	Concavity below left hilum	Left atrial appendage
	Level of left hilum	Left pulmonary artery
	Above left hilum	Aortic knuckle

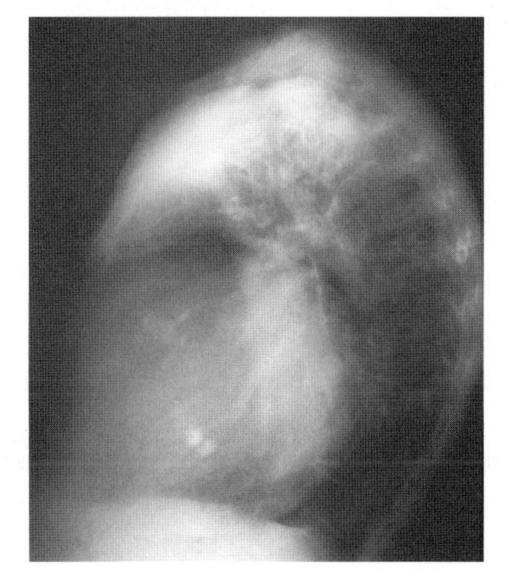

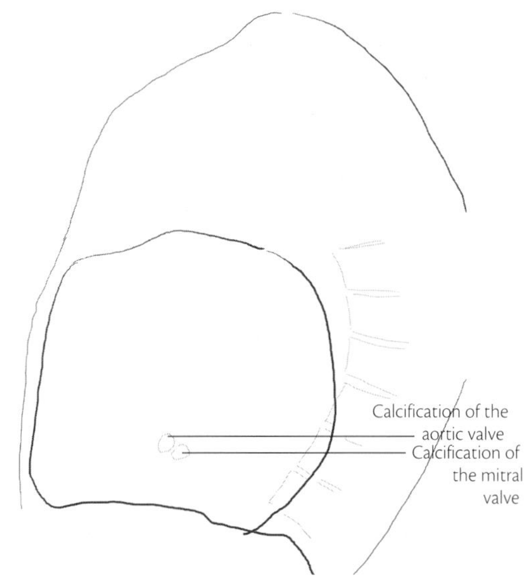

Fig. 16.14 Lateral chest x-ray Showing aortic and mitral calcification.

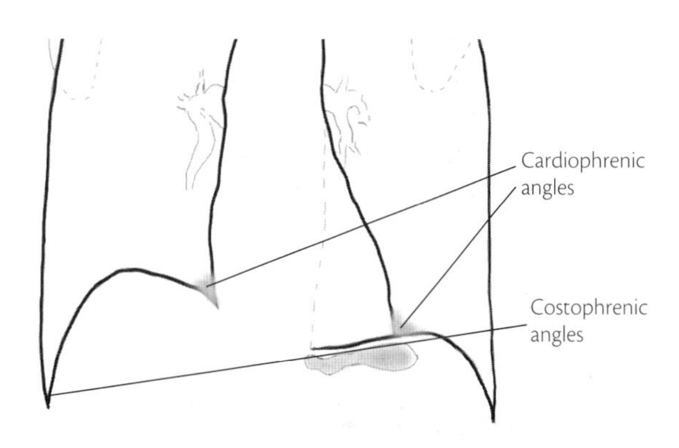

Fig. 16.15 Diagram of chest x-ray showing fuzzy areas.

(see Fig. 16.15). A hazy edge to any other parts of the mediastinum suggests a problem with the neighbouring lung (either collapse or consolidation). The mediastinum may be widened: causes include mediastinal tumours, mediatinitis, pleural effusions, and lymphadenopathy.

Hilar regions

8. Hilar regions.

These are due to the pulmonary arteries and upper lobe veins. They should be of equal density and size with concave borders. The left hilum (*high-lum*) is usually 1 cm higher than the right (see Figs 16.1 and 16.2).

Lungs

9. Lungs.

Radiologically the lungs are divided into zones. Each lung has three zones:

(1) **upper zone**—from apices to anterior rib 2;

(2) **middle zone**—from anterior rib 2 to anterior rib 4;

(3) **lower zone**—from anterior rib 4 to diaphragms.

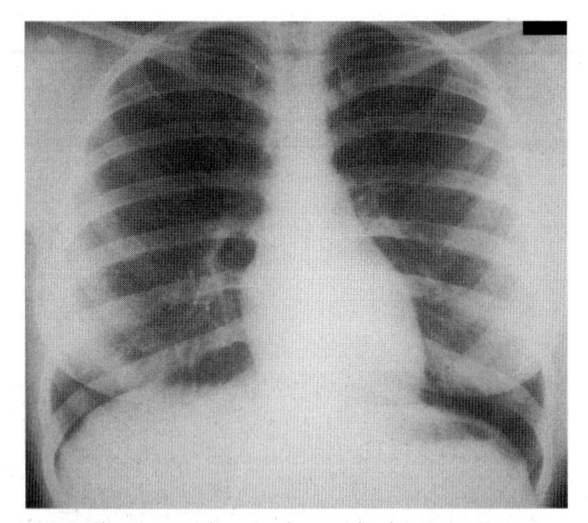

Fig. 16.16 Chest x-ray showing breast shadowing.

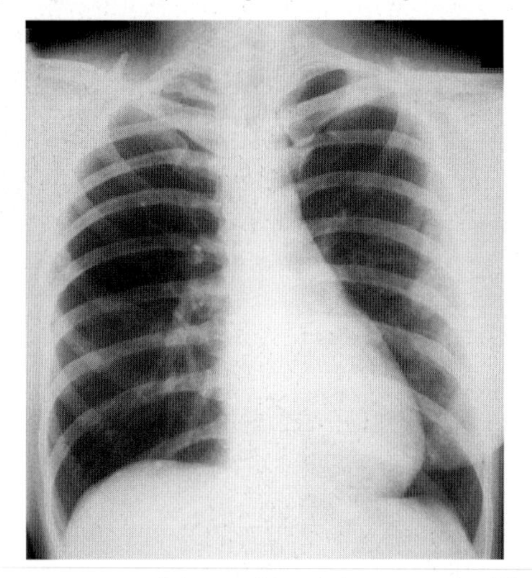

Fig. 16.17 Congenital absence of the right breast. Note the darkened lung field on the right compared to the left (and Fig. 16.16).

Remember, anatomically the right lung has three lobes and the left lung only two (see Fig. 5.8). When interpreting the CXR you should talk in terms of zones. The lungs should be of equal translucency. The only structures that can be visualized within the normal lungs are the blood vessels, the interlobar fissures, and the walls of large bronchi seen end on. Blood vessels can be seen because they are relatively opaque when compared with the surrounding air-filled, radiolucent lungs. If the alveoli become filled with fluid, then they will become opaque and also any mass lesion will be opaque. Similarly, breast shadows will cause the lower lung zones to appear more opaque (see Figs 16.16 and 16.17). So, it is important to compare not only one zone with its opposite counterpart, but also to compare zones on the same side.

Fissures

10. Fissures.

The interlobar fissures are the anatomical markings of the lobes of the lungs. On the PA view only the right horizontal fissure is seen. It runs from the right hilum to the sixth rib anteriorly in the axillary line. It divides the right upper lobe from the right middle lobe. The oblique fissure is only present on the right side dividing the right middle lobe from the right lower lobe. It tends to be only seen on the lateral CXR. Accessory fissures are occasionally seen—the azygus (*as-eye-gus*) and the left horizontal fissure. See Fig. 16.18.

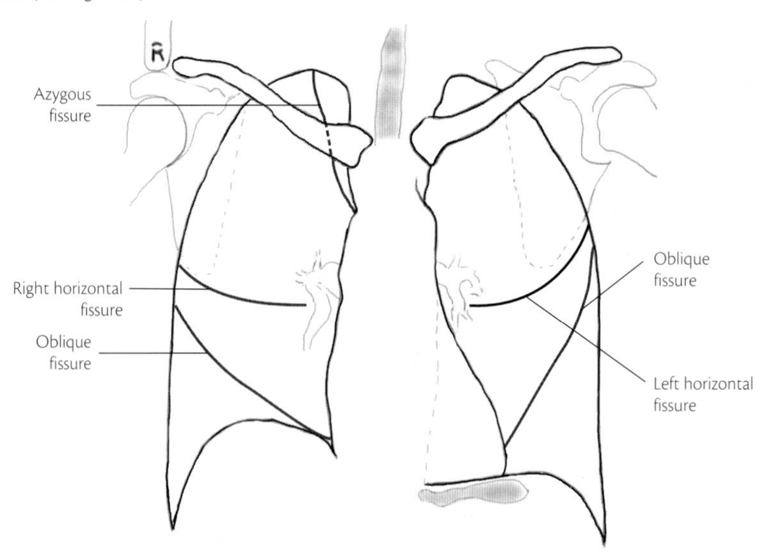

Fig. 16.18 Lung fissures.

Diaphragm

11. Diaphragm.

The diaphragm should have a smooth outline and be convex upwards. Loss of the outline implies lower lobe infection. The dome of the right hemi-diaphragm is 2 cm higher than the left and on full inspiration lies at the 6th rib anteriorly. The highest point of the right hemi-diaphragm is in the middle of the right lung field, the left hemi-diaphragm tends to lie more laterally in the left lung field (see Figs 16.1 and 16.2). There may be a fat pad adjacent to the cardiac border in obese people.

Soft tissues

12. Soft tissues.

Look for the normal breast shadowing in women. Watch out for the patient who has had a mastectomy—

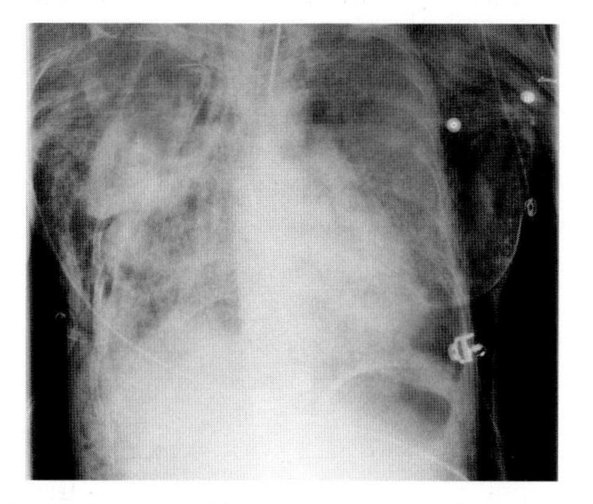

Fig. 16.19 Chest x-ray with surgical emphysema. There are widespread black streaks in the tissue indicating the presence of air.

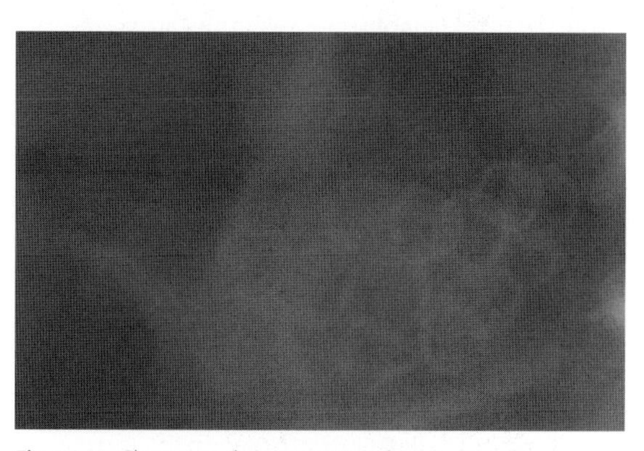

Fig. 16.21 Chest x-ray demonstrating radio-opaque gallstones.

(a)

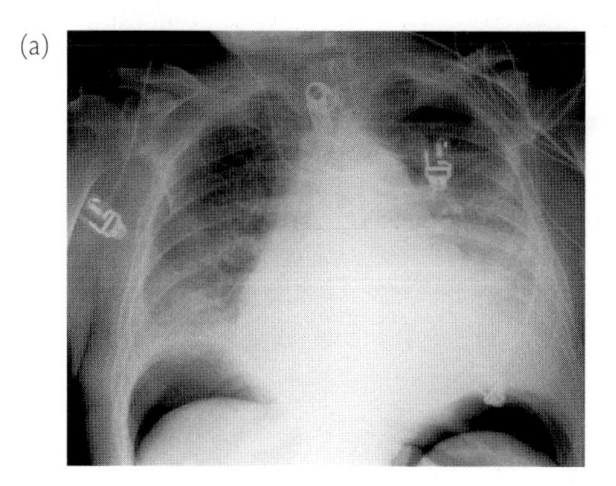

(b)

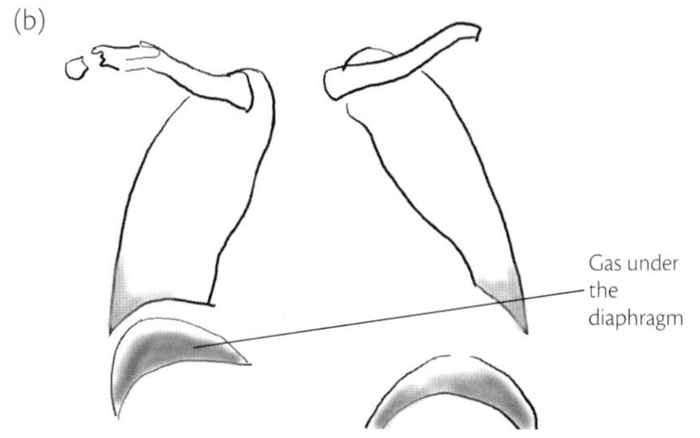

Fig. 16.20 Chest x-ray showing pneumoperitonium. Note the coincidental fracture of the right clavicle, suggesting that trauma played a role in the genesis of this condition.

(a)

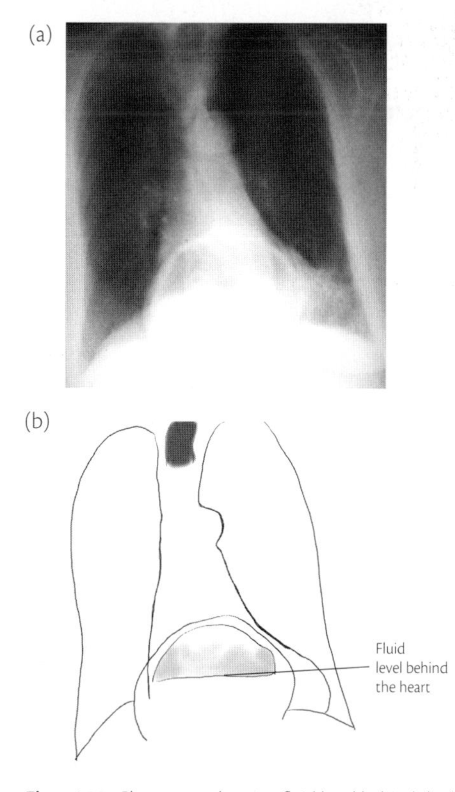

Fig. 16.22 Chest x-ray showing fluid level behind the heart. This is a hiatus hernia.

this is an examination favourite! The soft shadowing will be absent on the side of the mastectomy and is easily missed unless you are actively looking for it. Also look for air within the soft tissues characteristic of surgical emphysema (*em-fi-seem-ia*). This looks like black streaks within the tissues (see Fig. 16.19).

Below the diaphragm

13. Below the diaphragm.

Most CXRs will demonstrate gas in the stomach—the gastric bubble (see Figs 16.1 and 16.2). Only the upper border of the diaphragm is normally seen. If there is air in the abdomen (pneumoperitonium) (*new-mow-perry-toe-knee-um*) from say a perforation of viscera, then air will be seen below the diaphragm, but only if the film is taken as an erect CXR (see Fig. 16.20).Occasionally, you may see gallstones (see Fig. 16.21).

Hidden areas

13. Hidden areas.

Areas that are often forgotten are the lung apices and behind the heart. Remember to scan these areas, especially if you have not found any pathology. A fluid level behind the heart could represent a hiatus hernia, or achalasia (*ay-ka-lazia*).

Abnormalities within the chest x-ray

This section will take you through the common and important pathologies that can be identified on a plain CXR. The white lung field, the black lung field, the heart, the hilum, and CXR emergencies will be considered.

White lung field

There are many causes of white lung fields on a CXR. The most common will now be discussed.

Pleural effusion, collapse, and consolidation

Differentiating between these three pathologies can be difficult. They all cause an area of the lung to become white. See Figs 16.23–16.25 and Table 16.4. Air bronchograms are useful. In consolidation, the alveolar (*al-vee-owe-lar*) air spaces become filled with fluid, whereas

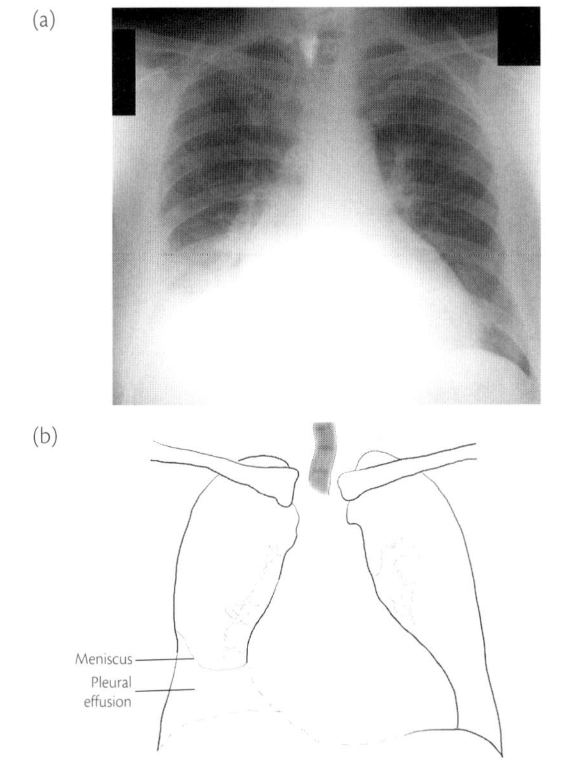

Fig. 16.23 Pleural effusion. The right hemidiaphragm is obscured and the clue to the aetiology is the concave meniscus which indicates fluid.

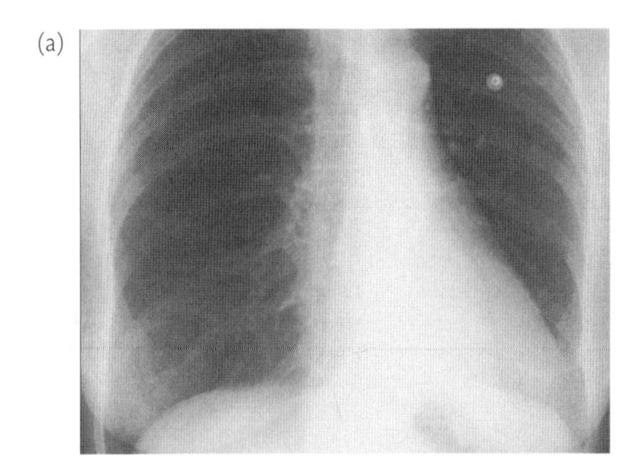

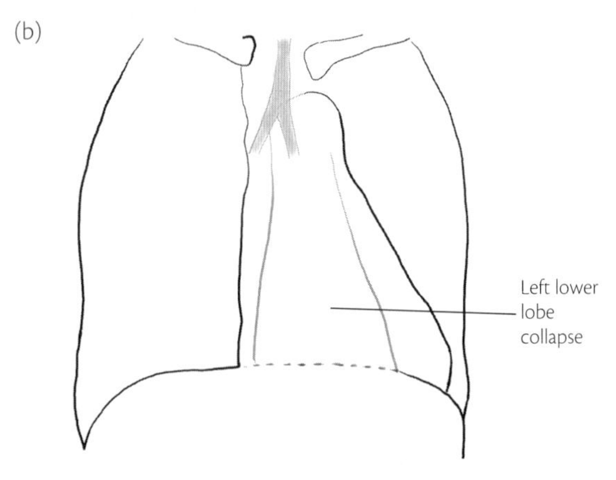

Fig. 16.24 Lobar collapse. A triangular shape behind the heart obscures the medial portion of the left hemidiaphragm.

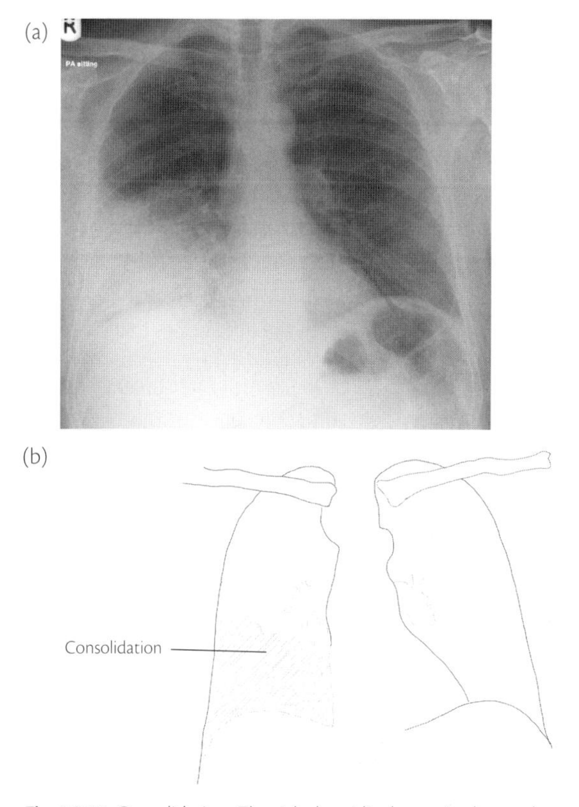

Fig. 16.25 Consolidation. The right hemidiaphragm is obscured but unlike Fig. 16.23 the superior edge of the opacity is ill-defined (without a meniscus).

TABLE 16.4 Contrasting the differing characteristics of effusion, collapse, and consolidation

Pathology	Characteristics
Effusion	Homogeneous (*hu-mo-jen-us*) shadowing,* meniscus (especially on lateral chest x-ray), lateral peak (a raised hemi-diaphragm will have raised central peak), mediastinal shift away from effusion, look for causes of the effusion (cardiomegaly of heart failure, lung masses/metastases)
Collapse	Mediastinal shift towards the collapse, distortion of radiological landmarks (movement of fissures, loss of volume of a lung), trachea deviated towards side of collapse, homogeneous shadowing*
Consolidation	Heterogeneous (*heh-to-roger-nuss*) shadowing†, air bronchograms, similar changes on previous chest x-rays implies fibrosis

* In homogeneous shadowing the area concerned will look completely white.

† In heterogeneous shadowing there will be small areas of blackness.

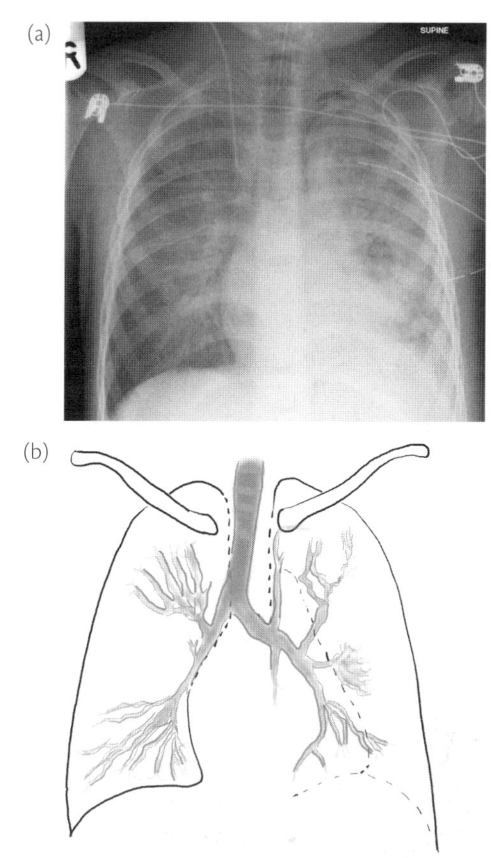

Fig. 16.26 Air bronchogram: due to extensive consolidation in both lungs.

the airways do not. So, you will see small black airways against a white background (see Fig. 16.26). Because consolidation involves the collection of alveolar fluid, the denser shadowing representing fluid will be found at the bottom of an area of consolidation. Consolidation always requires follow up CXRs. CXRical resolution lags behind clinical resolution. Therefore, a follow-up CXR should be done after a month to check if the CXR has cleared. If it has not further investigations are required to rule out an underlying cause such as cancer.

Pneumonectomy

In clinical practice, you will know from the history that a patient has had a pneumonectomy (*new-mow-neck-tummy*). Examinations unfortunately are not always real life! Essentially there will be one white lung field. The remaining lung herniates to the other side, pushing with it both the trachea and the mediastinum. Some of the ribs on the side of the pneumonectomy will have been cut and removed. See Fig. 16.27.

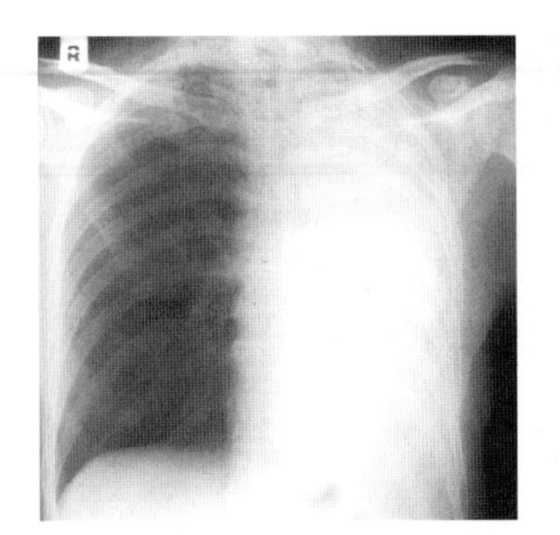

Fig. 16.27 Left pneumonectomy. Other possibilities for this appearance include a large left pleural effusion (with associated lung collapse to explain the lack of deviation of the trachea to the right) or extensive consolidation of the left lung.

(a)

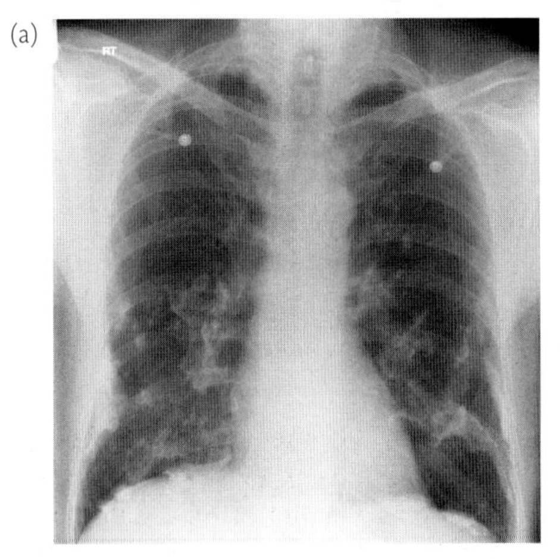

(b)

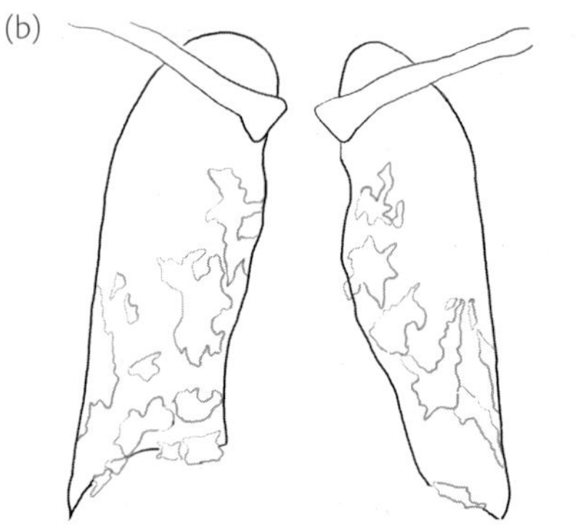

Fig. 16.28 Pleural plaques. In (b) they look almost 'holly-leaf' like in appearance and cross lung fissures.

Asbestos

Asbestos exposure was relatively common 20 or more years ago. Because of the natural time lag to disease presentation, asbestos-related pathologies will become increasingly common in the future. Asbestos can cause

- asbestos plaques
- mesothelioma (*me-sew-thee-li-owe-ma*)
- asbestosis
- bronchogenic lung cancer.

They can all cause a white lung field. Only asbestos plaques and mesothelioma will be considered here.

Asbestos plaques

See Fig. 16.28. These are benign areas of pleural thickening. They occur anywhere in the lung zones and can even be seen as diaphragmatic plaques. When they are projected face on, they look like 'holly leaves' and have well-defined edges. When seen at the edge of the lung, they look like thickened lines. They cross lung anatomy, such as fissures (anything following lung anatomy originates from the lung itself and should make one suspicious of malignancy). They are usually bilateral; reconsider the diagnosis if they are not. The white appearance is patchy. Remember to look at (or ask for) old CXRs. Asbestos plaques are slow growing and will often be present on previous X-rays.

Mesothelioma

See Fig. 16.29. Mesothelioma is a malignant tumour of the pleura that is associated with asbestos exposure. As

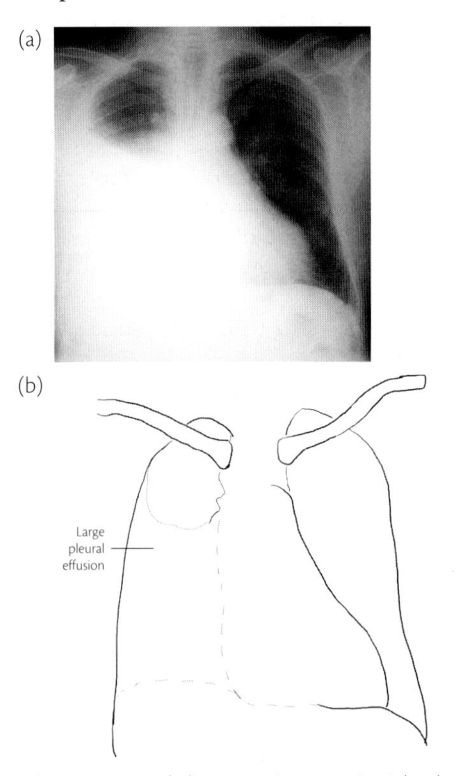

Fig. 16.29 Mesothelioma: causing a massive right pleural effusion obscuring the right hemidiaphragm and right heart border.

it is pleural pathology, it will have the characteristics of pleural shadowing (similar to asbestos plaques). Remember, it is not of lung origin and therefore will cross lung fissures. Its malignant nature will be apparent as the affected areas will be thickened and irregular and it will lead to a reduction in lung volume. Another feature is the development of large pleural effusions.

The coin lesion

Coin lesions are exactly what their name suggests. They are large, discrete, often round, white lesions found anywhere in the lung zones. They are significant because they usually represent cancer (either primary lung cancer or metastatic deposits). There are other possible causesn:

(1) **benign tumour**—benign hamartoma (*hammer-toe-ma*);

(2) **infection**—causing a focal area of consolidation;

(3) **infarction**—pulmonary embolism (PE);

(4) **granuloma**—rheumatoid nodule (note Caplan's syndrome (*Anthony Caplan (1907–1976), English physician*) of pneumoconiosis associated with rheumatoid nodules in the lung).

Metastatic deposits to the lungs are a frequent cause of malignant coin lesions. They are called 'cannon ball' lesions and typically arise from a primary tumour of the kidney. Certain radiological characteristics of coin lesions help in determining the cause (but the history and examination are more helpful). For example, consider a young female with a severe symmetrical deforming arthropathy. She is likely to have rheumatoid nodules in the lung, whereas an elderly, cachectic life-long smoker is likely to have a primary bronchogenic lung carcinoma. The following characteristics indicate the following causes:

(1) spiculated, irregular, lobulated—malignancy;

(2) calcification (dense white within the lesion)—benign;

(3) cavitating (darker centre)—tuberculosis (TB);

(4) air bronchogram within the lesion—consolidation;

(5) multiple coin lesions—metastases;

(6) associated with lymphadenopathy or bony metastases—malignant.

The cavitating lesion

These are hollow coin lesions. Essentially you will see a coin lesion with a dark centre representing air/fluid. You may detect a fluid level within the lesion. Rarely

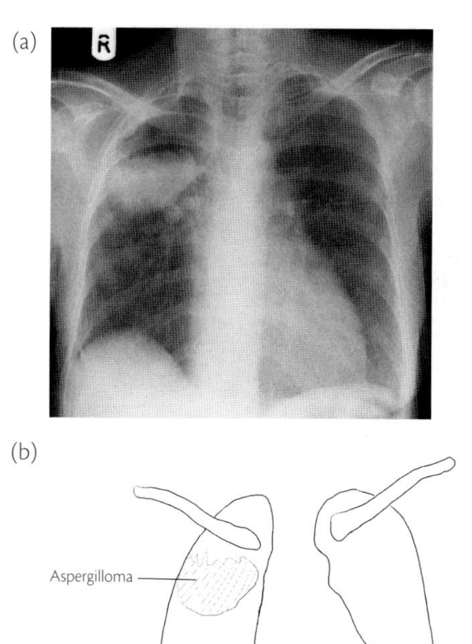

Fig. 16.30 Aspergilloma. The fungal ball occupies the TB cavity.

you will detect a white ball within the cavity; this is pathognemonic of an aspergilloma (*ass-per-jill-owe-ma*) (an aspergilloma is a benign tumour formed by a ball-like collection of the fungus *Aspergillus fumigatus*) (*ass-per-jill-us-fume-I-gart-us*) (see Fig. 16.30). The causes of cavitating lung lesions are

(1) **infection**—abscess, especially *Staphylococcus aureus* (called pneumatoceles) (*new-mat-owe-seals*);

(2) **true cavitation**—TB;

(3) **tumour**—malignant;

(4) **infarction**—PE, with a central area of necrosis within the coin lesion.

Again look at all the old CXRs to decide the rate of growth. Also, consider the clinical scenario. Patients with staphylococcal lung abscesses are systemically unwell. See Fig. 16.31.

Left ventricular failure

The author guarantees that during your first general medical take, you will admit a patient with acute left ventricular failure. You will have to diagnose and treat it. Often, the patient is too unwell to give a history, so

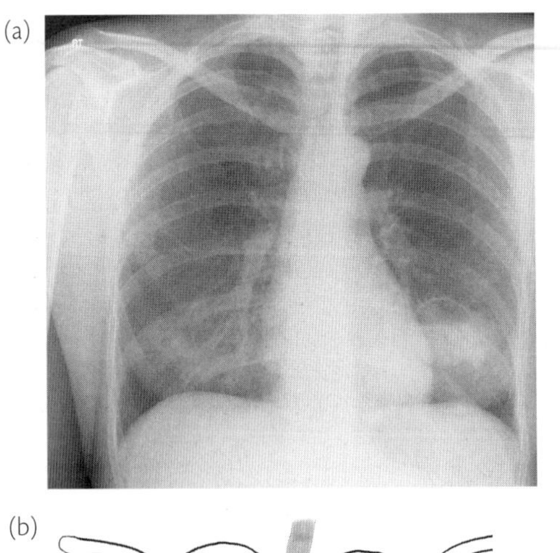

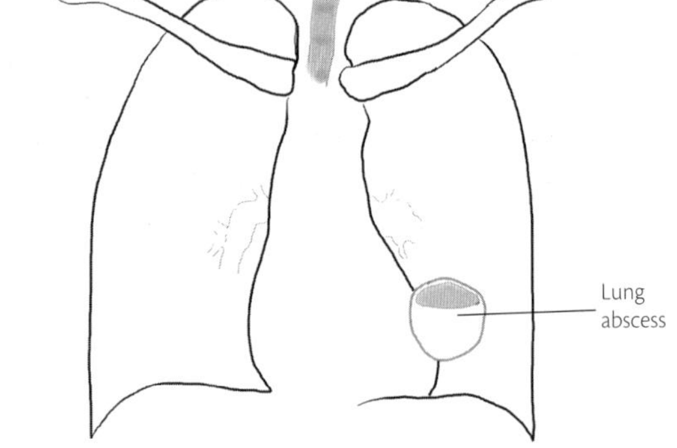

Fig. 16.31 Lung abscess.

you will rely heavily on the examination and results of investigations. The CXR will be crucial to your diagnosis. Remember left ventricular failure is only one cause of pulmonary oedema. A CXR of left ventricular failure will show the following (see Fig. 16.32).

1. **Upper lobe diversion.** Normally, the upper lobe blood vessels are narrower than those of the lower lobe. So if they are the same width or larger, then this is upper lobe diversion. This only applies if the film is taken erect—upper lobe diversion is normal on supine films. Upper lobe diversion arises because the lower lobe alveoli become hypoxic, thus causing vasoconstriction.

2. **Cardiomegaly.** Measure the cardiothoracic ratio as described earlier.

3. **Kerley (*curly*) B lines.** (*Peter James Kerley (1900–1978) Irish neurologist with an interest in radiology.*) These are small, horizontal, non-branching white lines seen at the periphery of the lower lung zones (see Fig. 16.33).

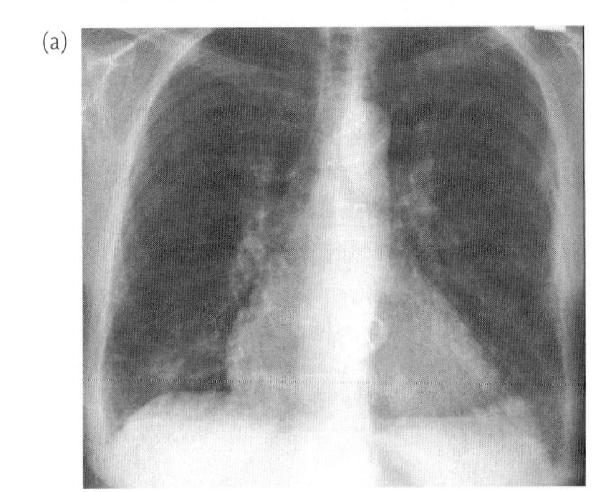

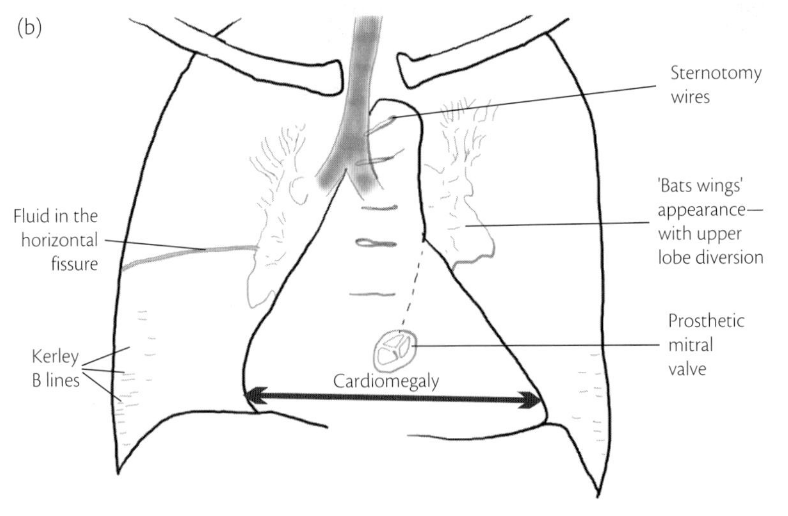

Fig. 16.32 Left ventricular failure.Note the prosthetic mitral valve indicating previous valvular heart disease.

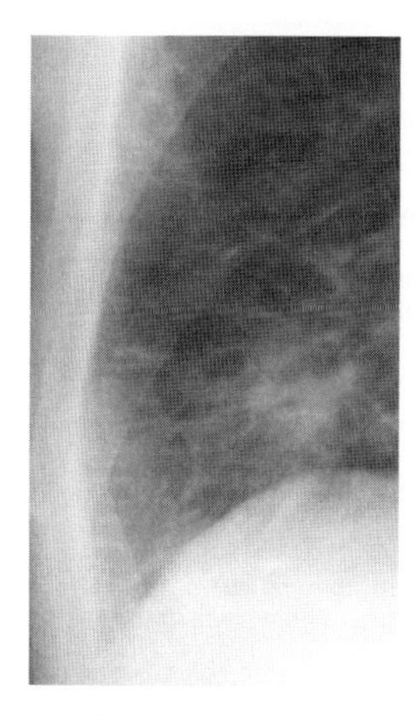

Fig. 16.33 Close-up of Kerley B lines.

4. **Bat's wing appearance.** Only in severe left ventricular failure will you see this white wing-shaped appearance spreading from the hilar regions. It represents alveolar oedema.

Bronchiectasis

If your teaching hospital incorporates a regional cystic fibrosis centre, then beware! CXRs showing the brochiectasis (*bron-key-eck-ta-sis*) of cystic fibrosis will appear along with the patient in Finals. You will see both ring and tramline shadows on the CXR. See Fig. 16.34. Ring shadows are diseased bronchi seen end on, whereas tramlines are bronchi seen side on. The bronchi may be filled with secretions, so that when seen side on, the tramline shadows become tubular shadows. Groups of tubular shadows form glove finger shadows. The gold standard radiological investigation for bronchiectasis is the computed tomography (CT) scan. A normal CXR does not exclude bronchiectasis. The causes of bronchiectasis are shown in Table 16.5.

Lung fibrosis

Lung fibrosis is a less common cause of a white lung. It is a chronic process, so you can see it in a series of CXRs. It causes shrinkage of the lungs. Often the fibrosis is bilateral and basal. It may be unilateral, if so it will cause

(a)

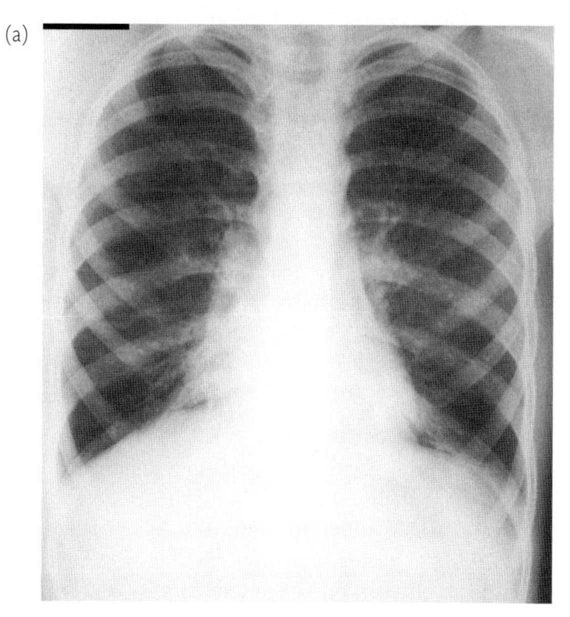

(b)

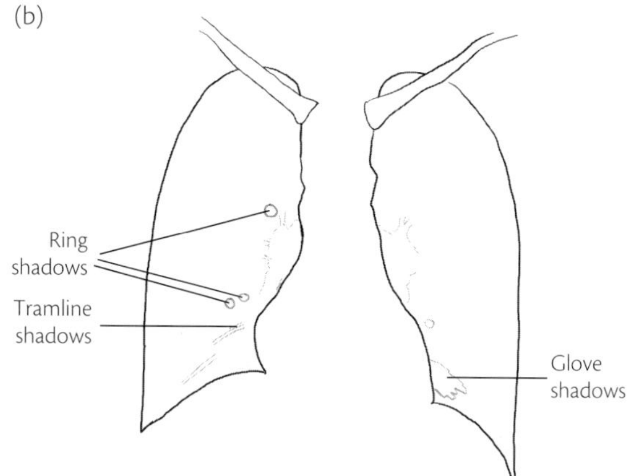

Fig. 16.34 Bronchiectasis.

TABLE 16.5 Causes of bronchiectasis

Congenital
Cystic fibrosis
Kartageners (*carter-jenners*) syndrome*
Hypogammaglobulinaemia
Acquired
Infections
After childhood whooping cough
Tuberculosis
Pneumonia
Allergic broncho-pulmonary aspergillosis

*Manes Kartagener (1897–1975), Swiss physician.

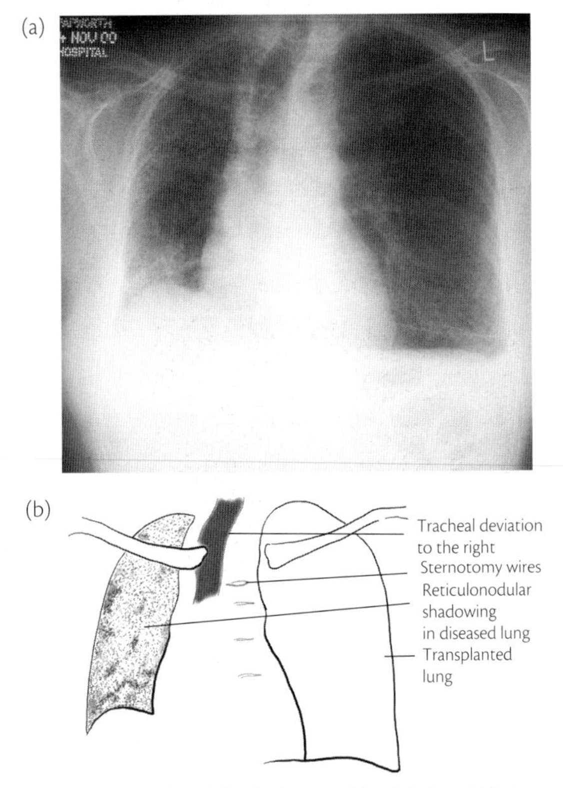

Fig. 16.35 Reticulonodular shadowing of the right lung. N.B. the patient has had a left lung transplant.

the mediastinum to be pulled across to the side of the fibrosis. CXRically, lung fibrosis is described as being 'reticulonodular'. This really means a meshwork of lines and rings (see Fig. 16.35). The reticular nodular appearance may be very fine giving a 'ground glass' appearance. In the later stages, the lung becomes 'honeycomb' in appearance (see Fig. 16.36). Coal miners with pneumo-

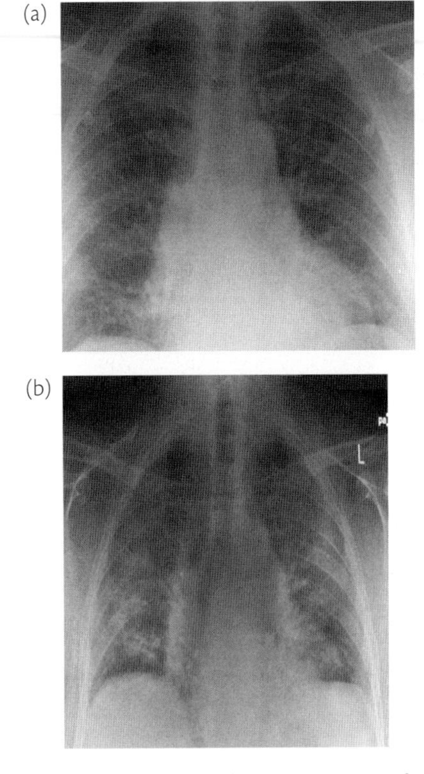

Fig. 16.36 Chest x-rays showing progression of interstitial lung fibrosis. (b) Seven months later. Note the developing 'honeycombing' of the lung.

coniosis (see Fig. 16.37) may develop 'progressive massive fibrosis' (see Fig. 16.38). There will be large areas of well-defined fibrosis on a background of smaller nodular opacities. There are many causes of lung fibrosis. A few are shown in Table 5.16.

Multiple small opacities

There are only a few causes of multiple small white nodules scattered throughout the lung fields. You should always consider miliary tuberculosis, which is easy to miss and fatal if untreated. Some people who have suffered from chicken pox pneumonitis may develop this appearance. These CXRs will show many areas of microcalcification (see Fig. 16.40).

Black lung field

You will be pleased to know that there are fewer causes of a black than white lung field. Four causes will be discussed here. An ordinary lung field on a CXR is dark shade of grey. However, sometimes it is jet black when compared to other zones on the same CXR or to another CXR. When considering how black a lung field is,

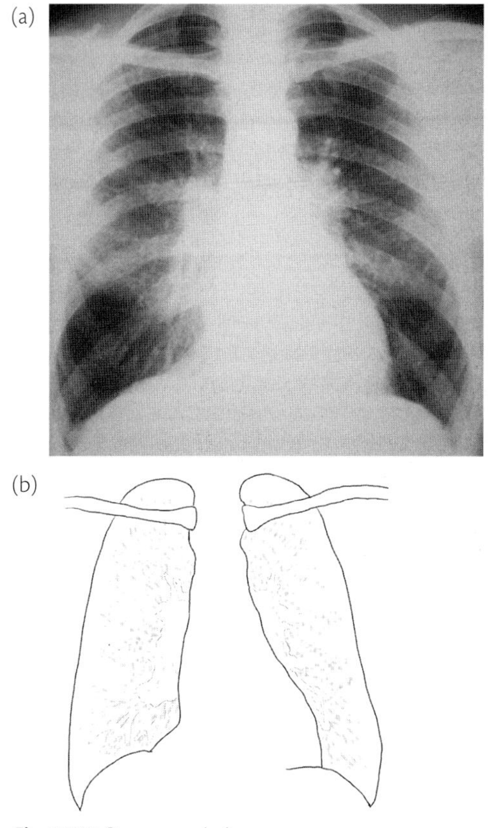

Fig. 16.37 Pneumoconiosis.

remember that the penetration of the CXR is important. If the penetration is satisfactory, the most likely cause is chronic obstructive pulmonary disease (COPD). This is bilateral, whereas pneumothoraces (*new-mow-thor-a-seas*) and PE tend to be unilateral.

Chronic obstructive pulmonary disease

See Fig. 16.41. Patients suffering from COPD have hyperexpanded chests. So if you count the number of ribs anteriorly above the diaphragm there will be more than seven. Similarly, there will be 10 or more above the diaphragm posteriorly. The diaphragms will be flat. If you hold a ruler across one hemi-diaphragm, drawing an imaginary line between the costophrenic and cardiophrenic angles, then the highest elevation of the

> **Tip**
>
> Check to see if the patient is rotated (see p. 435 earlier). The rotation can lead to one side of the chest being closer to the CXR source and therefore more penetrated (and hence more black), while the other side is further away, less penetrated (and less black).

(a)

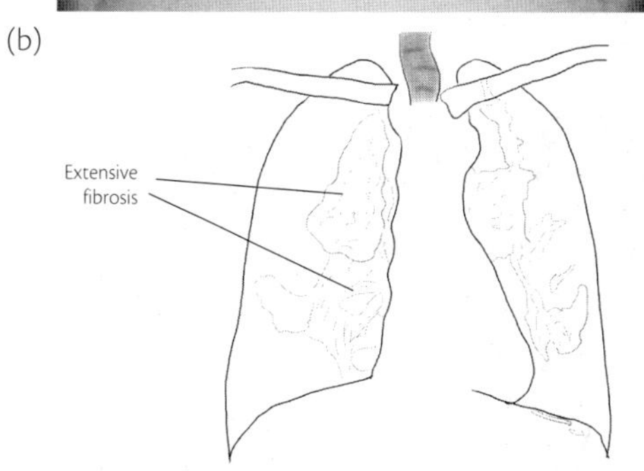

Fig. 16.38 Progressive massive fibrosis.

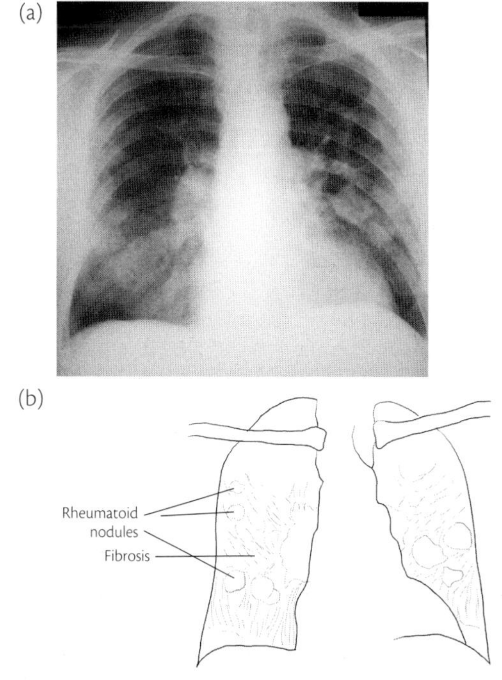

Fig. 16.39 Caplan's syndrome. There are multiple rheumatoid nodules on a background of fibrosis. The nodules can easily be mistaken for multiple metastases (compare with Fig. 16.53).

(a)

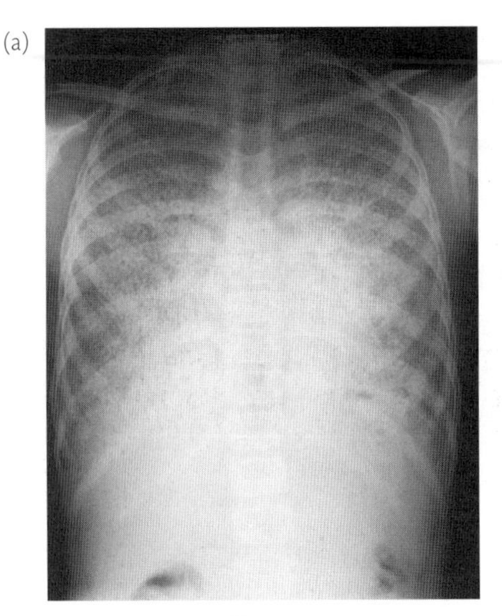

(b)

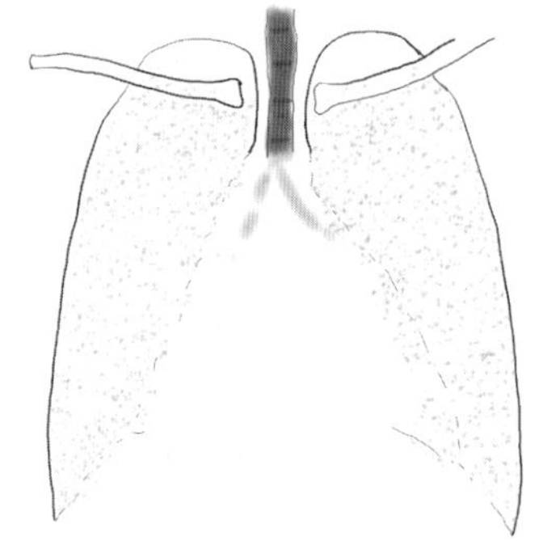

Fig. 16.40 Chest x-ray showing microcalcification.

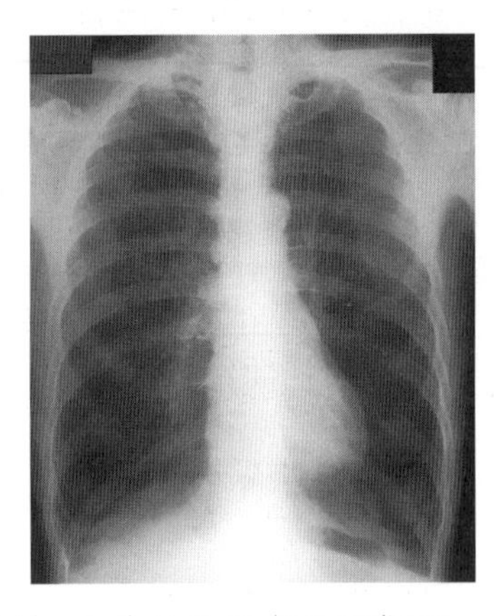

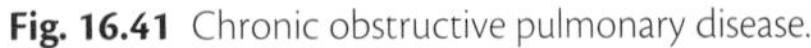

Fig. 16.41 Chronic obstructive pulmonary disease.

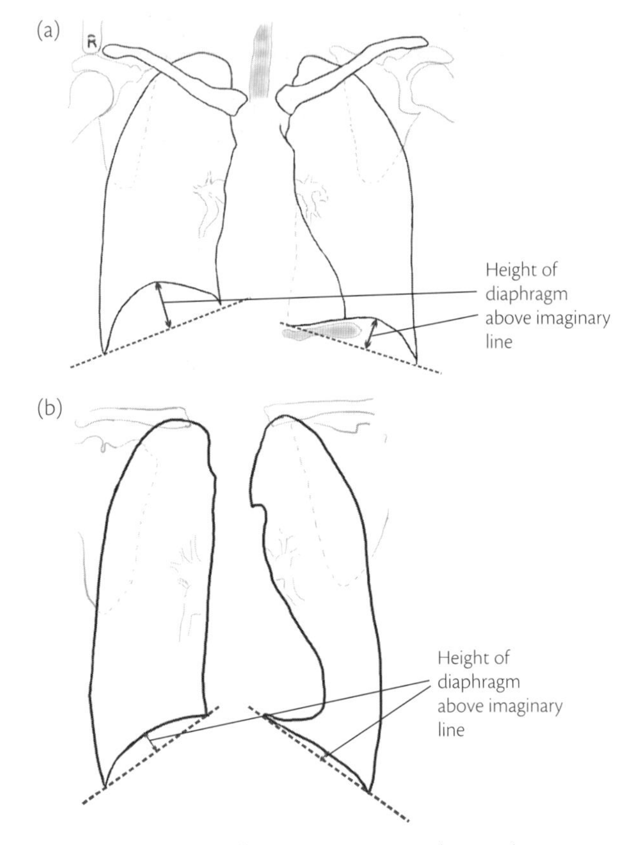

Fig. 16.42 Diagram demonstrating imaginary lines used to assess normal and flattened diaphragms. (a) Normal diaphragms and (b) flattened diaphragms.

dome of the diaphragm above the line should be no more than 1 cm if the chest is hyperinflated (see Fig.16.42). The heart will look small and thin in the context of an over-expanded chest. However, if the heart looks normal in size or is enlarged, you should consider heart failure associated with the COPD (cor pulmonale is right ventricular failure secondary to COPD). Bullae (*bully*) may be present on the CXR. These are round, dense, black areas surrounded by a thin line.

Pneumothorax

See Figs 16.43 and 16.44. A unilateral black lung field is an important finding. It often indicates a pneumothorax. Unfortunately, pneumothoraces can be very small and very difficult to visualize. For this reason, if you suspect a pneumothorax and it is not apparent on the provisional film, then an expiratory film will make it stand out. On expiration the lungs shrink so the pneumothorax becomes more prominent. Check all areas of the lung including the hidden areas. (It is a good idea to check and then recheck). A large pneumothorax will be immediately visible. The side with the pneumothorax will have no lung markings. Look for the edge of the collapsed lung. Air forming the pneumothorax will tend to accumulate in the apices first. This produces a vertical white line. Ask the examiner if you may turn the CXR horizontally to search for these vertical lines

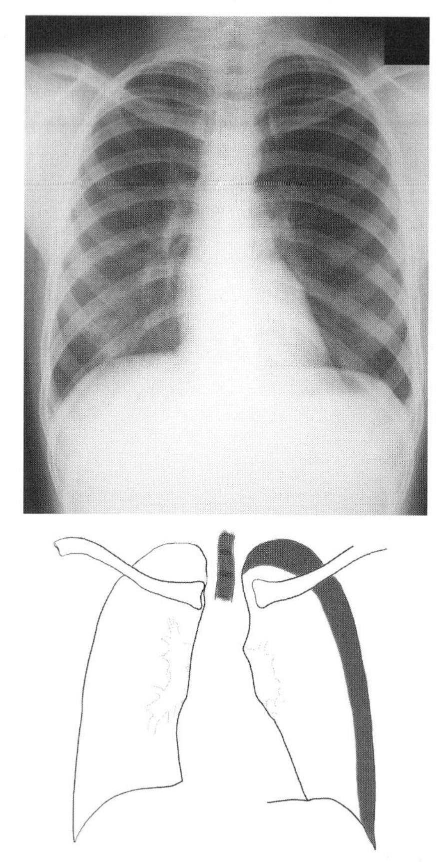

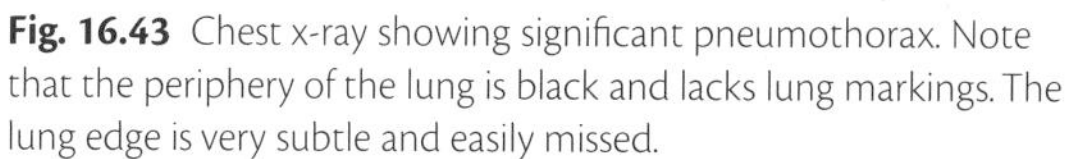

Fig. 16.43 Chest x-ray showing significant pneumothorax. Note that the periphery of the lung is black and lacks lung markings. The lung edge is very subtle and easily missed.

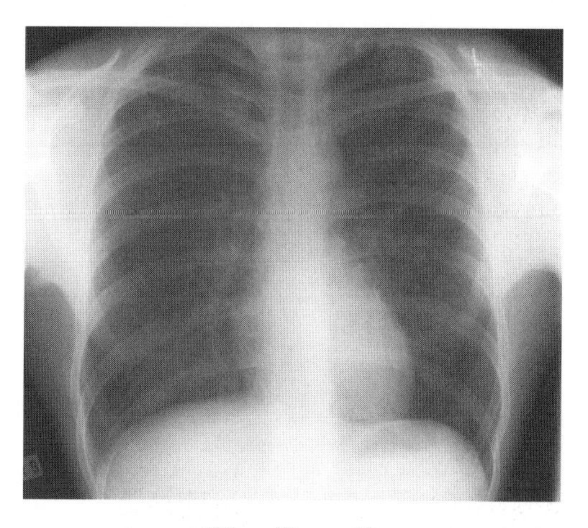

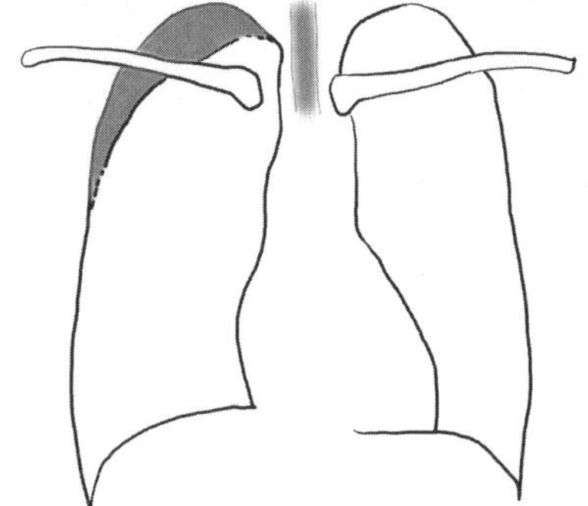

Fig. 16.44 Chest x-ray showing small apical pneumothorax. The same features apply as in Fig. 16.43 except this is even harder to spot.

suggesting a pneumothorax. Sometimes a bulla can mimic a pneumothorax, but there are often lung markings passing through a bulla. Causes of a pneumothorax are

- spontaneous
- trauma, for example, from central venous line insertion or pleural aspiration
- cystic fibrosis
- Marfan's (*mar-fans*) syndrome (*Antoine Bernard Jean Marfan (1858–1942), French paediatrician*)
- Ehlers–Danlos syndrome.

Pulmonary embolism (PE)

See Fig. 16.45. The CXRical changes associated with a PE are subtle. The CXR is usually normal. Occlusion of a pulmonary artery by a thrombus may result in an oligaemic (poorly perfused) segment of the lung (Westerman's sign). So the black area will be anatomically defined. Try to exclude COPD and a pneumothorax first as these are more common causes of a black lung. Other changes such as acute dilatation of the proximal site of the affected pulmonary artery (Pallas sign), dilatation of the right atrium and ventricle, and a compensatory over-perfusion of the rest of the lung should be left to the specialists! Once the PE is established and there is infarction of the lung, secondary changes will occur. You may see a small ipsilateral pleural effusion, wedge-shaped shadowing, or a raised hemi-diaphragm (see Figs 16.46 and 16.47).

MacLeod's syndrome

This is congenital hypoplasia (under-development) of the pulmonary vessels. It is unilateral and causes the whole of one lung field to become black. It is best seen on an expiratory film and is very rare!

Heart

Mitral stenosis

Mitral stenosis causes left atrial dilatation (see Figs 16.10). This can be seen on the CXR as a bulging convex left atrial border and a double right heart border where

(a)

(b)

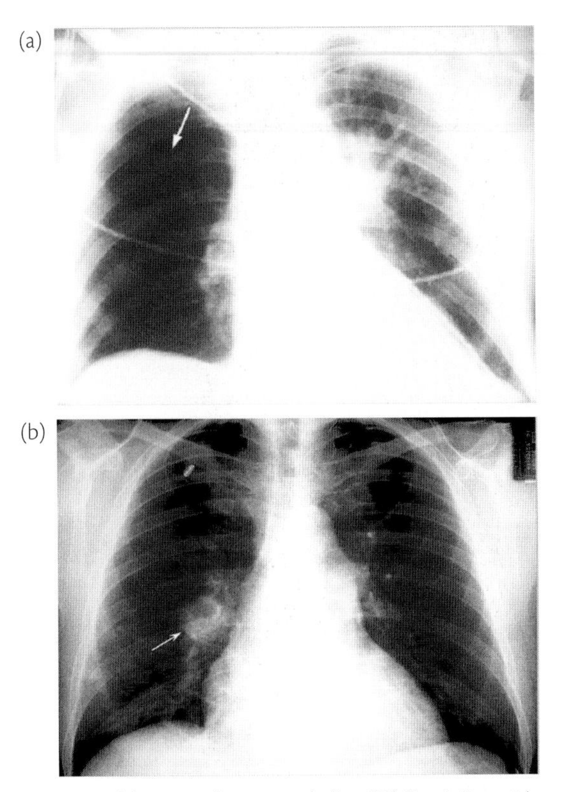

Fig. 16.45 (a) Acute pulmonary embolism (PE) (focal oligaemia). The arrow is pointing to an area of focal oligaemia (Westerman's sign). (b) Acute PE (dilatation of right pulmonary artery) compare with the opposite side. The arrow is pointing to the enlarged right pulmonary artery (Pallas sign).

the left atrium extends across the heart. The carina will become wider and is greater then 90°. If you look closely, within the heart shadow you may see the calcified mitral valve. Remember that mitral stenosis can also present with pulmonary oedema.

(a)

(b)

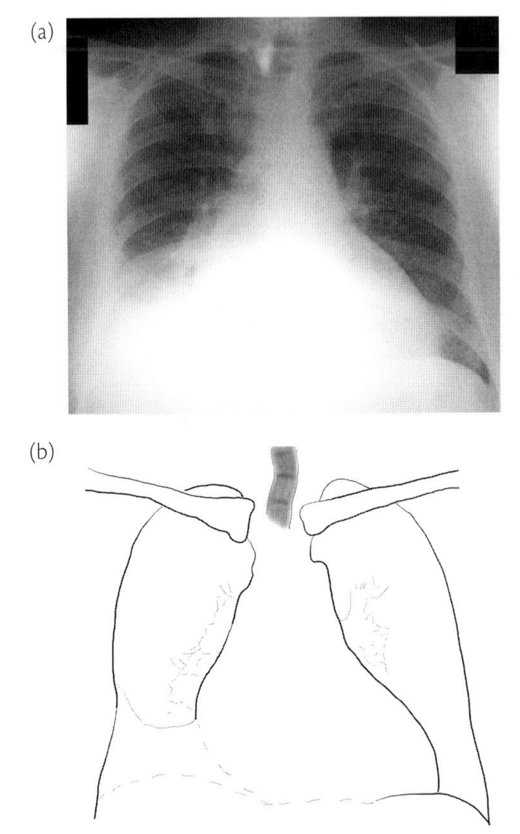

Fig. 16.46 Pulmonary infarction early. Note moderate right pulmonary effusion and perhaps some increased shadowing just above the meniscus adjacent to the right heart border.

Left ventricular aneurysm

See Fig. 16.48. You should see bulging of the left border of the heart and there may be calcification within it.

(a)

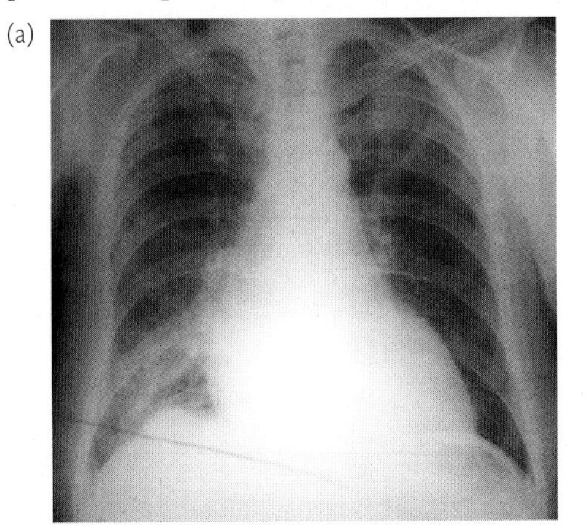

(b)

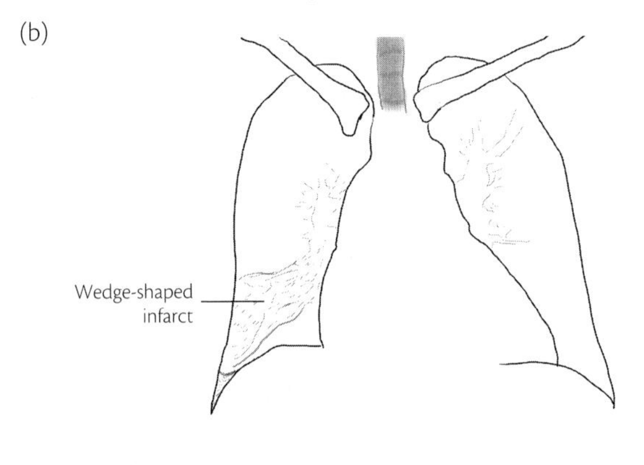

Fig. 16.47 Pulmonary infarction late. Two months later there is a wedge shaped infarct in the right lower zone (and the suspicion of another infarct in the left upper zone.)

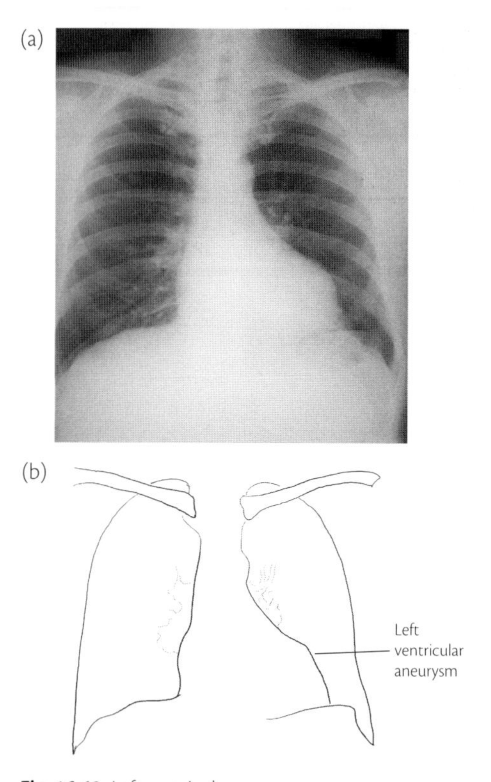

Fig. 16.48 Left ventricular aneurysm.

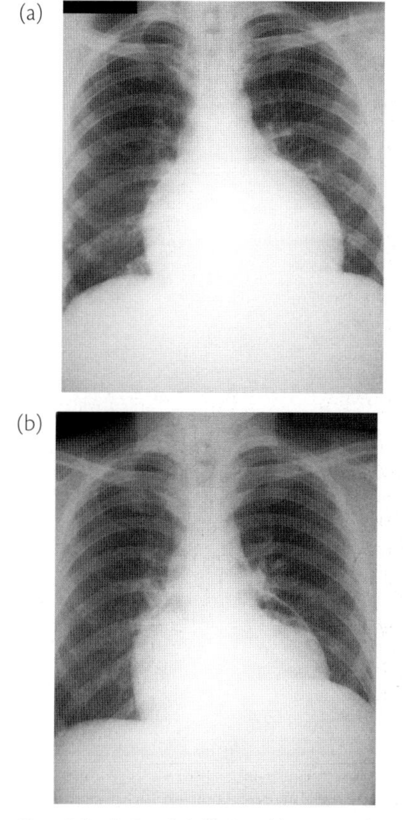

Fig. 16.49 Pericardial effusion. (a) Note cardiomegaly with the characteristic globular shape of the heart (b) Appearance following pericardiocentesis (a pericardial tap). Air has now been introduced into the pericardial sac.

Pericardial effusion

See Fig. 16.49. Pericardial effusions surround the heart, so a generalized (as opposed to a specific area of the heart) enlargement should make you suspicious of a pericardial effusion. A pericardial effusion develops quickly, so look at old films for comparison.

Hilum

When the hilum (Figs 16.50–16.51) is enlarged you should consider:

(1) bronchogenic lung cancer;

(2) **hilar lymphadenopathy**—due to malignancy, lymphoma, and infection;

(3) **vascular shadowing**.

The affected hilum will look larger and denser. It will have lost its normal concave shape. However, you may mistake hilar enlargement if the film is rotated, so review the old films. Bilateral hilar enlargement can also be due to vascular markings, cancer, or lymphadenopathy. Characteristically, sarcoidosis causes bilateral hilar lymphadenopathy (see Fig. 16.51).

Chest X-ray emergencies

There are many CXR emergencies; these include

- acute left ventricular failure
- tension pneumothorax
- PE
- dissecting thoracic aortic aneurysm.

The CXR is used in a large proportion of emergencies. There are a few situations whereby prompt action is needed to save lives. Acute left ventricular failure and PE have been covered earlier. You must be aware of the tension pneumothorax.

Tension pneumothorax

See Fig. 16.52. Whenever you see a pneumothorax you must ask yourself, is this a tension pneumothorax? The area of black lung will be large—often the size of one hemi-thorax. The mediastinum will be shifted away from the pneumothorax. The edge of the pneumo-

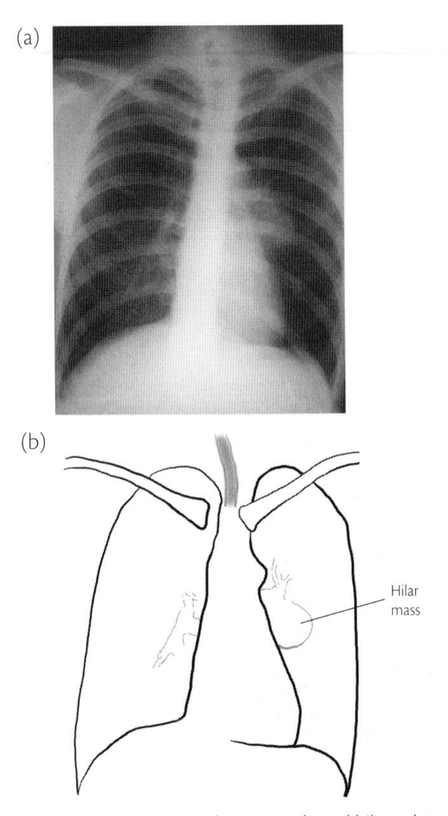

Fig. 16.50 Chest x-ray showing unilateral hilar enlargement, due to malignancy.

(a)

(b)

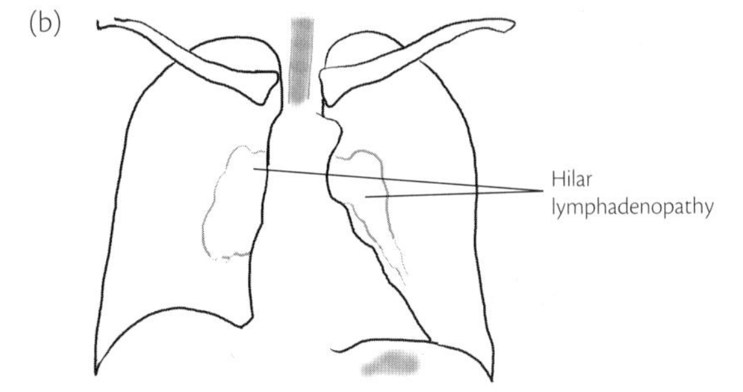

Fig. 16.51 Bihilar lymphadenopathy due to sarcoidosis.

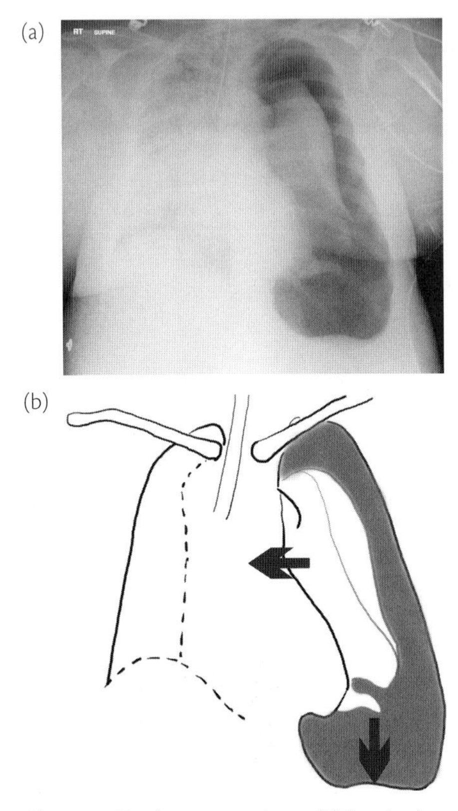

Fig. 16.52 Tension pneumothorax. (b) Despite the poor film this is one occasion where repeating the film would cost the life of your patient. There is enough information here allied to the clinical condition to make the diagnosis. There is mediastinal shift to the right with depression of the left hemidiaphragm (indicated by the arrows). This needs urgent decompression with a chest drain.

> **Tip**
>
> If a patient is mal-aligned during a CXR, any rotation will cause the mediastinum to look wide. So, check the technical quality of the film.

> **Tip**
>
> For any lung pathology try and obtain any old CXRs. They will let you know if the abnormality is new or old and how the abnormality is progressing.

thorax abutting the mediastinum will be concave to the side of the blackness.

Dissection of the thoracic aorta

The normal thoracic aorta is not visible on a PA CXR. When the thoracic aorta is aneurysmal, then it causes the mediastinum to widen. This in conjunction with a history of sudden, tearing chest pain should make you suspicious of a dissection. A pleural effusion containing blood may accompany it.

Examination favourites

The following films (with explanations) are some of the examination favourites that appear year after year.

1. **Fig 16.53.** Lung metastases in the presence of a mastectomy (absence of one breast shadow) in the examination would suggest metastatic breast carcinoma.
2. **Fig 16.54.** This picture is characteristic of old TB.
3. **Fig 16.55.** Apical pneumothoraces can be very difficult to identify.
4. **Fig 16.56.** If the thyroid enlarges significantly and passes behind the sternum, it will produce a mediastinal shadow.
5. **Fig 16.57.** A fluid level, corresponding to that of the herniated stomach will be seen behind the heart.
6. **Fig 16.58.** You will see notching of the ribs due to increased blood flow in the arteries running in the groove below the ribs.
7. **Fig 16.59.**

Presentation

Presentation is very important. If you were asked to comment on the CXR in Fig 16.60, you would say the following. 'This is a plain, PA chest X-ray of Mr Clause taken on the 25th December at the North Pole General Hospital. The most obvious abnormality is the appearance of cardiomegaly. I will focus on this after I have firstly studied the X-ray systematically. The X-ray is cor-

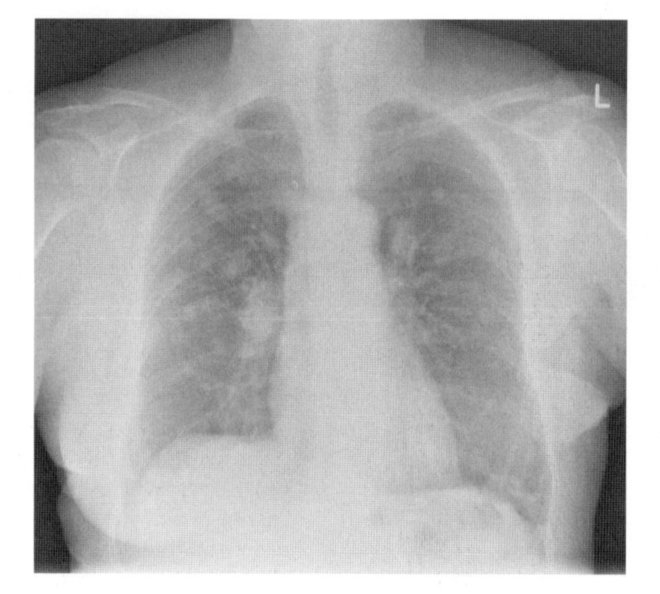

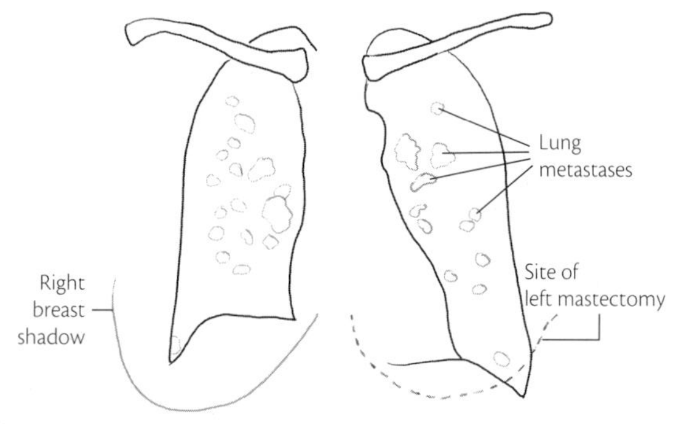

Fig. 16.53 Breast cancer with mastectomy and lung metastases.

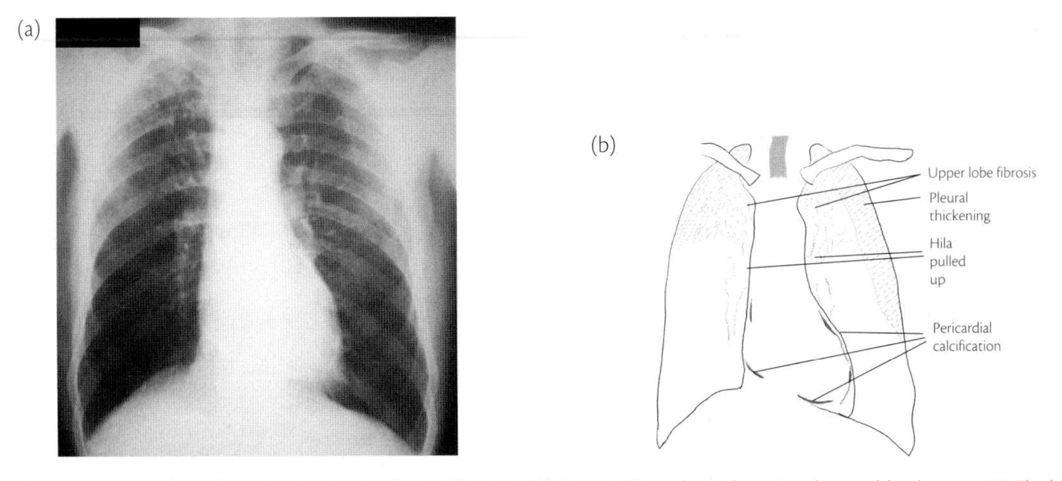

Fig. 16.54 Bilateral apical scarring (and pericardial calcification). (b) There is bilateral apical scarring due to old pulmonary TB. The hila are pulled up and there is thickening of the pleura especially on the left. If you observe the heart closely you can see curvilinear streaks of calcification outlining the pericardial sac.

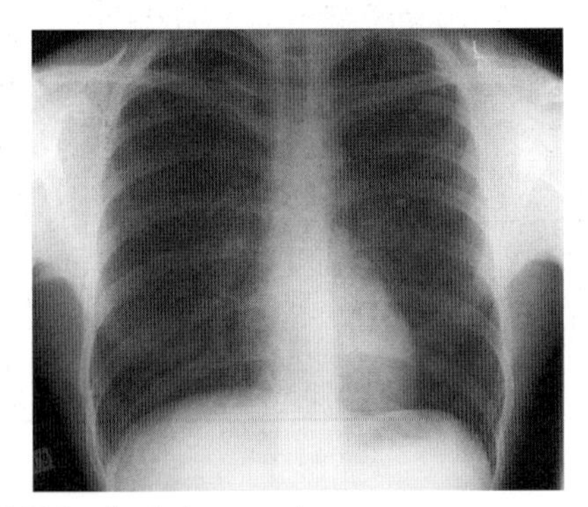

Fig. 16.55 Small apical pneumothorax.

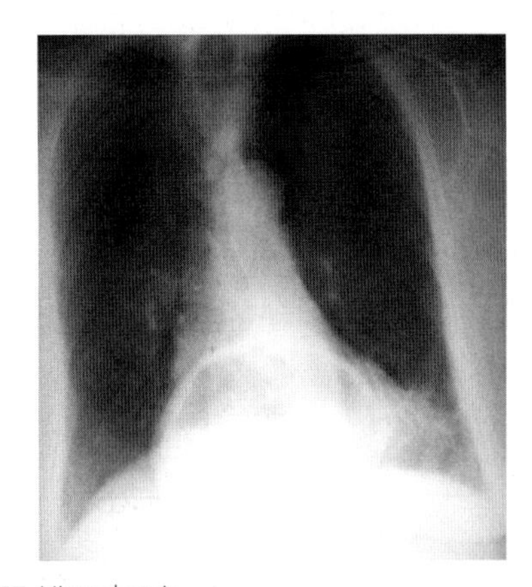

Fig. 16.57 Hiatus hernia.

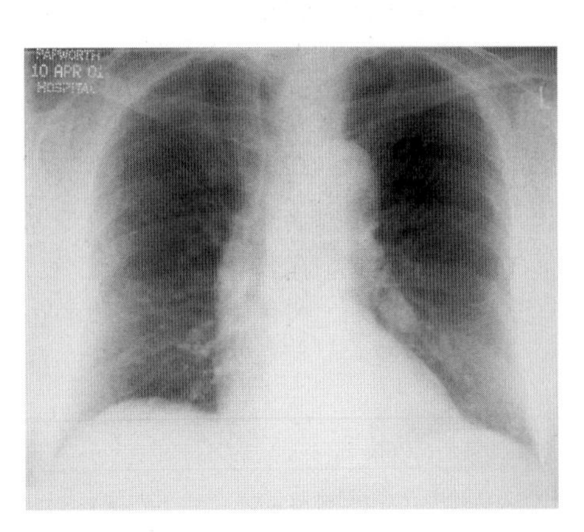

Fig. 16.56 Retrosternal thyroid.

rectly orientated and the exposure is satisfactory. The patient is not rotated. There are no obvious abnormalities within the bones. The trachea is not deviated. The mediastinum has clearly defined borders and there is no enlargement or change in density of it or the hilar regions. There is no CXRical pathology in the lungs and they are expanded normally. The diaphragms are clearly seen although there is blunting at the right costophrenic angle with a meniscus suggesting a small effusion. There are no abnormalities below the diaphragm or within the soft tissues. The cardiothoracic ratio exceeds 1:2. As this is a PA film, this confirms the heart is enlarged. With regards to the cardiomegaly, four causes are ischaemic heart disease, valvular heart disease, pericardial effusion, and cardiomyopathy.'

(a)

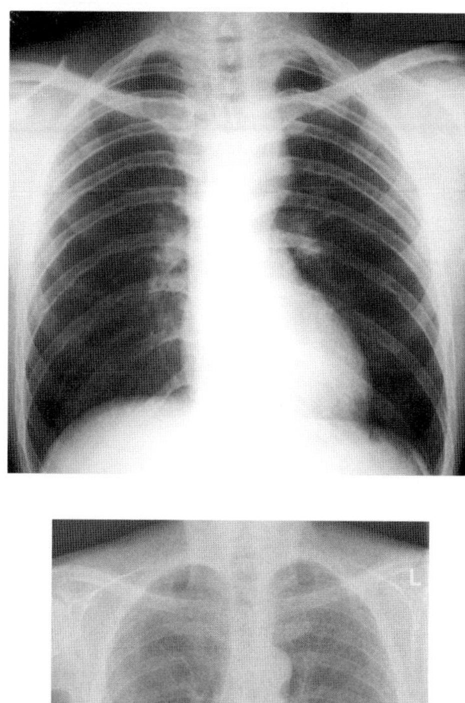

(b)

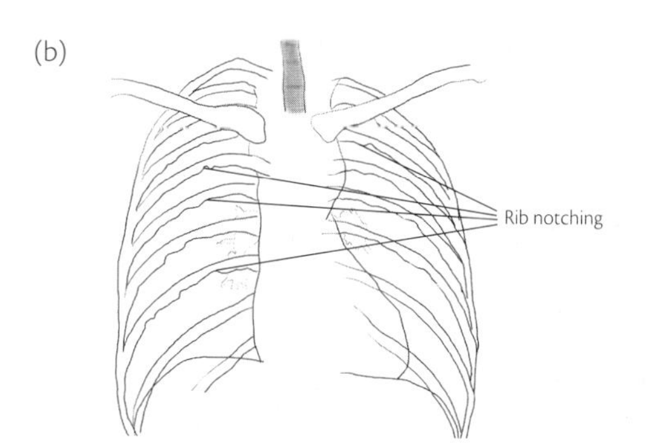

Fig. 16.58 Coarctation of the aorta.

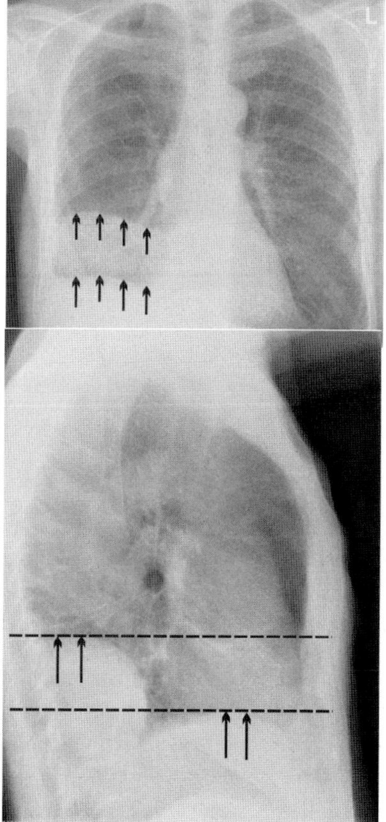

Fig. 16.59 Empyaema. (a) This PA film is unusual in that it shows two fluid levels on the right side. This can only occur if fluid is trapped in a pocket i.e. loculated between parietal and visceral pleura. This is illustrated by the lateral film which shows encysted fluid posteriorly producing the second fluid level. This is more likely to occur with viscous fluid like pus.

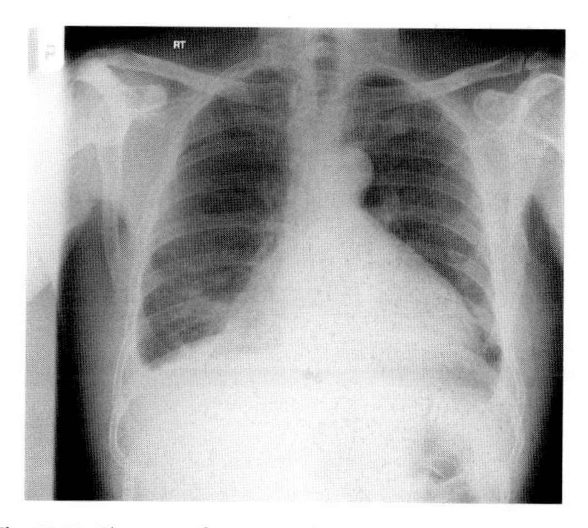

Fig. 16.60 Chest x-ray for presentation.

Further reading

Corne J, Carrol M, Brown I, Delaney D. *CXR made easy*. Edinburgh: Churchill Livingstone; 2002.

Harvey CJ, Roberts HRS, Shaw RJ. *Radiology casebook for the MRCP*. Oxford: Oxford University Press; 1999.

Kausik RK, Ryder REJ, Wellings RM. *An aid to radiology for the MRCP*. Oxford: Blackwell Science; 2002.

Scalley P. *Medical imaging, an Oxford core text*. Oxford: Oxford University Press; 1999.

CHAPTER 17

Practical procedures

Chapter contents

Introduction

The focus of this chapter is on the practical skills you will be expected to acquire before you finish your training (in readiness for your house jobs). House jobs have changed dramatically in the last few years. With the drive to reduce junior doctors' hours and their punishing workload, some of the tasks have been taken over by phlebotomists (blood takers) and nurse practitioners. Although the volume of tasks have decreased you will still need to be proficient in these skills because

(1) not all hospitals have nurse practitioners;

(2) not all hospitals have a phlebotomy service that covers weekends;

(3) you may be asked to do the 'difficult' patients that the practitioners cannot do;

(4) there may not be adequate cover when these staff go on leave or are off sick.

So! As with any skill that you have been trying to master, **practice is the key!**

Venepuncture

This is the art of blood taking. Practise when you can on the wards, but if you are having difficulty do not have more than three attempts on the patient before seeking help.

Venepuncture checklist

1. Get your equipment ready. (including sharps bin)
2. Identify the patient.
3. Introduce yourself to your patient and inform them of what you intend to do.
4. Wash your hands and put on gloves.
5. Apply tourniquet to the arm.
6. Find a suitable vein.
7. Swab the area.
8. Warn the patient you are about to inject the needle.
9. Insert the needle and withdraw blood.
10. Apply swab to puncture site for approximately 1 min.
11. Fill bottles (if not using the vacutainer system) and label them.
12. Dispose of needle in a 'sharps' bin.

Venepuncture in detail

1. Get your equipment ready. (including sharps bin)

Find a receiver (a disposable hospital bowl) and place in it a syringe, needles, mediswabs, blood bottles (each hospital will have colour-coded bottle for the type of blood sample you require), and some gloves. Have your tourniquet ready. There are two types of syringes, the old-fashioned syringe with the hand-drawn plunger and the newer vacuum collecting system. The vacuum system uses a number of colour-coded tubes, which are vacuum sealed. The needle is specially designed with a central prong at its opposite end. This prong inserts into the rubber cap of each sample tube (thereby keeping an air-tight seal). Blood then flows into each tube by virtue of their vacuum. With the old-fashioned syringe the size you use is determined by how many samples you need and the volume of blood each requires. For example, a full blood count only requires a 5 ml syringe, whereas a full blood count, a urea and electrolytes (U&Es), and clotting may require a 20 ml syringe.

2. Identify the patient.

This sounds self-evident but mistakes have been known to happen. So take care! Make sure the name on the blood card matches the name on the bed. Always ask the patient who they are also. It has been known for confused patients to sit by other patients' beds. Extremely confused patients may even admit to being somebody else, so be on your guard. Identification is particularly important with regards to cross-matching blood for transfusion. With other blood samples, bleeding the wrong patient can still be dangerous, so if you discover you have sent the wrong sample make sure you inform a doctor immediately! Never get complacent!

3. Introduce yourself to your patient and inform them of what you intend to do.

Be confident in your approach to the patient (even if it is your first attempt) because there is nothing more nerve wracking for a patient than seeing a trembling doctor approach them with a needle. Say something like,'I am Willam Osler, a medical student and I have come to take your blood.' Some people when they hear the word student will ask, 'Have you done this before?' If you **are** inexperienced, try and maintain a calm, unruffled demeanour (even though you may be shaking like a leaf inside) and say you have. Nobody likes having blood taken, especially by a novice (except perhaps a masochist).

4. Wash your hands and put on gloves.

This stage is essential to minimise the risk of cross-infection and the transfer of organisms from yourself to the patient (and subsequent patients) and from the patient to you. The gloves will help protect you from serious blood-borne diseases such as hepatitis B, C and HIV. Most patients with these conditions will usually be made known to you but there is always a small chance that you may encounter a patient in whom the diagnosis has not been made yet. Be suspicious if the patient is a known intravenous drug abuser, if the patient is of no fixed abode or has the hint of a suspicious background, or patients from abroad who come from areas where specific blood-borne diseases are endemic. If you are unsure, inform a doctor. If the doctor feels that a blood-borne disease is possible they may need to test for these viruses following counselling and consent (especially for HIV). These samples will need to be labelled 'danger of infection'.

5. Apply tourniquet to the arm.

Apply this to the upper arm just above the elbow. Some tourniquets simply wrap around the arm and fasten with velcro. Others are so fiddly they seem to require a training course all of their own. Keep the tourniquet on until a vein becomes apparent (this can take up to a minute). While you are waiting is a good time to get your blood bottles ready. Remove their caps and place them upright on the bedside locker: if using the vacuum system.

6. Find a suitable vein.

The best place to find a vein is in the antecubital fossa near the crease of the elbow. Tapping gently on your

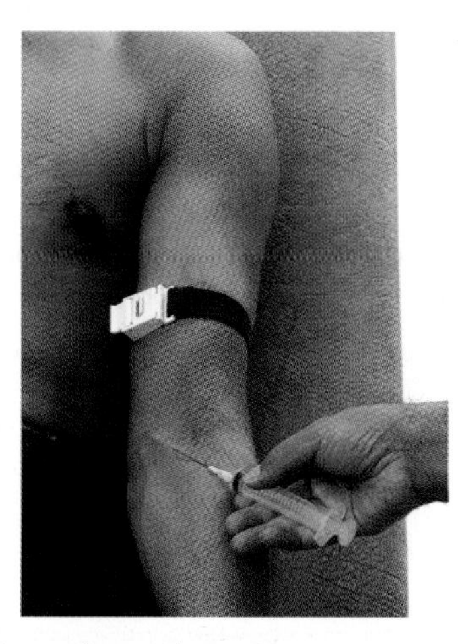

Fig. 17.1 Picture of arm with tourniquet.

target vein (or stroking it) can make it stand out more. Sometimes you cannot see the vein and you have to feel with your fingertips. This takes some practice. You need to build a mental picture on the skin surface of where you feel the vein is running. See Fig. 17.1.

7. Swab the area.

Simply tear open the mediswab packet and wipe the target site with the swab (do this scrupulously for blood cultures to prevent contamination from the patient's skin commensals).

8. Warn the patient you are about to inject the needle.

This is vital. There is nothing worse than having meticulously lined up your vein and having your patient jerk their arm, amid loud shrieking (your patient might shriek too!) Be warned! There are patients, who despite your warnings, may still jump. They tend to be the confused patients or the very anxious (you will develop a knack for spotting these people). People with a real dread of needles may tell you up front that they have a problem. If you have any doubts, get help from a friendly nurse or a fellow student and get them to hold the arm steady for you.

9. Insert the needle and withdraw blood.

Before insertion, the authors use the index finger of their non-dominant hand to retrace the path of the target vein. Then they gently pull back on the skin to put it under tension (they find the needle penetrates more easily and is less painful). Now go for it! Your syringe should be almost parallel to the forearm (too steep an angle and you could go right through the vein. If you are successful you will get a flashback in the plastic barrel above the needle indicating that you are in the vein (a flashback is a tiny reflux of blood into the needle barrel). If you do not get a flashback do not panic as you may have only missed the vein by millimetres. Just hold the syringe steady and with your left hand feel for the vein again. By changing the direction of the needle slightly and aiming toward your finger, you may be able to gain access into the vein (this obviates the need for a further painful injection). Once you are in the vein, hold the syringe in place by pressing it lightly against the forearm of your patient with your left hand. You now need to learn the skill of squeezing the plunger up with the fourth finger of your right hand, while you are holding it. Once the plunger has moved up about 2.5–5 ml or so, there should be more of it available for you to get a better grip and aspiration of blood becomes easier (so long as you remain within the vein). With the vacuum system you do not get a flashback and you have to judge that you are in the vein by developing 'a feel'. Once in the vein the vacuum draws up the blood and once you have sufficient for a sample, simply remove the tube and put the next one in its place (while keeping the needle still). See Fig. 17.2.

10. Apply swab to puncture site for approximately 1 min.

Now remove the tourniquet and apply a swab or cotton wool ball to the puncture site. Press down with your finger until the bleeding has stopped. If your patient is not confused it is reasonable to ask them to do this for you. Some people instruct patients to bend their arm up to 90°, trapping the swab in the elbow crease, with the resulting pressure between the biceps and forearm acting to staunch the flow of blood. However, some patients lose concentration quickly and forget to keep their arms bent fully. This can lead to continued bleeding or the formation of a bruise.

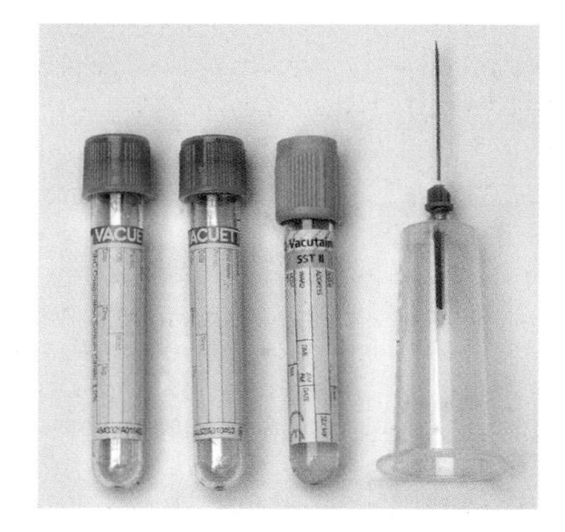

Fig. 17.2 The vacuum collecting equipment.

Tip

If you are taking blood for clotting, check to see if the patient is on warfarin or heparin on the blood card. If your patient is on either their clotting will be prolonged and you will have to press on the puncture site for much longer.

11. Fill bottles (if not using the vacuum system) and label them.

Fill the bottles on the bedside locker with the correct amount of blood. Take care not to spill any. Now label the bottles. You can use the sticky labels provided in the patient's case notes. If you are hand writing the patient's details for the cross-matching of blood, **make sure** that you **always** put the **patient's hospital unit number** on the bottle (and on the blood card). Finally, if the patient is known to have a blood-borne disease, a hazard warning label should be placed on the bottle and on the request card so that the technicians analysing the blood can take the appropriate precautions.

12. Dispose of needle in the 'sharps' bin & wash hands.

This is vitally important. In the excitement of getting your blood (or being a busy doctor) you can forget about disposing of sharps. However if you leave them lying about or dispose of them in an ordinary bin, if someone is pierced by your sharps (this is called a needle-stick injury), they have to go through rigorous investigations to make sure that they are not at risk of any blood-borne disease. Believe me, those moments while waiting for the 'all clear' can be very anxious ones. So tidy up after yourself! Now wash your hands!

Femoral stab

This is a technique to use if you are having difficulty getting blood from the more orthodox sites on the arm or hand. The technique can also be used for getting blood gases. It is a blind technique, that is, you cannot see the blood vessel that you are aiming for. It can be used to take blood from the femoral vein or the femoral artery. You may not use this technique much during your student days but it is very handy skill to know about because as a house officer you will be expected to get blood even in difficult circumstances.

CASE 17.1

Problem. When you insert the needle you get a flashback but you are unable to aspirate any blood.

Discussion. This happens frequently. Sometimes as you insert the needle you inadvertently pass through the vein. The flashback tells you that you have been inside the vein at some point. All you need to do is to withdraw the needle slowly, pulling back on the plunger as you go. With any luck a stream of blood should rush into the syringe. Once this occurs, hold the syringe in position and collect the remainder of your sample.

CASE 17.2

Problem. You have successfully entered the vein but after a few millilitres, you cannot get any more blood out.

Discussion: It is very easy for either you or your patient to move their arm a tiny fraction. This may be sufficient to push the needle into the wall of the vein (or through it, or back out of it). Pull the needle back a small way, pulling up on the plunger as you go. If this is unsuccessful try advancing the needle slowly back along the path you took during insertion, pulling back on the plunger in the usual way. Occasionally you may have to give up and start again.

CASE 17.3

Problem. After failing to get blood you remove the needle and a huge lump appears.

Discussion. This is a haematoma (a collection of blood in the subcutaneous tissues). It occurs because at some point you have gone through the vein or nicked it during insertion. The other factor is that you have not removed the tourniquet before removing the needle and blood is forced out of the vein under the increased pressure. If you produce a haematoma, press down firmly with a swab for about 2 min.

Tip

Always remove your tourniquet before taking out your needle.

CASE 17.4

Problem. Although the veins look juicy and easy to get, you cannot get blood from them.

Discussion. There are a number of possibilities here.

1. If you are a novice it could just be a matter of technique and it may be valuable to get a qualified doctor to watch you take blood for feedback.
2. You may just be anxious. You may have have done everything right, except at the critical moment anxiety makes you lose concentration as you start to insert the needle. The solution here is to relax as much as possible and remember that all qualified doctors struggle when they first start out.
3. Some people, particularly the elderly, have a lack of connective tissue support and the veins can squirm out of the way as the needle pushes against them (the author call these veins 'wrigglers'). You may be able to identify them prior to venepuncture with your finger as they tend to squirm away eel-like if you push them from side to side. To spear these wrigglers, the authors try to splint them with the left finger as far from the venepuncture site as possible. Then they insert the needle with a brisker action than normal (the idea being to penetrate the vein before the vein has time to move).
4. You may be having an off day. Even experienced doctors can miss for no discernible reason (a situation made embarrassing when another doctor comes and takes the blood first time and a situation made even more embarrassing if the doctor comments how easy those veins look). There is however, no real shame in missing the vein. If after three attempts you do not succeed as a student, ask for help.

Femoral stab checklist

1. Get your equipment ready including sharps bin.
2. Identify the patient.
3. Introduce yourself to your patient and inform them of what you intend to do.
4. Find the femoral artery.

CASE 17.5

Problem. You cannot see or feel a suitable vein in the antecubital fossa.

Discussion. There are a number of tricks you can try.

1. You can keep the tourniquet on a little longer than usual (up to 2 min). Watch out for the arm turning blue.
2. Get the patient to squeeze their hands into a fist repeatedly as the muscular effort can increase the venous engorgement.
3. Get them to hang their arm down by their side, as this will slow down the venous return to the heart.
4. There is no reason why you cannot use all three of the suggestions together.

CASE 17.6

Problem. Despite trying the measures in the last case, you still cannot find a suitable vein.

Discussion. You may have to look elsewhere for veins. Try the back of the hand but some facts need to borne in mind.

1. Taking blood from the back of the hand is more painful.
2. It is more fiddly than taking it from the elbow. You have to steady their hand by the fingers and you have no support for your syringe (you can rest your right hand on the forearm when taking blood from the elbow).
3. The veins are much closer to the surface than at the elbow and they are much smaller and thinner walled. Therefore it is very easy to rupture the vein if you are not careful.
4. Blood aspiration is much slower (because of smaller capacity) and therefore it is not a good route for getting vast quantities of blood (about 10 ml is a useful arbitrary limit). Any more than this and you run the risk of the blood clotting in the syringe or in those blood bottles where this is not desirable (for example, clotting or full blood count).
5. Hand veins are more likely to be wrigglers.

Tip

If you rupture a hand vein and can see another vein on the same hand you would like to attempt, try and get hold of a second tourniquet. Place your swab over the ruptured vein and tie your tourniquet over the swab and pull it tight. You can then put your original tourniquet on the same arm again without risk of worsening the bruising or producing a haematoma.

CASE 17.7

Problem. You cannot find veins at the elbow or the hands.

Discussion. This problem can occur with obese patients or those whose veins have been destroyed by repeated cancer chemotherapy. Try all the previous tricks listed in Case 17.5, including leaving the tourniquet on for longer, hand squeezing, and the arm hanging down but if these measures do not work, try soaking the hands in warm water for a minute with the tourniquet on (after giving the patient some time with it off). If this fails your next step depends on the need for the blood sample. If it is a relatively routine sample, it could be left for another day (discuss this with the doctor looking after the patient). If there is an urgent need for the blood then you could try a femoral stab (see later).

Keypoints

- Practice is the key to succeeding at venepuncture.
- Identify the patient.
- The best site for taking blood is the antecubital fossa.
- Be wary of blood-borne diseases and take precautions.
- A flashback signals that you have just entered the vein.
- Always remove the tourniquet before you remove the needle (to avoid haematomas).
- Label all bottles accurately (epecially blood for cross-matching).
- Label any infectious samples with a hazard warning sticker.

5. Wash your hands and put on gloves.
6. Swab the area.
7. Warn the patient you are about to inject the needle.
8. Insert the needle and withdraw blood.
9. Apply swab to puncture site and press firmly.
10. Fill bottles and label them.
11. Dispose of your sharps and wash your hands.

Femoral stab in detail

1. Get your equipment ready including sharps bin.

2. Identify the patient.

3. Introduce yourself to your patient and inform them of what you intend to do.

These steps are the same as in venepuncture except that if you are taking blood gases you will use a special blood gas syringe, which is heparinized and vacuum sealed. You will also inform your patient that you will be taking blood from their leg rather than their arm although the discomfort is about the same.

4. Find the femoral artery.

Whether you are taking an arterial or venous sample you have to identify the femoral artery. Move over to the side of the bed near the leg you are going to take blood from. Feel in the groin near the edge of the pubic hair until you feel pulsation of the artery. If you want blood from the femoral vein you need to go medial to the artery (a good way of remembering the neurovascular structures in the groin is **van**; the femoral **a**rtery being lateral to the vein, and the femoral **n**erve being the most lateral of the three). To locate the target area for the vein, simply roll your fingers medially in small

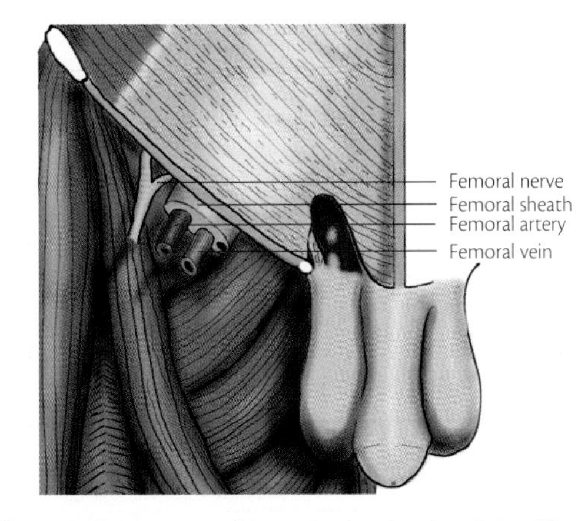

Fig. 17.3 The anatomy of the groin, showing the relationship between vein, artery, and nerve.

increments, monitoring the pulsations as you go. Eventually you will reach a point where the pulsations disappear as you leave the medial edge of the femoral artery. Move your fingers a few millimetres in the same direction and stop. Separate your index and middle fingers as they will act as target markers for the vein. See Fig. 17.3.

5. Wash your hands and put on gloves.

6. Swab the area.

7. Warn the patient you are about to inject the needle.

These steps are the same as for venepuncture.

8. Insert the needle and withdraw blood.

You will have to quickly find the artery again. Separate your index and middle fingers over the area of maximum pulsation for an arterial sample. If you are using the blood gas syringe, hold it vertically and aim it between your two fingers. Insert the needle slowly keeping the syringe vertical and watch for a spurt of blood into the syringe. When this happens hold the syringe still and the vacuum and arterial pulsation will fill it very quickly. If you are taking blood from the femoral vein, locate the vein as in Step 4. This time you will be using an ordinary syringe. Aim between your fingers and insert the needle vertically. Pull up on the plunger by squeezing up with your fourth finger as you insert the needle. Insert the needle slowly and watch for the blood rushing into the syringe. When this happens hold your position (you can now use your guiding hand to stabilize the syringe), while you aspirate blood with your right hand).

9. Apply swab to puncture site and press firmly.

For a femoral artery stab you need to press firmly for at least 2–3 min. Always check the site for signs of a haematoma as you may need to continue pressing for longer. For a femoral vein stab you will only need about 1 min.

10. Fill bottles and label them.

Tip

If you are performing a femoral stab for blood because you cannot get it elsewhere, it does not matter if you penetrate the femoral artery by mistake as the blood can still be analysed. You should however press on firmly with a swab for longer if you suspect you have done this. It does matter however if you stab the vein instead of the artery if you are taking a blood gas sample. Suspect this if the blood oxygen pO_2 is much lower than you are expecting clinically (or is incompatible with life).

Keypoints

- A femoral stab is a blind procedure.
- It can be used if blood taking is difficult elsewhere or for blood gas sampling.
- Finding the femoral artery is the key to this technique.
- The femoral vein is always **medial** to the femoral artery.
- If you have taken blood from the artery press down with a swab for at least 2–3 min.

Cannula insertion

A cannula is an essential tool for managing sick patients. It is a small tube which is inserted into a vein to give access to the circulation. The ability to insert a cannula is one of the most important techniques for a house officer to acquire.

Cannula insertion checklist

1. Get your equipment ready including sharps bin.
2. Identify the patient.
3. Introduce yourself to your patient and inform them of what you intend to do.
4. Wash your hands and put on gloves.
5. Apply tourniquet to the arm.
6. Find a suitable vein.
7. Swab the area.
8. Warn the patient you are about to insert the cannula.
9. Insert the cannula.
10. Cap off the cannula and secure it in place.
11. Dispose of your sharps and wash your hands.

Cannula insertion in detail

1. Get your equipment ready including sharps bin.

Get a receiver and place in it some mediswabs, gloves, *a vapour permeable clear dressing* and your choice of *cannula*. A venflon is essentially a plastic cannula with a needle

Tip

Use a blue or pink cannula for blood transfusions.

introducer running down its centre. It also has a colour-coded port with a cap, through which drugs can be injected. The colours correspond to the size of the venflon, with the smallest being blue or pink and the largest brown. Use the smallest cannula available for your intended purpose. Use brown or green cannulas in urgent situations where large volumes of colloid or blood are required very quickly, for example, bleeding aortic aneurysm (in practice browns are rarely used because they are so hard to get in especially when a patient's veins are 'shut down'). Most of the time a blue or pink cannula will fulfil most functions.

2. Identify the patient.

3. Introduce yourself to your patient and inform them of what you intend to do.

4. Wash your hands and put on gloves.

5. Apply tourniquet to the arm.

These steps are the same as for venepuncture except you will say something like, 'I need to put a little needle into your arm. It will stay in your arm so that we can give you drugs into your blood on a regular basis. It stops you having to have needles every time you need the drug.'

6. Find a suitable vein.

When finding a vein for a cannula, your requirements are different from that of venepuncture. You need a position where there is little movement from joints, which could bend the cannula and occlude it. Therefore the antecubital fossa is a last resort. The best site is the radial aspect of the forearm. If at all possible insert it into the non-dominant arm, so that if the patient is requiring a drip, they will still be able to use their dominant arm.

7. Swab the area.

8. Warn the patient you are about to insert the cannula.

These steps are the same as for venepuncture.

9. Insert the cannula.

See Fig. 17.4. Take the cannula out the packet and remove the white cap; place it by the bedside where you can reach it within arm's reach of the patient (you will see why later). Now place the thumb of your right hand against the back of the cannula and grasp the perspex wings with your index finger and middle finger at either side of the cannula. You should find that you can push forwards with your thumb and the force can be countered by your index and middle finger pushing backwards. In this way you can exert a good deal of fine control in guiding the cannula. Aim for the vein as you do with venepuncture at an angle almost parallel to the

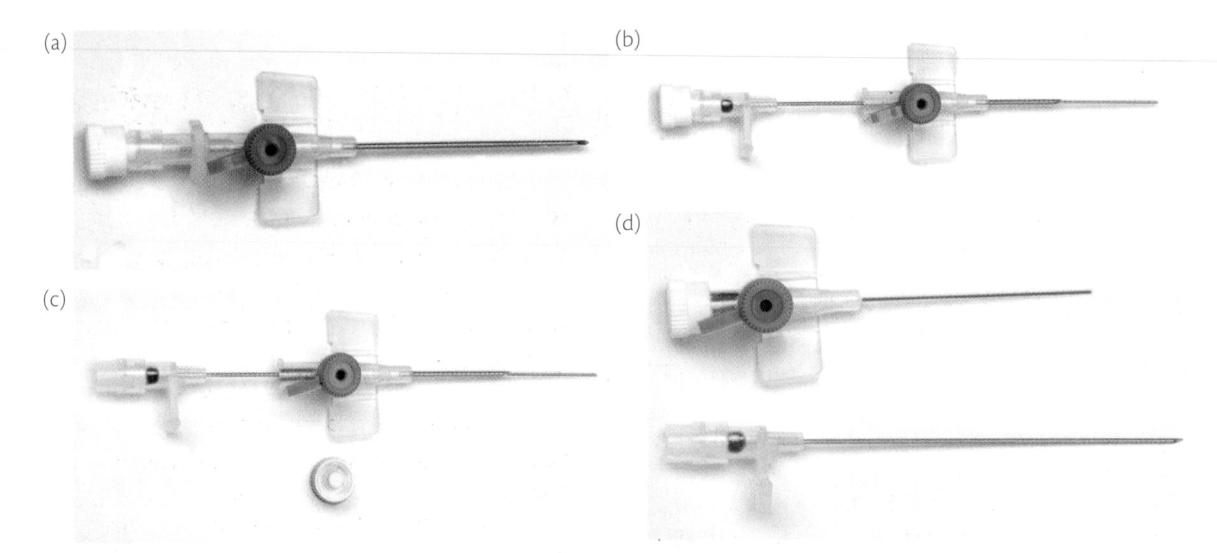

Fig. 17.4 Sequence of events for cannula insertion. (a) The complete cannula. (b) The cannula is inserted and the cannula is advanced a few more millimetres after the flashback of blood is seen. Then partly withdraw the introducer. (c) The cap can be removed at this stage and the cannula advanced fully. (d) The introducer is removed, the cap placed quickly over the end of the cannula and the cannula can be secured in place.

vein. If you are successful you will see a flashback near the back of the cannula. At this point, advance the cannula a few more millimetres. Now hold the plastic part in place while you withdraw the introducer a little and see if blood runs into the cannula. If this happens you can advance the cannula fully into the vein and remove the introducer and place it safely to the side. If you did not get a flashback, do not panic. Withdraw the cannula as far as possible without taking it out. Feel for the vein again and angle your cannula in its general direction and have another go. Poking around in the subcutaneous tissue is less painful than stabbing the skin again.

10. Cap off the cannula and tape it in place.

If you are successful, you will see blood oozing down the cannula towards the open end. At this stage remove the tourniquet and quickly reach for the cap that you put aside earlier and 'lock off' the cannula. Now secure the cannula with your clear dressing (those of you who forgot to bring tape will regret having to search for some and finding the cannula has dropped out in your absence). Position the dressing where you want it then peel off the backing while pressing down. The sticky underside of the dressing will keep it in place.

11. Dispose of your sharps and wash your hands.

It is very easy to forget the discarded introducer as you concentrate on securing the cannula. They have been known to turn up in bed linen (or more seriously, stabbing patients or nurses who have been making up the bed).

Many of the cases discussed in the 'Venepuncture' section in terms of finding a vein are relevant to cannula insertion.

Blood gas sampling

Blood gases are usually taken from very sick patients especially those who are breathless. They give information on the level of oxygen and carbon dioxide in the blood. The partial pressures of these gases are usually measured in millimetres of mercury (mm Hg) or kilopascals (kPa). Information is also available on the

Tip

You can remove blood from the cannula by engaging a syringe in the open end of the cannula (sometimes this leads to haemolysed blood and a falsely raised potassium).

CASE 17.8

Problem. As I remove the introducer from the cannula, blood always rushes out staining the bed sheets, the patient, and myself.

Discussion. There are a few things you can do to stop this.

1. Once the cannula is in the vein, remove the tourniquet.
2. Remember to remove the cannula cap early and have it close by so that you can quickly fit it to the end of the cannula. A lot of people forget the cap until the introducer is out and end up having to remove it under pressure, while blood starts running from the cannula.
3. The most important thing to stop blood loss is to press on the vein. However where you press is vital. Many people make the mistake of pressing on the vein directly over the cannula and no matter how hard they press the cannula will remain patent and blood will escape. The trick is to 'eyeball' the length of the cannula and try to imagine how far it extends within the vein once it is sited. What you aim to do is to press down on the vein **in front of** the cannula tip. Press the vein there and you should be able to dam back the blood long enough for you to put the cap on (or withdraw blood).

Keypoints

- There are various sizes of cannulas (blue or pink should be the most commonly used).
- Use a blue or pink cannula for blood transfusion.
- Insert the cannula in a vein away from a joint and preferably in the non-dominant arm.
- Look for the flashback and then advance the cannula a few more millimetres.
- Always withdraw the introducer partially to make sure that blood runs into the cannula.
- Remove the tourniquet before removing the introducer completely and press on the vein immediately in front of the cannula to achieve haemostasis.
- You can remove blood from the cannula.
- Always dispose of your sharps.

CASE 17.9

Problem, After I get a flashback, when I withdraw the introducer partially, no blood appears.

Discussion. You may have simply gone through the vein. All you need to do is to withdraw the plastic cannula slowly. At some point you will get a rush of blood into the cannula. At this moment advance the cannula and if you are lucky it will run into the vein smoothly and blood will continue to ooze towards the end of the cannula when you remove the introducer (and the tourniquet). If, when you advance the cannula, it feels rough and grating and no blood comes back, the chances are you have torn the vein. Take the tourniquet off, remove the cannula, and try elsewhere with a fresh cannula.

CASE 17.10

Problem. After the flashback you remove the introducer but when you advance the cannula, you feel a grating resistance and no blood comes out of the cannula.

Discussion. You are guilty of rushing here, plus there is a subtle detail about the cannula structure that you are not *au fait* with. If you look at the cannula, you will notice that the introducer needle protrudes a few millimetres from the cannula tip (see Fig. 17.5 for a close-up of a cannula tip). Many students fail to take this difference into account. Consequently when they see the flashback, they hold the cannula still thinking the cannula is in the vein. In actuality the introducer is in the vein (providing the flashback) but the cannula tip is either in the wall of the vein or just outside it. So, when you advance the cannula, the tip runs up the venous wall, tearing it and producing a haematoma. The important step here is, once you see the flashback, advance the whole cannula a few more millimetres before partially removing the introducer. Always check that blood enters the cannula before you advance it fully and remove the introducer.

acid–base status of the body (the majority of sick patients are acidotic). Taking blood gases is a difficult procedure and requires a lot of practice. Blood gases are usually taken from the radial artery (which is readily accessible). They can also be taken from the brachial or the femoral artery. This is less accessible but easier to obtain (see p. 462).

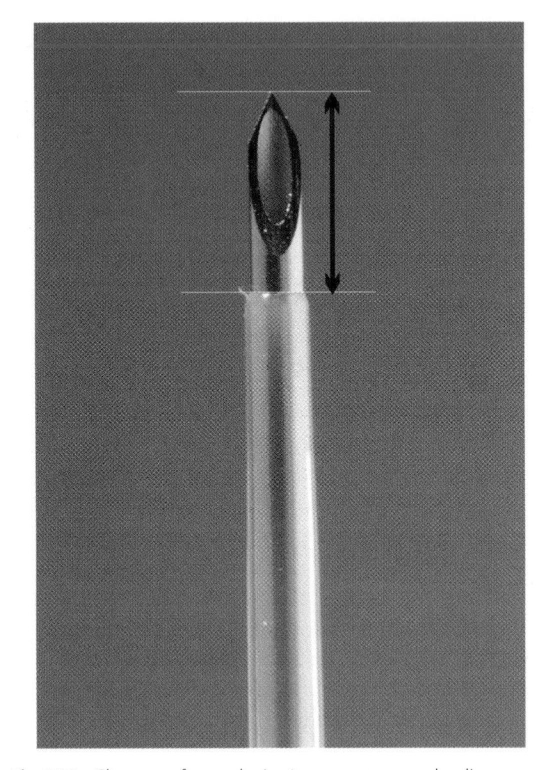

Fig. 17.5 Close-up of cannula tip. Arrow represents the distance between the tip of the introducer and the cannula.

Blood gas sampling checklist

1. Get your equipment ready including sharps bin.
2. Identify the patient.
3. Introduce yourself to your patient and inform them of what you intend to do.
4. Find the radial artery.
5. Wash your hands and put on gloves.
6. Swab the area.
7. Warn the patient you are about to inject the needle.
8. Insert the needle and withdraw blood.
9. Apply swab to puncture site for 2–3 min.
10. Bag the sample with the request card.
11. Dispose of your sharps and then wash your hands.

Blood gas sampling in detail

1. Get your equipment ready.

Fill a hospital receiver with a blood gas syringe, medi-swabs, and a specimen bag. (If your blood gas has to be transferred to another hospital for analysis, get some ice and put it in the bag. This is because the oxygen continues to be metabolized by cells in the blood and will lead to a falsely low result. The ice slows this process down.)

2. Identify the patient.

3. Introduce yourself to your patient and inform them of what you intend to do.

These steps are the same as for venepuncture.

4. Find the radial artery.

This is easy to do. You are simply looking for the pulse at the wrist. The difference is, you will be looking closely at the position of your finger over the pulse and making a mental note.

5. Wash your hands and put on gloves.

6. Swab the area.

7. Warn the patient you are about to inject the needle.

These steps are the same as for venepuncture.

8. Insert the needle and withdraw blood.

Place the back of the patient's hand on the bed and find the pulse again. The index finger of your left hand will be used as a marker. Now hold the blood gas syringe as you would a pen and at the angle you would write at normally (this is much easier than holding it vertically as is often taught). Aim close to your index finger and insert the needle slowly. Watch for the surge of blood and hold the needle steady. The vacuum and the arterial pressure will fill the syringe quickly. If you miss the artery, do not withdraw the needle fully. Feel for it again, redirect your needle towards it, and try again. See Fig. 17.6.

9. Apply swab to puncture site for 2–3 min.

Once you have your sample withdraw the needle and press firmly with your swab for 2–3 min. After this time, review the site and make sure that bleeding does not continue or a haematoma forms. If this occurs, press firmly with your swab again.

10. Bag the sample with the request card.

Put the sample in the specimen bag with the ice. Add the request card. Some hospitals have their own blood gas analyser for urgent samples in which case this step is not necessary.

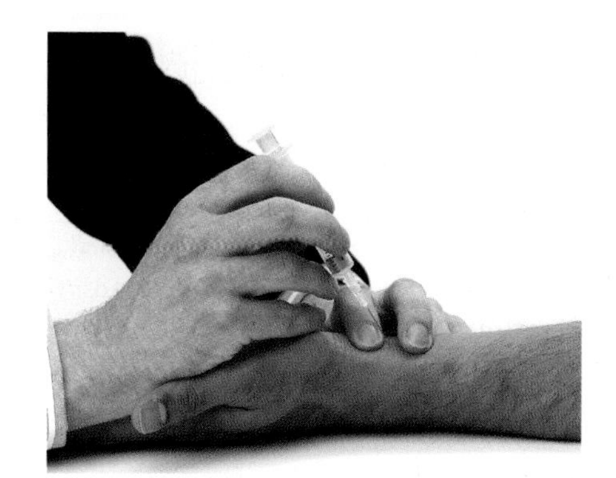

Fig. 17.6 Radial artery puncture for blood gases.

11. Dispose of your sharps, then wash your hands.

Tip

If there are no blood gas syringes available you can make your own. Get a 5 ml syringe and draw up 1 ml of heparin. Pull the plunger right out to the end to coat the inside of the syringe with the anti-coagulant and then push it back in and expel about 0.5 ml of the heparin. Use a green or orange needle. As there is no vacuum, you will need to pull up on the plunger when you take the blood gas.

Keypoints

- Blood can be taken from the radial, brachial, or femoral artery (the radial is used most commonly).
- It is easier to get blood gases from the femoral artery.
- If the sample has to travel a long way then pack the sample with ice.
- Always press with a swab for at least 2–3 min after taking the sample.

Intravenous drug adminstration

You will be pleased to know that this skill is very easy compared to what you have learned so far. The only thing required here is a careful and meticulous approach.

Intravenous drug administration checklist

1. Get your equipment ready.
2. Draw up 5–10 mls of normal saline.
3. Draw up the prescribed drug.

4. Identify the patient.
5. Introduce yourself to the patient and inform them of what you intend to do: check for allergies.
6. Check the cannula site and then give the drug.
7. Flush the cannula and then sign for the drug.
8. Dispose of your waste and wash your hands.

Intravenous drug administration in detail

1. Get your equipment ready.

Look at the drug chart and see what medication has been prescribed and the time it is due (some drugs are written as 'stat', which means it should be given immediately. They are usually written in the 'once only' column. Have a receiver handy, with syringes and needles (as you get experienced you will be able to choose the appropriate syringe for the drug prescribed).

2. Draw up 5–10 mls of normal saline.

You will use this to to check the patency of the cannula.

3. Draw up the prescribed drug

How you do this depends on the drug. Some can be drawn up straight from the vial. Others need reconstituting with sterile water. The instructions that come with the drugs will tell you the amount of water required (and hence the size of the syringe). Add a needle to the syringe and open the sterile water (flick the top of the vial to remove any drops lodged there). Draw up the water. Now plunge the needle in the rubber seal at the top of the drug bottle. Push the plunger down, while applying some downward force to the syringe itself. This is because you are injecting a given quantity of fluid into an enclosed space and this increases the pressure within the bottle, which tries to force the fluid back into the syringe. If you are not aware of this phenomenon, the needle can shoot back as you depress the plunger and you can spray the drug everywhere including your face. Once all the water is in the bottle, remove the syringe quickly, while still maintaining downward pressure on the plunger. Shake the drug bottle and allow sufficient time for the contents to dissolve. Now push the syringe and needle back into the drug bottle (hold both the bottle and the base of the syringe by your left hand) and the increased pressure should expel some of the contents into the syringe. Your right hand is free to pull back on the plunger to remove all the drugs. Remove the needle and point the tip of the syringe toward the ceiling. Flick the barrel a few times to induce all the air bubbles to rise to the tip. Expel the air by depressing the plunger carefully.

> **Tip**
>
> Some drugs can be drawn up into small (100 ml) bags of normal saline. They can be infused over a short time and can be set up by a nurse. So check with pharmacy.

4. Identify the patient.

Do this as before.

5. Introduce yourself to your patient and inform them of what you intend to do: check for allergies.

Say something like, 'Hello I am James Parkinson a third-year student and I am going to give you an injection of your regular medication.' If you are giving an antibiotic, particularly penicillin, check if the patient has any allergies. The original prescriber should have done this but it is good to have a safety net just in case.

6. Check the cannula site and then give the drug.

Before injecting, look at the cannula site. Does it look normal or does it look red suggesting phlebitis (the area will also be painful). Is there any pus/discharge suggesting infection. If the site looks normal open the coloured port of the cannula and engage the end of the syringe. Depress the plunger and inject about 2–3 mls of saline. If this causes pain, you should consider siting another cannula. If the saline flows freely without pain you can proceed to administer the drug. Sometimes the cannula is connected to a drip. If this is the case, turn off the drip before you inject the drug or the drug will shoot back up the giving set.

7. Flush the cannula and then sign for the drug.

Use the remainder of the normal saline in the syringe to flush the cannula. As a medical student you cannot sign for a drug. This should be done by a qualified doctor who has observed you and can take responsibility for your actions. Signing is important becsuse if there are any adverse events later down the line, the prescription chart can be used as evidence.

8. Dispose of your waste and wash your hands.

> **Tip**
>
> Another method, which is frequently used with a drip, is to twist and then pinch the tubing tightly as you inject the drug. This method has the advantage of allowing the drip to resume at its original speed once you release the pressure.

CASE 17.11

Problem. When you try to inject the drug there is resistance and you cannot get the drug into the vein.

Discussion. There can be a few reasons.

1. If the cannula is near a joint it could be kinked, so get the patient to straighten the joint before trying again.
2. The cannula could have clotted off. Press the plunger more firmly and maintain some downward pressure (to stop the drug spraying you or your patient) and this may be sufficient to dislodge the clot (the clot is too small to have any clinical significance).
3. The cannula may be incorrectly sited. Press the plunger more firmly but watch the area around the cannula. If you see a swelling forming, the drug may be going into the subcutaneous tissue. You will have to resite the cannula.
4. The cannula may have 'tissued' (see Case 17.12). This will be painful when you try to inject.

CASE 17.12

Problem. The patient experiences pain as you inject.

Discussion. Some drugs are irritants when injected. If this is the case, inject more slowly. The other reason can be that the cannula has 'tissued', which is the slang term for a local thrombophlebitis. An inflammatory reaction to the cannula occurs and you can see this if you inspect the cannula site, which will be swollen, red, and tender. The only recourse is to resite a cannula.

Keypoints

- Check the drug chart for the medication and the time prescribed.
- Draw up the drug according to the instructions.
- Identify the patient carefully (also double check for allergies).
- Inject the drug into the cannula port (watch for pain).
- If the patient experiences pain check to see if the drip has 'tissued'.
- If the cannula has a drip attached, either switch off the drip or pinch the tubing until you have injected the drug.
- Sign for the drug (as a student, have it countersigned by a qualified doctor).

CHAPTER 18

Finals

Chapter contents

Introduction

Congratulations! You have managed to get this far. Now only one obstacle remains, your exit examination. For the umpteenth time you find your heart in your mouth but never fear because here are some reassuring facts.

1. You have been preparing for this moment ever since starting medical school and you **are** ready.
2. If you have used this book throughout your undergraduate years you will have prepared solid foundations for the examinations and beyond.
3. If you are sensible you will have revised and practised all aspects of the examinations.
4. Believe it or not, most examiners are on your side.
5. Very few students fail their final examinations.

Most final examinations will have a written and a clinical section. The written section tends to be multiple choice questions (MCQs) or extended matching questions (EMQs). The clinical section is changing in the UK with the traditional Finals (that is, long cases, short cases, and vivas) being replaced by the objective, structured, clinical examinations (OSCEs). As a few UK medical schools and other international schools are still using the traditional finals examinations, both clinical formats will be covered.

Written examination

Multiple choice questions and extended matching questions

What are they all about?

Multiple choice questions and EMQs are two papers commonly used for finals examinations. You may have done these types of questions before, in other examinations such as paediatrics or psychiatry. Multiple choice questions and EMQs are a popular way of examining medical students as they test knowledge across many topics and as they are marked by computers, examiners love them! Whether you have come across similar examinations previously or whether this is all new to you, this chapter aims to help you prepare for these papers and show you how to approach them on the day.

What are multiple choice questions?

Multiple choice questions involve a stem and five related questions. Each of the five questions requires a **true** or **false** answer. For example,
In type 1 diabetes mellitus,

(a) metformin is the first line drug of choice

(b) HbA_{1b} is useful for monitoring control

(c) necrobiosis lipoidica can occur

(d) there is less concordance in identical twins than there is in type 2 diabetes

(e) urine dipstick for glucose and ketones is the best way to assess daily sugar control.

(a)–(e) each require a **true** or **false** answer.

What are extended matching questions?

Extended matching questions involve matching a stem to the most appropriate answer from a list of choices. Here is an example.

1. Blood gases. Below are a group of patients that have all had an arterial blood sample taken (on room air). Select the most appropriate ABG result for each patient. Use each answer only once.

(1) A drowsy 25-year-old diabetic man found by his mum. She says he hasn't been taking his usual injections for 2 days because he's got a cold and hasn't been eating.

(2) A 79-year-old woman, 4 days after AP resection for malignancy. She was talking to her daughter and suddenly became short of breath. She clutches her chest and looks very unwell.

(3) A 55-year-old former smoker with home nebulizers and oxygen presents with green sputum, pyrexia, and worsening shortness of breath.

(4) A 26-year-old goalkeeper has an ABG taken at the end of a football match.

(5) An anxious 27-year-old woman presenting with tingling around her mouth saying she just can't get her breath.

(6) A 70-year-old woman presents with a 3-month history of progressive vomiting and weight loss. Upper GI endoscopy reveals a mass in her pylorus.

(7) A 92-year-old man who is difficult to get a sample from, as his pulse is weak. The PRHO manages to get a sample but notices the blood doesn't shoot up the tube as fast as it normally does.

(8) A 39-year-old woman who says she has taken 57 aspirin tablets after a row with her boyfriend. She took the tablets 2 h ago. She has a raised respiratory rate and says she doesn't feel well.

Ranges

pH	7.35–7.45
pCO_2	4.7–6
pO_2	10.5–14
plasma	HCO_3 22–28
O_2 saturation	95–100%

For this question, you have to match (1)–(8) with answers (A)–(H). In this example, there are the same number of stems as there are answer options. This is not always the case, you often get more answer options than you can use. The question should say whether you can use each answer option once or more than once.

(A)	(B)	(C)	(D)
CO_2 11 O_2 6.2 O_2 saturation 81%	pH 7.48 CO_2 3.78 O_2 16	pH 7.43 CO_2 5.23 O_2 13.74 HCO_3 23	pH 7.15 CO_2 2.9 HCO_3 12 BE −6
(E)	**(F)**	**(G)**	**(H)**
pH 7.345 CO_2 9.1 O_2 7.4 HCO_3 35 O_2 saturation 91%	pH 7.451 HCO_3 38 CO_2 8.2 $O_2$13.6 BE +7	pH 7.51 CO_2 3.8 HCO_3 24	pH 6.98 O_2 6.19 CO_2 4.6 HCO_3 8 O_2 saturation 83%

Revising for the examinations

Start early! You need a good, broad knowledge base to do well on these papers. Even though the answers are there on the question paper, you need to be confident in your knowledge because the questions can trip up the unsuspecting or semi-prepared candidate.

Once you have got the knowledge base, the best way to prepare for the MCQ examination is by practising other MCQs. Many MCQ sources are widely available, from past papers to published MCQ books and internet question banks. Ask students from the year above where they got practice questions from. You can never do too many practice MCQs. The best way to use MCQ books is to take a topic, for example, stroke disease and do as many questions on stroke as you can find. You may see a similar pattern in the questions or notice frequently asked facts. If you learn anything from the explanations given with the questions, remember it and use the MCQs to enhance your knowledge.

Past EMQ questions are a bit more difficult to get hold of as they have not been in use for as long as MCQs. Books of questions are starting to be published though so you should be able to find them.

Most people seem to find MCQs harder than EMQs as you have to know if something is right or wrong on an MCQ paper whereas on an EMQ, you have to match the question to the answer.

The run up to the examinations

Keep up the practice questions! Try to set yourself a realistic time limit to do the same number of questions as there will be in your examination, so you can get a feel for the pace. The MCQ and EMQ papers are often done together, in the same examination. You need to find out if your examination is going to be negatively marked. Very few medical schools use negative marking these days, but you need to check. Make sure you know

(1) whether the examination is in the morning or afternoon;

(2) how long it will last;

(3) how many questions there will be;

(4) whether you will be given both the MCQ and EMQ at the start of the examination or whether you have allotted time for each, after which that paper is handed in;

(5) whether you will be given normal reference ranges;

(6) your seat number;

(7) whether candidates can leave before the end of the examination if they have finished.

Make sure you have a watch if possible, as the clock can be a long way from your seat. All this sounds like common sense but it will reduce your stress on the day!

The big day!

Attempt to go to bed at a humane hour the night before the examination. You are not going to learn very much the night before an MCQ/EMQ as medicine is far to broad to be done that late! Eat something before the examination. Do not drink excess caffeine on the morning of the examination, it will not improve your answers and you will need the toilet. Go to the toilet **before** the examination. People get panicky before examinations. Try not to get involved with the hype of it all, just be focused on going in and getting on with it. Avoid known panickers! **Read the instructions** on the front of the examination papers. Do exactly what the instructions tell you.

Most people find they have too much time in an MCQ paper, so pace yourself, do not rush. The EMQ may take more time than you think. Looking back at the blood gas EMQ questions above, this would have taken time to sort out. If you have both papers to do within the time limit, you need to really watch the clock.

For the MCQ, read every stem twice and every question twice. Then, and only then, answer '**true**' or '**false**'. The importance of reading the questions twice cannot be over-emphasized. It is very easy to misread the question or to not notice finer points. Look back at the diabetes MCQ question at the start of this chapter. Did you notice HbA_{1b} which should be HbA_{1c}? If you rush over the questions and only read them once, you may misread them and miss out on marks. Some people find it useful to underline important words in the questions too.

For the EMQ, read all the stems and all the answer options twice. Try not to be phased by all the answer options available. Some questions will give you more answer options than you need and some of the options in front of you should be obviously wrong or ones that you can be sure you are not going to need.

Examinations usually have a question paper and an answer paper with boxes on. Once you have decided on your answer, put it on the answer sheet straight away. **Do not leave this to be done at the end of the examination.** If you think you will scribble your answers on the question paper and then transfer them on to the answer sheet towards the end of the exam, what happens if the time runs out? The examination will end and all your answers will be stuck on the question paper as you hand in a blank answer sheet. This has happened frequently. Do not let it happen to you.

If you cannot do a question, be careful to leave a gap on the answer sheet to fill in later otherwise all your subsequent answers will be marked against the incorrect question number.

However the answer sheet is to be filled in, for example, filling a box or putting a cross, **make sure its legible**. Most of these examinations are marked by computers who cannot make allowances for candidates who do not fill in the boxes properly. Do not lose marks!

Look out for clues in the MCQ questions. From experience, the author has found that there are a few words such as 'may' and 'sometimes' that are used in MCQs and these often hint towards a **true**. 'Always' and 'never' in questions often hint towards **false**, as little in medicine is that black and white. These are by no means hard and fast rules but they may be little hints that are worth bearing in mind. Use your common sense when answering the questions. If you cannot remember something, look through the rest of the paper—is there something to jog your memory? Is there another question that uses the fact you cannot remember? Perhaps something on the EMQ paper will jog your memory?

Once you have decided on your answer and have written it on the answer sheet, move on. Experience shows your first answer is more likely to be correct than any re-think. Be firm. Do not be swayed by temptation to change your answers.

Once you have finished and checked your answer sheet correlates with the correct question number, you need to do **two** more things before you leave. The first thing is to have another peak at the back sheet of the question papers and be absolutely sure you have not missed questions by forgetting to turn over. The other thing is to double check you have put your name and other requested details on the relevant answer sheets and question sheets. These two little jobs take seconds but can stop you being the one that fails.

After the examination

Try to put it behind you. Possibly easier said than done, but try to move on. Many students 'post-mortemize' MCQ questions, but chances are you have other examinations ahead so focus on them, not on what is done. You need to remember that these two papers have questions of a variety of difficulty as they need to divide students into distinction or honours candidates, pass candidates, and fail candidates. You are therefore not going to be able to do every question with ease! There are bound to be a few questions that stick in your mind afterwards as being particularly difficult. It is worth remembering though that for every one you remember as being particularly hard or that you are sure you have got wrong, you have no doubt answered many with ease (and cannot even recall doing them.)

Good luck!

PS

Multiple choice question on diabetes

(a) **False.** Metformin? **No**! Read the question—type **1**. You know that is insulin dependent. Metformin is used in type 2 diabetes.

(b) **False.** Read the question. HbA_{1c} is used for monitoring.

(c) **True.** Have a look at a dermatology picture of this and then you will remember it.

(d) **True.** This is one of those annoying questions you either do or do not know. Epidemiological-type questions like this lend themselves well to MCQs as they give a clear yes/no answer. Doing lots of past MCQs should help you get better at this type of question.

(e) **False.** This is not the **best**. Blood samples from the fingertips are much better for glucose values. Urine testing like this is occasionally used by some people with diabetes but rarely by those who are insulin dependent. Urine testing for ketones is useful if concerned about diabetic ketoacidosis (DKA).

Extended matching question on blood gases

(1) **D.** The history tells you this is a classical case of diabetic ketoacidosis.

(2) **H.** Massive post-operative pulmonary embolism causing metabolic acidosis.

(3) **E.** Infective exacerbation of chronic obstructive pulmonary disease. Note the former smoker, home nebulizers, and oxygen—all clues of a question involving chronic lung disease.

(4) **C. Normal!**

(5) **B.** Tingling lips and anxiety are good clues for the diagnosis of hyperventilation. Respiratory alkalosis.

(6) **F.** This woman has gastric outflow obstruction caused by her mass. Metabolic alkalosis.

(7) **A.** Thrown in to catch out the unwary! This is a venous sample, not arterial! Blood not shooting up the gas tube was the giveaway. It can happen in patients who are particularly difficult.

(8) **G.** This is respiratory alkalosis associated with **early** salicylate overdose. Remember that acidosis comes later.

Clinical examinations

The Objective Structured Clinical Examination (OSCE)

This format is rapidly replacing the short case, long case, and viva and has become a feature of postgraduate training. The examination consists of around 20 themed stations, such as history taking, systemic examination, pictures of clinical signs or equipment, radiology, data interpretation, and role play. Each on average lasts 6 min, with a longer time allocated to communication stations. Rest stations are interspersed and are of the same duration. As the name suggests assessing is objective and the style has proved to be reliable and valid.

Tips

General tips include being confident and positive. Always consider your answer rather than blurting out the first thing that comes to mind. Speak clearly in an unhurried and assured manner. Avoid mentioning extremely rare conditions first when the blatant diagnosis is of a common complaint. Although modern examiners tend not to ritually humiliate candidates, digging equipment may be required. Never argue with an examiner. Finally, even if the buzzer goes, the examiner decides when you should go. Leave quietly! Practice makes perfect. If this overused cliché could be applied to one situation it would be the OSCE. Each station is timed and so rehearsing obvious scenarios such as history taking and examinations is vital. Some of these may be core stations, for example, history and examination stations, so not to perfect these is ritual suicide.

Candidates may panic if they run out of time on a station and this may affect their subsequent performance. If you do run out of time on a station, move to the next station with a clear mind. Use the rest stations to gather your thoughts and if there is time, complete a written question that you were unable to finish earlier. Remember that pacing is crucial and comes only with practice.

Rare examinations such as per rectum, fundoscopy, and auriscopy can be included. Real people may not be available or in the case of per rectum, unwilling, but rest assured plastic mock-ups can be brought in. Remember to treat the plastic model as if it were a real patient.

Radiology for undergraduates usually consists of common chest, abdominal, or orthopaedic conditions and is often straightforward. Sources include databases, textbooks, and obviously the relevant wards. Clinical signs and data stations (especially blood results) can vary in difficulty and tend to distinguish candidates.

The assessor's mark sheet consists of statements or actions needed to score points, so for example to score highly on a cardiovascular history taking station, the examiner would expect questions scrutinizing the finer aspects of chest pain, exercise tolerance, risk factors for ischaemic heart disease, and other relevant information. Extra marks are awarded for being erudite and slick. Examiners have a fine eye for spotting those who have learned only from textbooks.

You may be asked for a diagnosis and subsequent plan. Organize your information and provide a differential diagnosis. Always mention the fact that you would undertake a full history and examination. If you think that the case warrants emergency treatment do not forget basic and advanced life support. When asked about investigations, start with standard blood tests progressing to more complex blood tests and relevant imagery and pathology. Remember that elderly patients tend to get routine electrocardiography and chest X-rays.

The traditional examination

The long case

The long case is the one section of the clinical examination that closely resembles the way in which doctors work. It is essentially the clerking of a patient with an added time pressure. You have an hour to take a history and examine your patient (do not forget fundoscopy or urinalysis). I would recommend that you leave yourself 10 min before the end of your examination. This gives you enough time to gather your thoughts and work out what you are going to say to your examiners. Hopefully you will have recorded your findings and rehearsing them should be a formality. Make sure that you have taken a full social history. At this stage if you have forgotten any aspect of the history or examination you still have some time to check this with the patient. Now concentrate on what you think the diagnosis is (or a reasonable differential diagnosis). Consider what investigations you would do and what management would be appropriate. Do not restrict treatments to drugs. Think about physiotherapy, visual aids, walking aids, home helps, and financial benefits, particularly for the elderly patient.

Examiners vary in what they expect from you. Some will sit back and listen to you recite every fact you have unearthed, before asking you straightforward questions about management. Others will only ask for a diagnosis and be oblivious to all your hard work before going off at tangents, asking in-depth questions that test your knowledge (and sweat glands). It is this variability in student experience that has led to the (justified) charge of unfairness

The short case

This format is intimidating because you have trained eyes scrutinizing how you examine patients. A pair of examiners will lead you round a number of clinical cases and give you verbal instructions. In some cases these commands can cause confusion (areas of confusion and tips are a feature of the Finals section at the end of most chapters). A slick examination is always desirable but beware of rushing without processing your findings. Never finish examining a patient until you are sure of a particular sign. If not, your indecision can be exploited to devastating effect by a sharp-eyed examiner. In Finals you will usually be given barn-door cases so the signs should not be ambiguous. Only when you are ready, let your examiners know that you have finished and let them know what supplementary examination or signs you would normally perform, for example, per rectum examination, blood pressure, and so on. Then give a diagnosis with supporting findings (if you can) or give your findings and some sensible differential diagnoses. Some people state that the more cases you see the greater your chances of success. There is a grain of truth in this, however, you can rush through seven cases, do them badly, and fail and equally you may see only four in-depth cases, perform well, and pass.

The viva

This can be one of the most harrowing sections of the clinicals because you come face to face with your examiners and you can be asked **anything** medical under the sun (and how can you revise for this unpredictability?). Fortunately the vast majority of examiners will ask you basic questions that you should be able to answer so long as you have revised thoroughly and have your wits about you.

Nowadays vivas may be restricted to either a pass/fail or an honours variety. These test students at the extremes of performance. Those who are on the pass/fail borderline can expect straightforward questions that students are expected to know. If your examination performance was down to bad luck, this will be a welcome second chance. For those on the threshold of honours, the questions will be more searching. Try to relax and show them what you know because you have earned the right.

I find that questions are usually of two types—the closed/specific type and the open/general type. The specific question has a well-defined answer and does not usually cause problems, for example, 'Tell me how you manage hypoglycaemia.' The open question is more problematical. Many students can freeze if faced with such a question because the topic is so huge they do not know where to start, for example, 'Tell me about myocardial infarction.' It is fair to say it is better to say something than to remain gob-smacked. The examiners will often ask supplementary questions if they feel you have gone off the beaten track. Rather than trust to luck, the authors tend to try and structure their answer to this type of question, using headings including 'definition' (of myocardial infarction), 'aetiology', 'incidence' (do not worry if you cannot remember these), 'clinical features', 'investigations', 'treatment', and 'complications'.

Although the clinical section has been separated into the OSCE and the traditional examination, you should find that a number of tips will be relevant for either.

Good luck!

APPENDIX

Medical students: distinguished roll of honour

Michaela Quinn. *Medicine woman* (TV series starring Jane Seymour).

Leonard McCoy. Dr McCoy (*Star trek*— 'Its life Jim but not as we know it').

William Osler. Canadian physician and teacher remembered for eponymous conditions, for example, Osler–Weber–Rendu syndrome and Osler's nodes.

Friedrich Wegener. German pathologist noted for the description of Wegener's granulomatosis.

Berkeley Moynihan. British surgeon, Leeds-trained authority on abominal surgery.

Marjory Warren. British surgeon who ironically founded the modern specialty of geriatrics.

James Parkinson. British physician who described the condition known as Parkinson's disease.

Maurice Raynaud. French physician remembered for Raynaud's phenomenon.

Joseph Babinski. French neurologist who described a number of conditions of which the Babinski (plantar) reflex is the most recognized.

John Hughlings-Jackson. British neurologist famous for his descriptions of epilepsy and other nervous system disorders including the eponymous Jacksonian epilepsy.

Marie Curie. Polish scientist who was a pioneer of radioactivity and won two nobel prizes.

Abraham Colles. Irish Surgeon who is famous for the description of the Colles fracture of the wrist.

Index